What Works for Whom?

*A Critical Review of Treatments
for Children and Adolescents*

Peter Fonagy
Mary Target
David Cottrell
Jeannette Phillips
Zarrina Kurtz

with contributions from
Arabella Kurtz, Kathy Leach, and Liz Allison

THE GUILFORD PRESS
New York   London

© 2002 The Guilford Press
A Division of Guilford Publications, Inc.
72 Spring Street, New York, NY 10012
www.guilford.com

Paperback edition 2005

Printed in the United States of America

This book is printed on acid-free paper.

Last digit is print number: 9   8   7   6   5   4   3   2

Library of Congress Cataloging-in-Publication Data
is available from the Publisher.

ISBN 1-57230-751-X (hc)   ISBN 1-59385-166-9 (pbk)

About the Authors

Peter Fonagy, PhD, FBA, is Freud Memorial Professor of Psychoanalysis and Director of the Sub-department of Clinical Health Psychology at University College London. He is Director of the Child and Family Center at the Menninger Foundation, Kansas. He is also Director of Research at the Anna Freud Centre, London. Dr. Fonagy is a clinical psychologist and a Training and Supervising Analyst at the British Psycho-Analytical Society in child and adult analysis. He has published over 200 chapters and articles and has co-written and co-edited several books, including most recently, *What Works for Whom?: A Critical Review of Psychotherapy Research* (1996) and *Attachment Theory and Psychoanalysis* (2001).

Mary Target, PhD, is a Senior Lecturer in the Sub-department of Clinical Health Psychology at University College London, and Deputy Director of Research at the Anna Freud Centre, London. She is trained as a clinical psychologist and psychoanalyst. Her research areas are in child psychotherapy process and outcome research, and in personality development and attachment in both adults and children.

David Cottrell, MA, FRCPsych, holds the Foundation Chair in Child and Adolescent Psychiatry at the University of Leeds. He is Director of Learning and Teaching at the School of Medicine, and an Associate Professor of Psychology. He is a practicing consultant child and adolescent psychiatrist and a qualified systemic family therapist. Dr. Cottrell has a longstanding interest in learning and teaching and in medical undergraduate and postgraduate education. His main clinical interest is in the adaptation of children and families to chronic illness and disability in childhood.

Jeannette Phillips, MB, BS, MRCP(UK), MRCPsych, MRCPCH, is a consultant psychiatrist in Dartford and Gravesham, where she and her team are working to rebuild a community service. She trained at the Bethlem Royal and Maudsley Hospitals and is a member of the Royal College of Paediatrics and Child Health.

Her previous work includes the literature search for *Services for the Mental Health of Children and Young People in England* (Z. Kurtz, R. Thornes, & S. Wolkind) published by the Maudsley Hospital and South Thames Regional Health Authority (1994), and the literature review for Professor Robert Goodman's document, *Help for Troubled Children*, published by the Institute of Psychiatry (1997).

Zarrina Kurtz, MB, BS, MSc, FRCP, FRCPCH, FFPHM, is an independent consultant in public health and health policy. As a senior lecturer in pediatric epidemiology at the Institute of Child Health in London and as Medical Adviser to the former Inner London Education Authority, she conducted child health services research and policy analysis. In recent years, she has focused on the development and implementation of policy and service evaluation in child and adolescent mental health. She has acted as the lead adviser and investigator of the Audit Commission National Project on Child and Adolescent Mental Health Services (1999), and led Department of Health funded national studies on the mental health needs of young people in the secure care system (1998), and on the health needs of school age children (2000).

Acknowledgments

Completion of this work was greatly facilitated by support from the United Kingdom's Department of Health grant no. MCH 17-33, which was awarded to provide a systematic review of child mental health treatments. The project team would like to acknowledge the contribution of Arabella Kurtz in the initial stage of the project and in the development of the conduct disorder chapter in particular, and the editorial work of Kathy Leach and Liz Allison.

Contents

WHAT WORKS FOR WHOM?

1

Introduction and Review of Outcome Methodology

The Importance of Outcome Measurement

EVIDENCE-BASED MEDICINE AND ITS JUSTIFICATIONS

Evidence-based medicine is founded on an ideal—that decisions about care of individual patients should involve the conscientious, explicit, and judicious use of current best evidence. The arguments in favor of this approach are that (1) it makes more effective use of resources, (2) it enhances the clinician's knowledge, (3) it improves communication with patients, and (4) it allows the best-evaluated methods of health care to be identified and enables patients and doctors to make better-informed decisions. All these are good reasons, but all were as relevant to medicine in the past as at present. So why the current emphasis?

The real driving force behind evidence-based medicine is unlikely to be solely concern for the quality of care but rather economic considerations and the hope that health care organizations may be able to reduce escalating costs by focusing on the most cost-effective option, given a range of treatments.

The health economist Martin Knapp (1997) provided a helpful overview of both latent and manifest factors that have impacted on young people's mental health services over recent years, leading to an increased emphasis on the demonstration of the cost-effectiveness of the mental health care provided. The latent demands all entail scarcity of resources of some kind and may be summarized as follows:

1. The growing prevalence of most types of childhood disorder, including depression, suicide, alcohol abuse, drug dependency, and juvenile crime.
2. The gap between need and the capacity of the delivery systems (Kurtz, Thornes, & Wolkind, 1994).

3. Cultural, social, and economic changes, adding up to heightened strain experienced by families (Diekstra, 1995).
4. Changed social and family expectations, placing more importance on the mental health of youth (Parry-Jones, 1995).
5. Market forces and pressures, with payers demanding better value for their money (Fuller, 1995).

These latent demands have become manifest as explicit requests in a number of contexts. These were usefully summarized by Knapp: (1) The demand by purchasers to know that they are obtaining the best treatment for the price (Yates, 1994); (2) the sharp increase in the cost of mental heath care falling to employers and other payers arising out of perverse incentives (supplier-induced demand or indulgence of users' wishes) (Bickman et al., 1996); (3) the establishment of quasi-markets in the United Kingdom and the emergence of managed care (health maintenance organizations) in the United States (Subotsky, 1992); (4) the wish to develop policies that limit the damaging consequences of the fragmentation of children's mental health services (Hoagwood & Rupp, 1995; Jaffa, 1995); (5) the wish to evaluate new treatments, care settings, or new ways of organizing delivery (Kazdin, in press-a); and (6) the wish to justify and promote the purchase of new pharmaceutical treatment products (Freemantle & Maynard, 1994).

The upshot of these demands has been general acceptance of greater accountability of professionals to the funders and purchasers of health care. The emphasis on outcomes is a direct consequence of this shift in power. Pressures associated with reimbursement, managed care, and fiscal stringency in general, exercise a powerful influence on clinical practice and practice guidelines. Governments and health funders are attracted to the notion of allocating health resources on the basis of evidence.

SOME PHILOSOPHICAL CONCERNS ABOUT EVIDENCE-BASED MEDICINE

Evidence-based medicine is a practical example of "consequentionalism," that is, the proposition that the worth of an action may be assessed by the measurement of its consequences. There are several problems with the consequentionalist argument, most significant of which is the difficulty of measuring outcomes.

Many important outcomes of any medical treatment are not quantifiable. Evidence-based medicine claims to provide a simple, logical process for reasoning and decision making: (1) systematic scrutiny of the available evidence, (2) drawing appropriate conclusions leading to (3) a clinical decision as to the appropriateness of a treatment. Within this framework, for any decision to be balanced, all relevant consequences of a treatment must be considered. Unfortunately, given the current methods for child psychiatric measurement, many important outcomes can only be indirectly or inadequately measured. Child psychiatry concerns complex internal states in developing individuals, such as the degree of distress or pain experienced by a child. Often these complex states are reduced to simpler, easily quantifiable, subjective reports, such as experiences related to depression (Kovacs, 1985), anxiety (Papay & Spielberger, 1986), or total symptomatology (Achenbach, 1991a). If such measures are used without sophistication, they may become reified, causing researchers or users of research to conflate the measure with the phenomenon it aimed to quantify. Thus, the Children's Depression Inventory (CDI) score is not childhood depression and the total internalizing score of the Child Behavior Checklist (CBCL) is not equivalent to psychological distress. Similarly, the Parenting Stress Index (Abidin, 1997) does not capture in its entirety the guilt-ridden family's struggle to cope with an oppositional child. Exclusive reliance on these measurements may fail to do justice to the complex cognitive, affective, and physiological processes implicated by these terms.

Better measures will be developed for many of the domains of outcomes entailed in the treatment of child mental health problems, but other aspects, such as a "dignified childhood," a "sense of purpose," or "ethical childcare," are probably inherently unmeasurable. Even more troublesome are key domains that are not even well defined, let alone measurable. One such is the often cited "quality of life." Many attempts have been made to provide a metric for this in the adult physical and mental health literature (e.g., Dijkers, 1999), yet in the absence of a general consensus as to what a reasonable quality of life might entail for an adult, let alone a child, it is hard to imagine how meaningful measurement is possible.

There is a clear danger that a therapy "without substantial evidence" will be thought by all to be "without substantial value" (Evidence Based Care Resource Group, 1994). Once this idea is allowed to flourish, a cultural change becomes inevitable, which at least temporarily has the power to stop funded research and the development of potentially valuable approaches. It would be regrettable if uncritical reading of the evidence base were to lead to a series of self-fulfilling prophecies.

As we have said, the driving force of the recent upsurge of interest in outcomes assessment is more likely to be the motivation to impose social and political controls on the professional practitioner rather than simply to bring about improvements in patient care. Yet this is not to say that insistence on treatment programs "of known effectiveness" is an adverse outcome of social and structural changes in the field of mental health. There have been major shortcomings in systems of care delivery that can be clearly linked to the absence of adequate interest in research findings. The hospitalization of children may have been driven more by the perverse incentives for providers than by the known benefits of inpatient care. Most pediatric psychopharmacological treatments have not been thoroughly evaluated, and many are still not FDA-approved for use with children (Spencer, Wilens, & Biederman, 1995[vi]*). Many treatments in common use are, in all probability, not efficacious. It is an illusion that clinical experience can tell us what is effective. Historians of medicine could give dramatic counter examples of ineffective and even iatrogenic treatments that were warmly embraced by the profession (such as insulin

---

*See page 39 for description of categories of evidence.

coma therapy or the use of the centrifuge in the treatment of schizophrenia); this, unfortunately, is not just an issue of yesteryear. Ethically and professionally, it is essential to eradicate treatments that are likely to waste scarce resources.

Most would agree that, notwithstanding genuine scientific and clinical considerations, the interactions between social anxieties and professional concerns, public demand, and clinical opinion will determine whether certain interventions continue to be offered. For example, interventions for substance misuse and self-harm are not particularly effective (Committee on Child Health Financing and Committee on Substance Abuse, 1995), yet their elimination would create an intolerable clinical gap and potentially undermine the possibility of discovering new interventions and effective management strategies. We shall return to the key issue of the dialectic between petrification consequent upon rigid implementation of evidence-based practice, and a free-for-all where outcome information is generally ignored.

WHAT IS "OUTCOME"?, OR WHOSE OUTCOME IS IT ANYWAY?

The Complexity of Outcome Measurement

Child mental health outcomes cannot be considered in absolute terms, yet a range of fundamental questions that have practical implications are rarely asked. For example, when is the preservation of a family unit a positive outcome, or, rather, for whom is that outcome positive—the child, the parents, the clinician, or the purchaser who would be required to fund alternative care? What if the outcomes diverge—if what is optimal for the child is less favorable to other members of the family or to the service provider? We should be aware of the adage: "In many instances the most cost-effective intervention is to do nothing."

A possible practical problem arising out of this conceptual issue is the frequent low level of agreement between informants about the child's symptomatology or adaptation. Even at the level of symptoms, teachers, mothers, and fathers appear to share little more than 10% of variance concerning the child's internalizing symptoms (Achenbach, 1995). It cannot be assumed that parents" perceptions will accurately reflect the child's feelings and needs. A mother's mental health is a good predictor of the accuracy of her perception of the degree of her child's disability, even when this is of a physical nature (Jessop, Reissman, & Stein, 1988). Strikingly, children's views concerning their own treatment are rarely taken into serious consideration (House of Commons Health Committee, 1997), and indeed very little is known about children's understanding of mental health (Chesson, Harding, Hart, & O'Loughlin, 1997). Our understanding of this issue is increasing (Harris, 1989), but very little of this new knowledge has found its way into the treatment evaluation literature.

Psychotherapy researchers are particularly conscious of the danger of imposing ethnically rooted cultural biases on the definitions of "needing treatment" or a "good outcome" (Bernal, Bonilla, & Bellido, 1995). For instance, the achievement of selfhood through the separation–individuation process (Mahler, 1971) is one of the cornerstones of psychodynamic psychotherapeutic interventions, and yet is Lasch (1978) not correct that the emphasis on individual achievement in Western culture is excessive, and that an appropriate submission to the goals of the family and community may be a better indicator of healthy adaptation? Such considerations are particularly pertinent to the area of parenting practices, where legitimacy for harsh, even cruel disciplinary methods is sometimes eloquently claimed on the basis of cultural specificity. Rogler (1989) outlined some of the practical steps that culturally sensitive outcome research requires. In particular, interventions ought to be consonant with the subjective culture of the ethnic group to which they are applied, and the instruments used should be able to integrate cultural meanings with the pertinent scientific categories.

A further consideration complicating the issue of outcomes for childhood interventions is the developmental framework that now dominates child psychiatry and psychology (Cicchetti & Toth, 1995). Developmental psychopathology implies that symptoms cannot be considered the sole, or even the most important, criterion of treatment effectiveness. If psychiatric disorder is not just the end result of a series of interactions of biological, social, and psychological characteristics across time, but is itself part of a complex transactional causal chain, good outcome might sometimes be an increase rather than a decrease in symptomatology. We raise these issues to draw the reader's attention to a major limitation of this volume and other similar attempts at integrating information concerning treatment efficacy. Evidence is not absolute. Inevitably, its significance is determined by the cultural context that demanded it and gives it meaning. The results reported in this review should be considered within this relativist framework.

Levels of Outcome Measurement

A further complexity of outcome measurement concerns the range of domains that may be considered pertinent to the evaluation of specific programs. Distinguishing these domains is obviously a heuristic exercise. In this book, we broadly follow a classification proposed by Hoagwood and Jensen (Hoagwood, Jensen, Petti, & Burns, 1996) and Kazdin and Kendall (Kazdin & Kendall, 1998), differentiating five levels of outcome:

The Symptomatic or Diagnostic Level

A child is referred to treatment because of dysfunction in a specific domain. Both researchers and clinicians are most likely to focus on the child's presenting problem and target complaints. In most studies *symptom reduction* is the primary criterion for a good outcome (Kazdin, 2000c). Current measurement of child mental health outcomes is most sophisticated at this level. Both categorical (Angold & Costello, 1995) and dimensional checklist-based (Achenbach, 1991a) assessments may be achieved reliably with relative ease. The computerization of such assessments will overcome many remaining practical problems. Outcome studies frequently use a range of symptom measures; they vary in length, ease of administration, and qualit of standardization. The best-validated checklist measure, by some margin, is the CBCL (Achenbach, Howell, McConaughy, & Stanger, 1995a; Achenbach, Howell, McConaughy, & Stanger, 1995b; Achenbach, Howell, McConaughy, & Stanger, 1995c), which has parent, teacher, and self rating forms.

As symptom measures require informants to "aggregate" their observations of the child's behavior over a period of approximately 4 weeks to 3 months, relatively short periods of care (particularly in inpatient settings) require measures sensitive to changes over shorter intervals of perhaps no more than a few days. Studies that contrast structured respondent-based interviews and checklists tend to find that both have reliability and validity, although checklists take far less time to complete (Boyle et al., 1997). Nevertheless, the agreement between these methods of measurement is only moderate; consequently, the usual advice to researchers is to obtain multiple measures from different informants (Verhulst & Koot, 1992). Because multiple measurement inevitably reduces error through aggregation, this approach tends to lead to more robust findings (Fergusson, Horwood, & Lynskey, 1995[v]).

This approach raises the aforementioned concern of the low level of observed agreement between informants, especially concerning internalizing behaviors (Simonoff et al., 1997). Commonly, parents, but not teachers, note changes in the child's behavior; this is problematic, particularly when parents, but not the teachers, are active participants in the treatment, raising obvious questions of biased reporting. A further problem is that the data from different informants often fail to overlap, causing difficulties in the interpretation of results (Eaves et al., 1997). There are a number of possible explanations for the poor agreement between informants, including the lack of knowledge of one or both parents or the contextual dependence of the child's problem behavior, implying that a more balanced view will be provided by two informants. Ways of dealing with the disagreement include counting a symptom as present if it is reported by either of the informants (e.g., parent or child; see Angold, Erklanis, Costello, & Rutter, 1996) or using structural equation modeling to derive a latent variable (Fergusson et al., 1995[v]). Achenbach (1995) offered a decision tree approach for making taxonomic assignments from multiple sources of data. This approach, if applied, would enable the researcher to distinguish three reasons for such disagreements: (1) the contextual dependence of the child's problem, (2) comorbidity or multiple syndromes, and (3) distorted perception on the part of some informants. The relative value of these approaches to outcome measurement remains to be explored.

A broad range of symptomatic assessments is essential, because about half of individuals in community samples who meet diagnostic criteria for a DSM-IV disorder are likely to meet criteria for another disorder as well (Bird et al., 1988). In clinical samples the prevalence of comorbidity is likely to be even higher (70–75%; see Kazdin, 1996a[vi]). Some of this overlap may be the consequence of measurement problems and errors in prevailing psychiatric concepts (Rutter, 1998). Nevertheless, comorbidity may be meaningful in that problems tend to go together because they are causally linked. For example, delinquency is commonly associated with drug abuse (Ketterlinus & Lamb, 1994). They go together either because they serve similar functions in relation to development and adaptation (drug abuse and delinquency may both be understood in terms of attachment-related considerations; see Fonagy et al., 1997), or because one represents a risk factor for the other (e.g., reading retardation may be a risk factor for conduct problems: see Kazdin, 1995b[vi]), or because both are independent consequences of high levels of adversity. Without evaluating the full breadth of an individual's symptoms, we will have limited information on the effectiveness of a treatment, except for its impact on the individual's primary diagnosis.

The assessment of treatment inevitably involves repeated assessments. A recurrent feature in studies that use repeated ratings is that levels of psychopathology on the second occasion tend to be systematically lower than those in the first assessment (e.g., Boyle et al., 1997). This underscores the importance of using well-matched control groups as well as the importance of supplementing symptom ratings with other assessments. A further limitation of checklist and interview schedule-based measures is the rather obvious one, that they can tap only the constructs included in them. This is rarely a problem when the features to be measured are well-recognized, but may be an issue when the treatment of less well-studied conditions is explored. In these instances, important but uncommon problems may simply be missed. This argues for the use of investigator-based interviews that elicit descriptions of behavior, rather than yes or no answers to structured questions.

There are general limitations to a purely symptom-based approach to outcome assessment. Longitudinal studies of childhood disorders have shown that long-term outcomes are not well predicted by symptom severity alone (Rutter, 1999). For example, multiple social adversity can increase the chances of severe problems in adolescence almost a hundred-fold (Fergusson & Horwood, 1999[v]; Fergusson & Lynskey, 1996[v]). Symptoms may indicate the presence of pathological processes but say little about the nature of the problem or, indeed, the best course for resolving it (Cicchetti & Cohen, 1995). Focusing on symptomatic outcomes alone may reduce the scope of the treatment intervention in an undesirable way, leaving major child- or family-centered domains of dysfunction untouched, and increasing the chance of relapse or reducing the rate of change.

The Level of Adaptation

The second level of measurement concerns *adaptation* to the psychosocial environment. Mental health problems impinge on many domains of the child's functioning. Recent meta-analyses have demonstrated that evaluation of treatments solely in terms of their impact on core symptoms leads to a potentially misleading overestimation of the effect of such treatments, at least in terms of effect size (Weisz, Weiss, Han, Granger, & Morton, 1995b[ib]). The most likely reason for this is the high reactivity of many symptom measures. Often the originators of the treatment approach also develop the measurement technique (e.g., Beck, Ward, Mendelson, Mock, & Erbaugh, 1961), and therefore proximity (and even overlap) between the intervention and measurement domains should not surprise us. This may be inevitable to a certain degree, but treatments should not be evaluated merely in terms of whether they have modified the clients' response strategies to questionnaires.

We know that many treatments leave important areas untouched. For example, stimulants alone tend not to benefit the academic performance and peer relations of children with attention-deficit/hyperactivity disorder (ADHD) (Hinshaw, 1994). A well-planned study, comparing cognitive-behavioral therapy (CBT), family therapy, and supportive therapy in adolescents with major depression (Brent et al., 1996) showed CBT to be effective in reducing depressive symptoms but did not show parallel benefits for social functioning. An ongoing trial of hospital treatment contrasted with multisystemic therapy (MST) for adolescents with psychiatric emergencies has shown major advantages for MST in terms of symptom measures and hospitalization rates, whereas measures of self-esteem favored the hospital condition (Henggeler, Schoenwald, Rowland, & Ward, 1999).

Of course, assessing the quality of adaptation is tantamount in complexity to assessing the whole of the child's life. Several key aspects have provided appropriate foci for measurement, however. A treatment's effectiveness should be judged in terms of the extent to which it removes the impediment a disorder imposes on an individual's everyday functioning. In childhood and adolescence the critical dimensions include meeting the role demands of home and school, having adequate prosocial interactions with peers and adults, and not being restricted in the situations in which the individual can effectively function. Although level of adaptation generally correlates with symptomatology, it is also known to represent an important unique source of variance (Sanford, Offord, Boyle, Peace, & Racine, 1992). In particular, the likelihood that a child with symptomatology sufficient to meet diagnostic criteria will access mental health services has been predicted by the child's functioning in everyday life (Bird et al., 1990). Further, a low level of adaptation posttreatment often indexes a greater likelihood of relapse (Lewinsohn, Seeley, Hibbard, Rhode, & Sack, 1996b).

Where assessment of overall adaptation in children is concerned, our available measurement options are limited. The adult literature frequently uses the global assessment of functioning measure (GAF), based on the Health Sickness Rating Scale (Luborsky & Bachrach, 1974). The child equivalent of this is the Children's Global Assessment Scale (CGAS; Shaffer, Gould, & Brasic, 1983). The interrater reliability of this measure is known to be poor, at least in clinical practice (Steinhausen, 1987). Of course, many measures tap single dimensions of adaptation. For example, there are assessments of peer relationships based on the parent (Goodyer, 1989) or the child (Kernberg & Chazan, 1991) or peers (Asher & Dodge, 1986) as informants. A review of such measures is beyond the scope of this chapter. However, as the aim of such measurement is to obtain a profile of the child's adaptation across a number of areas, it is clearly preferable to obtain information concerning adaptation from a single measure. Target (Target & Fonagy, 1992), for example, has identified 14 dimensions in the Hampstead Child Adaptation Measure (HCAM) that may be reliably assessed on the basis of a parental interview. This was superior in reliability and validity to the CGAS (Schneider, 1999). An advantage of this measure is that it assesses variability across dimensions as one of the indicators of adjustment. Unevenness of adaptation may be particularly characteristic of clinical populations and has been suggested to be a risk factor for later pathology (Freud, 1965).

The presence of prosocial attributes may be particularly important in the comprehensive assessment of outcome. There are several operationalizations of this dimension. The Social Adjustment Inventory for Children and Adolescents (SAICA) is a semistructured interview-based measure that explores most key areas, including peer relationships, social functioning, prosocial competence, and academic functioning (John, Gammon, Prusoff, & Warner, 1987). Currently, the most widely used instrument is the Child and Adolescent Functioning Assessment Scale (CAFAS) (Hodges, 1995; Hodges, Bickman, Ring-Kurtz, & Rieter, 1991). This measure is completed by clinicians or independent raters based on interviews with an informant. It is also multidimensional and has very high reliability following a brief training. However, a strength of the HCAM relative to the CAFAS is the developmental anchoring of adaptation; anchor points are manualized for specific age ranges (2–3 years, 4–5 years, 6–9 years, 10–13 years, and 14–18 years, the latter rated from a direct interview with the adolescent) and can thus describe a child in terms of a clinician-rated developmental profile, highlighting areas of precociousness, immaturity, or age-appropriate functioning. Notwithstanding the availability of these and other instruments for measuring adjustment, few studies of outcome provide data on more than one or two dimensions of adaptation.

The Level of Mechanisms

The third level of outcome measurement concerns *mechanisms*, the cognitive and emotional capacities that probably underpin both symptomatology and adaptation. Cohen (1995) argued that outcome research must be grounded in a theory of both normal and abnormal child development as well as a theory of therapeutic action. More recently, Kazdin and Kendall (1998) stressed that the future of treatment development and outcome investigations lies in specifying the processes and mechanisms through which treatments achieve their effects, processes and mechanisms that relate to the development, onset, and escalation of the child's dysfunction. Such approaches imply that outcome measures should engage with the developmental theory within which a treatment is rooted, as well as satisfy the practical concerns of patients, families, clinicians, and funders.

Capacities important for the developmental outcome of psychological disorder include affect regulation (Eisenberg & Fabes, 1992), understanding of emotions (Harris, 1994), self-representation (Harter, 1988), understanding of mental states in self and others (Baron-Cohen, Tager-Flusberg, & Cohen, 1993), forming emotional bonds (Carlsson & Sroufe, 1995), making moral judgments (Fischer & Ayoub, 1994) and attributional biases (Dodge, 1991; Dodge, Pettit, & Bates, 1994b). The hypothesized dysfunction may also involve the parents—for example, the use of inappropriate discipline practices by the parents of children with conduct problems (Dodge, Pettit, & Bates, 1994a; Patterson, Reid, & Dishion, 1992), practices that parent management training has been shown to address successfully (Eyberg, Boggs, & Algina, 1995[ii]).

Although both symptoms and adaptation may be directly assessed from informants' reports or observation of behavior, capacities such as understanding of affect must be inferred from the child's performance on specially designed tasks. This creates measurement problems and challenges. For example, researchers are required to distinguish between competence and actual performance. What the child is capable of and what he or she tends to do are often rather different. An adequate demonstration of effectiveness must include a measurable change in those capacities (or mental processes) that the clinician believes may place the child at risk of symptomatology or maladaptation. Surprisingly, outcome studies measuring change at this level frequently fail to demonstrate that symptomatic change is associated with modifications of underlying mechanisms. For example, cognitive-behavioral therapy is sometimes successful without demonstrable changes in cognitive structures (Brent, Kolko, Birmaher, Baugher, & Bridge, 1999[i]). This is of more than passing significance in the evaluation of outcomes. Klein (1996) argues that if the Food and Drug Administration (FDA) were responsible for the evaluation of psychotherapy, then "no current psychotherapy would be approvable" (p. 84) because the FDA requires that the efficacy of *active ingredients* of any medication be demonstrated. As long as outcome studies cannot show that the changes observed are explicable on the basis of the hypothesized mechanisms of action, a key link in the chain of evidence will be absent.

Treatment studies provide an invaluable opportunity to explore causal mechanisms. Outcome gains should correlate with and be a function of changes in the postulated mediating mechanisms. Treatment studies, particularly those with random allocation, offer an opportunity to experimentally manipulate key variables of potential causal significance. Even within-group comparisons can yield important information concerning the relationship between the success of the therapy and the extent of change in key mediating variables. For example, the reliable observation that modifying parental reinforcement and disciplinary practices effectively tackles oppositional problems in the child contradicts recent assertions that parents do not matter for child development (Harris, 1998). Collecting information at the level of mechanism provides an important bridge between research on the causes of disorder and studies of treatment efficacy (Rutter, 1997).

The Transactional Level

The fourth level concerns *transactional* aspects of development. Child mental health professionals and developmentalists have traditionally been concerned with the contextual influences on the child's adaptation and generally see a progression and mutual accommodation between the individual and changing environments (e.g., Bronfenbrenner, 1979). Because developmental psychopathology posits transactional interactions between the mental state and behavioral predispositions of the child and the reactions of the environment to the child across time (Cicchetti & Toth, 1995), it seems essential that evaluators should assess the quality of these transactions. Research on conduct disorder over the past 20 years has indicated how risk factors such as temperament and parents' personal and interpersonal problems (e.g., maternal depression) may interact to cause elevated noncompliance (Webster-Stratton & Hammond, 1988). The caregiver's failure to cope with the oppositional behavior of the child may be further aggravated by the absence of social support (Webster-Stratton, 1985) and the high level of psychosocial stress associated with the environment in which the family lives (Rutter & Giller, 1983). Contextual influences on the child's problem include the parents, family relations, characteristics of the community, and the child's school, as well as more general cultural factors (Rutter & Smith, 1995a). Effective treatments address these risk factors, which must be evaluated alongside the child's characteristics.

Contextual or transactional measures of outcome could, in principle, involve an almost limitless range of measurement domains. Perhaps of greatest relevance, however, is the child's immediate context (parent and family functioning). Family dysfunction may be conceptualized in terms of psychiatric disorder among family members, a difficult marital relationship, or dysfunctional family dynamics—all of which have been shown to moderate and, in the case of family-oriented treatments, to mediate the effect of psychosocial interventions for children and adolescents. Contextual influences beyond family functioning encompass a myriad of life circumstances, including social stressors and enduring difficulties, socioeconomic status, and the general quality of the family's life. It should be noted that positive as well as negative aspects of the social environment impact upon treatment. Conditions that promote adaptation, such as the availability of confidantes and the amount of time the child receives from caregivers, particularly direct interaction time, impact powerfully on outcome.

Adequate global measures of family functioning are now available (Rey et al., 1997). Such measures, however, carry severe limitations: Considerable evidence now suggests that environmental effects are best considered in terms of the effect on individual children rather than as a family influence (Reiss et al., 1995[v]). Global measures are further limited in that family variables affecting one sort of outcome may not be the same as those influencing others (Rutter, 1985a). Furthermore, what appears, from correlational studies, to be an environmental effect may be at least partially mediated genetically (Plomin, 1994) or by gene–environment interactions (Kendler, 1995).

Family-based treatments of schizophrenia offer a good example of the pertinence of the transactional dimension for outcome studies. High levels of expressed emotion (parents' hostility, criticism, and overinvolvement) predict adolescent-onset schizophrenia (Doane, West, Goldstein, Rodnick, & Jones, 1981) and relapse after discharge (Vaughn & Leff, 1981). A number of well-conducted outcome studies have demonstrated that intervention programs addressing expressed emotion reduce the likelihood of relapse in adults on medication (Hogarty et al., 1986; Leff, Kuipers, Berkowitz, Eberlein-Vries, & Sturgeon, 1982).

Many effective interventions directly aim for change at the level of transactional processes. For example, parent training and social skills development programs for conduct problems of the kind described by Patterson and others (Patterson, 1982[vi]) are effective in improving child management skills (Barkley, Guevremont, Anastopoulos, & Fletcher, 1992), increasing prosocial behaviors (Webster-Stratton, Kolpacoff, & Hollinsworth, 1988[i]) and reducing behavioral problems in middle childhood (Bank, Marlowe, Reid, Patterson, & Weinrott, 1991[i]). A good illustration of the way transactional factors can moderate treatment outcome is provided by the "barriers to treatment" measure recently introduced by the Yale group (Kazdin, Holland, & Crowley, 1997[v]). This measure has been shown to be independent of other contextual dimensions known to complicate a child's treatment, such as parental psychopathology, socioeconomic status, and understanding of the treatment rationale. It provides vital information concerning the difficulties experienced by the caregiver in undertaking the practical and emotional burdens associated with engaging in the child's treatment.

Symptomatic improvements in the child can also bring about negative as well as positive changes in the family, school, or wider social environment. For example, Szapocznik and his colleagues (Szapocznik et al., 1989[ii]) compared structural family therapy with psychodynamic therapy in the treatment of conduct problems. On parent-rated measures of child behavior both treatments led to change that was maintained at one-year follow-up. However, the assessment of family functioning (transactional level) indicated that whereas family functioning had deteriorated in the individual group by the 1-year assessment, in the family therapy group it continued to improve. Thus, measurement at the transactional level may generate observations concerning outcome that are independent of both symptomatic and adaptational measures.

The Level of Service Utilization and Satisfaction with Services

The final level of outcome concerns the level and experience of *service utilization*. A number of interventions assume a reduction in posttreatment service utilization. For example, home-based preventive interventions implemented in early childhood may reduce childhood maltreatment, lessening the pressure on child welfare services. A number of studies have offered evidence that maltreatment can be prevented (Hardy & Streett, 1989; Olds, Henderson, Chamberlin, & Tatelbaum, 1986), although not all studies demonstrate significant benefit (e.g., Barth, 1991). The impressive series of investigations of MST in the treatment of delinquent youths (Borduin, 1999[vi]; Henggeler, Cunningham, Pickrel, Schoenwald, & Brondino, 1996a[vi]) consistently showed important reductions in arrest and recidivism rates in the young people participating in the program, with consequent substantial reductions in the use of juvenile justice and police services. A methodologically weaker study of multimodal treatment for ADHD (Satterfield, Satterfield, & Schell, 1987[iii]) demonstrated a fourfold reduction in felony arrests in a group of children offered such treatment in addition to stimulant medication 9 years posttreatment when contrasted with a comparison group who received medication alone. The successful treatment of antisocial behavior is not just directly related to health care, but impacts upon schools, social welfare agencies, the criminal justice system, and elsewhere.

Most children currently attending mental health facilities have multiservice needs (Burns et al., 1995). Service utilization data should therefore be comprehensive, longitudinal, and show frequency, intensity, and duration of receipt across a wide range of services (Burns et al., 1995). Many instruments have been developed to collect service utilization data. An instrument developed specially for mental health economic evaluations with a variant in the child and adolescent mental health field is the Client Service Receipt Inventory (Beecham, 1995; Beecham & Knapp, 1992). In the United Kingdom there is now an annual publication, *Unit Costs of Health and Social Care*, (Netten & Dennett, 1996). In the United States, a survey-based initiative is planned for a major multisite 5-year study of needs, service use, outcomes, and costs for children and adolescents with mental health problems. This survey will yield critical information concerning cost per service unit, total annual direct treatment costs, models of service organization and their respective costs, and the influence of insurance coverage.

Service utilization outcome may also be examined at the level of general service provision and the quality of integration of various services. Thus, an important outcome of intensive case management may be the better integration and greater accessibility of services relevant to child mental health.

Notwithstanding the self-evident usefulness of economic data, useful economic evaluations of child and adolescent mental health interventions are remarkably scarce. Obviously, until relatively recently researchers have not been interested in the health economist's perspective. However, as Yates (1994) pointed out: "The costs of clinical efforts are not mundane, unimportant, irrelevant, or too predictable to be of interest" (p. 729).

In addition to service use, outcome investigations frequently assess satisfaction with services. The social acceptability of the treatment offered may be a critical moderator of treatment success. For example, exposure treatment for children with obsessive–compulsive (OCD) symptoms may be highly efficacious, but it is also unacceptable to many (March, Mulle, & Herbel, 1994[iii]). An important outcome of childhood interventions may often be increased use of certain services. For example, some of the benefits of early home visitation may be mediated by the increased use made of a range of other pediatric medical services (Olds & Kitzman, 1993[ib]). Thus, increased service use, certainly in the short term, may sometimes indicate user satisfaction rather than failure of a treatment. This means that user satisfaction and service use measures should be looked at simultaneously.

The General Approach to Outcome Measurement

Multiple Levels of Measurement

The multiple-level outcome system described earlier has many features in common with the model advanced by Hoagwood et al. (1996) (Symptoms, Functioning, Consumer Perspectives, Environments, and Systems—SFCES) and the one proposed by Kazdin and Kendall (1998). The former workers, however, consider consumer satisfaction as a separate dimension of outcome, combining adaptational, cognitive, and emotional capacities into the single domain of functioning. The latter investigators group symptomatology with other aspects of adaptation under the heading "Child Functioning" and do not distinguish (although they forcefully imply) a separate level of measurement for the mechanisms and processes underpinning the child's disorder. Both systems highlight that outcomes should be considered across a range of domains and underscore ways in which the measurement of child mental health outcomes is more complex and yet less well developed than the assessment of adult functioning. Sophisticated evaluations of outcome are essential if we are to address the issue of the appropriateness of a particular treatment for a particular individual. Profiles of scores on the five dimensions cited above at baseline might predict the effectiveness of a treatment for particular groups of clients.

Broadening the scope of outcome batteries beyond the symptomatic level has been recommended by a number of authors (e.g., Kendall & Flannery-Schroeder, 1998, in the treatment of anxiety disorder). This is theoretically important because it may teach us about the interrelationship of these domains of functioning in the context of treatment intervention. In particular, a theoretical orientation may predict changes in some, but not other, domains. The discovery that individual child psychotherapy can lead to a deterioration in family functioning (Szapocznik et al., 1989[ii]) confirms the systemic nature of the child's psychopathology.

Beyond the theoretical benefit, the overall impact of a treatment may be erroneously evaluated as positive unless a sufficiently comprehensive evaluation of several domains of functioning is undertaken. Of course, some domains may be more relevant to some problems than others. For example, the transactional domain appears particularly relevant to conduct problems and may be less relevant to ADHD or autism. A further problem with multiple measurement across domains is the high likelihood that changes across domains correlate poorly with each other and that different children may show improvements in different domains following the same treatment. There are no generally agreed-upon methods for integrating outcome data across measures, let alone across domains. Using standardized scores presents no problems statistically, but conceptually such aggregate values may be very hard to interpret. The a priori establishment of a hierarchy may be critical to a conceptually sound integration of levels of measurements and methods of assessment.

Although there are no such agreed-upon hierarchies at the moment, they are not difficult to envisage. Present systems of service delivery implicitly prioritize symptoms and syndromes because access to services is based on measurement disorders at the level of symptoms and syndromes. A more rational prioritization might be based on long-term rather than short-term cost implications of outcomes and the best-validated predictors of these. This would imply the prioritization of the adaptational/functional and transactional domains. The ultimate criterion, the happiness and productivity of the child grown to adulthood, is not well predicted by any single measure and will not be part of outcome assessment, perhaps for years to come.

Clinically Significant Change

In attempting to identify effective treatment, it is important to consider to what extent changes on an outcome measure indicate a change that children and their families experience as meaningful. This dimension is frequently discussed under the heading of clinical significance.

A range of more or less psychometrically sophisticated approaches to this problem have been used. First, and most obvious, has been the use of standardized measures, which can demonstrate that the child, who had previously scored within a dysfunctional range, obtains posttreatment scores that are more likely to come from a normative population sample (Jacobson & Truax, 1991). This approach, of course, depends on knowing the distribution of both the normal and the clinical population.

A second approach sets a criterion for change in standard deviation units that exceed chance fluctuations, adjusted for the reliability of the instrument (Jacobson & Revenstorf, 1988). The disadvantage of this approach is that changes will depend not just on the effectiveness of the treatment but also on the reliability of the measure, although this may be considered a more general problem.

A third approach would label change clinically significant when a child no longer meets diagnostic criteria at the end of treatment. The problem here rests in the arbitrary nature of the diagnostic criteria. Westen and Morrison note in their meta-analysis (Westen & Morrison, in press) that although individuals receiving treatment for panic disorder may no longer meet diagnostic criteria, the average treated patient continues to panic only slightly less than once per week and endorses a total of four of the seven panic symptoms required for a DSM diagnosis of panic disorder. In contrast, a treatment for a disorder such as autism may make a substantial and meaningful impact on the child without effecting a change in the diagnosis. Others, considering similar issues, suggest that the extent to which participants return to within a normative range on important dependent measures after treatment should be used as the key criterion (Kendall, 2000[v]).

A fourth approach may be independent evaluation by an individual in contact with a client, who judges the change to be substantial enough to be regarded as clinically significant. This approach raises obvious concerns about subjectivity, particularly in relation to the biased perception of those who are in sufficiently intimate contact with a child to make such a judgment accurately. In a recent effectiveness study by Weiss et al. (Weiss, Catron, Harris, & Phung, 1999), psychosocial treatments delivered in a clinic setting were found to be ineffective in terms of standardized measures, yet parents considered the interventions helpful.

Finally, we may define clinical significance in terms of external criteria—the social impact of the behavior being measured (Kazdin, 1998). Recidivism in the treatment of delinquent youths is a good example of both the advantages and disadvantages of this approach. Although this measure is clearly of great social as well personal significance, it is also extremely sensitive to factors quite separate from the treatment of the disorder (e.g., changes in reporting and recording practices, current legislation, police practices, the geographical area in which the youth lives, the quality of policing, and the sentencing strategy of specific courts, etc.). Analogous considerations apply to other social impact measures, such as hospitalization, exclusion from school, truancy, and the like.

It should be noted that notwithstanding the limitations of each of these approaches, it is evidently desirable to go beyond the demonstration of statistical significance, which is the ultimate in arbitrary criteria. Rosenthal (1996) has pointed out, "God loves the .06 almost as much as she loves the .05." The risk of considering a change "clinically significant" merely because it has been labeled thus, by a statistical test or by any of the other more stringent criteria, is substantial. Although there is a rationale to each of the methods described, none have been validated in the sense of demonstrating that the change labeled "clinically significant" corresponds to a real and meaningful difference in the lives of the individuals who have participated in the treatment process. Currently, in identifying effective treatments, we are restricted by the psychometric or social impact measures used. Yet most of these instruments say too little about the way children and their parents experience their lives. In an ideal world, good outcome would identify those treatments that make the greatest and most profound contribution to the happiness and productivity of those involved in the intervention. We are still quite some distance from this ideal.

PROBLEMS OF EVIDENCE IN CHILD MENTAL HEALTH OUTCOMES

In this section we consider some of the central problems of collecting and interpreting evidence in the field of child mental health treatment. The coverage here is necessarily quite selective and limited. For a comprehensive, careful, and very accessible treatment of the methodological issues of interpreting evidence from outcomes research, the reader is referred to Alan E. Kazdin's (2000b) excellent monograph, *Psychotherapy for Children and Adolescents*.

Grouping Treatments by Diagnosis

The disadvantages of classification of psychiatric disorders are greatly outweighed by the advantages of using a reliable and valid system for grouping child and adolescent disorders. However, although the reliabilities of classification systems in current use are high if appropriate instruments are used for data collection (although this is true only for major categories of disorders (Shaffer et al., 1996)), the validity of these systems is questionable (Cantwell, 1996a). There are a number of disorders for which there is a satisfactory amount of external validation (e.g., attention deficit disorder [ADD], conduct disorder [CD], obsessive–compulsive disorder [OCD], autistic disorder), but for many disorders validation is less well developed. External validity studies do not necessarily imply homogeneity, and many disorders may have important subcategories. It is beyond the scope of this chapter to offer a comprehensive evaluation of the use of diagnostic systems in child psychiatry. Studies in the 1970s and early 1980s frequently focused on referral problems such as specific types of phobias, general problems of conduct, and specific fears such as public speaking anxiety. Treatment studies are now increasingly conducted on the basis of samples selected according to DSM (American Psychiatric Association, 1994) and, less frequently, ICD (World Health Organization, 1992a) criteria. Young people, however, even those with the same diagnosis, are not all the same (Kendall, 2000[v]). Variations in individual relations within families and cognitive levels of development are but two of the many important dimensions on which children differ, which will moderate their responses to a specific treatment. In a review such as this, we have no choice but to organize our material according to these diagnostic groupings and consider within each of these groupings the studies that focus on specific problems associated with each diagnostic group. Paradoxically, treatment studies tend to offer the most pressing indications that current systems are less than adequate. For example, not all children with ADD respond to stimulants, indicating an underlying heterogeneity in this group (Cantwell, 1996a). The issue of diagnosis will be taken up again in the context of the epidemiology of childhood disorders (see Chapter 2).

Randomized Controlled Trials

An issue that has, to some degree, polarized the field has been the controversy concerning the need for randomized controlled trials (RCTs). Many researchers in the field hold up the RCT as a "gold standard" of evaluation research and argue that observational methods "provide no useful means of assessing the value of therapy" (Doll, 1994). Some, particularly from a psychotherapeutic perspective, argue cogently against this (e.g., Chiesa & Fonagy, 1999; Fonagy & Higgitt, 1989; Garfield, 1996). The logic of RCTs is unassailable; their superiority to observational methods is so self-evident that alternative strategies can be justified only in terms of the limitations of RCTs. The limitations of RCTs can be seen as due either to the inherent nature of the method—this would be a *limitation in principle*—or to the conduct of the experiments—a *limitation of practice* (Black, 1996). Most objections to RCTs tend to concern procedural limitations which, at least in theory, may be overcome, yet these issues are frequently treated as if they were issues of principle. Limitations of principle may include the fact that in some circumstances the effect of an intervention is so dramatic that the likelihood of unknown confounding factors being important is appropriately considered negligible. Observational studies are adequate in such circumstances. A second limitation of principle may be that in some circumstances RCTs may be inappropriate—for example, when the phenomenon under observation is so rare that it is unlikely to occur in the context of a controlled trial, when the outcomes of interest are so far in the future that the question the RCT is designed to address may receive no answer within the time period within which the study takes place, or when random allocation cuts across the sometimes undeclared preferences of both clinician and patient, which may affect treatment administration: Built-in resistance to a new treatment may show the intervention to be less efficacious than it actually could be.

RCTs may also face practical obstacles. Sometimes clinicians may refuse to participate in an RCT because of a deep individual conviction that makes the clinician reluctant to alter his or her practice even though the profession as a whole accepts that the appropriateness of a specific intervention is questionable (Lilford & Jackson, 1995) Some ethical problems arise concerning RCTs—for example, the fact that a treatment (e.g., aversive conditioning of individuals with "challenging behavior") is proved to be effective does not necessarily make it right. Furthermore, RCTs require the clinician to act simultaneously as physician and research scientist: It is questionable whether the physician's moral responsibilities toward patients can be consistent with the recommendation that the patient should participate in a randomized controlled trial, particularly when such trials involve children. Beyond the question of ethics is the issue of the scope of the task. As there are at least 550 treatments for the more than 200 disorders of childhood mental health (Kazdin, 2000b), it is inconceivable that even a matrix of single types of therapy by types of disorder could ever be populated by appropriate studies (Goldfried & Wolfe, 1996). Simple arithmetic yields a figure of over 100,000 for the number of studies required. Not only are types of intervention large in number, but, moreover, most of these are "packages" of treatments with many components.

Finally, the generalizability and validity of RCTs cannot be unquestioningly assumed. RCTs are often regarded as inadequate in principle because their external validity or generalizability is low (Anonymous, 1992). This is a hotly debated issue in the field of psychotherapy and psychiatric research (Hoagwood, Hibbs, Brent, & Jensen, 1995; Olfson, 1999; Wells, 1999).

1. Participating *health care professionals* may be unrepresentative in terms of their enthusiasm for the treatment, the setting in which they work (e.g., university), their experience (either too senior or too junior), and so on. But although therapists in RCTs may be unrepresentative with respect to some characteristics critical to outcome, the field is some way away from identifying what these vital attributes might be. To some degree the operationalization of therapeutic procedures in manuals of psychotherapy mitigated this threat to external validity. Individual differences between therapists are reduced by manualization of treatments (Crits-Christoph et al., 1991).

2. A second threat to generalizability from RCTs is the unrepresentativeness of the *participants*. The strongest argument concerns the reduction of generalizability brought about by the greater severity and comorbidity of clinic rather than research cases. This has received some empirical support (Kazdin, Bass, Ayers, & Rodgers, 1990b; Weisz, Donenberg, Han, & Weiss, 1995a[vi]) in that participants in RCTs have fewer comorbid conditions, have less severe and chronic disorders, have parents with less psychiatric morbidity, stress, and impairment, and families are less dysfunctional and live in less disadvantaged environments. In one RCT of cognitive and systemic family therapy for children with major depression, those recruited by advertisement were significantly more likely to benefit than those presenting at the clinic, even though the disorders of the two groups were of comparable severity (Brent et al., 1999[i]). The scope and nature of the dysfunction in clinical samples may attenuate the impact of the treatment because of family characteristics, noncompliance, chronicity, and other negative prognostic indicators. Thus, it could be argued that research findings cannot be turned into clinical recommendations, as the research data pertain to a less challenging population of cases. Such an argument, however, presupposes an interaction between severity and the efficacy of specific modes of therapy. In our view, this interaction would need to be demonstrated before the argument could be accepted. Although there is good evidence for a "main effect" of setting, confirming the greater difficulties presented

by clinic-based populations, we know of no demonstrations of a significant interaction between type of therapy and setting that would substantiate the case for not being able to generalize from the findings of RCTs as a matter or principle. Nevertheless, it seems advisable for RCTs to make use of clinic-based samples as far as possible.

3. The third and final concern about generalizing RCTs is that the *treatment* offered may be atypical. In other fields of health care there is evidence that patients who participate in trials may receive superior care, regardless of which arm of the trial they are in (Stiller, 1994). A meta-analysis covering 20 years demonstrated that psychotherapy manuals, specially devised to asses treatment integrity in RCTs, had significantly decreased the variability of the therapist as a contributor to the variance in outcome (Crits-Christoph et al., 1991). The improvement in efficacy gained in the transition between the laboratory and the clinic is an issue of current concern to many researchers (e.g., Kendall & Southam-Gerow, 1995). There is strong indication that, at least for some therapies, the adoption of laboratory-based procedures in a clinical setting may be of great advantage to the patient (e.g., Henggeler, Schoenwald, & Pickrel, 1995). To argue against treatment manuals by asserting that ordinary clinical practitioners do not see things the same way as those working according to a manual seems to us quite unhelpful.

RCTs in child psychiatry are undoubtedly difficult to implement. The argument concerning generalizability ignores the rapidly growing body of RCT research that is based on services delivered to individuals seeking service at mental health facilities or clinics, and finds similar treatment outcomes for individuals who vary in the degree of comorbid psychological problems they have in entering treatment (Hunsley & Rumstein-McKean, 1999). Some recent reviews of the issue in general medicine take a more balanced approach to the relative merits of RCTs and observational designs (e.g., Ioannidis, Haidich, & Lau, 2001). It appears that empirical studies comparing RCT and observational methodology find comparable-sized treatment effects, which undermines the argument that only RCTs give the "true" assessment of treatment efficacy. Clearly, more studies that simultaneously use both approaches are needed in child psychiatry as elsewhere. Until such time that these studies are performed, we believe that findings resulting from RCTs provide the best option for clinicians who wish to base their practice on scientific data. Investigators should be encouraged to employ methodologies that allow their use in clinically relevant contexts, as such trials are often necessary for evaluating the efficacy of specific treatments. In combination with the readily available treatment manuals and training programs in empirically supported treatment methods, child mental health services can increasingly reflect efficacious patterns of care.

Problems of Evidence in Psychosocial Treatment Research

Psychosocial treatment is arguably the most rigorously evaluated of all medical interventions, and certainly this is the case for mental health interventions (Howard, Orlinsky, & Lueger, 1995). Weisz et al.'s (1995b[ib]) survey alone identified 150 outcome studies of child and adolescent psychotherapy collected since their earlier

1987 review. A review by Durlak et al., covering the period up to 1990, indicated that more than 1,000 empirical studies had been reported in the literature (Durlak, Wells, Cotten, & Johnson, 1995). Kazdin (2000a[v]) estimates that between 1990 and 1999 a further 500 empirical studies were completed. Studies continue to improve in quality, paying increasing attention to issues such as codifying treatment with manuals, treatment fidelity, and assessing the clinical significance of change and its stability after the end of treatment (Kazdin, 2000a[v]).

Problems of Evidence from Meta-Analytic Reviews

The limitations on the inferences that can be drawn from single studies have led reviewers to use meta-analytic methods to obtain assessments of treatment effects. Smith and Glass's (1977) seminal review of psychotherapy outcome studies was the first attempt to draw together a large number of outcome studies in order to obtain a reliable indication of the effects of specific types of interventions. For each study, they calculated the differences between the means of the treatment and control groups and, dividing this by the standard deviation of the control group, they obtained an indication of the magnitude of treatment effect independent of the measures used. This is the "effect size" (ES). By pooling ESs across studies, meta-analyses can generate estimates of overall treatment impact, compare outcomes among theoretically meaningful subsets of investigations, and explore client and therapist variables, therapy characteristics, or methodological moderators of treatment outcome. For example, by pooling ESs within categories of therapies, the authors could compare the relative sizes of expected effects. Following Cohen (Cohen, 1988), an ES of .20 is considered small, one of .50 medium, and .80 large. Meta-analytic reviews of the treatment literature (see review of meta-analyses by Kazdin, 2000b) suggest that the average ES of psychotherapy studies comparing treatment and no treatment is about .70 (between moderate and large). As an indication, an ES of .70 suggests that the mean of the treated group is at about the 76th percentile of the control group.

We know of four broad-based or inclusive meta-analyses of psychosocial treatments that together cover in excess of 300 separate treatment studies. The first (Casey & Berman, 1985) covered outcome studies published between 1952 and 1983, but limited its coverage to children under 12. The average ES was reported as .71 (medium to large), suggesting that 76% of children were better off than controls. The second meta-analysis (Weisz, Weiss, Alicke, & Klotz, 1987[ib]) covered the same period, but included children up to 18. The main ES was .79, indicating that almost 79% of treated children were better off than controls. A third meta-analysis (Kazdin, Bass, Ayers, & Rodgers, 1990a) included studies between 1952 and 1983, of children 4–18 years old. The ES was .88, suggesting that 81% of treated subjects could expect to benefit. The fourth meta-analysis (Weisz et al., 1995b[ib]) covered studies between 1967 and 1993 of children 2–18 years old. The mean ES was .71. In addition, there have been numerous meta-analyses confined to specific therapies (e.g., family-based interventions, see Hazelrigg, Cooper, & Borduin, 1987; Shadish et al., 1993[ib]) or specific problems (e.g., impulsivity, see Baer & Nietzel, 1991[ib]).

However, there are problems with the meta-analytic approach. First, it is not clear to what extent studies of different forms of treatment are comparable in terms of dependent variables, treatment standardization, average treatment length, the severity of disorders treated, and so on, yet such variables can either moderate or mediate the differences in effect size. For example, in one meta-analysis comparing behavioral and nonbehavioral psychotherapies, variables such as setting, measurement specificity, reactivity, and manipulability, as well as sample size, were found to be moderating variables, accounting for a substantial proportion of the differences in the effect size between these two forms of treatment (Shadish & Sweeney, 1991). The alternative is to restrict meta-analyses to studies that directly compare different treatments within the same study, using the same measures and controlling for treatment duration and other methodological features (Robinson, Berman, & Neimeyer, 1990; Shapiro & Shapiro, 1982b). Even here, there will be differences between the conditions in terms of therapist expertise and researcher allegiance (Luborsky et al., 1999).

A second problem with the approach of obtaining average ESs for treatments based on the categorization of studies concerns the way researchers arrive at such categories for treatment. Stephen Shirk (Shirk, 1998; Shirk & Russell, 1992), for example, reexamined the meta-analysis of child psychotherapy studies reported by Weisz et al. (1995b[ib]). He demonstrated that very few of the studies categorized by the original meta-analysis as psychodynamic could be seriously considered to be so. Less than a quarter of the studies met even rudimentary criteria, such as an established psychodynamic theoretical frame of reference or trained therapists. When pseudopsychodynamic studies were excluded, the observed ESs in the small number of studies remaining ($n = 4$) were comparable to those obtained in trials of cognitive-behavioral treatment.

Third, meta-analytic studies are prone to publication bias, a bias against negative findings that can have the effect of causing the support for a proposition in the published literature to seem stronger than it really is. Lipsey and Wilson (1993[vi]), in a meta-analysis of 92 meta-analyses of outcome research, found that average ES for published studies was .53, whereas in unpublished research it was only .39. More than 95% of published studies yield significant findings (Bozarth & Roberts, 1972; Sterling, 1959), yet it seems implausible that such a high percentage of research conducted actually confirms the hypotheses with statistical significance. Some have suggested that publication bias may be large enough to account for the generally positive findings of meta-analyses of treatment outcomes (Sohn, 1996). The quantification of the review process brings with it the potential for a reification of findings, which may encourage sophisticated reviewers to make inadequate use of their commonsense judgments as clinicians in drawing conclusions from the literature.

Finally, the comparison of average ESs for different classes of therapies aggregates significant differences in opposite directions. The problem arises because the hypothesis being tested is that the true ES for comparisons of treatments from two selected classes is zero, rather than the more appropriate hypothesis that the true ES for all comparisons between treatments is zero and any significant differences observed are chance observations (Type I error). Indeed, to exclude this possibility, an omnibus test of the differences between ESs needs to be performed—that is, the comparison of the mean differences in ES between treatments, relative to the variance within treatment categories, should be calculated (Wampold et al., 1997). When these methodological considerations are taken on board, the systematic differences between the ESs associated with different types of treatments evaporate (Wampold et al., 1997).

There are many further limitations. For example, meta-analyses do not include within-subject or single-case studies. They may include studies of questionable methodological adequacy. The current database of studies is unrepresentative in relation to what happens in clinical practice: There are few controlled evaluations of psychodynamic treatments, and behavioral and cognitive-behavioral studies are overrepresented. Studies that are not directly relevant to clinical issues, such as analogue studies, and trials of patients whose symptoms are not of clinically significant severity, may be included. Analyses can multiply sample measures taken from the same patient and from the same study, leading to ESs computed on the basis of dependent data. Using average Z scores assumes that outcome measures are appropriately measured on an interval scale, and that their distribution may be assumed to have significant skewness and kurtosis. Not all meta-analyses weight the means for sample size, yet small effects from a large trial are arguably more important then large ones from a small sample, and because the methodological decisions made by meta-analytic teams tend to vary, the comparison of meta-analytic results and comparisons of ESs are fraught with problems.

Kazdin (2000b) suggests that a balanced view should be taken of meta-analyses. Although he lists a number of limitations (those mentioned above and some others), he points out the advantages of the procedure in terms of providing a systematic base for literature review that make this explicit and replicable, summarizes the strengths and limitations of a body of literature (e.g., the general brevity of follow-ups, the smallness of samples), and permits the exploration of influences that would otherwise not be open to scrutiny. For example, meta-analyses by Luborsky et al. (Luborsky et al., 1999) demonstrated that the treatments favored by the investigator tend to produce larger effects than other treatments included in the study. The key problem with meta-analysis is the generality of the conclusions it tends to yield, namely, that treatment is more effective than no treatment, and much that is vital in understanding the value of a particular approach to a specific group of disorders is lost in the aggregation of outcome variables within a study and ESs between investigations.

Empirically Validated Treatments

There has been considerable debate in recent years concerning the evidence required to adequately evaluate a psychosocial intervention in the treatment of a particular mental health problem. The American Academy of Child and Adolescent Psychiatry, the American Psychological Association (APA) in the United States, and the National Institute for Clinical Excellence in the United Kingdom have attempted to identify guidelines for clinical practice with children so that decisions about funding various treatments should no longer be arbitrary. For example, the American Psychological Association Division 12's Task Force on the Promotion and Dissemination of Psychological Procedures set up working groups to identify psychosocial interventions for children with depression, anxiety disorders, conduct disorders, attention-deficit/hyperactivity disorder, and autism. It is suggested that by identifying effective psychosocial interventions for specific disorders "the Task Force could advance the science-based practice of clinical psychology and provide practitioners with the strongest justification for their services (e.g., for third-party payment)" (Lonigan, Elbert, & Johnson, 1998, p.141). As can be seen, economic considerations are not far from even the most professionally conducted reviews of outcome.

The criteria adopted by the Task Force of Clinical Child Psychologists were a variation of those used by the APA's Task Force on Promotion and Dissemination of Psychological Procedures (Chambless & Hollon, 1998; Chambless et al., 1996). In these reviews random assignment is considered an absolute criterion. The criteria for a well-established psychosocial intervention for childhood disorders include at least two well-conducted group design studies conducted by different teams of investigators; in which the treatment is shown to be superior to placebo or alternative treatment or equivalent to an already established treatment. Alternatively, 10 or more single-case design studies, with good experimental design and comparison with another treatment, would suffice. In either instance, a clear specification of the sample is essential and treatment manuals are preferred. The criteria for probably efficacious treatments are met when two studies show the intervention to be more effective than no treatment (control group) or superiority is demonstrated against placebo or alternative treatment with the studies conducted by the same investigator. A smaller number of single-case design studies ($n = 4$–9) would meet the same criteria. The criteria related to sample description and manuals apply equally to well-established and probably efficacious interventions. Manualization was not insisted on "because behavioral programs used with children use well-known social learning principles with no detailed treatment manual provided" (Lonigan et al., 1998, p. 141). The insistence on independent teams of investigators is imposed to counteract the potential bias from allegiance effects, which have bedeviled psychotherapy research (Luborsky et al., 1999). Treatments are regarded as empirically supported to the extent that studies are available that meet these prespecified criteria. Although identifying empirically supported treatments can discriminate between different treatment approaches and can often identify a treatment of choice, there is no implication, at least in principle, that the conclusions are not open to change. New evidence may emerge concerning existing treatments, new treatments may be introduced, limitations on the applicability of particular treatment approaches may be identified, or the criteria for empirically supported treatments may change.

What is the minimum period for which a treatment has to be effective in order to be considered efficacious? In the adult literature at least, there is ample evidence that even where brief manualized treatments have been shown to be effective, a significant percentage of clients remain symptomatic, many relapse, and others seek additional treatment. Empirical validation may risk conflating two radically different groups of treatments: those that have been adequately tested and found ineffective and those that have not been tested at all. Yet the reasons that a particular treatment has not been subjected to empirical scrutiny may have nothing to do with its likely effectiveness, but may rather be attributed to powerful factors such as the intellectual culture of practitioners, the availability of treatment manuals, and peer perception of the value of the treatment, which can determine the likelihood of both funding and publication. Defining treatments is as or more complex for establishing empirically validated treatments, as for meta-analyses.

First, the criteria specified by the Task Force are arbitrary. They have not been validated, and thus their mechanical application may, and in some places does, yield paradoxical findings. For example, treatments of evidently different value may be categorized under the same heading. Thus, problem-solving skills training (Kazdin, Esveldt-Dawson, French, & Unis, 1987b[i]) and a "time out plus signal seat" treatment (Hamilton & MacQuiddy, 1984) are both categorized as probably efficacious treatments for conduct problems. Yet they are obviously different in terms of their theoretical foundation, scope, and evidence base.

Second, the categorization of treatment is of limited help to clinicians attempting to choose the ideal treatment strategy. Requiring clear specification of sample characteristics recognizes that specific treatments may be effective only with a limited range of individuals, depending on age, ethnicity, severity of disorder, and so on (Kendall, 2000[v]; Weisz, Huey, & Weersing, 1998b). The categorization does not, however, answer the question, "What treatment works for whom?"

Third, the coding criteria are not available, so the user of the Task Force report has no access to information concerning the bases up which judgments such as "well-conducted group design" or "good (single-case) experimental design" were made (Kazdin, 2000b). In a similar vein, the definition of "established treatment" with which a new treatment is compared remains vague and leaves the door open to a circular definition of effectiveness. Further, the criteria specify a clear sample description but fail to be clear as to what constitutes such a description.

Fourth, the criteria do not specify what pattern of results might indicate that a treatment study showed that a treatment should be considered effective. For example, what is the minimum period for which the treatment has to be effective in order to be considered efficacious? In the adult literature at least, there is ample evidence that even where brief manualized treatments have been shown to be effective, a significant percentage of clients remain symptomatic, many relapse, and others seek additional treatment. Westen and Morrison (in press), in their meta-analysis of studies of anxiety and depression, found that roughly half the patients treated receive further treatment between termination and 2-year follow-up. Similarly, how many measures need to show significant effects for the trial to be considered successful? Most trials report significant differences on some measures (e.g., parent rating) but not others (e.g., teacher rating). Further, a study that shows marginally significant results is treated within this system as equivalent to a study with a large ES and high levels of statistical significance. Further, statistical significance is related to sample size, whereas ES will always be a function of the sensitivity of the instrument used (Kazdin, 2000b).

Fifth, the categorization conflates two radically different groups of treatments: those that have been adequately tested and found ineffective and those that have not been tested at all. Yet the reasons that a particular treatment has not been subjected to empirical scrutiny may have nothing to do with its likely effectiveness, but may rather be powerful factors such as the intellectual culture of practitioners, the availability of treatment manuals, and peer perception of the value of the treatment, which can determine the likelihood of both funding and publication. A different problem is presented by studies that show smaller effects or even "negative effects" relative to an alternative treatment. The binary categorical system does not recognize these subtleties.

Sixth, it is not self-evident whether two different implementations of a treatment program may be considered sufficiently comparable to be coded as the same and therefore merit the "empirically supported" badge. Alternatively, they may be considered to be tests of different treatments, and therefore both may merit only the "promising" label. For example, there are at least four forms of parent training currently validated. If these had been taken together as one form of intervention, then parent training for conduct problem children would have received full endorsement as an empirically supported method. As it was, these treatments were considered by the Task Force to be different, and therefore only two of them, which had been replicated on other sites, were considered to have been empirically supported. In brief, defining treatments is as or more complex for establishing empirically validated treatments, as for meta-analyses.

Seventh, the issue of the focus on technique raises a final and most serious problem (Kazdin, 2000b). Not only is there inherent ambiguity concerning when a particular technique was genuinely applied in a setting other than the one in which it was invented, but such a focus implicitly reifies psychosocial treatments, assumes that a treatment will produce equivalent effects regardless of therapist characteristics, the qualities of the setting, the developmental level of the child, the quality of the relationship established with the therapist, the level of family dysfunction, and so on. It is quite possible that certain treatments, deemed to be empirically supported, are so only given the constellation of moderating variables in place at the time of their assessment.

In general, empirically supported treatments cannot and should not be treated as assurances of efficacy in any clinical setting. As we shall see later, there is considerable doubt as to whether treatments originating in research laboratories can work effectively under conditions prevailing where most mental health professionals work. Of course, a complementary issue raised by Kazdin (2000b) is that there may be clinical interventions that are perfectly efficacious in practice settings but appear to be ineffective when examined under laboratory conditions. The dichotomy of *empirically supported or not* appears inadequate to the complexity of the problem of garnering supportive evidence. A lack of subtlety is quite directly implied by the imbalance between the number of empirical studies of psychological therapies in the literature (perhaps as many as 1,500) and the number of therapies that have received the badge of recognition from the APA Task Force (about two dozen).

Efficacy Meets Effectiveness

In any case, the applicability to patterns of service delivery of such global claims concerning effectiveness is problematic because of the discrepancy between the efficacy of psychological therapies as evaluated in formal outcome studies reviewed by evidence-based panels such as the APA Task Forces, and their observed effectiveness in naturalistic settings such as community clinics, health centers, or homes (Weisz & Weiss, 1993; Weisz, Weiss, & Donenberg, 1992).

Weisz et al. (Weisz et al., 1995b[vi]) used a meta-analytic strategy to explore why "research therapy" appears more effective than clinical practice. They identified studies that involved treatment of clinic-referred children, carried out in service-oriented clinics or agencies by practicing clinicians, with treatment done as part of the normal service delivery of the clinic. The ESs in these studies suggested negligible effects. The features of research therapy that appear to account for their superiority include behavioral methods, the use of focused treatment, and preplanning and structure. It is not inevitably the case that naturalistic settings reduce effectiveness, however. Multisystemic family intervention has achieved remarkable success in a naturalistic setting involving home, school, and community (e.g., Borduin et al., 1995[i]; Henggeler et al., 1995). Similarly, parent management training can be more successful in a community setting than in clinic-based applications (e.g., Cunningham, Bremner, & Boyle, 1995[i]).

There are other well-known differences between clinic-based studies and the world of service delivery. Important features of clinical samples include greater severity of problems, lower levels of motivation for treatment in both child and parent, inclusion of complex or difficult cases (children in foster care, children with substance abuse problems), high levels of comorbidity, and so on. Treatments designed in the laboratory are frequently simply unsuitable for implementation in the field. Treatments in clinics are mostly shorter than specified in manuals, primarily because of high rates of unnegotiated dropouts (Weisz & Hawley, 1998). Experimental studies are uninformative about the effects of the first half, or even the first quarter, of manualized treatment.

The term *effectiveness research* is used to describe outcome investigations that test the impact of a treatment in a naturalistic setting, as distinct from *efficacy research*, which is concerned with "laboratory"-based experimental treatment trials. The crucial distinction between efficacy and effectiveness has been carefully elaborated in the recent literature (Kopta, Lueger, Saunders, & Howard, 1999; VandenBos, 1996; Wells, 1999). The effectiveness model emphasizes the importance of researching treatments as they are applied in day-to-day practice. It aims to evaluate the extent to which specific treatments work as they are routinely delivered in the field.

An effectiveness design, such as large-scale surveys of subjects who have received or will go through psychotherapy, offers many advantages over randomized controlled trials in terms of external validity or generalizability. Unfortunately, most of these advantages also carry threats to internal validity in varying degrees. First, the sample is far more representative of the population that uses services in a given geographical area, giving the results of the study good external validity. However, samples are also quite heterogeneous, and therefore conclusions about specific groups may be difficult to draw.

Second, such large-scale studies yield a mass of multilevel information about both client and service characteristics that moderate outcome, which is extremely valuable to professionals, administrators, and policy makers in planning treatment provision. By the same token, they are limited to the populations currently receiving the service, and thus "cloning," the inadvertent perpetuation of existing patterns of referral and treatment, becomes inevitable. Third, naturalistic subgroups may be selected within the overall samples (e.g., clusters of different diagnostic categories), which would allow for internal comparisons, partially compensating for the lack of a control group. Unfortunately, these designs will, by definition, lack a no-treatment control group; early dropouts then frequently serve this role, but the assumption of comparability is doubtful even if there are careful efforts at matching.

Fourth, these studies may be far more cost-effective than randomized controlled trials. Efficacy trials take place in university hospital departments, which are unusual and expensive sites for treatment. Effectiveness studies are more likely to be mounted in community (public sector) settings, where services can be provided more cheaply. The cheaper service provision may, however, entail a compromise of the quality of service delivery. University evaluations are more likely to be rigorously controlled in terms of assessor blindness and the quality of measurements undertaken. On the other hand, laboratory-based measurement may be oversensitive and yield differences that are irrelevant to treatment choice. The lower cost of effectiveness studies enables large sample sizes. In contrast, as dropout rates tend to be high (Weisz & Weiss, 1989), what is gained in representativeness by large-scale recruitment to the study may be lost through selective attrition.

Fifth, efficacy trials examine discrete treatments, yet, clinically, treatments are usually given in combination (e.g., medication and psychosocial treatments). Effectiveness trials offer an opportunity to study treatment combinations, but only those combinations that naturally occur in clinical practice. These may not represent the optimal combinations. By the same token, the dose of treatment (i.e., treatment length or frequency in psychosocial treatments) is variable in effectiveness studies but rigidly controlled in efficacy investigations. The former offers information about optimal dose across large samples. This may be misleading, however, if larger doses appear to be ineffective because they are selectively offered to treatment-resistant individuals. Effectiveness trials further ensure the representativeness of treatments by not controlling how therapists participate in the trial work. Although this avoids the inevitable distortion that arises in examining the outcome of a treatment that will never exist in the real world, it also leaves uncontrolled the extent to which individual therapists do or do not adhere to specific treatment protocols. Efficacy trials may reflect an integration of services (e.g., child welfare and mental health) that is unlikely to occur in the "real world." In contrast, effectiveness interventions may identify certain treatment approaches as being ineffective, not because they are inert, but because of the absence of other service provisions necessary for the treatment to be successful (e.g., support for parents).

Effectiveness research cannot be seen as a panacea, and a combination of effectiveness and efficacy research will be required for us to comprehensively answer the outcome question of "what treatment works for whom." We raise these points here only to highlight the current tension between naturalistic assessments of treatment effectiveness and experimental measures of efficacy. Effectiveness studies will never be adequate substitutes for experimental investigations, yet they are increasingly seen as essential and complementary to RCTs (Wells, 1999). There is an inevitable dialectic between ambiguity and lack of relevance at these two poles of evaluating mental health treatment (e.g., Kopta et al., 1999). In general, it is likely that the rigorous application of the methodology developed in efficacy studies to naturalistic data collection will yield the highest dividends.

There are excellent models of such methodologically hybrid investigations under way in adult psychotherapy work (Wade, Treat, & Stuart, 1998) and, increasingly, also in child psychotherapy. For example, John Weisz (Weisz, 2000[v]; Weisz et al., 1998a; Weisz & Hawley, 1998), in the Los Angeles Mental Health Clinic Study, is attempting to test the value of experimentally developed psychosocial treatment approaches by randomly assigning clinicians to training in these methods or a nontrained control group, and monitoring their outcomes in clinical practice over subsequent years. Len Bickman (1996), in the Stark County System Coordination study, has examined the hypothesis that the coordination of child welfare services (e.g., through case management) improves the outcome of childhood psychiatric disorders. So far there appears to be no impact on outcome (Weisz, Han, & Valeri, 1997a). Scott Henggeler and his group are assessing the value of a comprehensive psychosocial treatment model MST when offered to families whose child is about to be hospitalized (see Chapter 5 and Henggeler et al., 1999; Rowland, Henggeler, Pickrel, & Edwards, 1999). Children (n = 113) in the process of inpatient admission, "on their way to the hospital," were randomly diverted to MST. At 4 months, youths who received MST demonstrated fewer externalizing symptoms and reduced alcohol use, had improved family structure and cohesion, and spent more time in school than the hospitalized youths. Hospitalization was more effective than MST in improving the young people's self-esteem. MST prevented any hospitalizations in 57% of the participants in the MST condition and reduced the overall number of hospitalizations by 72% and other out-of-home placements by 49%. The same group is bringing an effectiveness model to the problem of dissemination. Twenty-six agencies across the United States are implementing this treatment approach, but its effectiveness varies across sites. The effective sites may be distinguished from the ineffective ones in terms of the culture of the organization, the flexibility of the workplace, and the responsivity of the leadership.

There are impediments to the dissemination of research findings into clinical practice that reflect the dialectic between effectiveness and efficacy research. Weisz (2000[v]) put it eloquently: "Researchers have given a party, but clinicians and families have stayed home" (p. 837). Research-based treatments are often perceived as irrelevant by clinicians, perhaps because manualized treatments are perceived to be rigid (Addis, Wade, & Hatgis, 1999) and clinicians may feel colonized by researchers. Clinicians may well be right in thinking that these research-based treatments are irrelevant, although for rather different reasons. For example, researchers' understanding of the parameters and constraints of clinical practice has been limited in the past. Moreover, cost concerns currently loom large in clinical practice, producing a situation where many treatments, although empirically supported, cannot be implemented for lack of funds. It is clear that research and evidence-based treatment development, if it is to be implemented on a large scale, will have to occur in the context of a partnership between researchers and clinicians (Weisz, 2000[v]). Although such models of partnership have been extensively discussed (e.g., Roth, Fonagy, & Parry, 1996), they have not yet evolved in a coherent way on either side of the Atlantic. For this to happen, new treatment models should be developed in the context of service settings rather than simply through the modifying of laboratory-based approaches. Studies of the treatment process must happen alongside the assessment of effectiveness so that clinicians obtain immediate and complex feedback about how they can modify their therapeutic work, rather than receiving a simple prescription for particular procedures. This argument has been powerfully made by Kazdin (2000a[v]). We know all too well that dissemination is more than publication, but this realization has taken some time to be translated into action. The issue of training is critical; research supporting a particular psychosocial treatment is of limited value unless therapists in other settings and other countries can be trained, cheaply and effectively, to carry out this treatment.

There are several novel approaches to integrating efficacy and effectiveness data. Westen and Morrison (in press) propose a hybrid concept of "effective efficacy." Effective efficacy refers to the proportion of patients encountered in clinical practice who are likely to respond to empirically supported psychosocial interventions. So whereas the efficacy of a treatment is indicated by the proportion of those patients undergoing the treatment who manifest clinically significant improvement, effective efficacy refers to the range within which a treatment may be expected to be effective in clinical practice. Thus effective efficacy adjusts success rates for the number of patients excluded from efficacy trials, using the correlation across studies between exclusion rates and success rates. One review of psychosocial treatments for adult psychosocial disorders arrived at the conclusion that the more complex the clinical presentation the lower the success rates tended to be (Roth & Fonagy, 1996). Thus, the stricter the criteria for entry into a particular trial, the larger the exclusion rate and the higher the likely estimate of efficacy. However, clinicians working in the field cannot exclude such complex cases from their practice. The average child in a child-outpatient community clinic has more than 3.5 diagnoses (Weisz & Hawley, 1998). Thus, a better estimate of expected success would be given by effective efficacy, which takes exclusion rates into account. In the Westen and Morrison meta-analysis of recent controlled studies of psychosocial treatments of depression, panic, and generalized anxiety disorder (GAD), the intent-to-treat improvement rates were 37% for depression, 54% for panic, and 44% for GAD. When these figures are adjusted for those not treated because of exclusion criteria (principally comorbidity), these improvement rates could become 14% for depression, 19% for panic, and 10% for GAD. The true improvement rate for a clinic population is likely to be somewhere in between.

A fundamentally different approach to the dialectic of effectiveness and efficacy was proposed by Kazdin and Kendall (see Kazdin, 1998, 2000a[v], 2000b, Kendall, 2000[v]). These authors suggest that rather than simply seeking and testing treatments so that criteria for empirical support can be met, researchers should identify and target the core psychological processes involved in a disorder and test variations of duration, intensity, and focus with systematically varied populations in order to approximate more closely an answer to the "What treatment works for whom?" question. They outline a seven-step approach, moving from the conceptualization of the dysfunction and research on processes related to it, through to a conceptualization and specification of the treatment for the dysfunction that has its underpinnings in theory and research. Tests of effectiveness should not stop tests of treatment outcome. The question of whether intervention techniques actually affect those processes that are considered to be critical to the treatment model also need to be answered. There are some sobering lessons in the literature concerning this issue. In their thoughtful meta-analysis, Durlak et al. (Durlak, Fuhrman, & Lampman, 1991) found that changes in cognition were not significantly related to changes in behavior. Recent research on cognitive therapy for depression suggests that adherence to a manual may actually be negatively correlated with outcome (Ablon & Jones, 1998; Castonguay, Goldfried, Wiser, Raue, & Hayes, 1996). The variables hypothesized to produce change are not the ones associated with change when transcripts of psychotherapy process are coded. Finally, the limits and moderators of effectiveness need to be established. Diagnosis is an important beginning to answer "What treatment works for whom?" However, as this review will reveal, there are numerous child, parent, family, and other factors with which the effective elements of psychosocial treatments interact.

How Representative of Clinical Practice Is the Current Database of Studies?

The generalizability of the current body of child and adolescent psychosocial treatment research is severely limited by the absence of studies investigating the effectiveness of more traditional approaches such as psychoanalysis, psychodynamic therapy, client-centered therapy, and even family therapy. In the most recent meta-analysis (Weisz et al., 1995b[ib]) of 244 ESs, 50% were derived from behavioral treatment, 16% from cognitive or cognitive-behavioral therapy, 15% from parent training approaches, and only 11% from nonbehavioral treatment. Of this 11%, more than a third were from non-theory-driven discussion group "therapies" normally included in studies as a control group. Only 4% of the 244 ESs were from insight-oriented and 2% from client-centered therapies. Yet there is evidence to suggest that these traditional treatments represent a significant proportion of psychosocial treatment practice (Kazdin, Siegel, & Bass, 1990). In addition, there are many new therapies that have not been subjected to any kind of empirical study. The portfolio of psychosocial research on children provides a poor match with clinical practice.

A related problem concerns so-called mixed or integrated treatments. As we have seen, perhaps more than half of child mental health clinicians using psychosocial treatment are inclined to use a mixture of techniques, claiming to use "whatever works" with a particular child (Garfield & Bergin, 1994). The empirical base of such mixed strategies is limited. Nevertheless, there is a growing recognition that if research treatments are to be of relevance to clinical practice, evaluated strategies should include multimodal treatment approaches administered component-by-component on the "as needed" principle. Good examples of this approach include interventions with disruptive disorders (Henggeler, Melton, & Smith, 1992[i]; Henggeler, Melton, Smith, Schoenwald, & Hanley, 1993[v]) and studies with ADHD (Abikoff & Hechtman, 1996). It will be important to specify an algorithm that enables clinicians to administer treatment components in the most efficacious sequence, but to achieve this, much further research is required.

The Problem of Follow-Up

Most psychosocial treatment studies have not included long-term follow-ups. A review by Jensen et al. (Jensen, Hoagwood, & Petti, 1996[ib]) identified no more than two dozen recent studies with a follow-up of 6 months or greater. In studies that report follow-ups, the modal length from termination is 4–6 months (Weisz & Weiss, 1993). Most authors in the APA review of empirically supported psychosocial treatments noted the scarcity of long-term follow-ups. Even when longer-term follow-ups are available, there is no comparison with a control group. Long-term follow-up is, in any case, hard to interpret because of the high likelihood of additional therapeutic input.

Yet long-term follow-ups are essential in all evaluation research, particularly in studies of children. There are good reasons for assuming that treatment effects are less likely to be maintained for children and adolescents than for adults. A child-focused treatment may succeed in altering the child's behavior in the short term, but once discontinued the child again comes under the influence of adverse transactional processes (family, school, peer group) that may not have been adequately addressed as part of the treatment package. Children are less in control of their environment than adults, and this presents specific obstacles for favorable outcome in the long term.

Second, the impact of treatment may not be obvious immediately upon termination. For example, a young child may benefit from cognitive interventions in terms of a long-term modification of important schemas, but these changes may not manifest until the child's cognitive maturity permits for such schemas to be reliably and regularly used. Child treatment occurs during a period of rapid cognitive change, and cognitive development is likely to interact with treatment inputs; however, the results of this interchange may not be evident within the 6-month lag of the vast majority of follow-up assessments.

Third, some treatments, particularly psychodynamic ones, tend to focus less on symptomatic outcome than on addressing risk factors and vulnerabilities in the child. Long-term psychodynamic treatment of severely disordered children explicitly focuses on facilitating the development of mental capacities, which are expected to enhance the child's resilience to psychosocial stress from a variety of sources (family, peer group, etc.) (Fonagy & Target, 1996). Given the ambitious goals of such treatment, outcomes will be evident only in the context of a long-term developmental, perhaps life span, perspective.

All childhood interventions have a preventive component that will become apparent only through very long-term follow-up. Epidemiological studies that demonstrate the association of childhood psychopathology and adult adjustment problems (e.g., Champion, Goodall, & Rutter, 1995) pose an appropriate challenge to childhood psychosocial treatment research. Ultimately, effective childhood interventions are those that set a child on a developmental path comparable in risk to those without significant childhood disturbance. Thus, it may be suggested that, given the extremely limited time span covered by most treatment studies, the true effectiveness of most child mental health treatments is unknown. Most of the conclusions concerning effectiveness we shall be able to draw in this volume are based on treatment effects assessed at termination.

It should be borne in mind that the importance of follow-up varies considerably according to the nature of the disorder under scrutiny. In general, for disorders that have a time-limited course (e.g., enuresis), long-term follow-ups may not be necessary. In contrast, with disorders that are chronic with a poor prognosis (e.g., autism or childhood-onset conduct disorder), long-term follow-ups are essential, as relapse may mean a gradual reversion to type.

The Failure to Match Treatments to Cases

Outcome research should identify those characteristics of children, parents, and families that might make them particularly well suited to specific treatment approaches (Kazdin, 1996c), yet, in general, individual differences are rarely considered in experimental outcome studies (Morrow-Bradley & Elliott, 1986). There are also particular categories of disorders for which psychosocial treatments have not been thoroughly examined. This may be understandable in the case of relatively rare disorders (e.g., gender identity disorder, tic disorders, psychosis) but is harder to understand for some relatively common problems such as childhood maltreatment (Cicchetti & Toth, 1995) and somatization, anorexia and bulimia (Diamond, Serrano, Dickey, & Sonis, 1996).

In their focus on the internal validity of research designs, outcome studies have failed to pay adequate attention to the ecological validity of the treatments subjected to investigation. For example, ethnicity and cultural background of patients participating in trials is rarely reported (Weisz, Valeri, McCarty, & Moore, 1999) and almost never tested as a moderating variable. Currently, the assumption that evidential support for many treatments can be appropriately generalized to ethnic groups other than North American Caucasian samples is largely untested. It should be remembered that the proportion of those with clinically significant disorders who are referred for treatment is low (10–20%) (e.g., Kolko & Kazdin, 1993; Pavuluri, Luk, & McGee, 1996) and dropouts from treatment are relatively high (Kazdin, 1990b; Weisz & Weiss, 1989). This may be due to the inadequate attention paid to the match between users' expectations and researchers' goals and the somewhat artificial social situations that many psychosocial interventions create.

Psychosocial interventions sometimes foster an implicit blaming attitude. Inevitably, interventions address complex developmental transactional processes that are inconsistent with the simple linear models of causality underlying many psychosocial treatments and that make any attempt at attributing blame a meaningless exercise. Yet treatment programs of all orientations necessarily work with somewhat reductionist, implicit etiological models, which are sometimes explicitly and sometimes more subtly communicated to children and caregivers. Although psychodynamic approaches perhaps most clearly exemplify this problem (e.g., Bettelheim, 1967, and the notion of a "refrigerator mother" in autism), many behavioral techniques such as parent management training or social skills training for disruptive disorders may be argued to have similar implications. Low rates of take-up for experimentally validated treatments should be seen in this light.

Summary and Conclusions

The limitations listed here, when taken together, easily account for practicing clinicians' relative lack of interest in the findings of psychosocial treatment research. Clinicians often do not consider such findings to be of relevance to their day-to-day work (Cohen, Sargent, & Sechrest, 1986; Morrow-Bradley & Elliott, 1986) and tend to demonstrate this lack of concern by reading very few (fewer than one per year) research reports, although this situation may be gradually changing with the economic pressures on clinicians to demonstrate evidence-based practice. Integrating findings from psychosocial treatment research, either in meta-analyses or by defining criteria for evidence-based treatments, is complicated by the methodological shortcomings of both these approaches. The experimental model of the RCT may be difficult to apply to the testing of psychosocial treatments. Effectiveness research brings with it its own problems. The dialectic between internal and external validity is a current focus for investigators but has yet to be thoroughly addressed in empirical studies. The current database of outcome investigations is also unrepresentative in terms of clinical orientations and has inadequate follow-ups, relatively superficial exploration of individual differences in treatment response, and other methodological limitations (e.g., small sample sizes and inconsistent age ranges).

It seems that questions such as "What works for whom?" are inherently impossible to answer in the context of a review of outcome investigations. The number of disorders is too large, the number of psychosocial interventions too great in number and too heterogeneous in implementation, the number of contextual (moderating) factors to be taken into account too many and too difficult to specify for the field to yield definitive answers to an inquiry as crassly empirical as the "Who is likely to benefit?" question. Kazdin (2000a[v]) suggests the questioning should start with understanding the mode of action of therapy and the role of moderating factors beyond noting their empirical reality. A note of caution is sounded by those who warn that empirical support for beneficial outcomes must be sought prior to the search for process factors (Kendall, 2000[v]).

Problems of Evidence in Psychopharmacology Research

The Current Status of Practice

Psychotropic drugs are prescribed to children and adolescents with increasing frequency (Jensen, Vitiello, Leonard, & Laughren, 1992; Safer & Krager, 1994; Zito & Riddle, 1995). Just as research on adult psychosocial treatment is some way ahead of child and adolescent studies, so research in pediatric psychopharmacology has lagged behind the adult field (Jensen, Ryan, & Prien, 1994; Jensen et al., 1992; Vitiello & Jensen, 1997). With the exception of stimulants, which have been extensively studied, the label for most psychotropic drugs remains "safety and efficacy have not been established in children." The absence of outcome data has resulted in the "off-label" use of these drugs in the United States (American Academy of Pediatrics Committee on Drugs, 1996). As psychopharmacological agents are becoming more widely accepted in child psychiatry in the United Kingdom, the urgency for clinical trials is increasingly felt. Physicians and families have expressed concern about the use of untested treatments (e.g., clonidine in ADHD: see Swanson et al., 1996). Many children with severe behavioral or emotional problems might benefit from already available treatments but for the lack of research into indications and parameters of use. Conversely, the widespread use of psychotropics raises the possibility that some children may be inappropriately placed on medication when other forms of intervention (social or psychosocial) may be more desirable. However, in the United States a number of initiatives have been undertaken to address the scarcity of adequate outcome data, including the prioritization of pediatric psychopharmacology in the National Plan for Research on Child and Adolescent Mental Disorders (Committee for the Study of Research on Child and Adolescent Mental Disorders, 1995). We can therefore realistically anticipate a genuine explosion of data in this field. Rigorous, relevant, multisite work is somewhat easier to undertake in pediatric psychopharmacology than it has been in the psychosocial domain. In the remainder of this section we shall briefly review some of the outstanding issues facing outcome research in this area.

Developmental Considerations in the Safety and Effectiveness of Psychotropic Medication

Both the FDA and its British equivalent (the Committee on the Safety of Medicines) permit the generalization of evidence concerning efficacy to children from adult data if there is proof of an analogy between psychopathological features and psychopharmacological response across these groups (Food and Drug Administration, 1994). However, continuity of pharmacological response clearly has to be empirically established and cannot be based on similarities of presentation or even similarities of biological signs. For example, whereas biological indices of depression in childhood are similar to those in adults (Emslie, Rush, Weinberg, Rintelmann, & Roffwarg, 1990; Ryan et al., 1987), tricyclic antidepressants are notably more effective for the latter than for the former, for reasons that are poorly understood (Jensen et al., 1992). Some medications that are safe in adults are known to produce adverse effects in children. For example, phenobarbital is known to delay intellectual development (Farwell et al., 1990). Little is known about the chronic administration of medication, or even the long-term effects of acute treatment. It is perfectly possible that long-term use may yield long-term benefits and improve prognosis. Conversely, longer exposure to treatment may have negative influences on development. More information is needed on the impact of these preparations on cognitive development as well as their impact on behavior and physical growth (Vitiello & Jensen, 1995).

Data are particularly sparse with regard to polypharmacy (Rapport, Carlson, Kelly, & Pataki, 1993; Wilens, Biederman, Geist, Steingard, & Spencer, 1993), which, given the high prevalence of comorbidity in childhood disorders, is relatively common (e.g., Connor, Ozbayrak, Kusiak, Caponi, & Melloni, 1997b[iv]). The efficacy and safety of commonly used combinations should be established. We cannot assume that effective and safe combinations administered to adults have the same benefits for children. Even less is known about the combined effects of physical and psychosocial treatments, which, from a clinical point of view, may be the most pertinent information. These are underresearched areas even in the adult field (Roth & Fonagy, 1996); we may have to wait some years before comprehensive child data become available.

Methodological Limitations of the Psychopharmacology Outcome Literature

A range of methodological problems have plagued the literature on pediatric outcome studies. Although there is considerable heterogeneity among studies, depending on the agent and the condition, the following issues are repeatedly highlighted in reviews (e.g., Campbell & Cueva, 1995b; Campbell & Cueva, 1995a[ib]; Vitiello & Jensen, 1997).

The *sample sizes* of most studies are lamentably small. For example, only four of a dozen or so placebo-controlled studies of tricyclic antidepressants enrolled more than 15 patients into each treatment arm (Jensen et al., 1992). There may be several reasons for this. For example, parents may be resistant about accepting the possibility of placebo treatment for their child. Many children do not qualify for trials because of comorbidity or because a very high clinical severity threshold is set. Such restrictions not only have an impact on recruitment but also affect generalizability. It is also likely that pediatric psychopharmacology trials receive less support from practitioners and health maintenance organizations (HMOs) than do other pharmacology trials (Fava, 1996; Vitiello & Jensen, 1997).

The *age ranges* employed in studies are inconsistent. In some studies preschoolers (3–6), elementary schoolchildren (6–12) and early adolescents (12–16) are combined. Yet it is known that this wide age range encompasses qualitatively different phases of both physiological and psychological development. There is no generally accepted grouping of children according to age for the purposes of psychopharmacological research. Pharmacokinetic studies reveal important differences between newborns and infants, and early and late adolescents (Gibaldi & Perrier, 1982). Late adolescents tend to resemble young adults in pharmacokinetic studies (Geller, Cooper, Schluchter, Warham, & Carr, 1987).

Many of the problems of *outcome measurement* in children, outlined earlier in the chapter, are particularly pertinent to psychopharmacological studies. Some authors have suggested that the failure to demonstrate the effect of tricyclic medication on major depression in children could be related to the absence of a developmentally appropriate self-report measure of change. It has been pointed out (Fava, 1996) that most of the instruments used in pediatric psychopharmacology trials were developed and validated with adults and may fail to include symptoms characteristic of childhood disorders. The requirement for the use of multi-informant, multisetting assessments sensitive to changes in the phenomenological manifestation of psychopathology with age has been sadly ignored in many studies.

Treatment integrity poses a specific problem in this field. The identification of a clinically effective dose is often an empirical issue, although physicians tend to apply various algorithms involving age, height, and body weight. Because trial and error dominates clinical practice, fixed doses used in efficacy trials can appear somewhat arbitrary. Adherence to a treatment regimen may be another problem with disorganized, dysfunctional families. Compliance (concordance) has to be monitored, particularly in adolescence.

A major issue rarely considered systematically even in the adult psychopharmacological literature concerns the control condition: the *inert placebo*. An appropriate definition of a placebo is a preparation that contains no medicine related to the complaint, administered to cause the patient to believe that he or she is receiving treatment. If an inert placebo can yield an improvement rate of about 30% in a condition such as depression, then it seems highly likely that a tablet that can be felt or seen to be doing something is likely to increase the expectations of therapeutic efficacy (Thomson, 1982). There is general agreement that *active placebos* are more powerful than inert placebos. A meta-analysis of antidepressants under genuinely double-blind conditions using active placebos shows that effect sizes decrease to between a half and a quarter of those obtained when using inert placebos (ES = 0.19–0.25) (Greenberg, Bornstein, Greenberg, & Fisher, 1992; Moncrieff, Wessley, & Hardy, 1998). On balance, the research on active placebos places a major question mark over the objectivity of trials as they are currently practiced (Fisher & Greenberg, 1997). The effects of active placebos in the context of pediatric psychopharmacology trials are unknown. The frequently observed vulnerability of children to authoritative suggestion should make researchers particularly alert to this problem (Ceci & Bruck, 1993; Ceci, Huffman, Smith, & Loftus, 1996).

There are specific *legal and ethical issues* concerning psychopharmacological research with children, particularly with regard to the use of placebos, complex consent procedures, and inherent resistance to psychopharmacological studies in children. Fully informed consent cannot be obtained from children, but children with a mental age greater than 7 can assent to participate. Clearly, there are many important specific concerns about asking children and families to take part in psychopharmacology trials (Arnold et al., 1995; Glantz, 1996). Ethical concerns are even greater when administering a treatment without adequate knowledge of its likely effects.

Although all is clearly not well in the field of pediatric psychopharmacology, it should be noted that a number of trials that take on board these and other considerations are under way and many important results are about to be reported. Moreover, rigorous, relevant, multisite work has been easier to undertake in the field of physical treatments than in the equally important psychosocial domain.

THE CURRENT REVIEW

Methodology of the Review

The search strategy for this project was similar to those undertaken by several recent reviews and consisted of a combination of computer-based and hand searches. In our computer search of all the major databases, including MedLine and PsycLit/PsycInfo, we used 100 terms referring to different aspects of child and adolescent mental health and combined the results of these searches with 22 terms describing treatments. The terms used are listed in Appendix 2 (Appendix 1 provides a glossary of psychopharmacological treatments). In addition, we reviewed the articles included in large meta-analyses of child treatments and examined the bibliographies of reviews and primary studies. The computer search identified 5,375 abstracts, which were reviewed. From this corpus 743 papers were selected. We then amended this coverage with a hand search, which yielded a large number of further studies, particularly through the follow-up of bibliographies in primary studies and review papers. Overall, 830 primary studies were identified, as well as 648 further reports that either reviewed the treatment literature, reported clinical experience, or offered advice and opinion pertinent to child psychiatric treatments in the areas covered. The search covered the period up to the end of 1998. Only hand searches of major journals covered the most recent period (1999–2000). A significant number of early studies were reviewed but discarded when methodological improvements in the more recent literature made these findings obsolete.

To be included in the review, reports of research had to satisfy criteria of relevance, outcome, and design.

1. *Relevance.* Studies that reported evaluations of interventions with one or more of the target disorder populations of children and adolescents were reviewed. We included only interventions that fell in the domain of the health service or services accessible to health service providers. Macrosocial, legislative, and economic interventions, for example, were excluded.

2. *Outcome.* Studies were selected only if they reported outcomes that were either directly related to the disorder (e.g., symptom reduction) or related to intermediary variables. In the latter case, the reviewers had independent evidence of an impact on mental health associated with the outcome (e.g., major risk factors such as educational progress in conduct-disordered children) or an impact on mental health was plausible (e.g., family dysfunction). The reviewers were inclusive in their approach. Emphasis was placed on interventions that examined the direct impact on mental health or the intermediate (preventative) impact on risk factors, but studies with less well focused outcome information were also frequently covered.

3. *Design*. The review focused on studies that used an experimental or quasi-experimental study design. Observational studies such as cohort or case studies were also considered for review, but possible effects of this bias are indicated throughout the volume. This was a necessary relaxation of normal exclusion criteria because a preliminary exploration of the available evidence indicated that the exclusion of poorly controlled studies would drastically curtail the available database to a point where the meaningfulness and relevance of the review might well be seriously jeopardized. Our initial plan to exclude studies that did not meet the criteria specified by the Cochrane collaboration (Clarke & Oxman, 1999) proved impractical. To maintain maximum comparability between our work and theirs, however, we reviewed all the available evidence, highlighting in the review the methodological shortcomings and cautioning readers to interpret the results with appropriate care.

Initially, then, the selection criteria for studies to be included in the review were (1) group design involving random assignment, (2) well-documented treatment procedures, (3) uniform therapist training, or clear manualization of the protocol for administering medication, and evidence of adherence, (4) clinically referred samples of treatment candidates, (5) outcome assessment, including at least two outcome levels (e.g., level of symptoms, adaptation, mechanisms, transactions, or service utilization), (6) tests of clinical significance (see earlier discussion), (7) assessment of long-term outcome (follow-up greater than 6 months). We realized that these criteria were unrealistic when preliminary coding revealed that only 7.4% of studies in child and adolescent mental health met the first of these criteria, rigorous randomization.

Hence, the key selection criteria for acceptance into the review were finalized as follows:

1. A clear description of the patient population in the study, either in terms of diagnosis or in terms of specific problems addressed in the treatment. Disorders were categorized into the following groups:

   - Disruptive behavior disorders (e.g., oppositional defiant disorder, conduct disorder, delinquency, and criminal behavior)
   - Attention-deficit/hyperactivity disorder
   - Emotional disorders (e.g., depression, anxiety disorders)
   - Disorders involving serious self-harming behavior (e.g., eating disorders, repeated suicide attempts, substance abuse)
   - Psychosomatic and somatoform disorders, and physical symptoms exacerbated by emotional state (e.g., chronic pain or asthma exacerbated by stress, somatizing symptoms)
   - Psychoses (e.g., bipolar disorder, schizophrenia, neurologically based psychotic states)
   - Pervasive developmental disorders (e.g., autistic disorder, Asperger's disorder)

- Specific developmental disorders and delays (e.g., language delay, specific learning disorders)
- Tourette's disorder and related diagnoses

2. The study was reported in the English language.
3. The study had a group design or an experimental single-case design.
4. There was a systematic effort at the measurement of outcome, including at least pre- and posttest measurement on an objective instrument.

Other reviews of this literature have been forced to make similar compromises. For example, the American Psychological Association's Division 12 Task Force on empirically supported treatment for children and adolescents was not able to apply fully the criteria of the Chambless Task Force on promotion and dissemination of psychological procedures developed for an adult patient population, simply because in many areas the study design, particularly the size of experimental groups, was not up to the task. The Chambless Task Force specifies 30 per group as the minimum size for an adequate trial. A very small proportion of the current database, less than 10% of studies, would have met this criteria. The Division 12 Task Force (Lonigan et al., 1998) excluded all studies from consideration that did not involve random assignment. Although these criteria may be appropriate in evaluation of psychosocial treatment for a number of disorders—for example .conduct problems—they would have excluded the open trials of a number of drug treatments that we considered to be extremely relevant to current practice.

In line with the standard procedure for conducting such reviews, a hierarchy of evidence has been developed to distinguish studies according to their susceptibility to bias (Sheldon, Song, & Davey-Smith, 1993). Evidently, randomized controlled trials with manualized treatments and homogeneous samples are more reliable than trials where randomization was not possible and the treatment could not be described. The hierarchy of evidence is in line with generally accepted criteria described in the *Cochrane Reviewers' Handbook* (Clarke & Oxman, 1999) and other publications (e.g., Rosenthal, 1995; Woolf et al., 1990). The broad categories are as follows: (i) randomized controlled trials; (ib) systematic reviews and meta-analyses; (ii) other trials: a controlled trial without randomization, a quasi-experiment, or a failed randomization; (iib) experimental single-case designs; (iii) cohort studies, preferably from more than one center (a cohort allocates by exposure to treatments and looks for differences in outcomes), (iv) case–control (retrospective) studies, preferably from several centers (allocates by outcome and looks for differences of exposure—in terms of treatment); (v) large differences reported in comparisons between times and/or places, with or without interventions; (vi) opinions of respected authorities based on clinical experience, descriptive studies, uncontrolled studies, and reports of expert committees. As this review will highlight, for the treatment of some conditions there is an absence of good quality outcome research, and so clinical opinion is the only information available. We rated each citation in the treatment section of each chapter in terms of the broad categories of evidence (i)–(vi).

It was decided to organize the review according to type of disorder (rather than, for example, treatment type) because this followed the structure of the great majority of published works. Further, we felt that this approach may be most helpful to those concerned with identifying effective treatment for particular cases or in a particular clinical setting. To indicate the likely demands on services implied by this review, we offered epidemiological data, where it was available, concerning the prevalence of the disorder. Each chapter on each of the types of disorder has the same structure, to facilitate access. We begin with a definition and description of the clinical disorders covered, and consider epidemiological evidence on prevalence. The section on clinical presentation includes natural history and known risk factors, as well as an indication of the social costs of these disorders, particularly in the context of long-term outcome. The largest part of each chapter consists of evidence on the efficacy and effectiveness of psychosocial treatments, physical therapies, and, where appropriate, interventions at the level of consultation and training of non-mental health professionals. Each chapter concludes with a summary of the evidence and a statement of key implications. The final chapter summarizes our conclusions in a form intended to afford ready accessibility to the widest range of purchasers and providers of child mental health care. It also integrates the evidence for effectiveness for each type of intervention across disorders, in order to assist service planners and commissioners of services in identifying the specific interventions that are empirically supported and to which training funds may be appropriately directed.

Limitations of This Review

There are several important limitations to this review. First, although we aimed for exhaustive coverage of the literature, no doubt key contributions have been missed for a variety of administrative and practical reasons. Second, literature not published in the English language was not accessible to review. Third, anecdotal case reports, which represent a large proportion of the psychodynamic literature, were not included. These reports almost inevitably failed to meet the criteria of clear description of the case and rarely included objective measures of outcome. Fourth, we did not aggregate the studies using meta-analytic strategies. Earlier in this chapter the limitations of this approach were discussed. The central problem, from the point of view of identifying evidence-based practice, is the assumption that all the treatments being compared are homogeneous and therefore comparable, which must be made in meta-analyses. In our view, there are too few studies using genuinely comparable treatment procedures for such aggregation to be justified. Nevertheless, the review pays careful attention to the findings of meta-analytic reviews in the literature, and critical distillations of their findings are included. In most areas, however, the primary studies on which meta-analyses were based were individually scrutinized.

Fifth, although we paid careful attention to moderating variables in our attempt to identify specific client groups for which treatments were effective, and others for whom the treatments were not, in most cases we were unable to identify with sufficient clarity findings that unequivocally pointed to the appropriateness of specific treatment methods to a particular population. Finally, as with any review, the conclusions can be based only on the evidence that is available; in many instances, we identified dramatic gaps in the evidence base. It is easy to confuse the absence of evidence of effectiveness with absence of effectiveness per se. The conclusions we have arrived at may change dramatically as new data are introduced into the research literature. The review should, nevertheless, be helpful in identifying those areas where research is most urgently needed, even if the current state of evidence fails to point clearly to effective treatments.

2

Epidemiology

DEFINITION

The scope of epidemiological study of children's mental health broadened considerably during the 1990s, in terms of the type and differentiation of disorders, the risk factors associated with developing disorders, and the age span covered under the terms "childhood" and "adolescence."

Key to this broadening has been the improvement in clarity and validity of classification of mental health disorders, with the 10th revision of the World Health Organization's *International Classification of Diseases* (ICD-10; 1992a) and the third revised (DSM-III-R; 1987) and fourth (DSM-IV; 1994) editions of the American Psychiatric Association's *Diagnostic and Statistical Manual of Mental Disorders*. Both classifications are multiaxial and based on patterns of symptomatology. They take into account research findings and consensus on etiology, psychosocial risk factors and prognosis. These systems, which are more directly comparable than previous versions, constitute the "official" classifications of psychiatric disorders. They were developed from the DSM-I (1952) and the ICD-8 (1967), which originally "covered quite a range of disorders in adult life but included no more than a few token categories applying to childhood" (Cantwell & Rutter, 1994, p.3).

The earliest epidemiological studies (reviewed by Brandenburg, Friedman, & Silver, 1990) did not differentiate disorders, reporting instead on global conditions such as *maladjustment* or *maladaptation*. They focused on school-age children, did not distinguish age-specific features, and examined relatively undifferentiated environmental associations such as urban/rural differences.

The epidemiological features of individual psychiatric disorders in children and young people are described in later chapters. This chapter discusses the epidemiology of child mental health and disorders in general, focusing on features that are particularly important for treatment planning and evaluation, and including examples related to particular disorders where this is pertinent.

PREVALENCE

Even the earliest systematic studies, carried out in the mid-1950s in Buffalo, New York, showed a high frequency of emotional and behavioral problems among 6- to 12-year-olds (Lapouse & Monk, 1958, 1959, 1964; Lapouse, 1965a, 1965b). The studies carried out by Rutter et al. (Rutter, Graham, & Yule, 1970a; Rutter, Tizard, & Whitmore, 1970b) in the Isle of Wight in the mid-1960s estimated an overall prevalence of 6.8% among children aged 10–12 years, using multiple sources of information and social functioning to make diagnoses. Rutter (1989) has since stated, "For the most part, the Isle of Wight data were applied to rather broad psychiatric groupings of emotional and conduct disorders, rather than to the more specific diagnostic categories of psychiatric classification systems such as DSM-III-R and ICD-10" (p. 635). Nevertheless, this study showed the association of physical, intellectual, and educational impairments with psychiatric disorder and made clear that only a small proportion of affected children received specialist mental health services.

The Ontario Child Health Study (Offord et al., 1987) found a prevalence of disorder of 18.1% among 4- to 16-year-olds. This rate lies between those found in studies in Britain that compared the Isle of Wight (no large urban areas; prevalence 12%) with an exclusively urban inner-London borough (prevalence 25.4%: see Rutter, Cox, Tupling, Berger, & Yule, 1975). Differences in the populations studied and the coverage and measurement of disorders make it difficult to compare these studies. A recent cross-cultural review of childhood disorders (Bird, 1996) indicates that prior to 1980, studies differed markedly in the age groups included and in methodologies, and that the measures of psychopathology were neither based on a diagnostic viewpoint nor empirically grounded. These studies' estimates of the prevalence of childhood psychopathology ranged from 6.6% to 37%, with an overall estimate of disorder of 16% (Gould, Wunsch-Hitzig, & Dohrenwend, 1981).

Bird (1996) goes on to describe the findings from more recent studies carried out in different cultural settings that used similar methods, notably the Child Behavior Checklist (CBCL; Achenbach & Edelbrock, 1981, 1983a) and the parallel instruments for teachers (Teacher's Report Form [TRF], Achenbach & Edelbrock, 1986) and for young people themselves (Youth Self-Report [YSR], Achenbach & Edelbrock, 1987). These instruments are designed for use with children at different developmental stages, for girls or for boys. Bird refers to data from Chile, the Netherlands, Thailand, Australia, Puerto Rico, Kenya, France, Jamaica, Belgium, Greece, Germany, and China. Reported samples in the United States are used as a reference for the findings in each setting, with two exceptions: either the original norms published for various versions of the checklist (Achenbach & Edelbrock, 1981, 1987, 1986), or their most recent revisions (Achenbach, 1991a, 1991b, 1991c).

Verhulst and Achenbach (1995) provided a comprehensive summary of the findings from 11 studies reporting CBCL cross-cultural comparisons. Nationality differences were observed in mean CBCL scores, ranging from a low of 20.0 in the U.S. East Coast sample to a high of 35.4 in Greece. Against the United States as the standard, the greatest variation was found in Puerto Rico, with medium size effects in Australia and Greece, and small effects in Thailand and France. Comparisons with Chile, the Netherlands, Kenya, Jamaica, Belgium, Germany, and China were not statistically significant. In spite of observed differences in mean total problem scores, the rank order of item scores was found to be very similar across nationalities. Data from the TRF in six studies (in the United States, Jamaica, the Netherlands, Puerto Rico, Thailand, and rural and urban samples in China) gave mean scores ranging from 17.6 for the Dutch sample to 39.0 in the Chinese rural sample. On both the CBCL and TRF there were more items showing similar item scores across cultures than items with scores that were different in different settings. Only two reports (from the Netherlands and Puerto Rico) compared the YSR with the United States results. In both instances, the self-report findings showed significantly higher scores in the United States.

In Japan, China, and Korea, behavior problems in primary school children were surveyed using Rutter's parent and teacher questionnaires, developed for the Isle of Wight study (Matsuura et al., 1993; Rutter et al., 1970a). The prevalence of deviance in children as assessed by both parents and teachers was lower in these three countries than in other studies using the same instrument, that is, in Mauritius, Uganda, and New Zealand. Bird (1996) concludes that although there may be differences in rates of symptomatology, these cross-cultural comparisons indicate great similarities in the characteristics of psychopathology manifested in different settings. However, the use of standardized checklists to compare different settings limits the report of symptoms and behaviors to the items and wording on these instruments and may fail to record problems that particular cultures perceive as significant. Littlewood (1990) has reviewed the development of cross-cultural psychiatry and explored Kleinman's (1977) original challenge to the assumption that depressive reactions were identical across different cultures. Kleinman criticized the assumption that Western diagnostic categories were themselves culture-free entities, rather than explanatory models specific to the Western context; culture was less something that shaped an already existing natural phenomenon than the context in which any idea of illness was conceived. Thus, comparison across societies needs to take into account the local meanings of any patterns together with a wide range of related behaviors. Littlewood (1990) further examines whether psychiatry may be said to constitute a racist ideology, referring particularly to the development of British transcultural psychiatry.

Bird (1996) also summarized 13 major epidemiological studies of school age children and adolescents that are grounded in the diagnostic tradition, carried out in Mannheim, Germany; upstate New York, United States; Dunedin, New Zealand; Zuid-Holland, the Netherlands; Ontario, Canada; Columbia, Michigan, United States; Pittsburgh, Pennsylvania, United States; Puerto Rico (in Puerto Rico the study was multicenter); Warren County, New Jersey, United States; Dublin, Ireland; Christchurch, New Zealand; Chartres, France; and Western North Carolina, United States (the Great Smoky Mountains Study). The rates of disorders in the three studies using ICD-9 criteria were 12.4% (France), 25.4% (Ireland), and 51.3% (Germany), with an average of approximately 28%. The prevalence of DSM disorders (DSM-III or DMS-III-R) in the six studies that provided rates without taking severity or impairment into account, ranged from 17.6% in the 11-year old wave of the Dunedin study (Anderson, Williams, McGee, & Silva, 1987) to 49.5% in the Puerto Rico study (Bird et al., 1988), with a mean of approximately 29%.

Rates of Psychiatric Disorder According to Diagnostic and Clinical Significance Indicators

All of the 13 studies quoted by Bird (1996) refined their estimates of the prevalence of disorder by reporting the proportion of subjects whose disorder was of some clinical significance. Again, wide disparity was found in the rates of diagnosis (Bird, 1996; Bird et al., 1990). For the two ICD-9 studies reporting rates of clinically significant disorder (Germany and France), the average prevalence is approximately 12%, and an average of 14.3% is found for the DSM studies.

The assessment of clinical significance introduces another element of variability among different studies, as clinical significance may be indicated according to the severity of the disorder, by its pervasiveness, and/or by the level of associated functional impairment. However, a clinically based diagnostic system is likely to represent clinical practice better (Gould, Bird, & Jaramillo, 1993). As described earlier, the proportion of children meeting the criteria for diagnosis was remarkably similar across two somewhat different diagnostic systems—ICD-9 and DSM—as was the proportion of children with clinically significant disorder. Required impairment may lower the general prevalence rate of disorder, but Cantwell (1996b) states that it seems significantly to affect the rate for only some disorders, most notably anxiety disorders.

A review of eight studies by Brandenburg et al. (1990) gave a prevalence of disturbance based on severity rating scales, with or without a "need for treatment" criterion, as ranging from 5% to 26% for moderate and severe disorders. However, they point out the difficulties in drawing conclusions from the research literature because of inconsistencies between both individuals and centers in the way diagnostic criteria are applied and interpreted (Winokur, Zimmerman, & Cadoret, 1988). The potential for unreliability in the assessment of functional impairment appears to be even greater, given the vague use of terms such as "need for treatment" and "moderate or severe" in defining this aspect of psychiatric disturbance. Scales such as the Children's Global Assessment Scale (CGAS; Shaffer et al., 1983) define functional impairment more explicitly.

Among children attending a large health maintenance organization (HMO) in Pittsburgh, Pennsylvania, several impairment scales, including the CGAS (Shaffer et al., 1983), were used to assess the extent to which children appeared to be functioning in their roles at home and at school; only one in every nine children with a diagnosis did not have associated impairment (Costello et al., 1988). On average, children with a psychiatric diagnosis were rated as impaired in more than three areas of functioning, whereas those with no diagnosis on screening were impaired in only one area. A national survey of disability, carried out by the Office of Population Censuses and Surveys in Great Britain (Bone & Meltzer, 1989), found that mental health disorder was the single most prevalent disabling condition interfering with capacity to carry out daily activities, reported in 21 per 1,000 children aged 0 to 15 years. Virtually two-thirds of all the children with any form of disability (35 per 1,000) also had a disabling mental health condition.

Cantwell (1996b) reports the likely effect of the changing criteria (ICD-9 to ICD-10 and DSM-III-R to DSM-IV) on epidemiological studies. The recent series of National Institute of Mental Health (NIMH) studies using the Diagnostic Interview Schedule for Children (DISC) have used DSM-III-R criteria (Shaffer et al., 1996). Revision of the DISC for DSM-IV criteria may lead to different population prevalence rates for various disorders. The NIMH Methods for the Epidemiology of Child and Adolescent Mental Health Disorders (MECA) Study was set up to develop methods suitable for large-scale epidemiological and service studies of mental disorders in young people (Shaffer et al., 1996). The interesting initial findings from the MECA study, based on unreferred representative samples of 9- to 17-year-olds in four geographical areas in the United States (DeKalb, Rockdale, & Henry Counties, Georgia; 3 towns adjacent to New Haven, Connecticut; Westchester County, New York; San Juan, Puerto Rico) cannot, however, be considered representative of the general population. Prevalence rates of mood and disruptive disorders were in line with those reported in other studies (Costello, 1989a; Fleming, Offord, & Boyle, 1989; Kashani et al., 1987). Most young people with a psychiatric diagnosis showed evidence of impairment. However, the prevalence of certain anxiety disorders was very high and a substantial proportion of these subjects were seemingly unimpaired. If the diagnosis is made only when the anxiety symptoms create significant distress or impairment, as DSM-IV requires in contrast to DSM-III-R, prevalence rates fall dramatically.

Wolraich (Baumgaertel, Wolraich, & Dietrich, 1995; Wolraich, Hannah, Baumgaertel, & Feurer, 1996; 1998) has recently completed two epidemiological studies of attention deficit disorder (ADD) using DSM-III, III-R, and IV criteria, one in Germany and one in Tennessee. Teacher information was the sole source of data in both studies. In the German population, the prevalence figures for the primarily inattentive subtype, the primarily hyperactive impulse subtype, and the combined subtype were 9%, 3.9% and 4.8%, respectively. In the Tennessee population, the prevalence figures for the same three subtypes were 4.7%, 3.4%, and 4.4%. Using DSM-IV criteria led to an increase of 64% in total ADD prevalence as compared with DSM-III and DSM-III-R criteria. Comparison of the Tennessee and German rates suggests possible cultural, geographical, and ethnic differences in prevalence rates. DSM-IV has added a section in the description of each disorder specifically dealing with cultural factors.

A recent national study of psychiatric morbidity in children (aged 5–15 years) in Great Britain (Meltzer, Gatward, Goodman, & Ford, 2000) used random sampling of child benefit records (which include nearly all children in the United Kingdom) to recruit children. Specially trained interviewers interviewed the parents of 10,438 children (83% response) and 4,500 of the older children (aged 11–15) themselves. A postal questionnaire was sent to the teachers of all children who had participated in the survey. Diagnosis of mental disorder was based not just on symptoms but on evidence of distress or interference with personal function. A number of standardized instruments were used, including the Strengths and Difficulties Questionnaire, which assesses children's competencies as well as deficits (Goodman, 1997); also included were prompted questions from the interviewers about the impact of symptoms on children's lives. Some 10.4% of children in England, Scotland, and Wales were found to have some type of mental disorder, with no differences between the three countries' prevalence rates. In three broad groupings, 5.3% of children were found to have conduct disorders, 4.3% emotional disorders, and 1.4% were classed as being hyperactive. The less common disorders, for example, autistic disorders, tics, and eating disorders, were attributed to a half percent of the sampled population. Among 5- to 10-year-olds, 10% of boys and 6% of girls had a mental disorder. Among the 11–15 year olds, the proportions were 3% for boys and 10% for girls. As yet, figures for comorbidity have not been published. A strong association was found separately between social class and family income, and the mental health of the child. Children from families in social class V (unskilled occupations) were three times more likely to have a mental health problem than those from social class I (professionals). The association was found for all three groups of disorders. The prevalence of any mental disorder ranged from 16% among children living in families with a gross weekly household income of under £100, to 9% among children of families in the £300–399 weekly income bracket, and to around 6% in those families earning £500 per week or more. This trend was evident for all three groups of disorders.

Influence of Informants on Rates of Disorder

There is general agreement that most studies show acceptable reliability among researchers, for major psychiatric disorders. However, using the same diagnostic classification system, practicing clinicians are less reliable than researchers who are trained to make diagnoses in a standardized way (Prendergast et al., 1988). At least one reason for this is that data from multiple sources of information in the child assessment process often do not agree with each other. During the mid-1960s, Rutter (1967) found disagreement between teachers' and parents' assessments concerning children identified as having deviant behavior, and between the reports of mothers and their children. The prevalence data in the MECA Study show extremely limited overlap between parent and child reports of disorder. In almost all instances, the prevalence shown in using the combined data was equal to or greater than the sum of cases reported by parents and children separately (Shaffer et al., 1996). Good reliability has been shown when diagnostic information from parents alone is used and when information from parents and child are combined. When a child report alone is used, the results are not so good. Certain diagnoses such as attention deficit/hyperactivity disorder (ADHD) show much less reliability with child report alone. However, major depressive disorder is highly reliably identified with child report alone (Barrett et al., 1991; Cantwell, 1996b). Angold et al. (1987) showed that, certainly in teenagers, children were more likely to be aware of emotional problems than their parents, and in a study by Loeber, Green, and Lahey (1990), teachers were more sensitive than parents to internalizing symptoms in children. A recently published study from Finland (Puura et al., 1998) compared parent and teacher reports of depressive symptoms with self-report in a sample of 5,682 prepubertal children (Renouf & Kovacs, 1994). Parents and teachers readily saw and reported depressive symptoms in children, although each identified a different set of "diagnostic" behaviors. Psychiatric care had been sought or even considered for only a small minority of children with multiple depressive symptoms. Both parents and teachers had suggested seeking psychiatric help for an even smaller number of girls than boys, and help had been sought for those features that tend to irritate parents, such as disobedience and restlessness, or that may cause great concern, such as asthma and soiling. In the Dunedin follow-up, McGee et al. (1990) found that less than half of adolescents had their disorders confirmed by parental report, and that confirmation of disorders was more likely where the mother was depressed, there was poor social support for the family, and the adolescent was less socially competent.

Some disorders are situation specific, like separation anxiety or hyperactivity that becomes problematic only at school (Schachar, Rutter, & Smith, 1981). Parental accounts are essential for gathering information on the development of the child and on the type of behavior the child manifests at home (Achenbach, 1988). Information about the child's functioning can be obtained from teachers (Kolvin, Garside, Nicol, Leitch, & Macmillan, 1977; Rutter, 1967). The value of direct assessment from the child is increasingly recognized (Barrett et al., 1991; Rutter & Graham, 1968; Rutter, Tizard, Yule, Graham, & Whitmore, 1976). What the child thinks is likely to be a crucial influence on the mode and course of treatment, as well as on the primary outcomes to be sought. Rutter (1989), however, questions the clinical significance of depressive problems, reported at a much higher rate by adolescents than by their parents or other adults who interact with them. Despite the generally low correlation found between parent and teacher scales (Achenbach, McConaughy, & Howell, 1987), Brandenburg et al. (1990) support the view that synthesizing parent and teacher responses enhances the specificity of case definition. Data from multiple informants are required to indicate whether the disorder is pervasive or situation specific. The prevalence figure for pervasive disorders, reported by more than one source, tends to be lower; for example, Anderson et al. (1987) found a rate of 7.3% in 11-year-old children in Dunedin, as compared with an overall prevalence of DSM-III disorders of 17.6%.

Rise in Prevalence

There is considerable interest in whether psychiatric morbidity is increasing in young people. Achenbach and Howell (1993) reviewed problems and competencies reported by parents and teachers in a U.S. nationally representative random sample of 7- to 16-year-olds in 1989, compared with those reported by parents for a 1976 sample and by teachers for a 1981–1982 sample. All significant differences in problem items and scale scores indicated increased problems. All but one of the items (number of sports) indicated lower competence in 1989 than in 1976. The percentage of children classified within the clinical range increased, from 10.0% to 18.2%. The increases did not differ significantly according to age, gender, socioeconomic status, or ethnicity. The increases in problems and decreases in competencies were not overwhelming and were not concentrated in a particular area such as depression, but the consistency of the findings suggested real differences in parents' perceptions of their children's functioning in 1976 versus 1989. Competence and problems both contributed significantly to whether children were referred to mental health services. It is noteworthy that 8.3% of the 1989 sample were excluded from the study because they had received mental health services in the preceding year, as compared with 3% excluded from the 1976 sample. Thus, despite the increased percentage of children receiving services in 1989, more untreated children were considered to need help in 1989 than among the 1976 sample.

A major study of the time trends in psychosocial disorders in adolescence analyzed the scientific evidence from industrialized countries across the world (Rutter & Smith, 1995a) and concluded that there has been a real rise in all the conditions studied since the end of the Second World War: "The psychosocial disorders considered are ones that are common but involve a serious malfunctioning of individuals in their social setting; the disorders are those that tend to rise or peak in frequency during the teenage years: namely crime, suicide and suicidal behaviors, depression, eating disorders (anorexia and bulimia), and abuse of alcohol and psychoactive drugs" (Rutter & Smith, 1995a, p. 1). Not included were less common conditions that also increase in frequency during adolescence but that seem to represent qualitatively distinct disorders apparently less open to broader social influences, namely, major mental illnesses such as schizophrenia and organic brain disorders. Rutter and Smith (1995a) reported that with some disorders in young people, the rise seems to apply about equally to both sexes; with suicide and possibly depression, it has affected males more than females, and with crime, there has been a somewhat greater rise among females than males.

Following detailed and comprehensive analyses, Rutter and Smith summarized what can be learned about causal explanations for the time trends that have been established (Rutter & Smith, 1995b). They concluded that increased social disadvantage does not account for the rising levels of psychosocial disorder. Social disadvantage may increase other risk factors (such as family disorganization and breakup), the increasing levels of which may well have played a role in the rise of psychosocial disorders, but the effects on disorders are indirect. Unemployment does create psychosocial risks for individuals, but this explanation alone is not enough to account for the rise in disorders since the Second World War. Conversely, increasing affluence is likely to play a role in increasing substance abuse and opportunities for crime. An increase in people's expectations—coupled with difficulties in meeting them—may have played some part in the increase in psychosocial disorders.

Poor physical health is a risk to mental health, but physical health in the population has improved in this time period. The meaning of adolescence, and opportunities for young people, have clearly changed over time. It is not known how far such changes have led to an increase in psychosocial risks. It is most unlikely that the impact of the mass media (e.g., increasing violence on television) largely accounts for the rise in psychosocial disorders. However, the media may add to the effects of social change. Moral values have changed profoundly over the last half century (e.g., the growth in respect for individual beliefs). This may be connected with the increase in psychosocial disorders. Finally, although most psychosocial disorders have increased over much the same period, the evidence suggests that, to some extent, the explanations are different for different specific disorders.

AGE AND SEX

The study in inner London by Richman, Stevenson, and Graham (1975) clearly demonstrated the presence of psychiatric disorder in very young children; moderate to severe disorders were found in 7% of 3-year-olds, and mild disorders in 15%.

Overall prevalence varies according to the age distribution in the child population covered and, to some extent, by gender. In the Mannheim study (Esser, Schmidt, & Woerner, 1990), overall rates of moderate to severe disorders were 16.2% at age 8 and 17.8% at age 13. Between a quarter and a third of these children showed serious disturbances definitely requiring professional treatment. At the younger age level, only boys were found in this seriously affected group. In contrast to the Isle of Wight study (see below), the overall rates hardly increased during adolescence.

Higher rates of disorder, however, tend to be found in adolescents (Petersen & Leffert, 1995). When adolescents, as distinct from children, have been studied, despite differences in geographical location, year of survey, and general methodology, the results have shown remarkable convergence: about one in five adolescents is found to have some kind of mental health disorder. Krupinski et al. (1967) reported a prevalence of psychiatric diagnosis among 14- to 21-year-olds in Victoria, Australia, of 19% for boys and 22% for girls. Leslie (1974), in a study of 13- and 14-year-olds in Blackburn, United Kingdom, estimated that some 21% of boys and 14% of girls had a moderate to severe psychiatric disorder, and in the follow-up study on the original Isle of Wight sample, Rutter et al. (1976) reported a prevalence rate of 8% of the 14- and 15-year-olds, with a corrected prevalence estimate (taking account of those not selected on screening tests) of 21%. More recently, Offord et al. (1987) examined the 6-month prevalence rates for disorder in their 4- to 16-year-old sample from Ontario, Canada; for the age range 12 to 16 years, 19% of boys and 22% of girls were estimated to have a psychiatric disorder. In a sample of 14- to 16-year-olds in Columbia, Michigan, approximately two-fifths (41.3%) were found to have at least one DSM-III diagnosis, with a prevalence of 18.7% when "caseness" was restricted by the addition of measures of impairment (Kashani et al., 1987).

In a U.S. national sample of 5- to 17-year-old children attending school, boys outnumbered girls for most types of maladjustment, but McDermott (1996) raises the point that this may represent overuse of conduct disorder diagnoses, which are more commonly applied to boys. As with all studies of younger children, among 8-to 11-year-olds in the Eure-et Loire departement in France, conduct disorders were found to be more common in boys (9.3%) than in girls (3.2%), and emotional disorders more common in girls (6.3%) than in boys (5.6%) (Fombonne, 1994).

In Dunedin, New Zealand, the sex ratio was found to vary across different disorders, but in general DSM-III disorders were found to be more prevalent in boys, with a male to female ratio in 11-year-olds of 1.7:1 (Anderson et al., 1987). Both disruptive disorders and depression were more prevalent in boys than in girls. With the exception of overanxious disorder, anxiety disorders were more common in girls. In the same sample at age 15, a female to male prevalence ratio of 1.4:1 was found (McGee et al., 1990). In 15-year-olds in Christchurch, New Zealand, based on information from adolescents and/or parents, the rate was considerably greater in girls (32.9%) than in boys (21.6%). Anxiety disorders and mood disorders showed higher prevalence in girls, whereas ADHD was higher in boys. The expected higher rate of conduct disorder did not reach statistical significance, and there was a surprisingly significant higher rate of substance abuse/dependence in girls than in boys. Among 4- to 16-year-olds in Puerto Rico (Bird et al., 1988), a similarly higher prevalence was found in boys than girls, a difference that was driven by the predominance of disruptive disorders in boys. Although there were no general differences in the rate of disorder by age, there were age differences in specific disorders. ADD was equally common in middle childhood and adolescence, the prevalence of depression increased linearly with age, and separation anxiety was more common in the younger children. Similarly marked sex differences in the prevalence of deviance in primary school children, both at school and at home, were found by Matsuura et al. (1993) in Japan, China, and Korea.

NATURAL HISTORY

In young children, Richman et al. (1982) found a high level of persistence of disturbance. Overall, 61% of a large sample of 3-year-olds in London regarded as showing significant disturbance still had difficulties when clinically evaluated at the age of 8 years. In the Isle of Wight study, Rutter (1981) evaluated children at the age of 10–11 and again at 14–15. The overall persistence of disorder was estimated as 60%, with lower stability for emotional than for conduct disorders.

At younger ages, adverse familial conditions and specific learning disabilities emerged as relevant correlates of psychiatric disorders among German children (Esser, Schmidt, & Woerner, 1990). Out of a total of 71 children with psychiatric disturbances at age 8, one half were again rated as disordered at age 13. This group of 36 subjects with persisting disorders also constituted approximately half of the moderately or severely affected adolescents; the other half consisted of originally undisturbed children. Behavioral disturbances of adolescents were mainly determined by their psychiatric state, learning disabilities, and adverse family relations identified at the age of 8, and by the number of life events experienced in the preceding 5 years. In contrast to the Isle of Wight study, learning disabilities also kept their predictive power for psychiatric disorders of adolescence. The prediction of remission or late onset of psychiatric disorders proved more difficult. Subsequent development of disorders in initially healthy children was mainly related to prior learning disabilities and the occurrence of stressful life events. Conversely, the course of preexistent disorders was—as in the Isle of Wight study—determined by their specific diagnostic category and by an improvement of the psychosocial environment within the family. Rutter (1989) has pointed out, however, that improvements in family functioning do not necessarily result in remission in the children's disorders. He goes on to suggest that this could mean either that a greater degree of environmental change is needed to bring about remission, or that once a disorder is established, other factors lead to perpetuation of the disorder, or that the factors leading to onset of disorder differ from those influencing course.

The stability of disorders largely depends on their diagnostic category. In their follow-up of children from the age of 8 to 13, Esser et al. (1990) concluded that "the course of emotional disorders gave rise to a very promising prognosis" (p. 261). This was also shown clearly in the Oregon study of 14- to 18-year-olds, where the clinical consequences in those with pure anxiety were the least among all diagnostic groups (Lewinsohn, Rohde, & Seeley, 1995). A highly unfavorable prospect was noted for conduct disorders, and Esser and Schmidt (1987) showed four factors to be important: a severe hyperkinetic symptomatology at age 8, school problems, an increased number of life events, and a tendency toward worsened family conditions. Rutter and Sandberg (1985) noted that disorders that were pervasive over situations tended to be more persistent over time. This was also observed by Anderson et al. (1987): 11-year-olds with multiple disorders, particularly those with a combination of ADD and conduct and oppositional disorder, had a history of behavior problems from 5 years of age in parent and teacher reports.

Angold et al. (1999) have shown that impairment is as important as diagnosis in predicting future "caseness," whether this is measured by service use, impairment, diagnosis, perceived problem, or perceived need for help. Screening of a representative sample of 9-, 11-, and 13-year-olds in 11 countries in western North Carolina identified a sample of 1,015 young people, 90% of whom were followed up 1 year later. The sample subjects were assessed and reassessed for the presence of a DSM-III-R diagnosis of psychiatric disorder and independently for psychosocial impairment, service use, and parental perceived burden. Of the 1,015 subjects, on first assessment, 140 had both a diagnosis and an impairment; 143 had a diagnosis but were not impaired; and 205 had impairment but no diagnosis. Currently and at 1-year follow-up, rates of specialist mental health-related services, school-based mental health-related service use, parental perceived burden, parent or child perception that the child had a problem, and parent or child perception of need for help were higher in the symptomatically impaired group than in the no-diagnosis and diagnosis-but-no-impairment groups—significantly so in 8 of the 10 comparisons. Fifty-two percent of those using specialist mental health services in this Great Smoky Mountains study failed to meet diagnostic criteria for any of 29 well-defined DSM-III diagnoses. The larger portion of impaired but undiagnosed individuals had parent–child (overall weighted prevalence 3.6%), sibling (overall weighted prevalence 1.4%) and other (overall weighted prevalence 0.6%) relational problems. The overall weighted prevalence due to symptomatic impairment without a diagnosis was 9.4%, with 60% having impairment due only to disruptive behavior, 18% due to emotional symptoms, and 22% with both disruptive and emotional symptoms causing impairment. Subthreshold oppositional and conduct problems predominated.

Achenbach et al. (1995a) assessed the predictors of six signs of disturbance in 1992, in a nationally representative sample of children aged 9–18 years old who had been followed over the previous 6 years. The six signs were (1) received help for academic problems in school; (2) behavior problems in school, suspension, or expulsion; (3) received mental health services; (4) hinted, threatened, or attempted suicide or self-harm; (5) behavior that led to police contact; and (6) substance abuse (alcohol or drug problems). For each young person for whom at least one sign was reported, a "control" was selected from the study cohort, without signs of disturbance in 1992, and matched as closely as possible for sex, age, and ethnicity. Achenbach et al. reported that these signs

> were significantly predicted by various combinations of family variables, syndromes, competencies, stressful experiences, and reports of the signs themselves 3 years earlier. The predictive models accounted for a large percentage of variance in most of the signs for both sexes. Averaged across both sexes and different combinations of informants, rates for predicting which individuals would manifest each sign ranged from 69% to 77%. The overall predictive accuracy was similar for both sexes, but there were important sex differences in the specific predictors. The rates reached 83% for prediction of the use of mental health services among girls from combined parent and teacher data, and 82% for suicidal behavior among boys and for police contacts and mental health services use among girls from combined parent and self-report data. (p. 497)

Achenbach et al. (1995b) also defined eight syndromes with specific DSM counterparts and followed their course and relationships with later manifestation of syndromes and signs (see earlier). The delinquent behavior syndrome predicted more signs than any other syndrome, with attention problems predicting the second largest number of signs. The strength of these syndromes as predictors of signs of disturbance is borne out by similar findings in a Dutch sample (Verhulst, Achenbach, Ferdinand, & Kasius, 1993). Children who manifested several signs when young could be predicted to manifest the same signs when they were older. The percentage of children manifesting a sign in 1992, who had also manifested it 3 years previously, was as follows: police contacts, 13.6%; suicidal behavior, 24.1%; academic problems, 39.3%; school behavior problems and receipt of mental health services, both 40.1%. Thus, most signs reported in 1992 represented new onset since the earlier follow-up. Multiple other factors usually contributed more to the prediction of which young people would manifest each sign than the previous manifestation of the sign itself. This differs from the finding (Achenbach et al., 1995b) that most of the syndromes manifest in 1992 were predicted more strongly by earlier scores on the same syndrome than by other variables. Biederman et al. (1993a) in studying ADHD confirmed that significant associations have been found in research between syndromes and numerous other variables, such as DSM diagnoses.

The sex differences found in these studies in relation to risk factors, signs of disturbance, and the relationships between them suggest that the developmental course of problems in boys and girls should be differentiated. These problems include oppositional disorder in both genders and conduct disorder and major depression in girls. Major depression shows a pattern suggesting a role for the onset of puberty (Cohen et al., 1993b). Different approaches for each sex may also be needed in preventing and treating the conditions underlying specific signs. For example, Achenbach et al. (1995c) reassessed their national sample in young adulthood with respect to six syndromes derived from parent and self-reports and found strong predictive relationships between pre-adult and adult counterparts. There were important sex differences in the developmental pathways leading to young adult conduct problems: in males, these were primarily predicted by similar pre-adult syndromes, but in females, adult conduct problems were predicted by a variety of pre-adult problems. The attention problems syndrome also predicted more syndromes for adult females than for males.

Cohen, Cohen, and Brook (1993) studied the persistence and new onset of psychiatric disorder in a sample of 734 children from the general population. Diagnoses for six of the more prevalent disorders were generated from interviews with both the mother and the child when the children were 9–18 years old and again 2½ years later. Analyses demonstrated substantial levels of diagnostic persistence over the 2½-year period for all diagnoses except major depression. With few exceptions, persistence was roughly the same in young men as in young women and across age groups. These authors concluded that disorders assessed by structured interview of nonclinical samples of children cannot be dismissed as transitory.

The Dunedin Multidisciplinary Health and Development Study (Silva, 1990) gathered mental health data at ages 11, 13, 15, 18, and 21, in an unselected cohort that had been studied since birth in New Zealand. The prevalence of DSM-III-R disorders increased from late childhood (18%) through mid- (22%) to late adolescence (41%) and young adulthood (40%). At 21 years, 73.8% of those diagnosed had a developmental history of mental disorder, and the incidence of cases with adult onset was only 10.6%. Relative to new cases, those with developmental histories were more severely impaired and more likely to have comorbid diagnoses (Newman et al., 1996).

COMORBIDITY

Cross-sectional comorbidity is the occurrence at one point in time of two or more DSM-III-R disorders (Clarkin & Kendall, 1992). When one disorder is followed by the occurrence of another, different disorder, this is known as longitudinal comorbidity. To date, comorbidity has not been well addressed in scientific studies, but it poses the most difficult challenges in the treatment of psychiatric disorder in young people.

Diagnostic criteria for one disorder may not significantly discriminate it from another disorder. This may be true with depression and anxiety, and ADD and mania, which share the same symptoms. However, higher order, broader-based patterns (such as externalizing versus internalizing disorders) may represent more specific single-diagnostic entities. Where these higher-order disorders are artificially subdivided, high levels of comorbidity may result. In DSM-IV and ICD-10, for example, higher-order anxiety disorder is subdivided into multiple anxiety disorders (Cantwell, 1996b).

Andersen et al. (1987) showed that of eight categories of DSM-III disorders in 11-year-old children in Dunedin, New Zealand, 55% occurred in combination, and 45% as single disorders. The highest proportion of cases occurring as a single disorder were oppositional, conduct and ADD; the most overlapping category was depression/dysthymia, where only 3 of 14 children had a single disorder. Almost identical findings were obtained in Puerto Rico among the 4- to 16-year-old sample (Bird et al., 1988), although here, conduct/oppositional disorders most frequently overlapped with other diagnostic groups, a difference that the authors attribute to the different age compositions of the two samples. Follow-up of the New Zealand sample at age 15 showed about one in four adolescents having two or more DSM-III disorders (McGee et al., 1990). The greatest degree of comorbidity was found in those with depressive disorders; almost two-thirds had a coexisting disorder. The least overlap was in the case of conduct and oppositional disorder, and where there was comorbidity, it happened more frequently with a depressive disorder.

In a randomly selected community sample of 1,507, representative of high school students in western Oregon (ages 14–18 years), Lewinsohn et al. (1993) identified those with "pure" and comorbid forms of four major psychiatric disorders: depression, anxiety, substance use, and disruptive behavior. The young people were assessed by interview and questionnaire on two occasions, an average of 13.8 months apart. In 1987, 9.65% and in 1989, 7.8% had current psychopathology. In 1989, 42.8% had one or more lifetime (past or current) diagnoses. Major depressive disorder was found in 342 young people (205 with "pure" diagnoses); 124 had lifetime diagnoses of anxiety disorder, clustered according to DSM-III-R subdivisions (49 "pure" diagnoses); 148 had a lifetime diagnosis of substance use disorder (54 with substance use only); and 94 had a lifetime diagnosis of disruptive disorder (43 with only disruptive disorder). Eight hundred sixty-two had never been mentally ill, and 156 had two or more disorders. Forty-one of these had diagnoses in three or four of the disorders mentioned earlier. In 60.3% of those with comorbid conditions, these were found to occur together on the same occasion, but in the remainder, two or more disorders never met the criteria for more than one diagnosis at any one time. Females were overrepresented among those with pure depressive disorder and with pure anxiety. In the pure depressive group, the proportion of females was higher than in the depressive-plus-disruptive-behavior group; the pure substance-use group had a smaller proportion of females than did the substance-use-plus-anxiety group.

The young people with pure and comorbid disorders were compared on six clinical outcome measures: academic problems, mental health treatment utilization, past suicide attempts, role functioning, conflict with parents, and physical symptoms (Lewinsohn et al., 1995). Each was found to increase, in varying degrees, as a function of the number of psychiatric disorders. Comorbidity had its greatest impact on academic problems (showing a cumulative effect with increasing numbers of comorbid disorders), mental health utilization, and rate of past suicide attempts. Impact on poor global functioning and conflicts with parents was moderate; physical health was unaffected. Although some patterns of comorbidity were much more common in boys (e.g., substance use and disruptive behavior disorder) or in girls (e.g., depression and anxiety), the general impact of comorbidity on the clinical outcome measures was no different for boys and girls.

Russo and Beidel (1994) have reviewed the co-occurrence of childhood anxiety and externalizing disorders (i.e., attention-deficit/hyperactivity, oppositional, and conduct disorders), which, as these authors note, may seem counterintuitive. Among five epidemiological studies, substantial rates of comorbidity between anxiety and externalizing disorders of childhood were reported (Anderson et al., 1987; Bird et al., 1988; Bowen, Offord, & Boyle, 1990; Kashani et al., 1987; McGee et al., 1990). Age trends were also shown, in that adolescents diagnosed with anxiety show an increase in oppositional behavior, but in samples of younger children, an anxiety disorder is more likely to be given an externalizing diagnosis than the reverse. From the studies reviewed, it was noted that it is likely that there is a group of children that presents with three diagnoses—oppositional-defiant or conduct disorder (OD/CD), ADD, and anxiety—and that this group may manifest unique etiological and prognostic features. Studies of referred samples reviewed by Russo and Beidel (1994) confirmed considerably higher rates of comorbidity in younger children compared with adolescents, than is found in the studies of nonreferred samples. In children referred for anxiety, moderate rates of co-occurring externalizing disorders ranged from 2% to 21%, with the higher rates in the younger samples. However, children referred for behavior disorders have been found with rates of codiagnoses of anxiety disorders in the region of 40%. Higher rates were found in samples such as inpatients, who are likely to present with more severe disorders, even though these samples may contain a high proportion of adolescents.

Studies of the association between anxiety and conduct disorder, delinquency, or antisocial behavior have generally suggested that the presence of anxiety indicates a moderating effect on the severity of disruptive behavior. However, recent research on adolescent samples suggests that as children mature, those with high levels of aggression report significantly higher levels of anxiety than adolescents with lower levels of aggression (Newcorn, Sharma, Matier, Hall, & Halperin, 1992; Pliszka, 1989, 1992). In contrast, in one inpatient sample (Kazdin, 1992), there was an association between increased anxiety and covert (stealing) rather than overt (aggressive) antisocial behavior. Further, among a sample of incarcerated juvenile delinquents aged 12–18 years, increased substance abuse was associated with increased symptoms of conduct disorder, as well as anxiety and depression, and with an increased probability of multiple diagnoses (Neighbors, Kempton, & Forehand, 1992).

Robins, Locke, and Regier (1991), using the Epidemiologic Catchment Area Study, have shown that 60% of patients diagnosed with a single disorder had at least two other psychiatric disorders during their lifetime. They suggest that problems in children of disordered parents may be misattributed to a specific disorder when, in fact, comorbidity may be a relevant consideration in interpreting parental effects. Shared and overlapping factors (genetic and biological influences, and negative psychosocial and psychological similarities) may affect and generate compatibilities in children's adaptations despite the specific diagnoses that may have been assigned to ill parents.

Caron and Rutter (1991) have discussed three issues that are important with regard to the existence of comorbid conditions. First, the risk of development of one disorder may be increased by the presence of another particular disorder. Second, there may be overlapping risk factors. Third, comorbid syndromes may generate specific risks for prognosis and outcomes, and indicate specific treatment approaches. Young people with multiple diagnoses will be overrepresented in clinical practice; thus, it is important that interventions can address a multiplicity of problems. The observed patterns of comorbidity often involve combinations of "internalizing" and "externalizing" problems (Lewinsohn et al., 1995). This makes it important that the initial assessment is comprehensive and probes for disorders other than those suggested by referral. Lewinsohn et al. (1995) also suggest that the high rate of comorbidity in adolescents who are referred for treatment may at least partly explain why it has been difficult for clinicians to achieve treatment outcome results as good as those reported in randomized clinical trials (Weisz et al., 1992).

RISK FACTORS

Certain characteristics have consistently been associated with a higher prevalence of child and adolescent mental health disorders. Comparing findings from the Isle of Wight with those in a London sample, Rutter et al. (1975) showed that (1) rates of child psychiatric disorder were twice as high in the inner city, (2) that this difference could not be attributed to migration of those at higher risk into the city, and (3) that it could largely be explained in relation to the greater frequency of family disadvantage and discord in inner London. In 1989, Rutter affirmed that similar differences between metropolitan and rural areas were described by other studies, including the Ontario Child Health Study (Offord et al., 1987), and noted that higher psychiatric prevalence has not generally applied to nonmetropolitan urban areas, but may also occur in isolated communities, although then the risk did seem to be associated with psychosocial adversity. Offord et al. (1987) suggested that the urban/rural differences may predominantly be accounted for by the hyperactivity disorders. Cederblad et al. (Cederblad & Rahim, 1986; Rahim & Cederblad, 1984) followed changes in psychiatric prevalence in an area undergoing urbanization and found that despite improved physical health, psychological disturbance increased.

In upstate New York, Velez, Johnson, and Cohen (1989) showed that low socioeconomic status, especially the component of low maternal education, was a risk factor for all externalizing disorders and for separation anxiety disorder in children.

Family structure (never married) and parental sociopathy were risk factors for both conduct and oppositional disorders. A summary count of pregnancy problems was an important risk factor for all types of psychopathology presenting in young people at different ages. In the Ontario Child Health Study, family dysfunction and parental arrest had a strong independent relationship to conduct disorders. Family dysfunction and academic failure were associated with hyperactivity, and family dysfunction, parental psychopathology, and chronic medical illness were associated with emotional disorders. A history of physical abuse was associated with higher rates of psychopatholgy among 14- to 16-year-olds attending public schools in Columbia, Michigan (Kashani et al., 1987). From the Great Smoky Mountains Study, North Carolina (Costello et al., 1996), there is evidence that the impact of family and social adversity factors may differ among different cultural groups. Cherokee children—who had a slightly lower overall prevalence of disorder than white children—were slightly less likely to be exposed to family risk factors than white children but much more likely to experience social adversity. In the absence of either social adversity or family risk, rates were lower in both Cherokees and white children. However, the impact of social adversity in the absence of family risk factors was considerably more marked on white children than on Cherokee children.

Russo and Beidel (1994) reviewed the association between familial psychopathology and childhood psychiatric diagnoses, stressing that the relationship does not necessarily imply biological causality but may be the result of shared genetic makeup, social learning, or environmental influences. Although studies of the risk of children's developing schizophrenia when their parents have this disorder dominated the field until the mid-1980s (Garmezy & Masten, 1994), studies of depressed parents and of violent child-rearing environments have since established their importance in increasing the risk of mental health disturbance in children. These studies have led to detailed analysis of the complex of factors that place children of psychiatrically ill parents at risk of disturbance, especially the importance of parental discord and neglect of the infant's and young child's emotional needs. A number of studies have also established factors such as positive self-concept and school achievement that enable the child to show resilience in the face of a number of risk factors for psychiatric disorder (summarized in Garmezy & Masten, 1994).

A number of studies have reported an increased risk of externalizing disorders (ADD and ADHD) among children of mothers with internalizing disorders (anxiety and depression) (Keller et al., 1992a; Last, Hersen, Kazdin, Orvaschel, & Perrin, 1991; McLellan, Rubert, Reichler, & Sylvester, 1990; Silverman, Cerny, Nelles, & Burke, 1988). Barkley, DuPaul, and McMurray (1990b) have reported a distinction in the familial psychopathology between children with ADD with and without hyperactivity. In the former, there was a paternal family history of ADD with hyperactivity and a maternal history of substance abuse, and in the latter case, there was a significant maternal family history of anxiety disorder. Biederman et al. (1992) noted that the use of expanded DSM-III-R criteria for ADHD may lead to the finding of more accurate familial associations. These authors report that relatives of children with ADHD show an increased risk of numerous psychiatric problems, including ADHD, mood disorders, antisocial disorders, drug dependence, and anxiety disorders.

A meta-analysis by Loeber and Stouthamer-Loeber (1986) has shown the relationship between antisocial disorders in parents and psychiatric disorders in their children. Both risk and protective factors have been identified. A potential developmental progression toward delinquency and criminal behavior is found in children suffering a repetitive pattern of conflict between parent and child; the pattern of behavior includes neglect, familial alcohol and drug abuse, parental antisocial behavior, and a family climate of violence (Garmezy & Masten, 1994). A relatively weak hereditary influence has been shown for juvenile delinquency, but this may be stronger for antisocial behavior that extends into adult life. Protective factors serve to contain, overcome, and substitute prosocial behaviors for deviant ones.

In another study, Cohen, Velez, Brook, and Smith (1989), after 8 years, followed up a random sample of 976 families and children living in two upstate New York counties, first interviewed when the index child was 1–8 years old. Data on pre- and perinatal problems were linked to parent- and youth-assessed emotional and behavioral problems: attention deficit, conduct problems, opposition, anxiety, separation anxiety, and depression. For all six syndromes, there was a significant effect of early somatic risk factors, and it was significantly larger than that of pregnancy problems alone, which was also statistically significant for two of the six problems. Thus, major and minor illnesses of early childhood and childhood accidents were as predictive of late childhood and adolescent symptoms of psychopathology as were pregnancy and birth problems. For all three "externalizing" syndromes, there was also an independent effect of emotional problems in the mother during or related to the pregnancy. The specific intervening mechanisms of early risk were not identified in this study, but factors that should receive greater attention in primary prevention in the pre- and perinatal periods were clearly implicated: early emotional risk and postnatal early childhood illness experience.

The findings did not support any simple model that matches the type of syndrome with the type of early risk (Cohen et al., 1989). Overall, the pattern suggested that ADD may be similar in etiology to conduct and oppositional disorders, in that the emotional risk variable as well as somatic risk predicted later attention-deficit and hyperactivity symptoms. Syndromes conceptually linked to parental rejection or emotional problems—depression and anxiety—were not related to these antecedent risk factors. Cohen and colleagues point out that the findings should not be taken to mean that measured early risk is a strong enough predictor of later problems on an individual basis, but that they should increase general awareness of the early factors that can increase later vulnerability. Rutter (1994) writes:

> Causal inferences are strengthened when it can be shown that the effects are specific rather than undifferentiated and general. However, it is not uncommon for a single major risk variable to carry with it risks mediated by several different mechanisms. For example, Cadoret et al. [Cadoret, Troughton, Merchant, and Whitters] (1990), using an adoptee design, showed that antisocial personality disorder in parents carried a risk for similar disorders in the offspring that was mediated through genetic mechanisms and a separate risk for depressive symptoms in the offspring that was mediated environmentally. Similarly, parental depression may carry both genetic risks for depression in the offspring and environmental risks for conduct disorder because of the association between parental depression and family discord. (p. 936)

Studies have also shown that some supposed consequences of risk factors actually antedate the hypothesized risk experience. For example, Block, Block, and Gjerde (1986, 1988) noted that boys in families in which the parents subsequently divorced already showed particular behavioral features before the divorce. Similarly, data from the 1970 British birth cohort showed that children who were later placed in foster care differed from other children before their placement (St. Claire & Osborn, 1987). The implication is that much of the risk stemmed from the family discord and disorganization that preceded the divorce or parenting breakdown, rather than from the family break-up as an event (Rutter, 1989).

Children with other types of handicaps (chronic physical disorders, neurological disorders, low IQ) have high rates of psychiatric disorders (Cadman et al., 1986; Rutter et al., 1970a). In a national sample of children ages 0–15 years in Britain, disabilities that interfere with their capacity to carry out daily activities were found in 35 per 1,000; virtually two-thirds of these children also had a disabling mental health condition (Bone & Meltzer, 1989). Cantwell and Baker (1987) showed that among 600 children of mean age 5 years and 7 months, coming to a large community speech and language clinic in the greater Los Angeles area, between 31% and 73% suffered psychiatric disorders. The lower rate was found among children with pure speech disorder, and the higher rate (when corrected for age and IQ differences) among those with pure language disorder and those with speech and language deficits. Rutter (1989) suggests that the association between developmental disorders of speech/language and psychiatric disturbance is not an artifact and that longitudinal findings strongly indicate causal mechanisms. That associated social problems frequently persist many years after conversational fluency has been obtained also suggests that the psychiatric disturbance is not simply explained as a secondary reaction to the communication difficulties.

Specific learning disabilities have repeatedly been found to be associated with high risks of child psychiatric disorders (Graham, 1986). Similarly, poor school achievement is clearly linked with a high prevalence of deviant behavior (Kolvin et al., 1977; Matsuura et al., 1993).

A number of studies have shown that rates of behavioral disturbance and attainment in secondary schools are systematically linked to characteristics of the schools as social organizations, implying causal effects associated with school experiences (Gray, Smith, & Rutter, 1980; Rutter, Maughan, Mortimore, & Ouston [with Smith], 1979). Mortimore, Sammons, Stoll, Lewis, and Ecob (1988) presented evidence that the qualities that children bring with them at school entry are chiefly influenced by family background but that gains during the years that follow are more a function of the school attended.

A recent study in a deprived area of inner London described the mental health needs of children, encompassing manifest problems as well as risk factors (Davis, Day, Cox, & Cutler, 2000). Based on home interviews with mothers and children, nearly 72% of the children were found to have at least one moderate to severe problem, and nearly 37% had three or more. The most frequent difficulties were disruptive behavior, tantrums and eating problems in the 0- to 4-year-olds; anxiety, persistent lying, depressed mood, problem with temper control, and defiance in the 5–

10s; problem with temper control, depressed mood, defiance, food faddishness/eating problems, and father relationship problems in the 11–13s; and crime, school discipline problems, multiple sexual relationships, lying, high smoking/alcohol use, truancy, somatic anxiety, sleep problems, mood swings, temper control, and drug use in the 14–16s. Over 85% of the sample had at least one risk factor for child mental health problems, and over 51% had three or more. The most common risk factors included maternal and paternal mental health problems, environmental problems in relation to housing and neighbors, social isolation, chronic physical health problems in the parents, and trouble with the police. The number of problems per child was significantly correlated with the number of risk factors.

Most psychosocial risk factors have little effect when they occur on their own (Kolvin, Miller, Fleeting, & Kolvin, 1988; Rutter, 1979), an unusual circumstance in any case. There is now good evidence for a high prevalence of psychiatric disorder among groups of young people known to suffer particular and multiple risks. These groups have mostly not been included in population studies based on community samples such as the Ontario Child Health Study. McCann, James, Wilson, and Dunn (1996) reported a 67% prevalence of psychiatric disorder in adolescents in the public care of Oxford local authority, as compared with 15% in adolescents living with their own families; for adolescents in residential units, the rate was 96%. A finding of particular relevance is the rate of depression (23%) among this group of young people who, in England, traditionally have poor access to specialist mental health services. At the time of their entering local authority care in Glasgow, Dimigen et al. (1999) also found high levels of psychiatric disorder among 70 children ages 5–16 years. The most common disorders were conduct disorder (found in more than one-third) and depression, which was significantly more common among children entering residential establishments than among children in foster care. Comorbidity was found in over a third of the children. Children who are excluded from school (Barnes, 1998) and young people in the criminal justice system (Kurtz, Thornes, & Bailey, 1998) are also highly vulnerable to mental health problems.

SERVICE USE AND REFERRED POPULATIONS

Recent epidemiological studies indicate that only a minority of children with diagnosable problems have professional consultation (Bird et al., 1988; Offord et al., 1987). Information on certain aspects of treatment practice for children with psychopathology show that boys have higher rates of treatment in childhood and girls in adolescence (Bird et al., 1988; McCulloc, Henderson, & Philip, 1966; Rutter & Garmezy, 1983; Von Knorring, Andersson, & Magnusson, 1987). In a random sample broadly representative of adolescents living in the northeastern section of the United States, Cohen, Kasen, Brook, and Struening (1991) found (1) that many children with serious problems were not being seen by anyone regarding these problems, (2) that parents most commonly discussed the emotional or behavioral problems of their offspring with teachers, (3) that although a very high proportion of teenagers did see a physician during the course of a year, emotional and behavioral problems were rarely discussed with them, (4) that conduct disorder and oppositional/defiant disorder were most associated with treatment seeking, (5) that children with internalizing problems were relatively unidentified and unreferred, and (6) that there was no balancing tendency for mothers to seek advice regarding children with internalizing disorders from informal sources.

In Ontario, Offord et al. (1987) found that children with psychiatric disorders were four times more likely to use mental health and/or social services than their peers without disorder (Offord et al., 1987). However, five out of six children with disorders had not used specialized services within the previous 6 months. Children living in urban and rural situations did not differ significantly in their use of services, although for general community child health services—used by 50% of all children in the previous 6 months—there was less use by rural children. About twice as many children with psychiatric disorder were receiving special education services, as compared with children without disorder. A few years later, in Ontario, Whitaker et al. (1990) found that 35.1% of the students with a diagnosis of an internalizing disorder had used some form of services for their problems, as compared with 5.3% of those with none of the diagnoses considered.

A longitudinal birth cohort study in New Zealand—the Christchurch Health and Development Study (Fergusson, Horwood, Shannon, & Lawton, 1989)—found low rates of service utilization. Of the children meeting diagnostic criteria on the basis of mother or youth report, only 21% were in contact with any service for their problems or symptoms. Almost half of these had been in touch with mental health professionals, and 40% had received help from school counselors and 36% from other sources. Type of disorder and comorbidity seemed to be the major factors predicting service utilization. From the Dunedin study, McGee et al. (1990) also found that many adolescents with confirmed disorder had sought help from their school counselor and that nearly half of them or their parents had sought some kind of help. In particular, those with attention deficit problems often had a long history of referral to services. Many, however, with apparently significant parent-recognized disorders, had not made use of services. McGee et al. noted that it remains unclear whether the adolescents who had used the available services were any better off. Few adolescents were receiving prescription medication for mental health problems, and a relatively large number of adolescent girls, many with disorder, reported self-medication with alcohol or other drugs to make themselves feel better.

In the United Kingdom, studies by Garralda and Bailey (1986a, 1986b, 1989) have shown that about a quarter of children consulting in primary care have psychiatric disorders, although only between 2% and 5% attend with mental health problems as the primary complaint. Doctors in primary care settings vary widely in their identification of psychiatric disturbance. Identification rates are somewhat higher in pediatrically staffed clinics (Garralda & Bailey, 1989). Recognition is higher when children have severe, as opposed to milder, problems, and, accordingly, the more severely affected children are more likely to be referred to psychiatric services (Garralda & Bailey, 1990).

The four sites included in the MECA study differed in the reports of parents concerning the use of mental health or substance abuse services and the specific types of service used at each site, although the three mainland sites produced similar reports of overall service use (Leaf et al., 1996). Those in New York were most likely to have had some mental health-related services (18.1%), whereas youths in Puerto Rico had the lowest report of service use (7.4%). Sites differed significantly in the use of mental health specialists as compared with mental health contacts with general medical providers. Young people at the Connecticut site were three times as likely as those at the New York site to have a mental health-related contact in the general medical sector and 3.6 times as likely as young people in Puerto Rico.

Parents and young people frequently differed in their reports about the use of mental health services, but 14.2% of the combined four-site sample were identified by the parent or young person as having had an in-school mental health or substance misuse-related contact during the year prior to interview. Parents and young people together identified 12.9% of young people ages 12–17 as having had at least one mental health-related service contact out of school.

As with parent reports, significant differences were found in the likelihood of service use in the four MECA communities when reports from parents and young people were combined, but overall service use varied little in the three mainland sites—from 22.8% in New York to 23.8% in Atlanta. However, service use differed for those with a psychiatric disorder as compared with those not meeting criteria for a disorder, as measured by the DISC. At the three mainland sites, between 38.4% and 43.5% of all children meeting criteria for a psychiatric disorder in the previous 6 months also had some mental health-related contact in the year prior to the interview. Combining data from the four sites showed that young people with psychiatric disorders and poor functioning as measured by the CGAS were 6.8 times more likely to have seen a mental health specialist than were those without a psychiatric disorder and with a higher level of functioning. Rates of service use differed only for the children with a DISC diagnosis and a higher level of functioning (CGAS = 61 or more). The use of mental health specialists by young people with psychiatric disorders and significant dysfunction were similar in the four communities studied, although these communities differed in the percentage of children with a diagnosis who received mental health services and the percentage of children with a diagnosis and a CGAS score of 61 or greater.

Perceptions of the need for services have been shown to differ even among members of the medical profession. In Southwest Hertfordshire (United Kingdom) it was shown that 27 of 232 children, who were 8–14 years old and attending their general practitioner, had psychiatric disorder, assessed according to the Rutter parental questionnaire (Evans & Brown, 1993). The general practitioners, however, felt that a much lower proportion of children attending their clinics needed specialist mental health services, but were unsure about the specific number. Only 6 of the children assessed as having a psychiatric disorder, according to the Rutter questionnaire, had attended the child and family clinic. Overall, the parents of 28 of the children thought that their children would benefit from specialist mental health attention, but the children with high scores on the Rutter questionnaire and those whose parents thought they needed services tended to be different, with only 10 children in both groups. Four of these had had contact with the clinic. The other 6 children clearly had unmet needs. Another 17, with high Rutter scores, were assessed as likely to benefit from services, although their parents were not convinced of this.

SUMMARY

The prevalence of psychiatric disorders in community surveys is reported to be around 20–30% of school-age children, but this figure drops to 12–15% when only moderate to severe (clinically significant) diagnoses are considered. The prevalence estimates obtained depend on the informants asked and the instruments used to obtain the diagnostic information. Those investigations that use multiple informants to define caseness show greatest promise in identifying true cases in community samples, but there is no agreement on how information from multiple sources may best be integrated. Figures for overall prevalence are similar across cultures throughout the world, although there are substantial cultural differences in the types of disorders that are most commonly found. Characteristics of the parent, family, and the child or adolescent himself or herself determine whether the parent regards the child's behavior as being a significant problem. Parent confirmation that the child has a significant problem is not related to type of disorder but rather to the child's social competence, with the possible exception of aggressive conduct disorder. Many disorders have been increasing in the past decades, even when case identification methodologies are taken into account. Prevalence of the diagnosis of psychiatric disorders rises with age. The proportion of girls with psychiatric diagnoses relative to boys increases with age, although, overall, prevalence is higher for boys than for girls.

The stability of disorders depends largely on their diagnostic category. Overall, persistence of moderate or severe disorders at any age is about 50%, and a particularly high proportion of those with conduct disorders when young manifest similar disorders in adolescence. A high proportion of disorders are likely to persist or recur during the period of childhood and into adult life. This is dependent on the type of disorder and the age of presentation. Comorbidity is very common, particularly in referred samples. The natural history of child psychiatric disorder depends on the extent of comorbidity, which interacts with age, gender, and associated familial psychopathology. Children with comorbid conditions are particularly likely to have academic problems.

Poor-quality family, school, and neighborhood environments are risks for developing psychiatric disorders in childhood and are generally associated with poor treatment outcomes. Children with physical illnesses and other disabilities have an increased risk of psychiatric disorder, and those who care for them require special support. In general, there is poor correlation between specific risk factors and particular diagnoses. But exposure to a greater number of risk factors increases the likelihood of developing psychiatric disorder.

A high proportion of individuals with psychiatric diagnoses suffer from significant functional impairments. The concomitants and the sequelae of persistent childhood psychiatric disorder are profoundly serious with respect to adult life chances in a range of domains. Yet a significant number of children with relatively severe disorders are not in contact with mental health services. Children with certain problems, such as externalizing behavior, are more likely to be referred to services than others. Comparisons of community and clinic samples indicate that those who are known to services have more severe problems and poorer functioning. Functioning, but not severity of the disorder, predicts the likelihood that a child will be referred to child mental health services. There is evidence that poorly functioning children in contact with other services are less likely to be referred to mental health services.

IMPLICATIONS

The significant and growing proportion of children suffering psychiatric disorder indicates the need for considerable development in the level and type of services currently available. The evidence suggests that much child psychiatric disorder does not remit spontaneously, but becomes more complex and resistant to treatment with time, highlighting the importance of early effective intervention. Because children with mental health problems tend to experience numerous difficulties across different domains of their lives, which may present in a number of settings (e.g., school, home, social services), an integrated approach to children's welfare is necessary, ensuring coordination across services. Children with the most complex needs are the least likely to reach appropriate services. There is specific evidence that children whose parents have mental health problems are at significant risk, indicating the need for child and adult mental health services to be more closely integrated. In general, the challenge for service planning is how to address the difficulties in access to services for multiproblem families.

Because of the higher probability of comorbidity in clinic-referred populations, assessment needs to be comprehensive and not just targeted at presenting symptoms. A focus on treating impairment—relational and symptomatic—may be as effective as focusing on the diagnosis. In view of the evidence of persistence of disorders, it is important that facilities be made available for following up children who have been referred for psychiatric problems.

3

Anxiety Disorders

Anxiety disorders commonly present as part of a more complex picture, frequently including other disorders (e.g., Strauss & Last, 1993) and difficulties in adaptation such as shyness, academic underachievement, and unhappiness (e.g., Quay & LaGreca, 1986). Fears and worries are, of course, very common in normal development (e.g., Bell-Dolan, Last, & Strauss, 1990; Muris, Meesters, Merckelbach, Sermon, & Zwakhalen, 1998), and become diagnosable only where a persistent and disabling pattern has become established. Nevertheless, it has been shown that for children starting school, anxiety symptoms that do not meet diagnostic criteria are associated with academic impairment over the following years (Ialongo, Edelsohn, Werthamer-Larsson, Crockett, & Kellam, 1994, 1995). This chapter is concerned with treatments for symptoms that do meet the thresholds for at least one diagnosis.

DEFINITION

Anxiety disorders in children and adolescents include the syndromes described for the adult population, so the following categories from DSM-IV can be applied to children: generalized anxiety disorder (GAD), obsessive–compulsive disorder (OCD), agoraphobia, panic disorder, specific phobia, social phobia, and anxiety states due to either medical disorder or substance use. Certain important categories of disorder most commonly seen in childhood or adolescence in DSM-III-R, overanxious disorder (OAD) and avoidant disorder, were not retained in DSM-IV, as they were felt to be essentially similar to generalized anxiety disorder and social phobia, respectively. The only childhood emotional disorder that appeared in DSM-III-R and has been retained is separation anxiety disorder (SAD).

PREVALENCE

Overall figures from epidemiological studies (e.g., review by Bernstein & Borchardt, 1991) of children and adolescents spanning 4–20 years of age suggest that 8–12% of children in this age range suffer from one or more diagnosable anxiety disorder (earlier studies are reviewed by Costello, 1989b; Kashani & Orvaschel, 1990), making anxiety disorders the most common type of psychiatric disorder in children (e.g., Costello & Angold, 1995; Dadds, Spence, Holland, Barrett, & Laurens, 1997). Remarkably, Bell-Dolan et al. (1990) found that 10–30% of schoolchildren showed subclinical levels of OAD, whereas Dadds et al. (1997) found that one in six schoolchildren in their study had an anxiety disorder or features of one. Anxiety disorders are equally frequent in boys and girls until adolescence, after which there is a predominance of girls (Cohen et al., 1993c).

Children with emotional disorders are much less frequently referred for psychiatric attention than those with disruptive disorders (Beardslee et al., 1997; Beidel & Turner, 1997). In a sample of 6- to 19-year-olds (Keller et al., 1992b), 76% of children meeting criteria for anxiety disorders did not get treated. A longitudinal study of 776 adolescents presenting with a variety of disorders (Cohen et al., 1991) showed that young people diagnosed as suffering from OAD on DSM-III-R were not significantly more likely to be referred to a mental health professional than children in the rest of the population in the 2½-year period after diagnosis. Children with disruptive disorders were four to five times more likely than other children to be referred. It also found that parents were not seeking alternative advice (from teachers, friends, or relatives) about children with emotional disorders, whereas they sought this additional help when children were disruptive.

Certain disorders seem particularly likely to be unrecognized or untreated. An epidemiological survey by Flament, Whitaker, and Rapoport (1988) found a 6-month prevalence of OCD of approximately 1 in 200. Only 4 of the 18 children diagnosed as suffering from OCD were in psychiatric treatment. None of these had been recognized as showing OCD or offered treatment for it. The reasons for this may include factors specific to the condition (secretiveness and lack of desire to change) and insufficient awareness and treatment resources among mental health professionals. Jenike (1990) described OCD as a hidden epidemic. Epidemic is perhaps an exaggeration, but this disorder is very often hidden in children, as in adults.

There is some evidence on the demographic profiles of children and adolescents with different anxiety disorders. Those with SAD usually present at the youngest age and are more frequently from families with lower socioeconomic status or with single parents (Last, Perrin, Hersen, & Kazdin, 1992). Although SAD becomes less common in the older age group, GAD (or OAD) becomes more frequent (Westenberg, Siebelink, Warmenhoven, & Treffers, 1999), as does social phobia (Velting & Albano, 2001). OCD seems to present at two stages: in the early school years (modal age at presentation 7 years: see Swedo, Rapoport, Leonard, & Lenane, 1989) and in adolescence (mean age at onset 10 years in the same study, suggesting a bimodal distribution). Boys are more likely to present at the earlier age, girls in adolescence. There is evidence that panic disorder is rare before puberty (Klein, Mannuzza, Chapman, & Fyer, 1992), and an interesting study by Hayward et al. (1992) showed a clear relationship between onset of panics and stage of puberty, regardless of age. Anxiety disorders are more commonly treated among children in middle- to upper-class families (e.g., Francis, Robbins, & Grapentine, 1992), but these data should be used with caution because they may reflect referral patterns rather than actual prevalence.

CLINICAL PRESENTATION

The clinical picture in anxiety disorders varies according to the particular disorder and the developmental stage of the child involved. The common feature is anxious or fearful mood, which may be generalized or triggered by particular situations. The only anxiety disorder that DSM-IV (American Psychiatric Association, 1994) identifies as specific to childhood is SAD. The predominant symptoms vary according to the child's age; younger children show a wider range of symptoms, with anxiety focused more on possible harm to the attachment figures. Most children and adolescents with SAD (about three-quarters) show school refusal (Last, Hersen, Kazdin, Finkelstein, & Strauss, 1987a). GAD, previously diagnosed in DSM-III-R as OAD, involves excessive, unrealistic, and pervasive worrying (Strauss, Lease, Last, & Francis, 1988b). OCD, agoraphobia, panic disorder, specific phobia, and social phobia present in similar forms in children, adolescents, and adults. For instance, OCD involves repetitive, disabling intrusive thoughts or behavioral rituals associated with anxiety, and social phobia is marked by fear and avoidance in social situations, accompanied by pervasive functional impairment (Beidel, Turner, & Morris, 1999; Velting & Albano, 2001).

Comorbidity

One-third or more of children with one anxiety disorder also meet criteria for at least one other anxiety disorder (Strauss & Last, 1993), and about the same proportion suffer from major depression (Bernstein & Borchardt, 1991). Around 20% of children with SAD and OAD meet criteria for attention-deficit/hyperactivity disorder (ADHD) (Last et al., 1987a). Sixty percent of children meeting criteria for social phobia show another current Axis I disorder, most often another anxiety disorder (e.g., Beidel et al., 1999).

Natural History

The information available on the natural history of anxiety disorders has been summarized by Clark et al. (1994) and updated by the American Academy of Child and Adolescent Psychiatry (1997a) and by Kovacs and Devlin (1998). It is widely believed that these disorders often remit spontaneously. However, longitudinal investigations (e.g., Flament et al., 1990) and retrospective studies (e.g., Pollack et al., 1996) suggest that this is an over optimistic view (see review by Kovacs & Devlin, 1998).

To some extent, the natural history of different anxiety disorders varies. Although separation anxiety and early childhood phobias have a relatively benign course (Last, Perrin, Hersen, & Kazdin, 1996), OAD and panic disorder appear to be more chronic (Last et al., 1996) and to be associated with additional depression in adolescence (Strauss, Last, Hersen, & Kazdin, 1988a) and perhaps with generalized anxiety disorder in adulthood (Last et al., 1987a). A large-scale follow-up investigation (Cohen et al., 1993b) showed that 47% of children with severe overanxious disorder continued to suffer from the same disorder 2½ years later, almost all still at a severe level. Keller et al. (1992a) found that the mean duration of anxiety disorders at the time of first interview was 4 years, and it was estimated that 46% would be diagnosable for at least 8 years. Many children followed a relapsing course of illness.

Even disorders with a relatively good prognosis, such as SAD, may have an unstable rather than a benign course (Cantwell & Baker, 1989). There are indications that SAD is associated with difficulties with separation in adult life (see American Academy of Child and Adolescent Psychiatry, 1997a), continued SAD and neurotic depression (Flakierska, Lindstrom, & Gillberg, 1988), crises over leaving home or changing jobs (Werkman, 1987), work phobia (Coolidge, Brodie, & Feeney, 1964), and agoraphobia (Gittelman & Klein, 1984). In Cantwell's study (Cantwell & Baker, 1989), OAD had the lowest recovery rate after 4 years; 25% had the same disorder and 75% were still diagnosably ill with disruptive or emotional disorders. Similarly, social phobia has been shown to have long-term deleterious effects on adjustment in the areas of education, employment, and relationships, in addition to the raised risk of developing Axis I disorders (Velting & Albano, 2001).

Other studies have examined the persistence of OCD. For instance, Thomsen and Mikkelsen (1995) found that half of 23 children and adolescents treated as inpatients or outpatients for OCD still met criteria for OCD diagnosis at 3-year follow-up. Two-thirds of these had suffered from the symptoms continuously (the remainder showed an episodic course). In a very long-term follow-up, also by Thomsen (1995), 47 children admitted with OCD, followed up in young adulthood, were compared with matched comparison child psychiatric cases. The OCD group were significantly more likely to be still living with their parents, to be socially isolated, and to be registered disabled (because of continuing OCD, except for one person who had become schizophrenic). These and other studies confirm the common clinical view that untreated OCD is a complex and relatively intractable disorder in children, as it tends to be in adults.

Some evidence on the medium-term effects of anxiety disorders on general functioning is available. For example, Kashani and Orvaschel (1990) studied a community sample of 210 children and adolescents aged between 8 and 17 years. They found that children with anxiety disorders in each age group had higher rates of all other disorders than nonanxious children. They also showed that the anxious children failed to show the improvement with age in peer relationships seen in other children and that in the area of family relationships, the anxious children in the older groups showed an increasing frequency of problems. Other signs of poor adjustment were increasingly prevalent among the older anxious children. At 8 years, the anxious children had more symptoms than others, but were reasonably well functioning in other ways; by 12 years, they had more difficulties in school and poorer self-image; at 17 years, anxious children were more likely to be depressed, show behavioral disorders and somatic complaints, and have significantly poorer self-esteem than nonanxious peers. It seems that the impact of anxiety disorders is increasingly pervasive as the child gets older. A large (n = 330) longitudinal study (Cole, Peeke, Martin, Truglio, & Seroczynski, 1998) has shown that over 3 years, high levels of anxiety predict increasing depression (but not the other way around). Early adolescents with social phobia have been shown to be at risk for the development of substance abuse by mid- to late adolescence (Kessler et al., 1994); anxious children learn to medicate their anxiety symptoms, using alcohol or other substances that begin to be available in adolescence.

On long-term outcome, a recent, fairly small-scale (n = 44) study (Weissman et al., 1999) showed that prepubertal-onset anxiety disorders were associated with raised rates of mental health problems and service use 10–15 years later. Specifically, substance abuse and conduct disorder were more common, long-term service use was higher, and impairment was greater than among controls.

A recent study reported by Costello et al. (Costello, Angold, & Keeler, 1999) followed 300 7- to 11-year-old children into adolescence and examined the continuity in psychiatric disorder and its possible relation to functional impairment. They found that having an emotional disorder at ages 7–11 strongly predicted adolescent disorder in girls but not in boys. For girls, the likelihood of diagnosable psychiatric illness in adolescence was six times higher if the girl had had a diagnosable emotional disorder at elementary school age.

It is often thought that children who are younger at the onset of symptoms are more likely to "grow out of it." However, a well-designed prospective study of children presenting at an anxiety disorders clinic (Last et al., 1996) found that children whose anxiety disorder had started at a younger age remained ill longer.

TREATMENT

Physical Treatments

Benzodiazepines

Although they are fairly commonly prescribed (Riddle et al., 1999[ib]), there has been very little research on the efficacy of benzodiazepines, serotonin (5-HT) agonists, or "beta-blockers" for anxiety symptoms in children or adolescents. The earliest studies of pharmacotherapy for anxiety were of benzodiazepines, and the results were equivocal (see Allen, Leonard, & Swedo, 1995[ib]; Riddle et al., 1999[ib]). There have been a small number of noncontrolled studies of benzodiazepines since that time (e.g., Biederman, 1987[iii]; Kutcher & Mackenzie, 1988[iii]), and one small (n = 15) placebo-controlled investigation of the use of clonazepam with a variety of anxiety disorders (Graae, Milner, Rizzotto, & Klein, 1994[i]), which produced negative results and considerable difficulty with side effects. Similarly, a double-blind, placebo-controlled study (Simeon et al., 1992[i]) of alprazolam for 4 weeks, in 30 children with avoidant or overanxious disorder, found no significant difference between alprazolam and placebo, although there was a trend in favor of the active treatment (88% vs. 62% improved).

More recent work has focused on a range of drugs that in adults are most commonly used as antidepressants. The best-established role for medication in the anxiety disorders is in relation to OCD (see Grados & Riddle, 2001[vi]).

Tricyclic Antidepressants

Clomipramine is significantly more effective in the treatment of OCD than placebo, with 75% of children showing moderate improvement within 5 weeks. Both Flament et al. (1985[i]) and DeVeaugh-Geiss et al. (1992[i]) used double-blind, placebo-controlled designs in which clomipramine showed significantly better results than placebo. In the latter study, for instance, the active drug was associated with an average one-third reduction in symptoms. Clomipramine appears to be superior to other tricyclic antidepressants for OCD: Leonard et al. (1989[ii]) showed that clomipramine was superior to desipramine in a double-blind crossover trial, and the same group (Leonard et al., 1991[ii]) found that desipramine was significantly less effective when substituted (double-blind) during long-term treatment with clomipramine.

Tricyclic antidepressants have also been tested in the treatment of phobia and separation anxiety. Gittelman-Klein and Klein (1973[i]) were the first to conduct a double-blind, placebo-controlled study of the use of imipramine in treating 45 children. Both groups of children also received behavior therapy. School attendance and other measures of anxiety were significantly better after 6 weeks in the imipramine group, as compared with the placebo control (81% back at school vs. 47% in the control group). In several subsequent studies, results were very discouraging: Berney et al. (1981[i]) found no gain in using clomipramine over placebo for school phobia (51 children ages 9–14 years). It may well be that the clomipramine dose was below the therapeutic level in this study. Bernstein et al. (Bernstein, Garfinkel, & Borchardt, 1990[i]) found no additional benefit from either imipramine or alprazolam over placebo in a double-blind study of 24 cases of school refusal. When Klein et al. (1992b[i]) reevaluated imipramine for SAD (which had already failed to respond to behavior therapy), they did not find any superiority over placebo. The mixed results obtained in treatment studies for school refusal may well reflect the mixed etiologies underlying this symptom. Bernstein et al. (1990[i]) found that 65% of school refusers met criteria for both a depressive and an anxiety disorder, 23% met criteria only for depressive disorder, and the remainder had subthreshold depressive and anxiety symptoms; none met criteria for an anxiety disorder alone.

Bernstein et al. (2000[i]) have recently reported a double-blind randomized control trial (RCT), involving school-refusing adolescents, again with comorbid anxiety and depressive disorders. The study was designed to overcome previous limitations (in power, dosage, and monitoring of concurrent treatment) of the drug studies discussed earlier, which produced largely negative results. Sixty-three subjects began the trial and 47 completed treatment. All adolescents were treated with cognitive-behavioral therapy (CBT), while one group also received imipramine and the other received placebo medication. Assignment was random and school attendance was the major outcome measure. The outcome of the imipramine group was significantly better at the end of treatment, and improvement was also significantly faster. At the end of treatment, 54% of the imipramine group were attending school at least 75% of the time, whereas only 17% of the placebo group were (note, however, that even in the imipramine group almost half did not meet the criterion for remission). It is important to note that some subjects may have met the remission criteria before beginning the trial—subjects were required to show at least 20% absence to be included; anything up to 25% would have counted as a successful outcome. In addition, there was a nonsignificant difference between the groups at baseline, in school attendance (28% for the imipramine group and 17% for placebo). Although not significant, the level of attendance was already favoring the imipramine group; however, the difference in outcome remained significant even when baseline attendance was controlled for. Perhaps more serious, there was a significant difference in clinician-rated anxiety and depression scores at baseline, again with the placebo group being more symptomatic. Depression and anxiety scores were lower in the medication group than in the placebo group at the end of the treatment, but on three out of four measures, the difference between groups was nonsignificant.

A 1-year follow-up of the preceding study (Bernstein, Hektner, Borchardt, & McMillan, 2001[i]) raises worrisome concerns about the durability of gains from the treatment offered. Forty-one of the 63 originally randomized children returned for follow-up; this included 35 of the 47 completers and 6 of the dropouts. It could be that children were more likely to come for follow-up if their functioning remained impaired; however, in fact, comparison of the group who came for follow-up and those who did not showed that school attendance had been significantly better, at posttreatment, among those who presented for follow-up, and children were more likely to come for follow-up if they had been in the active treatment than in the placebo condition. There was therefore an overrepresentation of the successfully treated cases. At 1 year, 64% of the follow-up cases met criteria for at least one anxiety disorder and 33% for a depressive disorder (72% had at least one diagnosis). The imipramine group were no better off than the placebo group. Sixty-seven percent had been prescribed psychotropic medication (most often selective serotonin reuptake inhibitors, SSRIs). Twenty percent had been hospitalized, and 77% had received outpatient treatment. Unfortunately, records of school attendance were not available, but most cases had continued with some sort of education.

A serious difficulty in the use of tricyclics with children or adolescents is that they have been found to increase the (small but alarming) risk of sudden death from cardiac failure and the risk of long-term electrocardiographic changes. These side effects necessitate cardiac monitoring in this age range (for recent reviews, see Geller, Reising, Leonard, Riddle, & Walsh, 1999[vi]; Mezzacappa, Steingard, Kindlon, Saul, & Earls, 1998[vi]).

Selective Serotonin Reuptake Inhibitors

The other drugs that show promise in childhood anxiety disorders, newer and much less extensively evaluated so far in children than in adults, are the SSRIs (reviewed by DeVane & Sallee, 1996[ib]; Emslie, Walkup, Pliszka, & Ernst, 1999[vi]). They seem to produce different side effects than clomipramine and other tricyclics, which are almost certainly less serious. However, SSRIs do present some behavioral side effects (agitation and perhaps mania) in certain patients (see Emslie et al., 1999[vi]). These are being monitored as experience accumulates.

As to efficacy, Riddle et al. (1992[i]) reported a 20-week, double-blind, placebo-controlled crossover trial of fluoxetine in 14 children and adolescents with OCD. Children receiving fluoxetine showed a 44% decrease in obsessive–compulsive symptoms (on the Children's Yale–Brown Obsessive Compulsive Scale, CY-BOCS). There was a nonsignificant (27%) decrease among those receiving placebo medication. Several noncontrolled reports (e.g., a chart review of 38 cases by Geller, Biederman, Reed, Spencer, & Wilens, 1995b[iii]) have also suggested the effectiveness of fluoxetine for OCD. Fluoxetine may in addition be useful in the treatment of generalized anxiety. An open trial with 21 children with OAD (Birmaher et al., 1994[iii]) showed that 81% had moderate to marked global improvement within 2 months. This trial clearly needs to be followed by a controlled investigation. Another study (Black & Uhde, 1994[i]) reported the usefulness of fluoxetine in 15 children with elective mutism and either social phobia or avoidant disorder. This was a double-blind, placebo-controlled trial lasting 12 weeks. However, the results were inconclusive because the active treatment group dwindled to 6 subjects by the end of the period. There were no statistically significant differences in most ratings between fluoxetine and placebo; the children still had clinically significant symptoms, although there were signs of improvement.

Following an early encouraging open-label trial (Apter et al., 1993b[iii]) of fluvoxamine for OCD (n = 14) and depressive symptoms (n = 6), Riddle's group have reported a double-blind, placebo-controlled trial of fluvoxamine across 17 treatment centers (Riddle et al., 2001[i]). The subjects were 8- to 17-year-olds with OCD. One hundred twenty subjects were randomized, of whom 46 dropped out (19 from the fluvoxamine condition and 27 from placebo). Scores on the CY-BOCS, and on several other measures, were significantly lower for the children treated with fluvoxamine as compared with placebo, over a 10-week period. The mean reduction in CY-BOCS score was 24.6% for the fluvoxamine group, compared with 13.6% for the placebo group. Forty-two percent of the fluvoxamine group were considered to have responded to treatment (at least 25% reduction in CY-BOCS score), compared with 26% of the placebo group. Younger children were more likely to respond, which was unexpected and possibly accounted for by inadequate dosage of medication for the adolescent cases.

Alderman et al. (Alderman, Wolkow, Chung, & Johnston, 1998[iii]) evaluated sertraline as a treatment for OCD in 17 children ages 6–17 years. No other treatment was used for comparison. Medication continued for up to 5 weeks. Results showed that for the OCD group as a whole, there were significant reductions in symptomatology; for example, mean scores on the CY-BOCS were 50% lower at the end of treatment across the group (although it was not stated what proportion of children showed clinically significant improvement). It is not known whether the improvements were sustained. A similar study has been carried out using paroxetine in an open-label, uncontrolled trial with 20 outpatients with OCD (Rosenberg, Stewart, Fitzgerald, Tawile, & Carroll, 1999[iii]). There were promising, significant reductions in symptom severity (CY-BOCS) and no serious side effects. March et al. (1998[i]) carried out a large-scale multicenter RCT of sertraline, which produced results very close to those obtained for fluvoxamine by Riddle's group (see above, Riddle et al., 2001[i]).

Although the great majority of the studies of SSRIs for anxiety have been with OCD patients (as earlier), there are beginning to be studies of other anxiety disorders. For example, Renaud, Birmaher, Wassick, and Bridge (1999a[iii]) reported an open-label pilot study of the treatment of 12 children with panic disorder, using various SSRIs supported as necessary by benzodiazepines; two-thirds of the patients substantially improved. Carlson, Kratochwill, and Johnson (1999[iib]) have reported an interesting study of the efficacy of sertraline for selective mutism, using a single-case experimental design with five children. The study was double-blind and placebo-controlled, with a replicated multiple baseline design. The results were, unfortunately, less clear than the design; some children improved substantially and at the expected time after initiating active treatment, others either hardly improved or improved with placebo. Overall, the results were encouraging but far from conclusive. In addition, as the authors acknowledged, the pattern of symptoms and behavior changes in these children suggested that a behavioral approach could have been appropriate, either alone or in combination with medication.

Monoamine Oxidase Inhibitors

There is a possibility, based on evidence of some effectiveness with similar symptoms in adults, that the new selective reversible (safer) monoamine oxidase inhibitors (MAOIs) could be of use in childhood. However, there appear to have been no studies to date evaluating any kind of MAOI for childhood anxiety disorders.

Behavioral and Cognitive-Behavioral Treatments

The methods and rationale of behavioral treatments for childhood anxiety are fully described by King and Ollendick (1997[vi]; Ollendick & King, 1998[ib]), who also give a clear and comprehensive overview of studies of the cognitive-behavioral treatment (CBT) of childhood phobias. This form of treatment for anxiety disorders in general has been reviewed by Kendall (e.g., Kendall, 1993[vi]).

Phobias

The very early child CBT literature in this area consisted mostly of single-case reports of imaginal and *in vivo* desensitization for a variety of circumscribed phobias (see Morris & Kratochwill, 1991). Over time, more sophisticated designs involving small groups have been used in some studies, particularly a multiple baseline strategy (e.g., King, Cranstoun, & Josephs, 1989[ii]). In general, these studies, without a separate control group, suggested that behavioral techniques are worthwhile with many phobic children, though not all (Ollendick & King, 1998[ib]). Two general points seem to emerge: that it is important to enlist the support and participation of parents, particularly in the treatment of younger children, and for younger children *in vivo* exposure is particularly important (in contrast to imagery or other more cognitive techniques).

The most systematic early study (Hampe, Noble, Miller, & Barrett, 1973[i]; Miller, Barrett, Hampe, & Noble, 1972[i]) unfortunately gave inconclusive results; 67 children aged 6–15 years, with a variety of phobias (mostly school phobia), were recruited (not referred, but of "clinical severity"). They were then randomly assigned to systematic desensitization, psychotherapy, or a waiting-list control condition. Parents of the children in the two treatment groups were given behaviorally based advice on managing the child's symptoms. Both therapies were conducted three times per week for 8 weeks. Parental ratings of improvement showed that both active treatments were superior to the control condition, with no significant difference between them. However, ratings by a clinician (not the therapist, but aware of therapy assignment) showed no difference between the three groups. In fact, children in all three groups tended to improve over the therapy period; mean severity scores rated by the clinician fell by 45% in the desensitization group, 53% in the psychotherapy group, and 33% in the waiting-list group.

The strongest predictor of improvement was not treatment/control condition, but age: children under 11 years were significantly more likely to lose their phobic symptom. There were some indications of an interaction between age and treatment, in that 96% of treated children under 11 improved, as compared with 57% of the waiting list cases; for children over 11 the figures were 20% and 17%, respectively. At 2-year follow-up, those who had improved in therapy generally remained well, and those who had not responded at the time had also improved; only 7% remained phobic. Thus, it seems that both of these brief forms of therapy accelerated improvement in children of primary school age, whereas neither was effective for older patients.

Specific phobias (of dogs, dental treatment, small animals, etc.) are not a frequent cause of referral for treatment (Barrios & O'Dell, 1989[vi]), so the results of these studies are of greater theoretical than practical interest. Nevertheless, the conclusion of an authoritative review of behavior therapy for children's phobias by Ollendick and King (1998[ib]) is that imaginal systematic desensitization was found to be more effective than no treatment, in four between-group studies (Barabasz, 1973[ii]; Kondas, 1967[iii]; Mann & Rosenthal, 1969[i]; Miller et al., 1972[i]). However, these reviewers caution that two other studies demonstrated that *in vivo* desensitization was superior to imaginal desensitization for phobic children (Kuroda, 1969[ii]; Ultee, Griffiaen, & Schellekens, 1982[ii]) and that recent evidence supports emotive imagery as still more effective. The emotive imagery technique involves pairing frightening situations with an exciting story involving a hero figure, as opposed to pairing them with relaxation. A single-case design study (King et al., 1989[ii]) has provided evidence to support further evaluation of this technique with children.

Other behavioral techniques have also been evaluated in early group studies (see review in Ollendick & King, 1998[ib]). Studies have demonstrated the effectiveness of modeling, based on social learning theory (Bandura, 1977), for childhood phobias. It seems that either live or filmed modeling is beneficial, but that the most effective treatment is participant modeling, which involves *in vivo* exposure as well as modeling of exposure by others (e.g., Blanchard, 1970[ii]; Ritter, 1968[ii]). Similarly, contingency management (based on operant conditioning, or modification of the consequences of the child's behavior) has also been found to be effective for phobias in young children (e.g., Menzies & Clarke, 1993[i]).

Ungraded exposure treatment, or flooding via rapid return to school, can be successful in managing school refusal. Blagg and Yule (1984[ii]) conducted a study of 66 school refusers, mostly of secondary school age, comparing behavioral treatment (BT) with inpatient treatment and home tutoring of cases in a neighboring area. Children were not randomly assigned to groups, but were matched on relevant variables. Two important exceptions to the success of matching were that children in the BT group were significantly younger and had been away from school for somewhat less time. The BT involved careful assessment and preparation of all concerned, followed by flooding, that is, forced return to school, with escort as long as necessary.

BT led to very much better rates of maintenance in school in the year following treatment; 93% were successful, compared with 38% and 10% in the other two groups. Separation anxiety was also successfully treated, in that none of the BT cases showed separation anxiety at follow-up; hospital treatment also led to large improvements in this symptom, but two-thirds of the home-tutored children still showed significant difficulties with separation. The treatment was not only far more successful, but also very rapid (2½ weeks vs. about 1 year for the alternatives) and very much cheaper than the other forms of management.

More recently, King et al. (1998[i]) conducted an RCT in which 34 children, ages 5–15, with school phobia were randomly assigned to either CBT or waiting list control. The CBT condition involved six individual therapy sessions over a 4-week period, with gradual return to school. There were also sessions with parents and teachers to communicate the strategy being adopted and enlist cooperation. On ethical grounds, the waiting-list group was offered treatment rather than remaining untreated through the 12-week follow-up period, which, of course, limits the comparison of outcomes. There were no dropouts from either condition, and children in the CBT group showed significantly greater improvement during treatment (both statistically and clinically). Gains were generally maintained over the (brief) follow-up period.

Another study of CBT for school phobia was reported at the same time as the King study (Last, Hansen, & Franco, 1998[i]). This added an important feature: an attention-placebo as opposed to waiting list control. Fifty-six children and adolescents were randomly assigned either to CBT, involving graduated *in vivo* exposure and coping self-statements, or to an educational support (ES) control condition (which involved education about the nature and treatment of phobic disorders, together with therapeutic support such as reflective listening and clarification). There were two follow-up assessments, at 4 weeks posttreatment and 2 weeks into the next school year. Both treatments (CBT and control) were associated with statistically and clinically significant levels of improvement, which were maintained at the first follow-up but tended to fall off—in both groups—in the stressful period of beginning a new school year. It seems from this study that either the nonspecific factors (e.g., attention, education) were the effective agents in both treatments, or that the educational support protocol was an active treatment. Whichever may be correct, the finding has been replicated in a further, more recent study by Silverman and her colleagues (1999b).

Silverman and co-workers (1999b[i]) compared the relative efficacy of two treatments for phobic disorders, the first based on behavioral principles of operant conditioning, the second on a cognitive therapy model. The two active treatments were exposure-based contingency management (CM) and exposure-based self-control (SC), and these were compared with the same educational support (ES) control condition that was used in the study just described. All treatments continued for nine sessions. Follow-up assessment was carried out after 1 year. The study involved 104 children, mostly with diagnoses of simple phobias, and their parents. Seventy-two percent of the children had comorbid diagnoses. Treatment assignment was random, but with twice as many children referred to each active treatment as to the control group. Eighty-one children completed the treatment offered, with no differential attrition between groups. Analysis of the results was carried out only on these completers, not on all cases where there had been intention to treat. The results showed that both active treatments produced clinically significant improvements maintained at follow-up, but so did the control condition (educational support). This confirmed the surprising finding that the control procedure, which involved no element of exposure, was as effective as the two experimental conditions that share an important exposure element.

Kearney and Silverman (1999) have reported a very careful study of eight school-refusing children. Four received "prescriptive" (essentially behavioral) treatment, while the others received "nonprescriptive" treatment (relaxation and cognitive therapy without exposure). These treatments were individually planned following functional analysis of the symptoms. The children in the prescriptive condition improved a great deal more, and more rapidly, than those in the control condition, who were either still impaired or actually worse. The latter children were then given prescriptive treatment, which was successful. This study therefore supports the inclusion of behavioral prescriptions in addition to nonprescriptive anxiety management techniques for this serious problem.

Beidel, Turner, and Morris (2000[i]) have recently reported an RCT of Social Effectiveness Therapy for Children (SET-C). This therapy, for 8- to 12-year-old children, involves 24 sessions over 12 weeks and combines group social skills training, individual exposure, and homework assignments. At the end of treatment, 67% of the SET-C group no longer met diagnostic criteria, in comparison with 5% of the control group children, who had received nonspecific psychotherapy focused on test anxiety (no assessment of the credibility of this control condition was included). Treatment gains were maintained over 6 months.

Recently, several studies have investigated the efficacy of group CBT. First,

Mendlowitz et al. (1999[i]) examined this in an RCT with 62 7- to 12-year-old children with anxiety disorders. The cases were randomly assigned to a parent–child group, a children-only group, or a parent-only group. Some of them had to wait for a few months between assessment and treatment, and these were designated a waiting-list control group. The children in all three active treatment groups improved in rated anxiety and depression in comparison with the children waiting for treatment. Those who were in groups together with their parents showed more active coping strategies than the others. The authors acknowledged that the greater evidence of active coping in the parent–child treatment group might have been caused by the greater amount of therapeutic input in this condition and the parents' motivation to perceive benefits, among other possible biases. It would be very worthwhile to follow up these children to see whether the reported gains persisted after the end of the intensive treatment program.

Silverman and her group (Silverman et al., 1999a[i]) have reported an RCT examining the efficacy of group CBT (GCBT), as compared with waiting list, for 56 children ages 6–16 with a range of anxiety disorders as their primary diagnoses. At the end of the treatment (or waiting time), 14/17 treated children who had initially shown clinical-level Child Behavior Checklist (CBCL) Internalizing scores no longer showed them at posttest, whereas only 1/11 of the waiting children showed this improvement. (This indicates that only half of the children had been in the clinical range at the beginning.) Sixty-one percent of the treatment completers no longer met diagnostic criteria at posttest, compared with 13% of those in the waiting condition. Note that the analyses reported only involved children who completed their assigned condition, that is, 41 of the original 56 children; no intent-to-treat analysis was reported. At 12-months follow-up the gains were well maintained, although no comparison could be made between treated and control children at follow-up because all waiting-list children had by then been offered treatment. A weakness of waiting-list controlled studies of psychosocial treatments is, of course, that the parents and children providing ratings of symptom levels cannot be blind to whether the child has been in the active or control condition. This is where a convincing control condition, such as the educational support (ES) included in another of Silverman et al.'s recent studies (1999b[i]), is especially valuable.

A smaller RCT has been reported by Hayward et al. (2000[i]), who examined the efficacy of GCBT for adolescent girls with social phobia. Twelve received the CBT while 23 were offered no treatment. The group treatment was associated with significantly fewer diagnosable cases at the end of treatment, but not at 1-year follow-up. However, the combined risk of social phobia and depression was still significantly lower at follow-up in the treatment group, especially among those with a history of depression.

Another recent study, which directly compared group and individual CBT, was carried out by Flannery-Schroeder and Kendall (2000[i]). Participants were 37 8- to 14-year-old children referred for treatment of anxiety disorders, who were randomly assigned to individual CBT (ICBT), GCBT, or a 9-week waiting list followed by random assignment to one of the treatments. Eight further children were entered into the study but dropped out, half before starting treatment and half during treatment (all of these came from the ICBT condition). Outcome was analyzed both for completers only and by intent-to-treat. GCBT cases had (by chance) lower mean scores on anxiety measures, before beginning treatment, than did the children in the other groups. Those who dropped out were found to have been—at intake—significantly more likely to have a primary diagnosis of social phobia, had lower self-rated depression, and were rated by their parents as less anxious or better at coping. At the end of treatment, 73% of children who completed ICBT no longer met criteria for their primary disorder; 50% of those in the GCBT condition met these criteria, and only 8% of those in the waiting-list group (they were not followed at 3 months, because they were treated after their waiting time). Average effect sizes were 1.77 for ICBT and 1.55 for GCBT for those who completed treatment. Results were similar at 3-month follow-up. If an intent-to-treat analysis is applied to the diagnostic changes, then the improvement rates fall to 50% for ICBT, 46% for GCBT, and, again, 8% for waiting list. Although the differences between treated and untreated groups remain large, it must be said that this still leaves half of the children assigned to an active treatment retaining their primary diagnosis. As the authors conclude, this study supports the idea that CBT for childhood anxiety disorders can be delivered in a group as well as an individual format, but a larger study with a longer follow-up is now needed.

Generalized Anxiety

Although generalized anxiety states in children are a frequent cause of referral for treatment (Last, Hersen et al., 1987), treatments for this disorder were not evaluated with the use of behavioral or cognitive methods until their value had begun to be demonstrated with more circumscribed problems. However, Kane and Kendall (1989[iib]) reported a multiple-baseline design study of CBT with four children diagnosed as suffering from OAD, which gave promising results. Subsequently, Kendall (1994[i]) reported results of an RCT of a similar cognitive-behavioral program for 47 children ages 9–13 years, the majority of whom met diagnostic criteria for OAD, with the remainder diagnosed as showing SAD or avoidant disorder. A 16-session ICBT package was used, involving an educational phase followed by teaching of coping strategies and self-reward. This program was shown to be frequently successful, in that there were significantly greater improvements in the treated group than in the waiting-list group on most measures. Nevertheless, more than one-third of the treated children were still diagnosable after the course of treatment, and 22% of patients dropped out before it ended. The latter children were excluded from analyses of effectiveness; an intent-to-treat analysis would have been an important addition.

One caution in interpreting the results of this impressive study is the possibility of bias due to expectations. Although the ratings of parents and children showed a significant effect of treatment, obviously neither of these groups of informants was blind to the treatment condition. Behavioral ratings of anxiety symptoms were also recorded by blind raters and showed a similar impact of treatment, but it is likely that the children who had been through the program would be less anxious performing on video in the clinic setting, as this was an important part of the therapy procedure. Waiting-list subjects had presumably not had comparable rehearsals. A crucial question, therefore, is whether outside observers confirmed the improvement. Teachers were asked to rate the child's anxiety and other problems on the Teacher Report Form of the CBCL (Achenbach & Edelbrock, 1986), and their judgments unfortunately did not confirm the effectiveness of therapy. They judged all children to have improved, regardless of condition. Kendall (1994[i]) points out that not all children were rated as disturbed by teachers at the outset, but even when only cases initially rated as disturbed were included, there was no greater improvement among the treated group; in fact, scores on the relevant scale were lower in the waiting-list group.

An important sequel to the preceding study (Kendall & Southam-Gerow, 1996) showed that at a long-term follow-up (average 3.3 years from end of treatment), treatment gains in the Kendall sample had generally been maintained. However, because the waiting-list control was no longer available, and there is a tendency for anxiety symptoms to improve over time without treatment, these results remained hard to interpret with confidence. Fortunately, Kendall et al. (1997[i]) conducted a further RCT with 94 participants, which confirmed their earlier successful results. We can therefore conclude from these carefully designed studies that CBT can be very helpful to some overanxious children and that, for those who improve, the gains are well maintained at follow-up.

A small number of other studies have investigated the inclusion of families in CBT for children with anxiety disorders. Howard and Kendall (1996b[iib]) used a multiple-baseline design across six children (ages 9–13 years) suffering from diagnosable anxiety disorders. The treatment was a manualized 18-session, family-based CBT that included the elements of the Coping Cat program used in Kendall's individual treatment (Kendall, 1994[i]; Kendall et al., 1997[i]), but with an added dimension of family problem solving and understanding the function of the symptom(s) within the family. Four of the six participating children showed improvement during treatment, and these gains were maintained through a 4-month follow-up, except in the case of one child who had experienced negative life events in the follow-up period.

Barrett and her colleagues (Barrett, Dadds, & Rapee, 1996[i]) conducted a well-designed study, comparing individual CBT with individual + family cognitive-behavioral work. The results replicated those reported by Kendall et al. (Kendall, 1994[i]; Kendall et al., 1997[i]) and confirmed that adding family management increased treatment effectiveness still further. The CBT was an Australian version of Kendall's model. There was a waiting-list control group. In total, 76 children ages 7–14 were included and randomly allocated to one of the three conditions. CBT + family intervention led to significantly fewer children being diagnosable at posttest and at follow-up, in comparison with CBT only (57% were well after CBT, 84% after CBT + family treatment, compared with 26% in the waiting-list control group). As in the Kendall (1994[i]) study, it was not possible to compare treatment and waiting list at follow-up, as all children on the waiting list who remained symptomatic after 12 weeks were given the combined child and family intervention. However, the CBT + family condition remained significantly superior to CBT alone at 12-month follow-up (96% versus 70% well, respectively). Looking more closely at the treatment groups, it emerges that younger children (up to 10 years) benefited more from the additional family component, whereas the 11- to 14-year-olds did not.

Cobham, Dadds, and Spence (1998[i]) usefully extended the preceding study by evaluating one component of the family package: parental anxiety management (PAM), which was hypothesized to be important because of evidence (e.g., Last, Phillips, & Statfeld, 1987b) that many parents of anxious children themselves meet criteria for an anxiety disorder. Sixty-seven children ages 7–14 years, the majority suffering from generalized anxiety disorder (GAD), were assigned either to group CBT or to group CBT + group PAM. Families assigned to each treatment condition were stratified according to the level of parental anxiety (measured by the State–Trait Anxiety Inventory [STAI]; Spielberger, Gorsuch, & Lushene, 1970). The results confirmed the hypothesis, that the addition of PAM had an impact on outcome only where there was high parental anxiety, in which case child CBT alone was significantly less helpful (39% no longer diagnosable vs. 76% with CBT + PAM). However, this result held only at posttreatment; differences were reduced to nonsignificant trends at 12-month follow-up.

Obsessive–Compulsive Disorder

The status of treatment for childhood OCD was summarized by Flament and Vera (1990[vi]), and 32 studies of cognitive-behavioral methods were carefully reviewed by March (1995[ib]; March & Leonard, 1996[ib]; March & Mulle, 1995). March and co-workers (March, Franklin, Nelson, & Foa, 2001) have described the rationale and effective elements of CBT for childhood OCD, together with issues of assessment and research, in detail. Another survey is provided in the Practice Parameters of the American Academy of Child and Adolescent Psychiatry (1998c[ib]). March's conclusion (1995[ib]) was that "although empirical support remains weak, CBT also may be the psychotherapeutic treatment of choice for children and adolescents with OCD [as for adults]" (p.7). March and his colleagues repeated this view in a recent review paper (March et al., 2001); however, although work in the intervening period has strengthened the basis for this suggestion, the efficacy of medication remains much better established.

There were several early case reports (e.g., De Seixas Queiroz, Motta, Pinho Madi, Sossai, & Boren, 1981; Friedmann & Silvers, 1977[iib]) of successful treatment of children and adolescents with response prevention or thought stopping, often with simultaneous family therapy. In addition, Bolton, Collins, and Steinberg (1983[iii]) reported results from a series of 15 adolescents with moderate to severe, entrenched OCD; they were mostly tertiary referrals, with a history of failed attempts to treat their symptoms elsewhere, and they often needed to be treated as inpatients. The report retains relevance as a study of the kind of stubborn picture that often confronts the clinician. The adolescents were treated primarily with response prevention, with family therapy used to support this (focusing mainly on obstacles to the response prevention approach). Sometimes other treatments were required for associated symptoms (5 patients received clomipramine to ease depression or anxiety, with mixed effects on the OCD symptoms). Treatment lasted for up to 4 years, although the successful outcomes were generally achieved within 1 year.

In 8 of the 15 cases, symptoms were completely relieved at the end of treatment; 6 of these subjects remained well at follow-up (between 1 and 4 years later), while the other 2 had relapsed quite severely. Three cases showed no response to treatment lasting between 5 months and 4 years, and the remaining 4 showed partial improvement. The authors offered a useful discussion of the factors that appeared to affect response to treatment. To summarize, it seemed from this small sample that poor adolescent motivation, primary obsessional ruminations, conduct disorder, and obsessional slowness were associated with the bad outcomes.

Although the use of different combinations of therapies in this series makes the results hard to interpret in terms of the effectiveness of individual components, it is a useful account of the effectiveness of response prevention treatment with a difficult group of adolescents with severe obsessive disorders. Using such a sick group meant that the outcome could not ethically be compared with no treatment, but this naturalistic study with careful documentation of outcome, in the context of reasonably clear natural history, began to indicate that the treatment helps most cases at least partly, and to suggest factors associated with outcome.

Kearney and Silverman (1990[ii]) reported an interesting experimental single-case study of CBT with childhood OCD. They treated a 14-year-old boy with severe OCD (the major symptom was checking the window for bats, and his own body for contamination) and a moderate major depressive disorder. The symptoms had been severe for 2 months before referral. Treatment consisted of alternating response prevention (without exposure) and cognitive therapy, with the aim of treating both the obsessional symptoms and the depressive disorder. Both checking rituals were eliminated by the end of the 24-session program; the two rituals seemed to respond selectively to one or the other form of therapy. Rather surprisingly, anxiety symptoms were most responsive to cognitive therapy and depression to response prevention.

The authors regarded the treatment as successful, and the boy was clearly functioning more normally after treatment and at 6-month follow-up. However, careful reading of the results necessitates qualification of this view: (1) Scores on the Children's Depression Inventory showed no improvement at all during treatment, (2) self-esteem remained very impaired, (3) symptoms of anxiety and depression (Internalizing scale on the CBCL) had moved halfway back to pretreatment levels at follow-up, mainly due to the return of obsessive–compulsive features, and (4), most strikingly, the authors note that when either treatment was repeated for a second week rather than alternating, there were signs of deterioration. When response prevention was repeated in the middle of treatment, there was a dramatic relapse of anxiety and depression as rated by both parents and child. The authors suggest that this combined treatment works, but using consecutive weeks of the same approach leads to partial extinction! This study does *not* confirm the efficacy of either response prevention or cognitive therapy alone, but only of the two in combination.

Even then, there must be concern about the remaining depression and the tendency toward relapse of obsessional symptoms at follow-up.

March et al. (1994[iii]) advanced this area using a manualized CBT package, combining anxiety-management techniques designed to appeal to children and graded exposure with response prevention, in an open trial of 15 young people with DSM-III-R diagnoses of OCD. The treatment protocol used in this study introduced the important modification that exposure and goals were placed within the child's control; this seems likely to reduce the common problem of noncompliance with behavioral techniques among children. In their series of consecutive referrals, no patient refused treatment, although two did drop out before it was completed. Parents were heavily involved in the treatment regime, which was conducted on an outpatient basis for an average of 8 months. Interpretation of this study is obscured by the fact that all but one of the subjects were simultaneously treated with medication, and four subjects received either family or individual dynamically oriented therapy.

The group on the whole did very well: Nine of the 15 were well at follow-up, although booster behavior therapy was required to wean these children from medication without relapse. Of the remaining 6, 2 dropped out unimproved, 3 received prolonged treatment without benefit, and 1 was improved but still symptomatic. On average across the whole group, symptom ratings were halved between assessment and follow-up. Although the concurrent use of other treatments limits the clarity of these results, it appears that the combination was somewhat more effective than medication alone: In the multicenter child clomipramine trial, the average magnitude of improvement was 37% (DeVeaugh-Geiss et al., 1992[i]).

Franklin et al. (1998[iii]) also carried out an open trial of CBT (exposure and response prevention) with 14 children and adolescents who met diagnostic criteria for OCD. Half received intensive treatment (more or less daily sessions), the others weekly sessions, but the overall amount of treatment was equivalent; assignment to these conditions was decided by practical considerations. The treatment does not appear to have been manualized, but is described in some detail in the report. There was an average 9-month follow-up period. Twelve of the 14 patients responded to treatment with a reduction in symptom severity of at least 50%. These gains were well maintained at follow-up. Overall, the results for this treatment compared quite closely with those reported by March et al. (1994[iii]). Many of the patients were receiving concurrent antidepressant medication, but this did not make an obvious difference to the degree of improvement, nor did intensity of treatment. However, this was a small-scale, open study: The results justify a more rigorous test.

A promising comparative pilot study of 22 children is reported by de Haan, Hoogduin, Buitelaar, and Keijsers (1998[i]). The children were randomly assigned to either behavioral treatment (BT) or (open-label) clomipramine (CPI). Both treatment conditions were associated with large effect sizes (ESs) (1.58 for BT and 1.45 for CPI) after the 12-week study period; 8/12 BT cases responded, using the rather modest criterion of at least 30% improvement, compared with 5/10 CPI cases. It is reported that the mean dosage of CPI was below the therapeutically desirable level because of side effects. It is noticeable from the individual results that those children who did not respond at 12 weeks tended to show good results after a further 12 weeks of mixed treatment; it therefore seems important to continue with treatment in resistant cases. Again, a further investigation including larger groups and an untreated (or placebo) control is needed.

A recent report by March (1999) has recommended that the treatment of choice for childhood OCD should be a combination of SSRI medication and CBT. He is currently undertaking a trial in which 12 weeks of fluoxetine is followed by 6 weeks of drug + CBT, with a further 18 weeks of maintenance therapy. This regime is intended to be close to current clinical practice for child or adolescent OCD, and a recent small-scale study by Neziroglu, Yaryura-Tobias, Walz, and McKay (2000[i]) gives preliminary evidence that it may be effective, with improvement maintained at a 2-year follow-up.

The recent review paper by March et al. (2001) stated that although clinicians agree that CBT is usually helpful for OCD, they also say that patients will not comply with behavioral treatments and that parents claim clinicians are inadequately trained in CBT procedures. This report, from perhaps the foremost authority in this area, reminds us of the importance of three things: maintaining more than one psychosocial treatment approach, to provide options in cases where child or family does not comply; making sure that treatment manuals and procedures are well adapted to children so that compliance is more likely; and, of course, specific training for clinicians in the best-validated treatments.

A very important aspect of choice of treatment is maintenance over time. A recent and authoritative review by Foa and Kozak (1996[vi]) concluded that although the improvements seen with pharmacotherapy required maintenance medication, those provided by CBT were better maintained.

Other Anxiety Disorders

A small number of studies have evaluated cognitive and/or behavioral treatments for other anxiety disorders, but these are less fully developed than the programs already described.

Ollendick (1995[ii]) conducted a small multiple-baseline design investigation of CBT for panic disorder with agoraphobia in four adolescents. Results were promising, and the timing of improvement appeared to be related to the stage of treatment, as expected. However, this study clearly needs extension, because it was small and the therapist also acted as assessor, which may have produced pressure toward reporting improvement once treatment began.

Albano, Marten, Holt, Heimberg, and Barlow (1995[iii]) explored the effectiveness of group CBT (CBGT-A) for five socially phobic adolescents (a larger trial is in progress). The treatment incorporated education, skill building, modeling and role-playing, cognitive restructuring, and both within- and between-session exposure to anxiety-provoking social situations. Parents were also involved in the treatment. Although there was no control group, independent clinical assessment suggested that there had been remission of diagnosis and significant reduction in self-rated anxiety during treatment. A preliminary report (Tracey et al., 1999[i]) of their large-scale RCT of CBGT-A suggests that the treated youths improved, whether or not their parents were also involved in the protocol. The comparison with a waiting-list control group is not yet available.

Toren et al. (2000[iii]) have recently reported on an open trial of parent–child GCBT for preadolescent children with anxiety disorders (almost all suffered from SAD; half also showed OAD and/or phobias). Twenty-four children and their parents participated in 10 sessions of treatment following CBT principles. Half of the mothers had a diagnosable anxiety disorder, but only two of the fathers did. Ten children were assigned to wait for 10–15 weeks in a no-treatment control condition. However, it is not clear whether these children were (randomly?) selected from among the 24 and all were eventually treated (i.e., a multiple baseline design), or whether the 10 were additional to the 24 and not included in analysis of the treated group. Seventy percent of the treated children had ceased to meet diagnostic criteria by the end of treatment, and by 3-year follow-up, 91% were no longer diagnosable. Intriguingly, the children whose mothers met criteria for an anxiety disorder did better than those whose mothers were not anxious, even though the anxious mothers' own anxiety levels were not reduced during treatment. This small study strongly justifies extension and clarification, as it involved a relatively brief and low-cost treatment that appears to have been helpful with a challenging group: clinically referred children, most with comorbid diagnoses and half of whose mothers had similar symptoms.

Psychodynamic Psychotherapy

Psychodynamic psychotherapy is quite widely used in the treatment of anxious children, especially those with entrenched and complex problems, yet there have been few attempts to evaluate its effectiveness systematically. The attempts that have been made fall short of the methodological standards applied to evaluation of much briefer and more goal-directed therapies, partly because of the complexities of designing such studies and partly because of their much greater costs.

Preliminary evidence suggesting specific benefit for anxious children in psychodynamic treatment came from a chart review study carried out at the Anna Freud Centre in London (Target & Fonagy, 1994a[iv]). The parents were predominantly middle-class professionals. In this study, children with anxiety disorders (with or without comorbidity) showed greater improvements than those with other conditions, and greater improvements than would have been expected on the basis of studies of untreated outcome (see section on natural history). More than 85% of 299 children with anxiety and depressive disorders no longer suffered any diagnosable emotional disorder after an average of 2 years' treatment. Looking in more detail at specific diagnostic groups, it was found that phobias ($n = 48$), separation anxiety disorders ($n = 58$), and overanxious disorder ($n = 145$) were resolved in about 86% of cases. OCD was much more resistant, remaining at a diagnosable level in 30% of cases at the end of therapy. There are serious limitations to a retrospective study, and there was no control group or follow-up; however, these rates of improvement certainly appear to be above the level expected from longitudinal studies. A further finding was that children with severe or pervasive symptomatology, such as severe OAD or multiple comorbid disorders, required more frequent therapy sessions, whereas more circumscribed symptoms, such as phobias—even if quite severe, improved comparably with once- or twice-weekly sessions. These findings justify an RCT in which difficult cases, perhaps those that have not improved with briefer treatments, are treated with a well-defined psychodynamic approach.

Recently, controlled studies of psychodynamic psychotherapy for emotional disorders of middle childhood have begun to emerge. An important study from the University of Pisa (Muratori et al., 2002[ii]) looked at the effectiveness of an 11-session treatment program for 58 children with anxiety disorder or dysthymic disorder. The treatment was structured, focal psychodynamic psychotherapy, beginning with five sessions with the entire family, in which the relational basis of the child's symptoms was established. This was followed by five sessions with the child alone, in which the therapist helped the child articulate thoughts and feelings, memories and wishes, with the aim of helping the child to make connections between his or her feelings and unconscious conflicts about the relationship with the parents. The final session was a family meeting in which the therapist restated the dynamic formulation of the child's conflict based in family relationships. The control group was referred for community treatment, which often meant that they received no intervention, but it also included a variety of interventions, such as unstructured individual psychotherapy and supportive therapy for parents. Measures were taken at baseline, 6 months (end of treatment for the experimental group), and 2 years follow-up. The two key measures were CGAS (completed by a blind, independent interviewer who interviewed both child and parent), and CBCL completed by the parents. The results revealed a significant difference between the groups, only at follow-up, on both the CGAS and CBCL scales. Effect size was approximately 0.75 for both measures. There was a modest improvement on the externalizing scales of the CBCL, but both internalizing and total problem scores showed a dramatic decline, between end of treatment and follow-up, for the children in the psychotherapy condition. In addition, the authors report a significantly lower level of service usage in the experimental group during the follow-up period. This study is unique in providing a well-matched control group, in assessing the effectiveness of psychodynamic psychotherapy. However, there are several important weaknesses. These include an inadequate randomization procedure, where patients were allocated to treatment or control groups according to therapist vacancies; no training or assessment of treatment integrity (although the treatment was manualized and videotaped); lack of information about therapist experience; and relatively mild levels of disorder. Only around 60% were in the clinical range of the CBCL at the start of treatment. By follow-up this was reduced to 34% in the treated group, and increased slightly to 65% in the control group. Although this treatment includes a component of family diagnosis it is not assumed to be a family therapy, and the family work is there to help the therapist focus on helping the child to address a specific set of relationship issues.

In the past there have been indications that psychodynamic intervention was more acceptable to children and adolescents than a behavioral or cognitive-behavioral approach. Apter, Bernhout, and Tyano (1984[iii]) reported that some hospitalized adolescent patients with OCD refused to cooperate with behavioral treatment, but accepted and improved with supportive psychotherapy. This underlines the importance of trying to modify techniques, such as exposure to feared situations, so that they are not only effective but also acceptable to the patient. Some excellent manuals have now been written concerning children with particular disorders (see Kendall, 1994[i]; March et al., 1994[iii]), which present child-oriented strategies and explanations, rather than simply applying techniques developed for adults to children.

SUMMARY

Anxiety disorders are very common, but most cases go untreated. Different disorders have different prognoses, but moderate to severe cases are not likely to remit spontaneously, and when they do remit, it is quite common for other disorders to take their places. Anxiety disorders commonly evolve into other anxiety or depressive syndromes. Persistent anxiety disorders cause pervasive and lasting impairments. The high placebo response observed in child and adolescent patients makes demonstration of efficacy of all treatments problematic.

There has been very little research on the efficacy of benzodiazepines, SSRIs or beta-blockers for anxiety symptoms in children or adolescents, although they are fairly commonly prescribed. Such studies as there have been have given disappointing results. The best-established role for medication in the anxiety disorders is in relation to antidepressant medication for OCD. For this condition in children and adolescents, SSRIs appear to be significantly more effective than either placebo or tricyclic medication, although the effectiveness of clomipramine has also been demonstrated. Approximately half the patients with OCD in trials of SSRIs show clinically significant improvement. Imipramine may be helpful, in combination with CBT, in accelerating the improvement of school refusers; however, at follow-up the medicated group were no better off. Otherwise, there has been little evaluation of the efficacy of medication for childhood anxiety disorders, apart from OCD.

Behavioral techniques are often effective in the treatment of children with circumscribed phobias, especially younger children. OCD can be improved in some cases, though generally not eliminated, by a CBT approach. This approach has so far mostly been evaluated with concurrent medication, but there is some evidence that CBT makes a distinctive contribution. Certain CBT packages have been shown to be effective in the treatment of generalized and other anxiety disorders, and, for those who improve, the gains can be maintained. Exposure has been assumed to be a central aspect of the efficacy of CBT, but two recent well-designed studies of the treatment of school phobia found that therapeutic support without exposure was equally effective. Where exposure treatment is used, it may well be more effective, as well as humane, to use a gradual, rather than a "flooding," approach. There is accumulating evidence that CBT for childhood anxiety disorders can be delivered in a group as successfully as in an individual format. Adding a family component to CBT may well be valuable for younger children or for families where parental anxiety is also high.

There is some evidence that psychodynamic psychotherapy may be effective in the treatment of anxiety disorders, perhaps particularly if delivered in a structured and focused way. No studies have so far examined the effectiveness of family therapy for childhood anxiety disorders, other than CBT delivered in a family format.

IMPLICATIONS

Screening for undiagnosed anxiety disorders may be worthwhile, in view of their prevalence, their impact on social and academic functioning, and their tendency to develop into other disorders.

Given the evidence of effectiveness of certain medications for OCD, it is important that children or adolescents with this condition be seen by a psychiatrist familiar with this literature. As a substantial proportion (about half) of children with OCD fail to show clinically significant, sustained improvement even with the best-supported medication, there is a need for continued work on effective psychosocial treatments for this condition. Further research is needed on the efficacy of medication in other anxiety disorders.

It is a mistake to think of generic behavior therapy or cognitive-behavior therapy: There are particular packages that have been at least partly validated, for children with specific problems and particular developmental stages. Specialized training in these BT and CBT techniques for children is needed; such training is not widely available at present, so it is unlikely that clinicians are providing the treatments being validated by research. The replicated finding that therapeutic support is as effective as CBT, at least in the treatment of school phobia, challenges the general view that exposure is a central element in CBT for anxiety disorders; this assumption needs to be further tested.

Research is urgently needed on whether some children specifically benefit from systemic or psychodynamic psychotherapies, both approaches that are widely provided in clinics. For instance, those who are hard to help with the use of other treatments may be found to respond to one of these techniques, in which case it would be important to try to identify their effective elements and the groups for which they are most appropriate, in order to use available resources as efficiently as possible.

4

Depressive Disorders

The literature on interventions for childhood and adolescent depression has lagged behind the adult literature and the literature on most other common childhood mental health disorders. This may reflect both the general problem that internalizing disorders receive less attention than externalizing behavior, and a long-running dispute over whether children and adolescents can become clinically depressed. Then, in the early years of treatment evaluation, it was rare for referred children to be studied: Such outcome research as there was, was confined to community samples of youths showing subclinical levels of depressed mood. Generally, depression in children has been treated by adapting approaches used with adult patients, particularly medication and cognitive-behavioral therapy (CBT) (Kaslow & Thompson, 1998). However, gradually a more developmentally sensitive approach has been taken, leading to greater understanding of the different responses to these treatments. This approach also needs to be informed by the increasing evidence of the disturbed social contexts of depression in childhood and adolescence: not only the comorbidity and associated social and academic problems of the young people themselves (reported later in this chapter), but also the social and psychiatric problems of their parents and families (Hammen, Rudolph, Weisz, Rao, & Burge, 1999).

DEFINITION

Depressive disorders are partly defined by somewhat arbitrary thresholds on continua of sadness, lethargy, and pessimism. In children and teenagers, a diagnosis of major depressive disorder (MDD) requires a minimum 2-week period of pervasive mood change toward sadness or irritability, and loss of interest or pleasure (American Psychiatric Association, 1994). This needs to be a clear change in functioning, accompanied by impairment in social or other role performance. The symptoms must not be explicable by other influences such as other illnesses, substance abuse, or recent bereavement. Many children and adolescents have some depressed feelings, and they will not be diagnosed as suffering from depressive disorders unless these feelings become entrenched and relatively disabling. Diagnosis of major depression also requires the presence of some biological characteristics, such as loss of appetite, insomnia, reduced energy, or libido, in adolescents. Children and adolescents may show more anxiety and anger, fewer vegetative symptoms, and less verbalization of hopelessness than adults; however, the broad picture is now thought to be similar across the life span (American Academy of Child and Adolescent Psychiatry, 1998a).

The other depressive syndrome to be considered here is dysthymic disorder (DD). This is by definition a chronic condition, marked by depressed and/or irritable mood, which must be present on most days, for most of the day, for at least a year. In addition, at least two other symptoms of MDD must be present (American Psychiatric Association, 1994).

Bipolar mood disorders, which include depressive episodes, are included in Chapter 8, on psychotic disorders.

PREVALENCE

Overall figures from epidemiological studies of children and adolescents spanning 4–20 years of age (earlier studies reviewed by Costello, 1989b; e.g., Kashani & Orvaschel, 1990) suggest that depression and dysthymia both have point prevalence rates of about 2% among children and 2–5% for adolescents (see Birmaher et al., 1996a; Lewinsohn & Clarke, 1999[ib]). Findings in the Oregon Adolescent Depression Project show that the cumulative prevalence of MDD up to age 18 is 28%, 35% for girls and 19% for boys (Lewinsohn, Hops, Roberts, Seeley, & Andrews, 1993; Lewinsohn, Rohde, Klein, & Seeley, 1999). Depressive disorders are equally frequent in boys and girls until adolescence, after which (from age 14) there is a predominance of girls (approximately 2:1—see Lewinsohn, Clarke, & Rohde, 1994[ib]; Weissman, Warner, Wickramaratne, Moreau, & Olfson, 1997). This preponderance of depression among girls mirrors the gender gap seen among adults (see Cyranowski, Frank, Young, & Shear, 2000, for an ingenious suggested explanation). A recent study by Rao, Hammen, and Daley (1999) showed a 37% rate of first-time MDD among late-adolescent girls followed for 5 years into young adulthood. Overall, the rate of MDD—in this sample of 149 high school graduates who could be followed through the 5 years—was 47%; almost half of the group experienced a major depressive episode in the transition to adulthood. There is evidence from both clinic studies and population surveys that mild–moderate depressive disorder is both becoming more common and beginning earlier (e.g., Birmaher et al., 1996a; Kovacs & Gatsonis, 1989).

A longitudinal study of 776 adolescents (Cohen et al., 1991) indicates that young people diagnosed as suffering from major depression on DSM-III-R were not significantly more likely to be referred to a mental health professional than were children in the rest of the population, in the 2½-year follow-up period after diagnosis. This was in marked contrast to children with disruptive disorders, who were four to five times more likely than other children to be referred. The study also found that parents were not seeking alternative advice (e.g., from professionals such as teachers or informally from friends or relatives) about children with depressive disorders, whereas additional help was sought when children were disruptive. However, the community study by Lewinsohn, Rohde, and Seeley (1998) suggested that 61% of adolescents meeting criteria for MDD received some treatment, though this was usually brief and unsystematic (and not reflective of research evidence on efficacy).

Two recent studies (Wu et al., 1999; Oldehinkel, Wittchen, & Schuster, 1999) bear on this issue, although it remains unclear. Wu et al. used data from the National Institute of Mental Health Methods for the Epidemiology of Child and Adolescent Mental Health Disorders (MECA) study. In this report, the mental health service use of 1,285 children and young people (9–17 years) in the community was examined, focusing on a comparison between depressive disorders and disruptive disorders. Forty-four children in the sample were found to have depressive disorders without comorbid disruptive disorders. It was found that although children with depressive disorders perceived a need for help, they were significantly less likely to have received mental health service treatment, over their lifetimes, than were those with disruptive problems (38.6% versus 56.3%, respectively). However, when service use over the past year only was examined, depressive disorders and disruptive disorders were associated with similar rates of mental health service use (31.8% and 29.2%, respectively). These data may show that a current disruptive disorder is more likely to be associated with a history of emotional or behavioral problems leading to mental health service referral. The second paper, from the Max Planck Institute of Psychiatry (Oldehinkel et al., 1999), examined the prevalence, incidence, and outcome in a community adolescent sample ($n = 1,228$). Prevalence figures were similar to those reported previously. Over a 20-month follow-up, only about 10% of those showing a depressive disorder (3/4 moderate–severe) received any professional advice.

CLINICAL PRESENTATION

Clinical depression in children and adolescents goes well beyond ordinary and appropriate sadness. The contrast between the two parallels the contrast between adult depressive illness and sad or pessimistic moods that almost everyone experiences. Depression is rather rare in preadolescents, but when it occurs it tends to be expressed more through anxiety, frustration, or somatic complaints than is usual in adolescents or adults (e.g., Birmaher et al., 1996a; Kovacs, 1996). Depressed adolescents tend to show more biological symptoms and suicidal ideation and behavior than do younger children, and their functioning is likely to be more impaired. Thus, in many ways, they are more like adults with depressive episodes, but, in contrast, they are more likely than adults to show behavior problems. In a recent study of 74 male and female adolescents diagnosed with MDD, 85% of whom were being treated as inpatients, the great majority reported significant aggressive behavior, often unknown to their parents (Knox, King, Hanna, Logan, & Ghaziuddin, 2000). There was no difference according to gender. However, this finding needs to be understood in the context that an important criterion for inpatient admission might be aggressive or antisocial behavior.

DD again presents a fairly similar picture in children and adolescents as in adults: long-term low mood or irritability. It therefore tends to be a milder but longer-lasting disorder, which can probably be more disabling and destructive to social and academic functioning in the long-term (Kovacs, 1997; Kovacs, Akiskal, Gatsonis, & Parrone, 1994). This may be because it becomes a more entrenched maladaptive style and therefore appears to be part of the personality rather than a discrete episode of illness.

Comorbidity

For children and adolescents with a diagnosis of major depression, it has been estimated that 40–70% have a second psychiatric disorder, and at least 20% have three or more disorders (see Birmaher et al., 1996a). The most common comorbid disorders are dysthymia and anxiety disorders, followed by disruptive disorders, and the depressive disorder most often develops after the other disorders are established (e.g., Biederman, Faraone, & Lelon, 1995; Goodyer, Herbert, Secher, & Pearson, 1997; Lewinsohn, Zinbarg, Seeley, Lewinsohn, & Sack, 1997). However, conduct disorders can develop as a complication of a preexisting depressive disorder, sometimes persisting after the mood disturbance has lifted (Kovacs, 1996; Kovacs, Paulauskas, Gatsonis, & Richards, 1988). The association between a diagnosis of personality disorder (PD) and adolescent depression should be viewed with caution. Although some studies have reported that most depressed adolescents also show diagnosable PDs, these symptoms may no longer meet criteria for PD once the depression has remitted (Lewinsohn et al., 1997; Marton et al., 1989). The majority of children or adolescents diagnosed with DD also have other diagnosable disorders: 70% develop a major depression, 50% have other disorders such as anxiety, conduct, and elimination disorders, and about 15% have two or more comorbid disorders (Ferro, Carlson, Grayson, & Klein, 1994; Kovacs et al., 1994).

Natural History

The American Academy of Child and Adolescent Psychiatry (1998a) and Kovacs (e.g., Kovacs & Devlin, 1998) have expertly summarized the information available on the natural history of depressive disorders. Kazdin (1990a) characterized the picture shown by studies as demonstrating high rates of recovery from episodes, but with high rates of relapse, that is, it is a similar picture to the situation in adults (e.g., Coryell et al., 1989). This is illustrated in many studies included later in this chapter (Birmaher et al., 2000).

Kovacs and Gatsonis (1989) followed up a sample of more than 100 cases of children ages 8–13 with depressive disorders (DSM-III criteria) for a number of years. They found that although nearly all episodes had resolved within 3–4 years (median time to recovery 9.5 months), the majority had further episodes of major depression over the following 5 years. There was also a 20–30% risk of secondary anxiety, conduct, or bipolar disorder during these years. A similar pattern has been reported more recently for the 14- to 18-year-age group (Lewinsohn et al., 1994[ib]; Sanford et al., 1995). There is a great deal of accumulated evidence (see Birmaher et al., 1996a) to show that comorbid diagnoses worsen the prognosis for depressive episodes. Prospective studies have shown that even after recovery from a depressive episode, there tends to be impairment of adaptation, in terms of quality of relationships, self-esteem, and physical health (e.g., Rao et al., 1995; Rohde, Lewinsohn, & Seeley, 1994).

The median duration of an episode of major depression among children or adolescents referred for treatment is 7–9 months; among those in the community it is somewhat shorter (perhaps 2 months as a median, and 6 months' mean duration; see the useful review by Kovacs, 1997). About 90% of episodes will have remitted within 2 years. However, it is very important to note that this disorder tends to relapse after remission or successful short-term treatment: About 50% of sufferers will have a further episode within 2 years, and about 70% will have relapsed within 5 years (Kovacs, 1996; Rohde et al., 1994). Childhood DD has a mean duration of 3–4 years in both clinical and community samples (e.g., Kovacs et al., 1994), and this is further protracted if there is a comorbid disruptive disorder (Kovacs, Obrosky, Gatsonis, & Richards, 1997). Typically, a first episode of MDD occurs 2–3 years after the onset of DD, suggesting that the development of major depression may be prevented in such cases.

The recent large-scale study from the Max Planck Institute (Oldehinkel et al., 1999) demonstrated unexpectedly poor outcome of depressive disorders among this community adolescent sample ($n = 1,228$). Full remission over 20 months was seen in only 43% of MDD cases, 54% of subthreshold cases, and 33% of dysthymia cases. Higher age and more severe depression at baseline were associated with worse outcomes.

Depressive disorders in childhood and adolescence are linked with significantly greater risk of affective disorders in adulthood (e.g., Klein, Lewinsohn, & Seeley, 1997; Kovacs et al., 1997). The study by Harrington et al. (1994; Harrington, Fudge, Rutter, Pickles, & Hill, 1990, 1991), for instance, showed an association of depression in childhood or adolescence with relative risks of psychiatric treatment, hospitalization, and serious suicide attempts in adulthood three times higher than those found among matched nondepressed child psychiatric patients. There seemed to be a specifically increased rate of affective illness (both depressive and bipolar) rather than psychiatric morbidity in general. A more recent study ($n = 83$; Weissman et al., 1999) showed that prepubertal-onset MDD was associated with raised rates of mental health problems and service use 10–15 years later. Substance abuse, conduct disorder, suicide attempts, and bipolar disorder were more common, long-term service use was higher, and impairment was greater than among controls. The risk of further depressive illness has been found to be greater where there is dysthymia as well as the index episode of major depression ("double depression") (e.g., Klein et al., 1997; Kovacs et al., 1997). Similarly, the level of impairment among youths with dysthymia and major depression is higher (Goodman, Schwab-Stone, Lahey, Shaffer, & Jensen, 2000).

TREATMENT

The treatment of depression in children and adolescents has been reviewed by, among others, Harrington (1993[ib]; Harrington, Whittaker, & Shoebridge, 1998b[ib]), Birmaher, Ryan, Williamson, Brent, and Kaufman (1996b[ib]), the American Academy of Child and Adolescent Psychiatry (1998a), Lewinsohn and Clarke (1999[ib]), and Asarnow, Jaycox, and Tompson (2001[ib]).

Physical Treatments

This field has been recently and authoritatively reviewed by Ambrosini (2000) and by Wagner and Ambrosini (2001[ib]). The latter review has a particularly helpful discussion of the methodological differences and limitations of the pharmacological studies.

Studies of tricyclic antidepressants, with both children and adolescents, fairly consistently show superiority to placebo in open trials (e.g., Ambrosini, Bianchi, Rabinovitch, & Elia, 1993[iii]; Geller, Cooper, Chestnut, Anker, & Schluchter, 1986[iii]), whereas 10 out of 11 controlled, double-blind studies do not show a difference (e.g., Birmaher, Quintana, & Greenhill, 1998[i]; Geller, Cooper, McCombs, Graham, & Wells, 1989[i]; Kye et al., 1996[i]). The one exception (Preskorn, Weller, Hughes, Weller, & Bolte, 1987[i]) found a small superiority of tricyclic antidepressants over placebo on one measure of outcome. These negative results need to be qualified by some methodological considerations explored in more detail by Birmaher et al. (1996b[ib]); these include the relatively mild levels of depression among the children studied, small sample sizes, short periods of medication, and sometimes low dosages applied. Most of these studies probably had insufficient power to detect moderate differences in effect, given the high rate (50–70%) of improvement in children and adolescents given placebo medication. However, a study conducted by Birmaher and his group (1998[i]) that tested this possibility, using only cases of severe and chronic depression, also found no difference between amitryptiline and placebo, due to a very high rate of response in both groups. This study, like others before it, had a small sample ($n = 13$ and $n = 14$ in the two groups, respectively). However, this is not likely to account for the negative findings, because there was not even a trend toward greater improvement in the amitryptiline condition on any measure. The only difference approaching significance was that side effects were somewhat more severe in the active treatment group.

Despite these findings, some clinical observations suggest that some children respond better to tricyclic antidepressants than to alternative medications. One possible reason for the failure to establish efficacy is that trials have included children with mixed comorbidity. A small-scale study by Hughes et al. (1990[ii]) suggested that children with comorbid disruptive disorders showed a poor response, whereas those with comorbid anxiety did well on tricyclic medication. This was a double-blind, placebo-controlled study of 31 children, in which 57% of children with comorbid anxiety improved on medication and 20% on placebo, while of those with comorbid disruptive disorders, only 33% improved on medication and 67% on placebo! Of course the result would need to be replicated with a larger sample, but if confirmed the pattern could help to explain the puzzling and largely negative findings on tricyclic treatment.

A recently reported double-blind randomized controlled trial (RCT), involving school-refusing adolescents with comorbid anxiety and major depressive disorders (Bernstein et al., 2000[i]), was more fully described in the previous chapter (on anxiety disorders). All adolescents were treated with CBT, while one group also received imipramine and the other received placebo medication. Assignment was random and school attendance was the major outcome measure; however, depression was assessed by both self-report and clinician rating. Unfortunately, there was a significant difference in clinician-rated depression at baseline as well as at the end of treatment, with the placebo group being more symptomatic. Thus, although this study demonstrated a role for imipramine in the treatment of adolescent school refusal, it did not support it as a treatment for major depression.

A further important issue affecting tricyclic medication is the danger of serious side effects (see Chapter 3, on anxiety disorders). Some recent reviews offer detailed clinical guidance (Kutcher, 1997[vi]; Mezzacappa et al., 1998[vi]).

Initial findings on the efficacy of selective serotonin reuptake inhibitors (SSRIs) for child and adolescent depression were similarly negative. Although open trials reported high response rates of 70–90% for adolescent depression (e.g., DeVane & Sallee, 1996[ib]; Leonard, March, Rickler, & Allen, 1997[iii]), the results of the first controlled study were disappointing (e.g., a small double-blind, placebo-controlled study reported by Simeon, Dinicola, Ferguson, & Copping, 1990[i], on fluoxetine). However, a much larger double-blind randomized, placebo-controlled trial of fluoxetine in children and adolescents with depression showed encouraging results, with 96 outpatients ages 7–17 years (Emslie et al., 1997[i]). The two main outcome measures were the Clinical Global Impressions (CGI) scale and the Children's Depression Rating Scale—Revised (CDRS-R), which were administered weekly through the 8-week study. Twenty-seven of the children receiving fluoxetine and 16 of those receiving placebo were rated as "much" or "very much" improved according to the CGI. The CDRS-R scores were significantly lower for the fluoxetine group at week 5. Overall, the results suggested that fluoxetine was significantly more effective than placebo, but complete remission was rare. Two-fifths (40%) of the patients who received the active drug did not respond, and of those who did improve, more than two-thirds still reported significant depressive symptoms (i.e. CDRS-R score above 28).

There is a very important multicenter RCT being carried out currently: the Treatment of Adolescents with Depression Study (TADS). It is funded by the National Institute of Mental Health (NIMH) and organized by John March, comparing the efficacy of fluoxetine only, CBT only, the two treatments combined, and placebo only. The group hope to recruit more than 400 adolescents suffering from depression.

Ambrosini and his colleagues (1999[ii]) have recently reported a six-center, open-label trial of the efficacy of sertraline (another SSRI), using an initial 2-week assessment period of single-blind placebo administration. The trial took in 68 patients, of whom only 53 proceeded to the active treatment phase (the other 15 no longer met diagnostic criteria and therefore could presumably be thought of as having shown considerable improvement on placebo medication). Although an intent-to-treat analysis was carried out, only those patients who actually began active medication were included. The proportion of patients showing clinically significant improvement was greatest at 10 weeks, suggesting that this medication takes a considerable time to work, or that spontaneous improvements were occurring (as they had in the baseline phase) in addition to any due to medication. Estimates of improvement varied according to the measures used, but approximately three-quarters of patients who had begun on active medication and who continued until week 10 showed significant improvement by that time. However, as only 33 out of 68 patients were still in the trial by that stage, it is clear that the authors' conclusion that the medication was effective needs to be replicated in a placebo-controlled trial, with an intent-to-treat analysis, including all assigned patients.

A recent important international RCT examined the efficacy of paroxetine versus placebo for 286 adolescents (Milin, Simeon, & Spenst, 1999[i]). In this study, paroxetine was not found to be superior to placebo for adolescents up to 16 years of age (in fact, more responded to placebo in the younger age group), but 17- to 18-year-olds did respond more strongly to the active drug (the interaction with age was significant at the .002 level).

Hopes continue to be high for the efficacy of SSRIs for children and adolescents because of the doubtful effectiveness and the potential dangerousness of tricyclic antidepressants. So far, the evidence appears to be cautiously promising for the safety of SSRIs (e.g., Dittmann, Czekalla, Hundemer, & Linden, 2000[iii]).

Psychosocial Treatments

Cognitive-Behavioral Intervention

Programs have been devised for children and adolescents, initially using techniques adapted from cognitive therapy for depressed adults (see Brent et al., 1997[i]; Kendall, 1993[vi]; Lewinsohn, Clarke, Rohde, Hops, & Seeley, 1996a[i]). In their helpful discussion of factors affecting choice and effectiveness of particular therapies, Lewinsohn and Clarke (1999[ib]) indicate that developmental factors need to be taken into account in designing protocols and that more research is required to clarify how long treatments should be, how much structure is optimal, and whether individual treatment protocols can be successfully adapted for groups.

Reynolds and Stark (Reynolds & Coats, 1986[i]; Stark, 1990) described a package of procedures drawing on social learning theory and cognitive therapy. The program is administered to a group and lasts for 21 sessions. Stark, Reynolds, and Kaslow (1987[i]) compared the effectiveness of elements of this package, with 29 9- to 12-year-olds recruited from schools, who scored at least 16 on the Children's Depression Inventory (CDI) (a score of 13 or more is considered indicative of significant depression). One group of children received self-control therapy (modeled on the cognitive therapy approach with adults; Rehm, Kaslow, Rabin, & Willard, 1984); another group received behavioral problem-solving therapy, which focused on fostering skills for coping with difficult situations and increasing the frequency of pleasant or rewarding events in the children's lives (Stark, 1990). Children were treated in groups of five for 12 sessions. A third group of children were placed on a waiting list for 5 weeks, then offered the self-control therapy if they wished.

The results of this study are generally taken to show that children in both treatment groups showed significantly reduced depressive symptoms in comparison with those in the control group, and that these gains were maintained over an 8-week follow-up (see Harrington, 1993[ib]; Jensen et al., 1996[ib]; Kazdin, 1994[ib]). This was the case to the extent that, on individual *t*-tests, several comparisons of mean differences (for each measure, treatment condition, and pair of assessment points) were significant and favoured the two treatments over the waiting-list group. However, with such a large number of comparisons of related measures and no reported Bonferroni adjustments, the danger of Type I errors is considerable.

The other major analysis reported in this study, an analysis of covariance comparing scores between groups, controlling for pretreatment scores, is more robust and reliable. In this multivariate analysis, scores on only one measure (the CDI) confirmed the reported result to a significant degree. This study had a small sample size (9–10 per group at the outset, falling to 5 or 6 in the treatment groups at follow-up) and cannot be seen as providing strong evidence of the effectiveness of these forms of therapy.

Many early investigations used CBT for specially recruited children with mild symptoms of depression, not for clinically referred children or adolescents (e.g., Marcotte & Baron, 1993[i]; Liddle & Spence, 1990[i]; King & Kirschenbaum, 1990[i]; Jaycox, Reivich, Gillham, & Seligman, 1994[i]). They have produced mixed results on the efficacy of CBT approaches (see review by Asarnow, Jaycox, & Tompson, 2001[ib]). A well-designed example of a study using cutoffs on symptom rating scales, rather than diagnostic criteria, has been reported by Weisz, Thurber, Sweeney, Proffitt, and LeGagnoux (1997b[i]). In this study, 48 elementary school-children (3rd–6th grade) were selected by using rating-scale cutoffs comparable to clinical levels, and 16 of the children were treated using a brief (eight-session) CBT package aimed at enhancing "primary and secondary control." Thirty-two control children were untreated. There was a significantly greater improvement in depressive symptoms at both posttest and 9-month follow-up among the treated children. (However, only 60% of the children were available for follow-up; it is not clear whether the attrition was greater among treated or control children, but if evenly spread, given the small size of the treated group this would have meant 9–10 treated children followed up. Thus, the evidence of maintenance of gains needs to be treated with caution).

Lewinsohn, Clarke, Hops, and Andrews (1990[i]) took a step toward evaluating treatment for clinical symptoms. They evaluated a course of 14 2-hour group sessions for 59 adolescents who (although not referred) met DSM-III criteria or Research Diagnostic Criteria (RDC) for major, minor, or intermittent depressive disorder. The treatment was a modification of the Coping with Depression course designed for adults (Lewinsohn, Antonuccio, Steinmetz-Breckenridge, & Teri, 1984). One group of 19 received just the adolescents' group course; for a second group of 21, there was an adolescents' group course and a simultaneous group for parents. A third group of 19 were placed on a waiting list and treated later. Adolescents in both treated groups improved significantly more than those on the waiting list; 95% in the waiting-list group were still diagnosable at termination, in comparison with 57% and 52% in the adolescents-only group and adolescents-and-parents groups, respectively. The gains were generally maintained over a 2-year follow-up.

This careful study used clinically significant levels of depression, but caution is appropriate. Only half of the adolescents met DSM-III criteria for major depression, and most of the remainder (44% of the total group) met RDC criteria for intermittent depression; that is, they might well have improved spontaneously during the study. This relates to another (common) difficulty: Presumably for ethical reasons, the waiting-list group were treated after 7 weeks, so the untreated course cannot be compared with treated outcome, which was followed up for 2 years. Furthermore, although improvement was much greater in the treated groups, more than half of the treated individuals still met diagnostic criteria at posttreatment. Finally, although adolescent-report measures improved in both treatment conditions, parent-report measures improved (beyond the improvements found in the waiting-list group) only in the second condition, when the parents were also given intensive advice and support, raising the question of whether the reported improvements reflected attention as well as symptom change. Adolescents reported improvement when they were treated, parents reported improvement in adolescents when the parents were also helped, but not otherwise.

A further trial of this therapy introduced two modifications to the design of the first study and included 96 depressed adolescents (Lewinsohn, Clarke, & Rohde, 1994; Lewinsohn et al., 1996a). First, the treatment protocol was improved, particularly by making social skills training more integrated with the other cognitive and behavioral elements. Second, there were three alternative follow-up conditions, one involving booster sessions and follow-up assessments, and the other two involving either four monthly or annual follow-up assessments only, with no booster treatment. The two active treatment conditions (adolescent only and adolescent + parent intervention) were found to be comparably superior to the waiting-list control (ES = .39; this modest figure seems to have reflected the high recovery rate, 48%, in the control group, in comparison with 67% in the treated groups). Unexpectedly, the different follow-up arrangements did not have differential outcomes in terms of preventing relapse, possibly because subjects received other treatments during the follow-up phase. Adolescents with less severe symptoms and better initial adaptation tended to benefit more from the treatment. At the 2-year follow-up point, 97.5% of the adolescents who had received one of the active treatments no longer met criteria for a depressive condition.

There were some difficulties with these studies; in particular, they used nonreferred children, and they used group treatments, which are not always practicable in a clinical setting (Harrington, 1993[ib]). Nevertheless, they supported the possible usefulness of these forms of treatment in child and adolescent psychiatry.

A recent and important series of studies by Brent et al. (1997[i]) has compared the usefulness of CBT, systemic–behavioral family therapy, and nondirective support for 107 adolescents, two-thirds of whom were clinically referred (the remainder recruited by advertisement). CBT achieved the greatest improvement overall (Brent et al., 1998[i]), especially for adolescents with comorbid anxiety. This superiority was not eliminated when there were multiple adverse predictors. However, where the mother was herself clinically depressed, the outcome of treatment of the adolescent was worse, eliminating the general superiority of the CBT condition over the others. Brent et al. (1998[i]) therefore recommended that maternal depression should be evaluated and, if present, actively treated alongside adolescent depression. Family discord predicted slower recovery and higher chance of relapse. An analysis of types of response (Renaud et al., 1998[i]) showed that the rapid responders tended to have the best outcome during treatment and at follow-up. They also found that supportive therapy included the largest proportion of both rapid responders and nonresponders, and therefore suggested that it could be worthwhile to institute supportive therapy before more specialized treatments, in clinical settings.

Brent et al. (1998[i]) did not find specificity at the level of process mechanisms: CBT altered depressive cognitions more, but (at an individual level) this was not associated with better outcome. (The finding that improvement in CBT is not accounted for by a reduction in depressive cognitions is consistent with the results reported by Lewinsohn et al. (1990[i]).) There were interesting, strong differences between patients who had been referred and those recruited through advertisement. Initial severity did not differ, but referred youths tended to show more hopelessness. An important aspect of the Brent study is that it is one of very few to include a family intervention, although this was intended only as a control group.

A 2-year follow-up of the Brent study has been reported (Birmaher et al., 2000[i]; Brent et al., 1999[i]). The short-term superiority of CBT had not been maintained, in that subjects in all three conditions showed similar recovery and relapse rates (about one-third relapsed during the 2 years, and one-fifth showed persistent MDD throughout the 2 years). As with short-term outcome, the relapse rate was higher among the adolescents referred to clinics as opposed to the specially recruited—a difference not accounted for by greater initial symptom severity, family history, or duration. Further service use was similar across the three treatment groups, with more than half of all the adolescents in the trial entering further treatment, an average of 7 months after the trial started.

Wood, Harrington, and Moore (1996[i]) have reported a controlled trial of brief (five to eight sessions) individual CBT for children and adolescents (9–17 years) diagnosed with depressive disorder. The children were outpatient referrals with mild–moderate levels of clinical depression. CBT was compared with relaxation training, and there were 24 subjects per group. CBT produced significantly superior results at posttreatment on most of the outcome measures (e.g., an ES of 0.73 on the Mood and Feelings Questionnaire). However, these differences were mostly eliminated or nonsignificant at 6-month follow-up. Some of the CBT group had relapsed, and the relaxation group had generally continued to improve (however, the latter group had had more treatment during the follow-up period). It should also be noted that the significant difference was not found on parent-report measures, only on child-report measures. This detracts little from the value of the findings, however, because parent-reports are notoriously unreliable as a guide to depression (e.g., Harrington, 1993[ib]). The authors concluded appropriately that this short-term treatment has a short-term, specific benefit, not explicable in terms of greater attention. However, that specificity is lost during follow-up, perhaps because of the brevity of the two treatments, or because the relaxation group more often obtained other treatments during the follow-up phase (in itself an important outcome in favour of CBT). A further study by the same group (Kroll, Harrington, Jayson, Fraser, & Gowers, 1996[iii]) showed that monthly booster sessions of CBT greatly reduced the relapse rate, as compared with historical controls (20% relapse versus 50%, respectively).

Jayson, Wood, Kroll, Fraser, and Harrington (1998[iii]) studied the combined sample of adolescents given CBT in the Wood and Kroll studies, to look for predictors of good outcome. They found that younger patients and those less severely impaired had a better response. (Of course, it may be that these patients would have been more likely to improve with an alternative treatment or without treatment, so one cannot be sure from this study whether the result is specific to CBT.)

Vostanis, Feehan, Grattan, and Bickerton (1996a[i]) offered two to nine (an average of six) sessions of CBT, similar to that offered in the Wood et al. study, to children and adolescents aged 8–17 (n across groups = 56). The children had been referred for outpatient treatment. Of the children in the CBT group, 87% improved, but so did 75% of the children in the nonfocused intervention control condition. As a majority of the sample had been diagnosed with minor depression, it may well be that there would have been a very high recovery rate with no intervention, and thus the treatment was not given an adequate test. However, it may also be that the "nonfocused intervention" was helpful to many children: The authors suggest that, across conditions, "non-specific psychotherapeutic elements such as empathy, sympathetic listening, reassurance, reinforcement and indirect ways of achieving self-understanding and problem-solving may be involved in the recovery" (Vostanis, Feehan, Grattan, & Bickerton, 1996b[i], p. 199).

A recently reported study by Clarke, Rohde, Lewinsohn, Hops, and Seely (1999[i]) from the Lewinsohn research group extends the findings on booster treatment. The study recruited 123 adolescents and randomly assigned them to either group CBT, group CBT plus a parent group, or a waiting-list control. Subjects who received CBT were then further randomly assigned either to receive booster sessions or to receive only follow-up assessments. They replicated the findings of the earlier trial (Lewinsohn et al., 1990[i]) on posttreatment and follow-up improvements, although the size of the difference between treatment and control groups was narrowed because of higher improvement rates in the waiting-list group. The addition of parent involvement for adolescents did not provide extra benefit. Booster sessions did provide additional benefit, but this was largely through providing a longer treatment with faster recovery during follow-up among those who had not responded in the treatment phase.

Reinecke et al. (Reinecke, Ryan, & DuBois, 1998[ib]) carried out a meta-analysis of these studies of CBT for adolescent depression and found a robust ES of 1.02 at termination and .61 at follow-up. Harrington et al. (Harrington, Whittaker, Shoebridge, & Campbell, 1998b[ib]) have also carried out a very useful systematic review of all methodologically sound CBT outcome studies (n = 6) for childhood depressive disorder. Their pooled odds ratio was 3.2, with children receiving CBT significantly more likely to be in remission by the end of treatment. This odds ratio fell to 2.2 if a (very conservative) intent-to-treat analysis was applied (in which all dropouts from the control groups were counted as having remitted, and all those from the CBT groups as not having remitted).

Social Skills Training

Matson (1989[vi]) described the use of a social skills training program using individualized vignettes of difficult situations, and evaluated this program in two case reports of individual treatment of depressed children. Both improved substantially, but as there was no comparison condition and there were other treatment components, this report gave only weak support to social skills training.

Subsequently, Fine et al. (1991[i]) compared two group therapies for adolescents who met DSM-III-R criteria for either major depression or dysthymia. The patients were referred for outpatient treatment and then assigned to a 12-week therapy group using either "therapeutic support" (27 patients) or formal social skills training (20 patients). Forty-one percent of the patients were receiving other treatment: psychotherapy, medication, or both.

At posttreatment, adolescents in the therapeutic support group were significantly less likely than those given social skills training to be diagnosed as depressed and had significantly lower scores on the CDI self-report measure of depression. These group differences were no longer significant at follow-up (this appeared to be a result of diminishing sample size as much as a change in relative rates of depression). As the authors point out, in the absence of an untreated control group, it is not possible to assert that the two treated groups improved on the spontaneous remission rate; 68% of adolescents in the study were no longer diagnosable at 9-month follow-up, and in Kovacs and Gatsonis's (1989) study the median time to recovery was 9.5 months. This does suggest a benefit from therapy, but it is difficult to be sure how comparable the samples were. The high proportion of adolescents receiving other treatments also poses problems of interpretation.

Although this study was regarded by others as supporting the use of social skills training for depressed adolescents, the main finding was, in fact, the unexpected superiority of the therapeutic support group over the "active" treatment. Fine et al. (1991[i]) suggested, on the basis of process measures, that adolescents in the social skills training group were less engaged and more avoidant. They further suggested that social skills training may be too demanding for clinically depressed adolescents, but that they may be able to use some of the skills learned as they become less depressed (between posttreatment and follow-up). They suggested that a fruitful approach might be to offer therapeutic support that introduces social skills training at a later stage.

Interpersonal Psychotherapy

Interpersonal psychotherapy (IPT) is a brief treatment approach developed for adult patients (Klerman, Weissman, Rounsaville, & Chevron, 1984[vi]), which focuses on a specified range of interpersonal problems that may underlie the individual's depressed state. It has been tested in several clinical trials, notably the NIMH collaborative study of the treatment of depression (Elkin et al., 1989[i]). The approach has been adapted for adolescents (IPT-A; Moreau, Mufson, Weissman, & Klerman, 1991[iii]), and Moreau and colleagues first conducted a small, open trial using this modified manualized approach, with promising results (Mufson et al., 1994[iii]). More recently, a clinical RCT has been reported (Mufson, Weissman, Moreau, & Garfinkel, 1999[i]). This included 48 referred adolescents with MDD, of whom 32 completed the protocol. The majority of dropouts came from the control condition, which was "clinical monitoring," effectively, a waiting list. An intent-to-treat analysis showed that 75% of patients treated with IPT-A recovered, as judged by Hamilton Rating Scale scores, in comparison with 46% of those in the control group.

An interesting recent study of 71 Puerto Rican adolescents meeting criteria for MDD showed that both IPT and CBT were effective in reducing depressive symptoms (CDI and Child Behavior Checklist [CBCL]), but IPT was more effective than CBT in improving self-esteem (Piers-Harris Children's Self-Concept Scale) and social adaptation (Social Adjustment Scale for Children and Adolescents) (Rosselló & Bernal, 1999[i]). This study was the first to attempt to compare IPT and CBT; it needs to be replicated as soon as possible within other cultural groups, inasmuch as this study manualized the treatments to be specifically appropriate to Puerto Rican society.

Santor and Kusumakar (2001[ii]) have reported an important controlled study comparing 12 weeks of IPT with sertraline in the treatment of 49 moderately to severely impaired adolescents with MDD. The 25 subjects with IPT were compared with 24 who had previously been treated using sertraline, in an open trial. Thus, allocation was not randomized, but historical controls were matched for patient characteristics. The outcomes were compared on the Beck Depression Inventory, the Children's Global Assessment Scale (CGAS), and indication of clinical recovery. Both treatments led to significant improvement, but IPT was superior across all three measures. A notable feature of this study was that the IPT therapists had little or no previous experience with IPT, suggesting that the treatment protocol is relatively easy to transport from the development "laboratory" into clinical settings.

Family Therapy

Although there is ample evidence of the importance of the family context and parental psychological problems in relation to child and adolescent depression (see Asarnow, Jaycox, & Tompson, 2001[ib]), there have been very few studies bearing on the effectiveness of family therapy for depression. The conclusion of the Asarnow review is that although psychoeducation with families is helpful as an adjunct to CBT, extended family intervention has not yet been properly assessed. There have been very few studies on the effectiveness of family therapy for depression. In the Brent et al. study (1997[i]) described earlier, for example, systemic–behavioral family therapy was used as a control condition. It seemed that this form of family therapy could be beneficial, especially in cases where the mother was perceived to be controlling. In general, evaluation of family therapy has probably been hampered by the lack of a manualized version of the approach. However, Asarnow and colleagues (2001[ib]) report that three research groups are currently evaluating family therapy models, and they persuasively argue that the family component may be particularly important for preadolescent depressed children.

Psychodynamic Psychotherapy and Psychoanalysis

There is so far little research evidence on the effectiveness of psychodynamic therapy for depressive disorders in children. A chart review study of 763 patients who had been in intensive psychoanalytic therapy (Target & Fonagy, 1994b[iv]) included 65 children and adolescents with dysthymia and/or major depression, who had been treated for an average of 2 years. By the end of therapy, 82% of the subjects no longer had these symptoms, and in 75% of cases their global adaptation score (CGAS; see Shaffer et al., 1983) showed a reliable improvement. As major depression has been shown to run an episodic course, the absence of regular reassessment during and after treatment means that this study does not demonstrate the effectiveness of psychodynamic treatment for depression. However, one finding was that children and adolescents with depressive disorders appeared to benefit more from intensive (four to five sessions per week) than from nonintensive (one to 2 sessions per week) therapy, after controlling for length of treatment and level of impairment at referral. This is of some interest, given that the depressed subjects were mostly adolescents, who generally did not gain additional benefit from frequent sessions (Target & Fonagy, 1994a[iv]).

SUMMARY

Major depression and dysthymia both have point prevalence rates of about 2% among children and 2–5% for adolescents. Depression is equally common in girls and boys up to adolescence, but thereafter girls outnumber boys by two to one. The majority of clinically depressed children have other comorbid disorders, mostly anxiety and disruptive disorders. There is a high rate of recovery from episodes of depression (mean length, 9 months), but a high rate of relapse (50% within 2 years). Childhood or adolescent depression is associated with raised rates of depression and other psychopathology in adult life.

The approach to the treatment of depression in children has generally been to adapt approaches used with adult patients, particularly medication and CBT. Studies of the efficacy of medication have not yet supported the efficacy of tricyclic antidepressants, which also involve rare but serious risks; SSRIs show greater promise and, so far, fewer side effects. CBT appears to be effective, whether provided individually or in a group. However, it has mainly been tested with mildly–moderately impaired adolescents, rather than with either severe cases or (preadolescent) children. Family factors can reduce treatment response. CBT is not more effective in cases where there are greater cognitive distortions, and its benefits are apparently not explained by a reduction in such cognitions. Providing longer courses of CBT (or booster sessions) in cases of nonresponse to a standard length of treatment seems to hasten recovery. CBT seems to be more effective than tricyclic medication. However, it is less likely to be effective in more severe cases. Recent studies have confirmed that referred depressed adolescents are more difficult than recruited subjects to treat successfully, even when severity is comparable. As studies of the effectiveness of tricyclic medication for childhood depression have generally involved more severely impaired cases than have the studies of CBT, the apparent superiority of CBT may be partly accounted for by the selection of milder cases.

IPT, adapted for adolescents (IPT-A), appears promising for treatment of adolescent depression. Family therapy, or parent work in parallel with individual treatment for the child, has been included as a condition in four RCTs. Neither approach has been convincingly shown to be more effective than general support, or routine care, but family therapy in particular needs to be manualized. Social skills training and individual child psychotherapy have not yet been shown to be effective treatments.

As in outcome studies for many other disorders, outcome of the treatment of depression has generally been defined in terms of symptoms and diagnostic status, but other impairments, such as deficient social adaptation and academic performance, are also central.

IMPLICATIONS

The high rate of untreated depressive disorders, particularly in adolescence, and their high social and personal costs extending into adulthood suggest that more should be done to detect and offer help to young people with this disorder. Low-grade, chronic depressed mood (dysthymia), which is associated with episodes of major depression and with worse long-term outcome, should not be regarded as a minor problem.

As there is a high rate of remission among children in inactive control conditions, it may be wise to offer brief supportive therapy as the first-line treatment, followed by CBT or medication only if the child fails to improve. Psychosocial therapies, including both CBT and IPT-A, need to be made far more available through affordable, local trainings, so that validated treatments can be provided. At the same time, validation urgently needs to be extended (for a range of psychosocial therapies) to assessment of severe cases and younger depressed children.

Given the episodic nature of this condition and the possibility of increasing benefit over time with some forms of treatment, it is important to continue follow-up assessments for at least 2 years. The large difference in outcome between clinically referred depressed adolescents and those recruited through advertisement, not attributable to greater severity, indicates that findings on efficacy in nonreferred samples cannot confidently be extrapolated to clinical groups.

Research so far has shown a variety of treatment packages to be effective; further research will need to disentangle the elements of these packages, to identify elements that are most helpful in particular clinical situations, and to compare active treatments with each other rather than with inactive conditions such as a waiting-list control. As the benefits of CBT are apparently not attributable to a reduction in negative cognitions, the mechanisms of effectiveness need to be explored. Psychodynamic and family therapies need to be manualized as a step toward systematic evaluation of these widely used approaches. Outcome measures should cover more domains than symptomatology and diagnosis: A treatment may be more effective in the long run if it has a beneficial impact across other domains of functioning, even if the effect on symptoms is no greater. Family context is important in the development of psychopathology, and in supporting or thwarting treatment efforts.

The fact that 40–50% of the treated subjects, across trials of both medication and psychosocial interventions, generally do not respond and remain depressed clearly shows that we need to continue to develop more effective models of treatment, and that meanwhile a range of alternative approaches needs to be retained.

5

Disturbance of Conduct

PETER FONAGY
ARABELLA KURTZ

Disruptive behavior disorders are characterized by high rates of noncompliant, hostile, and defiant behaviors, often including aggressiveness and hyperactivity. DSM-IV (American Psychiatric Association, 1994) categorizes these behaviors under three broad headings: attention-deficit/hyperactivity disorders (ADHD, described in Chapter 6), oppositional defiant disorder (ODD), and conduct disorder (CD). Disturbance of conduct covers a wide range of behaviors manifesting somewhat differently at different ages in the same child across settings. A wide variety of treatment techniques have emerged in response to the diversity and prevalence of these problems. There have been a number of relatively recent summaries of these approaches (see, for example, Brestan & Eyberg, 1998[ib]; Kazdin, 1995b[vi]; Rutter, Giller, & Hagell, 1998[ib]). We will examine psychosocial interventions for child (3–10 years) and adolescent (10–17 years) conduct problems separately. Pharmacological treatments will be reviewed across the age span in terms of the agents used.

DEFINITION

Perhaps more than other problems of children and adolescents, disturbances of conduct are in the eye of the beholder. The "acting out" behaviors of these young people range from the irritating (yelling, whining, temper tantrums) to the frightening and terrorizing (physical destructiveness, interpersonal aggression, even murder). The literature on antisocial behavior is difficult to summarize because of conflicting definitions of the problem, often linked to the backgrounds of the scientists reporting the investigations. However, these heterogeneous behaviors appear to be elements of a complex syndrome. Accumulating epidemiological evidence suggests that the young child's annoying oppositional behaviors—for example, noncompliance and argumentativeness—are developmental precursors of more serious forms of antisocial behavior in adolescence.

CD and ODD are defined in DSM-IV. ODD must include a repetitive pattern of defiance and disobedience and a negative and hostile attitude toward authority figures of at least 6 months' duration. To meet the criteria, four of the following behaviors must be present: loss of temper, arguments with adults, defiance of or noncompliance with adult rules and requests, being a deliberate source of annoyance, blaming others for one's own mistakes, being touchy and easily annoyed by others, frequent anger and resentment, and spite or vindictiveness. These behaviors must be common and lead to impairments of academic and social functioning.

Although ODD and CD overlap in definition, CD, unlike ODD, entails the violations of the basic rights of others or of age-appropriate societal norms or rules. Three of the following 15 behaviors, categorized under four headings, must be present over the previous year to meet the criteria, with one present in the last 6 months: aggressiveness to people and animals (bullying, fighting, using a weapon, physical cruelty to people, physical cruelty to animals, stealing with confrontation of the victim, forced sexual activity); property destruction (fire setting, other destruction of property); deceptiveness or theft (breaking and entering, lying for personal gain, stealing without confronting the victim) and serious rule violations (staying out at night or being truant before age 13, and running away from home).

DSM-IV now distinguishes two subtypes of CD on the basis of age at onset. In *childhood-onset type*, at least one of the 15 behaviors must appear before the age of 10. In *adolescent-onset type*, none appear before age 10. Field trials have shown these definitions to be robust (Lahey et al., 1994), with evidence for the validity of childhood- versus adolescent-onset types (Waldman & Lahey, 1994). Comorbidity with ADHD, male gender, and high level of aggressivity appear to accompany CD of the childhood-onset type. Aggression rarely accompanies conduct disorder when the onset is later than 10 years; at this age the gender balance shifts somewhat toward girls, and fewer have family histories of antisocial behavior (Lahey et al., 1998). Some authors (e.g., Moffitt, 1993[vi]) have proposed a developmental taxonomy to distinguish the two subcategories of CD, viewing neuropsychological deficits as the primary basis of antisocial behavior emerging during childhood, with imitation of peer behavior seen as the principal cause of adolescent-onset antisocial behavior. However, others (e.g., Lahey, Waldman, & McBurnett, 1999b) propose that the strength of each of the multiple causes of antisocial behavior varies along a continuum of age of onset.

Statistical attempts to subtype disturbance of conduct tend to produce two bipolar dimensions distinguishing four groups. The first dimension distinguishes *covert* from *overt* problems (Loeber & Schmaling, 1985a), and the second distinguishes *nondestructive* from *destructive* behaviors (Frick et al., 1993). Destructive–overt problems are usually aggressive in nature (e.g., assault, cruelty, blaming others). Destructive–covert acts are, by and large, property violations (stealing, vandalism, fire setting). Overt, nondestructive acts reflect an oppositional pattern (anger, stubbornness, touchiness, defiance). Covert nondestructiveness is more serious, reflecting the status-violation aspect of conduct disorder (running away, truancy, substance misuse). It has been suggested that overt and covert conduct problems may represent distinct pathways to CD and delinquency (Loeber, Russo, Stouthamer-Loeber, & Lahey, 1994). Relatively more is known about overt than about covert disturbance of conduct. Stealing represents a considerable risk for adolescent delinquency, particularly when combined with social aggression (Loeber & Schmaling, 1985b). Lying is highly correlated with stealing, but appears earlier and the association becomes stronger with age (Stouthamer-Loeber & Loeber, 1986). Lying also correlates with some overt disturbance of conduct, particularly when it is also accompanied by stealing.

Most of the treatment studies considered in this chapter have not used formal diagnostic criteria. Selection criteria tend to vary from parental reports of conduct problems, to clinical status in outpatient or inpatient services, to court referrals. The formal diagnostic criteria may represent a convenient cutoff rather than a genuine threshold at which clinical dysfunction may be considered present (Kazdin, in press). Existing evidence indicates poor long-term outcome of the disorder even in children who do not meet diagnostic criteria, and treatment is both desirable and justified (e.g., Offord et al., 1992[v]). This chapter will therefore mainly discuss treatments of disturbance of conduct rather than treatments of ODD or CD specifically. We will use the terms ODD and CD where studies report that individuals met formal diagnostic criteria.

PREVALENCE

The prevalence of oppositional problems is quite high: 5–10% of nonclinical samples meet DSM diagnostic criteria. The more serious problems included in the diagnosis of CD have a more variable but comparable prevalence of 2–9% (Costello, 1990). Gender differences appear not to emerge until after the age of 6, but no firm conclusions can be reached about prevalence in relation to age (Loeber, Burke, Lahey, Winters, & Zera, 2000). Prevalence is higher in low socioeconomic status (SES) groups (Lahey, Miller, Gordon, & Riley, 1999a). There is some indication that disruptive behavior disorders are on the increase (Loeber, Farrington, & Waschbusch, 1998b; Rutter & Smith, 1995a). Disturbance of conduct represents the largest segment of most clinic caseloads (Kazdin, 1995b[vi]; Sholevar & Sholevar, 1995). Conduct problems are the most common reason for referring young children to mental health services (Reid, 1993[ib]). Thirty percent of primary care practitioner consultations involving children in the United Kingdom are for behavior problems, and 45% of community child health referrals are concerned with behavior problems (Herbert, 1995).

The prevalence of school-based disturbance of conduct (e.g., bullying) is also high. Studies across national boundaries indicate that 10–23% of children may be bullies or victims in any one year (Pepler, Craig, Ziegler, & Charach, 1993[vi]). The prevalence of childhood fire setting is also surprisingly high: as much as 35% among childhood psychiatric inpatients (Kolko & Kazdin, 1988) and 3–10% in epidemiological samples (Achenbach & Edelbrock, 1981; Heath, Hardesty, Goldfine, & Walker, 1983). The prevalence of adolescent onset disturbance of conduct is higher than that for childhood-onset disturbance of conduct: 24% and 7%, respectively, were found in the Dunedin Multidisciplinary Health Study (Moffitt, Caspi, Dickson, Silva, & Stanton, 1996).

Criminological statistics reflect these figures. Young people under the age of 18 years account for more than 30% of all arrests in the United States for index offenses, including 19% of arrests for violent crimes and 35% of arrests for property crimes (Federal Bureau of Investigation, 1996). Official arrest records show a substantial increase in rates of arrests of juveniles for violent crimes from 1984 to 1994, with no increase in arrests for property crimes (Snyder & Sickmund, 1995). Recent U.K. Home Office statistics show that in 1994 boys and young men between the ages of 10 and 20 committed 42% of all indictable offenses (Audit Commission, 1996[vi]). These figures greatly underestimate the prevalence of youth criminal activity (Loeber et al., 1998b; Rutter et al., 1998[ib]). A large number of offenses by young people are not reported and recorded by the police (Audit Commission, 1996[vi]). Young men who commit 50% of violent crimes constitute but 8% of the total population (Steiner & Stone, 1999). According to some studies, the rate of murders committed by 14- to 17-year-olds has increased 165% from 1985 to 1993 (Snyder, 1994). By the year 2005, the teenage cohort in the United States will increase by 25%, bringing further possible increases in violence rates unless appropriate interventions are found. There is indication that gender differences in delinquency have narrowed in recent years (Bjerregaard & Smith, 1993).

CLINICAL PRESENTATION

Comorbidity

Other Disruptive Disorders

Few studies provide evidence of comorbid disorders associated with ODD. An exception noted by Loeber et al. (2000) is the Smoky Mountains epidemiological study (Angold & Costello, 1996), which looked at ODD cases in a community sample. The comorbidity was 14% with ADHD, 14% with anxiety disorder, and 9% with depressive disorder. Comorbidity noted for CD is far more extensive. From the point of view of treatment, the association between ADHD and disturbance of conduct is most significant (Eiraldi, Power, & Nezu, 1997). ADHD normally precedes disturbance of conduct. In two separate well-controlled studies, children with ADHD were significantly more likely to meet criteria for CD or antisocial personality disorder (APD) at age 16 (27%–32% vs. 8%) (Gittelman, Mannuzza, Shenker, & Bonagura, 1985; Mannuzza et al., 1991). In a further follow-up of the samples, those who had ADHD in childhood had an 18% chance of being diagnosed with APD at the age of 26, as opposed to 2% in the controls. Impulsivity and hyperactivity have been described as "driving" early-onset disturbance of conduct, particularly in boys (Coie & Dodge, 1998; Loeber & Keenan, 1994; White, Moffitt, Bartusch, & Needles, 1994), but there is no evidence that the adequate treatment of ADHD can prevent CD. It should be noted that ADHD is more commonly associated with internalizing problems than with CD (Loeber et al., 1994). A number of studies find no elevation of antisocial behavior in later development associated with ADHD (Lahey, McBurnett, & Loeber, 2000). Girls with ADHD seem to be at higher risk of becoming conduct disordered than boys with ADHD (Loeber & Keenan, 1994). On the other hand, in preadolescent children, ADHD may cause the academic problems associated with disturbance of conduct (Hinshaw, 1992a, 1992b). Children with disturbance of conduct are likely to show academic deficiencies, particularly in reading (Kazdin, 1995b[vi]), and their interpersonal skills and relations are likely to be poor. In adolescence, academic problems, long-standing social difficulties, and ADHD are likely to play interacting roles. Comorbidity with ADHD is associated with worse quality of life (e.g., social withdrawal, lower self-esteem, higher anxiety, higher maternal pathology) (see Kuhne, Schachar, & Tannock, 1997). Notwithstanding the definitional problems associated with ADHD (reviewed in Chapter 6), clinicians should be alert to the possibility of dual diagnoses, particularly the presence of ODD, which may signify a more adverse course for the conduct problems of early childhood (Lahey et al., 1999).

APD or psychopathy may be related to disturbance of conduct. Among adolescent boys, those with a combination of hyperactivity, impulsivity, and attention and conduct problems resemble psychopathic adults most closely (Lynam, 1998). Studies of school-age children have identified modest correlations between disturbance of conduct and a personality type characterized by superficial charm, absence of concern and guilt, and lack of anxiety (Christian, Frick, Hill, Tyler, & Frazer, 1997; Frick, O'Brien, Wootton, & McBurnett, 1994). Quality of parenting seems to play a less central part in the etiology of young people with such traits, as they are thought to be impervious to socialization (Wootton, Frick, Shelton, & Silverthorn, 1997). Children with an ODD or CD diagnosis without callous and unemotional traits show deficits in verbal reasoning, whereas children with the same diagnoses who also have these traits do not (Loney, Frick, Ellis, & McCoy, 1998). Disturbance of conduct is quite highly correlated with anxiety, whereas psychopathy precludes this. However, psychopathic features identify a group of children with quite serious disturbance of conduct and predict the increased likelihood of contact with police.

Disturbance of conduct is a significant risk factor for substance use (Hawkins, Catalano, & Miller, 1992[vi]; Loeber, 1988), although by no means all young people with substance use problems have disturbance of conduct in their histories. The onset of minor delinquency appears to precede the use of alcohol (Loeber & Keenan, 1994). However, marijuana use often precedes the onset of more serious offending, as well as the onset of polydrug use. The comorbidity of substance use and delinquency is marked only at the more serious levels of both disorders. There is some evidence for a higher risk of substance use for girls with disruptive disorders.

Internalizing Problems

Childhood anxiety disorder on its own appears to protect against future conduct problems, but the presence of conduct problems increases the chance of an anxiety disorder diagnosis (Loeber & Keenan, 1994; Zoccolillo, 1992). Comorbidity of internalizing problems with disturbance of conduct is relatively common. Depression is frequently comorbid with ODD and CD (Zoccolillo, 1992). The onset of these problems is more consistent with a clinical picture of emotional problems arising as a reaction to disturbance of conduct (Loeber & Keenan, 1994). The likelihood of comorbid depression and CD in boys increases in preadolescence, but after a certain point in puberty boys are less likely to suffer from this comorbidity, whereas comorbid depression and CD become increasingly likely in girls. There is more evidence that depression exacerbates disruptive behavior over time than for the converse (Loeber & Keenan, 1994). In early adolescence, stable depressed mood occurs more often when boys advance in either overt or covert pathways toward CD than when they are involved in multiple pathways (Loeber et al., 1994). This may suggest that the multiple pathway group is more closely related to the callous unemotional subgroup of disturbances of conduct identified by Wootton et al. (1997). The prevalence of suicidality also increases with disturbance of conduct (Renaud et al., 1999b), especially for girls (Loeber & Keenan, 1994) and youths with a history of substance and physical abuse (Renaud et al., 1999). The high rate of comorbidity of depression and CD is of particular concern, because the joint presence of these disorders appears to increase the risk of serious outcomes such as substance abuse (Buydens-Branchey, Branchey, & Noumair, 1989) and suicide (Shaffi, Carrigan, Whittinghill, & Derrick, 1985).

Anxiety disorders also co-occur with disturbance of conduct in girls (Loeber & Keenan, 1994). Some studies suggest that anxiety is a relatively good prognostic indicator (Fonagy & Target, 1994[iv]; Walker et al., 1991). Anxiety may protect kindergarten boys from becoming delinquent (Ensminger, Kellam, & Rubin, 1983; Tremblay, Pihl, Vitaro, & Dobkin, 1994). In these studies, age at onset of both conditions appears to be influenced as to whether anxiety serves to increase or decrease the likelihood of developing comorbid CD. Other studies, however, either show no effect (Campbell & Ewing, 1990) or show that shy and withdrawn children with disturbance of conduct have a relatively poor life outcome (McCord, 1988; Serbin, Peters, McAffer, & Schwartzman, 1991). One explanation, for which evidence is available (Kerr, Tremblay, Pagani, & Vitaro, 1997), is that social withdrawal and a nonanxious preference for solitary activity (Rubin & Mills, 1988) may sometimes be mistaken for behavioral inhibition, yet represent a risk for, rather than a protection from, delinquency. Disruptive withdrawn boys appear to be at greatest risk of delinquency (Kerr et al., 1997; Ladd & Burgess, 1999). Withdrawal without aggression is neither stable nor predictive of ongoing difficulties (Ladd & Burgess, 1999).

There appears to be a high level of comorbidity between delinquency and posttraumatic stress disorder (PTSD). A study of 85 incarcerated boys documented a rate of up to 50% of active and partial PTSD (Steiner, Garcia, & Mattews, 1997). Somatization disorder may also be comorbid with disturbance of conduct (Lilienfeld, 1992). Somatization is more common in girls and disturbance of conduct in boys, yet this type of comorbidity appears to be more marked in boys than in girls (Offord, Alder, & Boyle, 1986). However, the data on the comorbidity of disturbance of conduct and somatization are relatively small and unconvincing (Loeber et al., 2000; Loeber & Keenan, 1994).

CD is strongly associated with later substance use disorder (Boyle & Offord, 1991). Early onset of substance use predicts later criminality (Hovens, Cantwell, & Kiriakos, 1994). It is likely that the relationship between CD and substance use is reciprocal, with each amplifying the potential for the other.

Natural History

In early childhood boys are far more likely than girls to manifest disturbance of conduct, but during adolescence the proportion of girls increases markedly. Epidemiological studies have shown that excessive disobedience in relation to adults is a key precursor to the development of full-blown CD (e.g., Frick et al., 1993), which underscores the importance of the nature of parent–child relationships in this disorder. Noncompliance also explains the academic and peer relationship problems that many of these children experience (Walker & Walker, 1991). A detailed review of the last decade's literature on ODD and CD (Loeber et al., 2000) has identified age at onset, severity, age and gender atypicality, overt versus covert disruptive behavior, the nature of aggression and the presence of early antisocial personality disorder-related symptoms as of prognostic importance. The Ontario Child Health Study 4-year follow-up found that 46% of children with CD at time 1 had another psychiatric disorder at follow-up (particularly hyperactivity and emotional disorder), compared with 13% with no disorder at time 1.

Aggression is another early sign of severe disturbance of conduct (Olweus, 1992[v]). Some distinguish between aggression that is "reactive" as opposed to "proactive" (Dodge, 1991), and others distinguish "affective" from "predatory" aggression (Vitiello & Stoff, 1997[vi]). In general, childhood aggression can be described as either hostile, reactive, defensive, impulsive, and covert, or instrumental, proactive, offensive, predatory, and controlled (Vitiello & Stoff, 1997[vi]). This distinction is important because certain treatments are applicable to only one type.

Reactive aggression is a defensive, explosive, and uncontrolled response to perceived provocation, accompanied by fear or anger. Proactive aggression provides a means by which the young person may obtain some self-serving outcome, but it is not accompanied by intense emotion. Affective–proactive aggression is more likely to be associated with neurotransmitter abnormalities (particularly 5-HT; see Unis et al., 1997) and consequently may be more likely to respond to pharmacotherapy (Malone et al., 1998[iv]; Stoff & Cairns, 1996). Indications of autonomic abnormalities have also been demonstrated in support of this distinction (e.g., Van Goozen et al., 1998). There is growing evidence of biological differences, such as higher adrenal androgen levels in children with ODD as opposed to both normal and other psychiatric groups (Van Goozen et al., 2000). Childhood aggression is a good predictor of delinquency and ODD and CD problems in adolescence (Pulkkinen, 1996; Vitaro, Gendreau, Tremblay, & Oligny, 1998). Well over half of future recidivist delinquents can be predicted at age 7 from their aggressive behavior, given that their families manifest ineffective child rearing practices (Farrington, 1995[vi]). Fighting correlates significantly with lying, and lying predicts stealing behavior, particularly in adolescence (Loeber & Schmaling, 1985a; Stouthamer-

Loeber & Loeber, 1986). Assaultive behavior in childhood predicts adult imprisonment, as does criminality in a biological parent. But CD on its own is not a perfect
predictor of adult criminality (Lundy, Pfohl, & Kuperman, 1993).

There is a strong linear increase from early childhood to the late teenage years
in the prevalence of nonaggressive antisocial behavior (Lahey et al., 1998; Loeber,
Farrington, Stouthamer-Loeber, & Van Kammen, 1998a). A number of longitudinal studies, however, reveal declining ratings of physical aggression as age increases
from 4 to adolescence (e.g., Stanger, Achenbach, & Verhulst, 1997). In contrast,
among some young people, the prevalence of serious physical aggression increases
with age (Lahey et al., 1998). It is possible that minor physical aggression declines
with age in the general population, but a small percentage of highly aggressive
youths follow a different course. Normative studies demonstrate that early disruptive behavior problems tend to improve without assistance over the first 10 years of
life (Campbell, 1995[vi]; Spieker, Larson, Lewis, Keller, & Gilchrist, 1999). In a
longitudinal study of 177 clinic-referred 7- to 12-year-old boys who were interviewed annually, a spontaneous improvement rate of 14 out of 86 was found by year
7 (Lahey, Loeber, & Burke, 1999). Recovery was associated with higher IQ and socioeconomic status, and with improvements in comorbid conditions (ADD, ODD,
and depression). This tendency is particularly marked in children of mothers with
low coerciveness, anxiety, and depression (Spieker et al., 1999). Two independent
population studies identified four prototypical developmental pathways for overt
aggression from kindergarten to middle-school years: two relatively high-aggression
and two low-aggression paths (Nagin & Tremblay, 2001; Shaw, Gilliom, Ingoldsby,
& Schonberg, 2001). Low maternal age and education, rejection of the child, and
apparent fearlessness of the child as an infant appear to distinguish the high-overt-
aggression group (representing 5% of the sample) whose aggression does not decline
over middle childhood (nondesisters) and those whose aggression starts high but
declines over this period (representing 30%). It is as yet unclear whether the observed decline is genuine or part of a change in pattern of aggression that is con-
flated with measurement methods. Aggression commonly shifts from a highly overt,
uncontrolled pattern in the early years that is easily noted by adult observers, to a
more covert, sneaky type of aggression that increases rather than decreases developmentally and is more obvious to playground observers than to parents or teachers
(Snyder, Suarez, & Brooker, 2001). In general, longitudinal studies have demonstrated the continuity of disturbance of conduct from early to later childhood
(Campbell, 1995[vi]), from childhood to adolescence (Lahey et al., 1995), and from
adolescence to adulthood (Farrington, 1995[vi]). There is also evidence that the
risks of disturbance of conduct are transmitted across generations (Huesmann,
Leonard, & Monroe, 1984). However, it seems that many of these continuities may
be moderated by intercurrent social experiences (Quinton, Gulliver, & Rutter,
1995), which underscores the possibility of effective treatment as a prevention
measure.

Psychiatric disorders that follow CD include alcoholism, drug dependence,
and antisocial personality disorder (Robins & Price, 1991). Other associated non-
psychiatric antisocial behaviors include theft, violence to people and property,

drunk driving and the use of illegal drugs, the carrying of illegal weapons, and group violence with vandalism (Farrington, 1995[vi]). Overall, 75% of 254 children with clinically significant CD, when followed up into adulthood, went on to exhibit pervasive and persistent social malfunctioning, although often below the threshold for diagnosis of personality disorder (Zoccolillo, Pickles, Quinton, & Rutter, 1992). There is high continuity between failure in school, associated with conduct problems, and adult unemployment (Rutter et al., 1998[ib]). The long-term outcome of conduct disturbances must be considered poor. A recent editorial (Harrington, 2001) pointed out "that the evidence that adult personality problems are clearly predicted by a child's anti-social behavior combined with difficulties in the family raises the possibility that such problems could be prevented" (p. 237).

ASSESSMENT

There is a rich and comprehensive literature on the clinical and research assessment of disturbance of conduct (see the summary in McMahon & Estes, 1997). The key areas of assessment are as follows: (1) The child's behavior in an interactional context. Assessment in this area needs to be a multimethod approach because the child's behavior may vary across settings, children tend to underestimate their own behavioral symptoms (Edelbrock, Costello, Dulcan, Conover, & Kala, 1986), and all informants are known to manifest significant bias. Structured interviews, with evidence for reliability and validity, are available for teachers (Breen & Altepeter, 1990) and parents (Forehand & McMahon, 1981[vi]). Behavioral rating scales are usually administered to parents or teachers, and direct behavioral observation, although time-consuming, provides a unique additional source of information. A recent review has evaluated current alternative methods (Reitman, Hummel, Franz, & Gross, 1998). The direct observation form of the Child Behavior Checklist (CBCL), for example, is relatively easy to use (Achenbach, 1991a). (2) The pertinent child characteristics. Among these are the possibility of neurological injury, the child's temperament, the presence of ADHD or internalizing disorders, and the child's social skills and academic achievement.

At least seven additional areas may also be relevant to the treatment of disturbance of conduct: (1) parenting practices (Arnold, O'Leary, Wolff, & Acker, 1993), (2) biases in the parents' perceptions of the child (Campis, Lyman, & Prentice-Dunn, 1986; Johnston & Mash, 1989), (3) parents' psychological status (particularly mother's depression), (4) parental antisocial behavior, (5) marital discord (Straus, 1990), (6) child-rearing disagreements (Jouriles et al., 1991), and (7) maternal isolation (Dumas & Wahler, 1983[v]).

Such comprehensive assessment aims to identify the child's status and progression on a particular developmental pathway and the likelihood of a favorable outcome. The assessment should also be contextually sensitive, inasmuch as treatment frequently addresses the context rather than the child. However, the results of the assessment are rarely relevant to the selection of treatment strategies. There is little evidence to direct clinicians to appropriate treatment strategies from specific assessment procedures. The "Summary and Implications" section of this chapter attempts to give some preliminary suggestions along these lines.

TREATMENT OF OPPOSITIONAL DEFIANT DISORDER AND CONDUCT DISORDER

Of all child psychiatric disorders, disruptive behavior disorders have been subjected to the most extensive set of evaluations. This review of treatment approaches will consider the evidence for psychosocial treatment strategies for children and adolescents, systemwide implementations, and studies of pharmacological interventions.

Psychosocial Treatment Interventions for Preadolescents

Family-Based Interventions: Parent Training

The parent training model is rooted in social learning theory. It is based on the assumption that many overt disturbances of conduct, including oppositional behavior and mild forms of aggression, reflect parental difficulty in adequately reinforcing socially appropriate forms of conduct, as well as a tendency to maintain inappropriate forms of conduct through coercive interactions (Kazdin, 1995b[vi]; Miller & Prinz, 1990[ib]; Patterson, 1982). The intervention is conducted with the parents, with limited therapist–child contact. Parents are encouraged to refocus on prosocial behaviors rather than on the elimination of conduct problems. The training component of the program is based on behavioral management principles drawn from social learning theory. It includes training in monitoring and tracking the behavior, using positive reinforcements, and training in extinction and mild punishment procedures (e.g., ignoring, response cost, and time-out). The aim is to reduce the inadvertent provision of any positive reinforcement (such as parental attention) for engaging in disruptive or defiant behavior, while simultaneously increasing the parents' reinforcement for prosocial or compliant behavior. Punishments are applied contingently on the display of unacceptable behavior, and parental use of consequences is made more predictable, contingent, and immediate. In most programs, only one parent (usually the mother) comes to treatment, partly because of scheduling issues but also because of the high rate of single-parent families among youth with conduct problems. Although there is little experimental research on this issue (Horton, 1984[vi]), the presence of both parents seems not to be needed for the intervention to be successful (Kazdin, 1997b[ib]).

Programs for young, mildly oppositional children require only 6–8 weeks, whereas clinically referred children with full CD diagnoses are usually offered 12–25 weeks. Program duration varies as a function of two competing demands. First, there is a tendency for increasingly cost-effective, and therefore briefer, interventions (Thompson, Ruma, Schuchmann, & Burke, 1996[ii]). On the other hand, treatment programs using parent training have become more complex, including components from a number of modalities, incorporating cognitive components such as the principles of problem solving and the delivery of clear instructions (Webster-Stratton, 1996a[vi]). Although programs vary in terms of the exact syllabus and the methods of delivering these contents, in all programs dyadic instruction is accompanied by other aids to learning, such as role-playing, behavioral rehearsal, and structured homework exercises. The programs have been successfully implemented in clinic, community, and home settings with individual families or groups of families. Guidelines are available for choosing between these parameters, but these are mostly based on clinical experience rather than formal comparative studies (O'Dell, 1985).

The effectiveness of behavioral parent training in producing short-term changes in parent–child behavior has been established since the mid-1970s (O'Dell, 1974[vi]). The generalization of these changes to other settings posttreatment, to nontargeted behaviors of the referred child, and to other children of the treated parents, is less well established (Estrada & Pinsof, 1995[vi]; Serketich & Dumas, 1996[ib]; Shadish et al., 1993[ib]). A review of psychosocial treatments for conduct problems by Brestan and Eyberg (1998[ib]) found 82 studies of parent training, which they evaluated according to the criteria developed by the American Psychological Association's (APA) Task Force on the promotion and dissemination of efficacious psychological procedures. Of the 82 studies identified, all but one had a comparison group; 75% used random assignment, but only 37% had at least 6 months follow-up and even fewer reported sample characteristics sufficiently to indicate with confidence the populations to whom the results could be generalized. The APA review identified only two interventions meeting the criteria set out by the APA, and both were parent training approaches: (1) the Oregon Social Learning Center program and (2) the videotape modeling group discussion program. A further 20 studies were identified as supporting the value of probably efficacious treatments.

Programs have focused on noncompliance in 3- to 8-year-olds as the target of their intervention. A number of research groups are working with slight variations of this approach. The most significant sets of contributions come from Forehand and McMahon (1981[vi]), Webster-Stratton (1996a[vi]), the Oregon Social Learning Center (Patterson & Forgatch, 1995[vi]), and Eyberg (1995[ii]). All these programs are clearly described, well-manualized treatments, but some require relatively elaborate procedures, more appropriate to university than clinic settings. Problems of generalization have led to an extension of the parent training approach beyond the original components outlined earlier. This extended form of treatment, often referred to as "behavioral family therapy" (Wells, 1985), incorporates distortions of parental cognitions concerning the child, issues raised by marital conflict, parental psychopathology, and the child's temperament and attributional style (Johnston, 1996[vi]; Miller & Prinz, 1990[ib]). In some programs (to be reviewed separately) parent training may be one module within a multimodal treatment package (as, for example, in Kazdin's [Kazdin et al., 1987a[i], 1992[i] combination of problem-solving skills training [PSST] with parent training, Henggeler and Bourduin's [Henggeler et al. 1992[i], 1993[v], 1986[ii]; Borduin 1999[vi] multisystemic therapy, or Chamberlain's foster care treatment for delinquent youths [Chamberlain, 1994[vi]; Chamberlain & Reid, 1994[vi]).

META-ANALYSIS

Two meta-analyses of parent training approaches have been reported. The first covered all family-based treatments (Shadish et al., 1993[ib]). The selection criteria were random assignment, clinically distressed subjects, and marital or family therapy as one of the treatment conditions. The sample identified 18 studies specific to conduct disorder. The effect size (ES) of family therapy was .53. Behaviorally-oriented treatment yielded an ES of .55 (n = 18) and systemic approaches an ES of .26 (n = 8). Eclectic therapies obtained an average ES of .57 (n = 7). Eleven studies specifically examined parent management training and obtained an ES of .41. Although containing some interesting indications (e.g., that studies using multiple behavioral strategies (n = 11) obtained considerably larger ESs [ES =.83]), this review included only studies from the 1980s and failed to differentiate adequately between the client groups addressed by the reports.

Serketich and Dumas (1996[ib]) reported a specific meta-analytic study of parent training. The review identified 117 (including 3 unpublished) studies of parent training applied to conduct problems. The criteria for selection from this sample were (1) at least one antisocial behavior to be included as entry criteria to the trial, (2) inclusion of training of parents in the use of differential reinforcement and/or time-out procedure, (3) preschool or elementary school age child, (4) one control group (no-treatment, placebo treatment, or alternative treatment), (5) minimum group size of five subjects, (6) outcome measure to assess the child's behavior at pre- and posttreatment. Only 26 out of the 117 studies that met criteria 1–3 met criteria 4–6. The studies yielded 36 comparisons between treated and untreated groups. Overall, 27 of the comparisons were for parental reports, 10 for teacher reports, 23 for behavioral observations, and 12 for parental adjustment. Two methodological indices were also calculated: (1) accuracy scores were highest when the ES calculation could be based on means and standard deviations and lowest if they had to be estimated from p values; (2) high-validity scores were assigned to studies that gave complete data for nonsignificant outcome measures and low-validity ones if the possibility of bias existed because means or standard deviations (SDs) were not supplied for insignificant comparisons.

The average ESs were .86 (overall), .84 (parent report), .85 (observer report), .73 (teacher report), and .44 (parental adjustment). Some of the overall results were promising: Seventeen of the 19 intervention groups that were above the clinical range on pretest measures dropped below this level on at least one measure posttreatment. Fourteen (73%) of the samples showed this kind of clinically significant change on all the measures applied.

A number of aspects of the findings give grounds for concern.

1. There was a significant negative correlation between ES and sample size, indicating that the largest effects were observed in the smallest studies.
2. The correlations between the accuracy and validity ratings and the ESs were very high and negative, suggesting that the larger effects were from studies with less claim to validity.
3. There was a significant positive correlation between the child's age and ES,

suggesting a substantial heterogeneity of treatment response related to the child's age, but in the opposite direction to that reported in the vast majority of individual reports.

4. There were insignificant correlations between ES and both socioeconomic status and single-parent status; these are both well-known moderators of the outcome of parent training. The fact that well-known associations between the effects of parent training and socioeconomic and single-parent status did not emerge, and that a counterintuitive positive association between ES and child's age did, raises general questions about the validity of the meta-analytic approach to this body of investigations. It is most likely that poorly controlled studies with major problems of internal validity have substantially distorted the ES estimates.

There are important differences between the practical demands of the various major approaches to parent training. We will review each of their respective evidence bases separately.

HELPING THE NONCOMPLIANT CHILD

The Forehand and McMahon program, Helping the Noncompliant Child, is an individual family-based program including didactic instruction, modeling, role-playing, and skills practice with therapist feedback from behind a one-way screen. Specific structured exercises ensure generalization to the home setting. In the initial phase of the program, the coercive cycle is broken by increasing social attention to the child, focusing on the child's socially appropriate behavior, and gradually learning to use social attention contingently with compliance. Structured homework exercises include increasing the frequency of at least two specified child behaviors. In the second phase of the program, parents are taught appropriate methods for instructions and commands, and instructed that if commands are not followed, a time-out procedure is initiated (a command-warning 3 minute time-out sequence). The program is structured in a stepwise, graded manner.

Six uncontrolled or minimally controlled studies show that progress made during the program is maintained (Baum & Forehand, 1981[ii]; Forehand & Long, 1988[ii]; Forehand, Rogers, McMahon, Wells, & Griest, 1981[iii]; Forehand et al., 1979[ii]; Long, Forehand, Wierson, & Morgan, 1994[iv]; Peed, Roberts, & Forehand, 1977[ii]). These studies taken together demonstrate that, relative to nonreferred ("normal") samples, the referred noncompliant group function well up to 14 years after the initial training. There is also evidence of generalization to nontargeted behaviors such as aggression, temper tantrums, swearing, and destructive behaviors (Wells, Griest, & Forehand, 1980[ii]). There is some suggestion that siblings of the referred child also benefit in terms of greater compliance to maternal directives (Humphreys, Forehand, McMahon, & Roberts, 1978[iii]). Two studies investigated whether the program generalizes across settings and found no evidence that classroom behavior either improves or deteriorates (Breiner & Forehand, 1981[ii]; Forehand et al., 1979[ii]).

Wells and Egan (1988[ii]) report a comparison study between this parent training program and systemic family therapy. Nineteen families with children with ODD diagnoses (ages 3–8) were randomly assigned. Both treatments were associated with some improvement on self-report measures of depression and anxiety in the parents and marital adjustment. Observational measures of parent–child behavior reflected significantly greater improvement associated with the parent training program. These findings are not surprising, given that parent training explicitly targets changes in these variables (e.g., providing positive attention, rewarding child compliance, etc.). The study included no measures of family functioning.

In an unpublished study, Baum, Reyna McGlone, and Ollendick (1986, November[i]) compared a group-based version of this parent training with a parent discussion group based on the Systematic Training for Effective Parenting (STEP) principles. Thirty-four highly noncompliant children (ages 6–10) were randomly assigned to one of three conditions: a basic group-administered parent training, a combined parent discussion and child self-control condition, and a combined parent training and child self-control condition. Treatment for all families involved eight weekly 75-minute sessions conducted in small groups. The targeted measures were the parents' report of the child's behavior, observed parent–child interaction during an analog task, and parental self-reports of self-esteem, anxiety, and depression. Outcomes were assessed posttreatment and at 6–8 months follow-up. The parent training conditions, with or without the child self-control component, were superior to the discussion control group and did not differ from each other at posttreatment. At 6–8 months' follow-up the parent training plus child self-control training was superior to parent training alone and to the control condition, based on observational measures of the child's deviant behavior and on child and maternal reports of adjustment. However, the absence of a group that received STEP but no child-oriented treatment in the trial is a clear limitation. The treatment groups were quite small, threatening external validity.

Sayger et al. randomly assigned 43 aggressive boys (7–10 years), selected on the basis of teachers' reports of classroom aggression, to either 10 sessions of parent training or a waiting-list control (Sayger, Horne, Walker, & Passmore, 1988[i]). At termination, significant differences were found in positive child behaviors at home and at school. Differences were also manifest in family cohesion, empathy, problem-solving efficiency, and total positive family relationships. Family conflict decreased. A further study (Sayger, Horne, & Glaser, 1993[iii]) reported that improvements were largely maintained at 9–12 months' follow-up and changes were generalized to school behavior. However, the waiting-list control group had been taken into treatment for ethical reasons and levels of disturbance were not high at the outset, so the generalizability of these findings is unclear.

There is evidence that mothers' perceptions of their children's behavior change in consequence of the program, with about a 2-month delay (Forehand, Wells, & Griest, 1980[ii]). User satisfaction has also been demonstrated (Cross Calvert & McMahon, 1987[iii]). Both the inclusion of self-control procedures for the child in the program (Baum et al., 1986, November[i]) and an expanded set of examples of parent–child situations that could lead to coercive interaction (Powers

& Roberts, 1995[ii]) enhanced the effectiveness of the program in the short term. The inclusion of components related to marital adjustment, parental personal adjustment, parental perceptions of the child's behavior, and the parents' extrafamilial relationships enhanced the maintenance of gains (Griest et al., 1982[ii]). McMahon et al. taught general social learning principles in addition to child-management techniques to 24 parents of young noncompliant children and found this a valuable adjunct, with better maintenance of improvements relative to baseline at 2-months follow-up (McMahon, Forehand, Griest, & Wells, 1981[ii]). In a study of 16 mothers, teaching the mother self-control strategies in addition to parent training (Wells et al., 1980[ii]) also strengthened maintenance of treatment gains, in terms of the mother's report of deviant behavior (although not in terms of direct observation).

VIDEOTAPE MODELING GROUP DISCUSSION

Webster-Stratton (1996a[vi]) described a 9–10-week group discussion videotape modeling program (GDVM) that uses a standard package of 10 videotapes (BASIC). The videotapes show 250 2-minute scenes in which parents interact with their children in both appropriate and inappropriate ways. After each scene, the therapist leads a discussion of the interactions and solicits parents' responses. Children do not attend the therapy sessions, but structured homework exercises for the practice of parenting skills ensure the generalization of the behaviors from the clinic setting. Parents are taught play and reinforcement skills, effective limit setting, and nonviolent discipline techniques, as well as problem-solving approaches.

A large-scale study that randomized a sample of 114 families with young (3- to 8-year-old) children with disturbance of conduct has been reported by Webster-Stratton (1989[i], 1990b[i]; Webster-Stratton, Kolpacoff, & Hollinsworth, 1988[i]). The four conditions were the BASIC GDVM program, a self-administered videotape modeling without therapist feedback or group discussion (IVM), group discussion alone (GD), and a waiting-list control condition. The study provided outcome data from changes at the level of symptoms (behavior problems), adjustment (deviance, school performance), transactional processes (parental stress, negative parental behaviors), and consumer satisfaction. All three treatment conditions appeared effective relative to the waiting-list condition. Improvements were maintained at 1-year follow-up. Only consumer satisfaction distinguished the combined treatment group from the other groups. At 3-year follow-up (Webster-Stratton, 1990b[i]), parents' reports of improvements in the problem behaviors of the child were maintained only in the BASIC GDVM condition. In contrast, parents in both the IVM and GD conditions reported significant increases in their children's externalizing behavior, although these still remained below the baseline levels. Even with the combined approach, more than a quarter of the children showed significant school problems at follow-up. Overall, 46.3% of mothers, 25.5% of fathers, and 26.5% of teachers reported behavior problems in the deviant or clinical range in the children's grade school years. However, the sample was predominantly middle class, with only 30% single mothers. More than one-third of the families continued to have concerns about their children's behavior problems, and 30% (those troubled by alcoholism, drug abuse, or depression) asked for further therapy either for their children or for themselves. Webster-Stratton (1996b[vi]) found no differences between the response of boys and girls to the BASIC program, although for girls severity of disturbance of conduct did not predict negative outcome, whereas maternal depression, negativity, and paternal life stress did.

A further report (Webster-Stratton, 1990a[i]) compared 43 families divided into three groups: videotape modeling, videotape modeling plus consultation, and an untreated control group. The sample was ages 3–8 years. Compared with the control group, those in both treatment groups reported a reduction in behavioral problems, reduced stress levels, and reduced use of spanking. There were relatively few differences between the treatment conditions, but at the end of treatment fewer children in the group that included two 1-hour consultations scored in the clinical range of the CBCL. No long-term follow-up was reported.

Webster-Stratton (1992[i]) also reported a study of a self-administered BASIC IVM program. One hundred families were randomly assigned to the program or to a waiting-list control condition. In total, 46% of subjects were self-referred and 56% were professionally referred. The mean age of the children was just over 5 years. Two-thirds (66%) of the mothers were married, but 27% of the mothers complained of spouse abuse; 69% of the sample were relatively well off (social class 1–3). Assessments included parent, teacher, and home observation measures. Only 69% of the treated mothers and 45% of teachers reported pretreatment CBCL externalizing behavior in the clinical range. Follow-up data were available on about 80% of the sample. The treated parents came to the clinic weekly to see 10 videotape programs. A manual was provided with each program, which described each of the scenes and asked open-ended questions about them. A written discussion of the author's interpretations was provided, but the parents were asked not to look at these until they had tried to answer the questions themselves. On average, parents completed the program in 10 hours. There were significant changes on many of the measures. Treated parents reported using significantly less physical punishment, and they perceived improvements in their children's behavior problems, as compared with control parents. During home observations, treated parents exhibited significant changes in at least two of four behavior outcome variables (e.g., decreased criticism). Changes were maintained or further improvements were observed at follow-up. However, more than half of the children in the clinical range on the CBCL remained so on both mothers' and teachers' ratings. Only 23% of the families requested further help for their child's behavior problems. Children of mothers with a partner, low levels of stress and depression, and relatively high IQ benefited most from the treatment. High negative life stress and depression in fathers correlated with more negative perceptions of the child's adjustment and increased deviance immediately posttreatment.

This team reported some important qualitative research on the problem of resistance to parent training (Webster-Stratton & Herbert, 1993[vi]). Participating parents appear to go through several phases in sequence, first acknowledging the problem, then being alternately hopeful and despairing, next accepting that total recovery is not possible, then working on fitting the program to their specific family situation, and finally coming to effective coping. Similar qualitative data describe the experience of families after the termination of treatment (Webster-Stratton & Spitzer, 1996[vi]). Qualitative data have also been collected to describe the therapists' tasks in relation to the expected reactions of the parents (Webster-Stratton, 1996a[vi]). These include the construction of a supportive relationship, the empowerment of the parent, didactic teaching, offering understanding of behavior, leading the family through patches of resistance, and anticipating complications, difficulties, barriers to change, and constructive moves forward.

Webster-Stratton (1994[i], 1996a[vi]) reported a refinement of the video-based treatment method with a similar set of outcome measures. Three months (12 sessions) of BASIC GDVM parent training was followed in one group by an additional 3 months of video-based ADVANCE treatment. The ADVANCE program involves six videotaped programs with therapist-led discussions focusing on the parents' interpersonal distress and the enhancement of parental interpersonal skills. This latter component dealt with teaching children to solve problems, problem solving between adults, anger management, self-care, family communication skills, depression control, and giving and receiving support. Seventy-eight families with a child diagnosed with ODD or CD were randomly assigned to either GDVM alone or GDVM + ADVANCE. The results partially supported the use of the ADVANCE treatment. There was observed benefit from the additional videotape component, in that parents' problem solving and quality of communication and collaboration skills improved (transactional level), as well as their child's problem solving and overall satisfaction with the program (consumer level). However, parents' self-reports of marital satisfaction, anger, or stress levels were not significantly different even at short-term follow-up. Parents in the ADVANCE program did not report enhanced improvement in their children's behavior, and independent observation of parent–child interactions in the home did not indicate significantly less deviance in the children of these parents.

Researchers at Arizona State University have reported a similarly designed study (Spaccarelli, 1992[ii]). Twenty-one parents were assigned to a problem-solving training group, which was an adjunct to parent skills training. Sixteen parents were assigned to parenting skills alone or waiting-list control groups. At posttest both treatments demonstrated significant improvements in parents' reports of child behavior problems. The problem-solving skills training had additional benefits in terms of changes in parents' perceptions of their own functioning as parents and their attitudes toward their child.

In another study Webster-Stratton and Hammond (1997) described a child social skills and problem-solving training intervention (KIDVID), which is also a videotape-assisted modeling program targeting problem-solving and social skills deficits, peer rejection, loneliness, and negative attributions. It includes empathy training, problem-solving training, anger control, friendship skills, communication skills, and school training. It is administered in small groups over 22 weeks. Each session lasts 2 hours. These components of the program were tested with 97 children ages 4–8 with disturbance of conduct. Adding this program to the two programs discussed earlier appears to enhance problem-solving skills and social competence. The program on its own, without parent involvement, also has a favorable impact, as compared with a waiting-list control group, in terms of symptomatic behaviors, adaptation, and problem-solving capacities. However, the combined parent and child intervention had the most robust improvements in child behavior at 1-year follow-up. Independently observed child deviance in the home that did not show a statistically significant reduction immediately posttreatment, was significantly reduced over time for all three treatment conditions, but particularly for the combined treatment. However, as the control group was subsequently treated, it is difficult to tell whether long-term changes were due to maturation or to treatment. A 30% reduction in deviant behaviors (of clinical significance) in mother–child interaction was observed in almost three-quarters of the child training group, in 60% of the parent training group, and in 95% of the combined treatment group. Earlier attempts at child training had not been particularly effective for this younger age group, perhaps because the programs were not developmentally appropriate. However, as in other combined therapies, the treatment dose was effectively doubled for the combined treatment (Kazdin, 1996a[vi]).

Webster-Stratton (1996c, 1998[iii]) extended the program to the school environment, exploring the value of specific parent training as an addition to the traditional Head Start curriculum. The study assessed the effectiveness of a parenting program for 394 mothers, 264 in the intervention group and 130 in the control group. The sample was disadvantaged; more than 50% were single parents, one-fifth were teenage mothers, 45% had been physically or sexually abused as children, and 20% had recently been involved with child protection services because of abuse or neglect. The intervention involved an abbreviated version of the BASIC program lasting 8–9 weeks. Weekly parent group meetings led by family support workers (30% with master's degrees) aimed to promote parental involvement in school activities. The teachers also received some special training in addition to the Head Start curriculum, which promoted the teachers' classroom management skills. In general, the program resulted in significantly larger behavior changes in both child and parent in the experimental group, but the results were mixed. At posttreatment, externalizing behaviors on the CBCL decreased significantly for both treatment and control groups. Only on the Eyberg Child Behavior Inventory (ECBI) was the decrease significantly larger for the intervention group. Not surprisingly, home observations of mothers' behavior favored the intervention group. The impact on the children's behavior was marked. Children's social competence improved in both mothers' and teachers' reports. There was no effect on teachers' reports of externalizing behavior. For both groups, there was a tendency for externalizing to get worse. For both the intervention and the control group, externalizing behavior continued below baseline on mothers' reports but was above baseline on teachers' reports. In terms of clinical significance, 69% of the mothers in the intervention condition and 52% in the control condition showed marked changes in their behavior. Correspondingly, 73% of children above clinical cutoff showed a 30% reduction in noncompliant behaviors in the experimental group, compared with 55% in the control. However, these group differences were no longer significant at 1-year follow-up for either mothers or children. It is not clear whether the limited success of this implementation was due to the higher level of deprivation of the sample, the relatively abbreviated administration of the program, or the nonclinical setting. A similar large-scale preventive implementation of parent training also failed in the Worcester Public School system (Barkley et al., 2000[i]).

The only non-U.S.-based study of this method of intervention was performed at the Institute of Psychiatry in London between 1995 and 1999 (Scott, Spender, Doolan, Jacobs, & Aspland, 2001[i]). The treatment was offered to 144 families meeting criteria, of whom 90 were assigned to parenting groups of 6–8 and 51 to waiting-list control. Follow-up assessment was at about 7 months for the treatment group and 4½ months for the control group. Eighty-one percent of the treatment group and 73% of the control group completed the trial. Outcome was assessed using the Parent Account of Child Symptoms, a semistructured interview. There were parent-report-based measures of outcome (CBCL) and direct observations of parenting in an 18-minute structured play time. The pre–post differences were impressive in the parents' accounts of the child's symptoms (ES = 1.1). Similar ESs were obtained for questionnaire measures. However, 50% of the treated group still met criteria for oppositional defiant disorder at the end of treatment, which nonetheless represented a reduction of 30% from pretreatment. The study is notable because of the high level of deprivation that characterized the sample, considerably more severe than in North American tests of this treatment. A limitation of the study was the exclusion of children with hyperkinetic syndrome or any other condition requiring separate treatment. The findings indicate that parent training using videotape modeling is a viable treatment in the United Kingdom as well as in the United States.

THE OREGON SOCIAL LEARNING CENTER PROGRAMS

The Oregon Social Learning Center (OSLC) programs address a somewhat wider age range of children (3–12 years rather than the 3–8 age group targeted by the two compliance-focused programs described earlier). The programs focus on aggression as well as noncompliance. They have been well manualized (e.g., Forgatch, 1991; Patterson, 1976; Patterson, Reid, Jones, & Conger, 1975). They usually commence with bibliotherapy, where the application of social learning principles to family life is outlined (Patterson, 1976). Initially, parents learn to identify and track various behaviors of their child. Parents normally identify two or three behaviors, often including noncompliance, that concern them, and then monitor these behaviors for daily 1-hour periods over seven days. Once the child's behaviors are reliably monitored, a positive reinforcement system is introduced, using points and backup reinforcers (privileges or treats) as well as social reinforcement (e.g., attention and praise). Once the positive reinforcement schedules are in place, a 5-minute time-out procedure for aggressive behavior and noncompliance is taught. Response cost (loss of privileges) and mild punishments (work chores) are also used. Parents are increasingly encouraged to be proactive in drawing up and implementing programs for specific desirable or undesirable behaviors. The program also includes a substantial component (up to 30%) in which problem solving and negotiation strategies are taught, to deal with marital difficulties, family crises, and parental personal adjustment problems (Patterson & Chamberlain, 1988[ii]).

The OSLC program is probably the most widely used parent training procedure, although not the most thoroughly evaluated. The first study (Patterson, Cobb, & Ray, 1973) reported the treatment of 13 consecutive referrals. Seventy percent of these families demonstrated at least a 30% reduction from baseline levels of deviant behavior. Several early studies replicated these findings. There is evidence from uncontrolled studies that treatment effects can but do not invariably generalize across settings, are maintained for up to 2 years posttreatment, benefit other children in the same family, and extend to deviant behaviors beyond those targeted in the course of treatment (Arnold, Levine, & Patterson, 1975[iii]; Firestone, Kelly, & Fike, 1980[i]; Horne & Van Dyke, 1983[ii]; Patterson & Forgatch, 1995[vi]; Wiltz, 1974[ii]). The program appears to be effective for children up to 12½ years of age. Fathers appear not to be necessary for parent training to be effective (Firestone et al., 1980[i]).

Studies with active control groups have yielded relatively promising results. In one study 19 families were randomly assigned to parent training or a waiting-list condition. The control group, however, turned into a treatment-as-usual contrast because 8 of the 9 families obtained treatment from various other sources in the community (which ranged from eclectic to behavioral in orientation). Treatment lasted an average of 17 hours. Home observations indicated a reduction in deviant behavior in the parent training group only, but parent-reported problem behaviors were reduced in both groups (Patterson, Chamberlain, & Reid, 1982[i]).

A larger study was reported (Patterson & Chamberlain, 1988[ii]) in which 70 families with children ages 6–12 years were assigned to parent training ($n = 50$) or a community-based eclectic family therapy program ($n = 20$). Unfortunately, the report includes findings based only on the first 34 families. The parent training group showed significant reductions in problem behaviors in the children and reductions in self-reported depression in the mothers. Further, only mothers in the parent training condition also demonstrated significant reductions in self-reported levels of depression. The review did not identify a follow-up report on the total sample from this study.

In an early study (Bernal, Klinnert, & Schultz, 1980[i]), 36 families of children with conduct problems were assigned to 10 sessions of parent training, client-centered counseling, or a waiting-list control group. Supervised graduates performed the treatment. At termination, the outcome from parent training was superior in terms of parents' behavior reports. At 4-month follow-up the parent training condition was no longer superior on parent report measures. Direct observation data showed no advantage of parent training over client-centered therapy or over waiting-list controls. The limited effectiveness of the parent training intervention was probably due to the relatively low level of intervention and the wide age range of the children studied (5–22 years).

Research by Patterson and Chamberlain specifically addressed resistance to parent training (Patterson & Chamberlain, 1994[ib]). Patterns of parent resistance interestingly correlate highly with coercive parenting discipline at home. It is argued that overcoming resistance by, for example, reframing can contribute to positive outcomes.

The original OSLC findings have now been replicated with socially aggressive children in other settings (Fleischman & Szykula, 1981[iii]; Weinrott, Bauske, & Patterson, 1979), including community-based group implementations (Fleischman, 1981). These adaptations of the OSLC program have halved the number of sessions necessary for effective implementation, from 31 to approximately 15, yet reported comparable improvements at posttreatment and 1-year follow-up.

PARENT–CHILD INTERACTION THERAPY

Parent–Child Interaction Therapy (PCIT) is a particularly successful version of parent training. It is based on the work of Eyberg at the University of Florida (Eyberg et al., 1995[ii]; Hembree-Kigin & McNeil, 1995[vi]). The therapy is designed to teach parents to build a warm and responsive relationship with their child and to teach the child to behave appropriately. The program has two phases. In the first phase (Child-Directed Interaction) parents learn nondirective play skills similar to those used by traditional play therapists. The aim is to change the quality of the parent–child relationship. In the second phase (Parent-Directed Interaction) the parent learns, within the play interaction, to direct the child's play with clear, age-appropriate instructions. The emphasis is on consistent consequences, praise for compliance, and time-out for noncompliance. Parents take turns to practice with their child behind a one-way mirror, and the therapist coaches the parent extensively through a "bug in the ear" earphone. Teaching takes place in the laboratory and is only gradually extended to the home.

Initial findings were encouraging (Eyberg et al., 1995[ii]). Mother's verbalization of praise rose from 2% at baseline to 23% after treatment, and parent negative talk fell from 6% to 1%. Although the amount of negative talk from the child did not change during treatment, compliance during mother–child interactions increased. Children's behavior problems in the treatment group fell from the clinical to the normal range. The waiting-list control did not change. Treatment effects generalized to siblings closest in age to the treated child. Classroom behaviors also showed indications of improvement.

In an early study (Zangwill, 1983[ii]), 11 families with 2- to 8-year-old children with conduct problems were randomly assigned to immediate or delayed treatment. Therapists were graduate students. The rate of punishments decreased, and the rate of reinforcements increased, together with the rate of compliance in the children. These findings were based on both home observation and parent reports. Thus, in most cases, there was generalization from clinic to home setting.

Schuhmann et al. (Schuhmann, Foote, Eyberg, Boggs, & Algina, 1998[i]) reported the interim results of a study of 64 clinic-referred families of children of preschool age who met ODD criteria. The families were randomly assigned to immediate PCIT or to a waiting-list control. Treated parents interacted more positively with their child and were more successful in dealing with their child's noncompliance than waiting-list controls. They also reported significant decreases in parenting stress and increases in internal locus of control. Parents in the PCIT group reported significant improvements in their child's behavior after treatment. The improvements were clinically significant and maintained at 4-months follow-up. Parents reported high levels of satisfaction with both process and content of PCIT therapy. A further demonstration of the effectiveness of a similar technique (McNeil, Eyberg, Eisenstadt, Newcomb, & Funderburk, 1991[ii]) not only reported change in directly observed home behavior, but also found generalization to the classroom, using both observational data and teacher ratings. Further support for the model was provided by the strong correlation between changes observed in the home and those noted at school. This method has also produced quite convincing demonstrations of generalization across siblings who were not involved in the treatment (Brestan, Eyberg, Boggs, & Algina, 1997[i]).

Further encouraging results were reported by Funderburk et al. (Funderburk et al., 1998[ii]). This study contrasted the long-term effects of a 14-week treatment of PCIT for 12 children with those of a comparison group of 72 children drawn from the classrooms of the treated children. Those in the comparison group were identified by the teacher as low problem, average problem, or severe problem children. The outcome variables included classroom observation and measures of social competence and school adjustment, as well as behavioral problems. Follow-ups were carried out at 12 and 18 months, although there was considerable attrition on some measures in the treatment group—for example, 42% on the ECBI. On measures of conduct problems, improvements were clearly maintained at 12-month follow-up and there was limited deterioration by 18 months. The percentage of appropriate behaviors on observational measures remained high at 1 year and dropped somewhat by 2-year follow-up. At 18-month follow-up the treatment group showed higher levels of inappropriate behavior than either the low or average problems comparison group and was comparable in terms of compliance and on-task behavior to the high problems group. Notwithstanding the relatively small sample size, this study is important in demonstrating both generalizability from parent training to school settings and reasonably robust maintenance of gain in long-term follow-up.

ADJUNCTIVE TREATMENTS

There have been a number of attempts to improve the generalizability of findings from parent training with various adjuncts to parent training programs. These adjuncts usually improved the effectiveness of the intervention. They have included cognitive adjuncts such as maternal (Sanders, 1982[ii]; Sanders & Glynn, 1981[v]) and child (Baum et al., 1986, November[i]) self-control and problem-solving training (Webster-Stratton, 1994[i]).

In a relatively large early study, Martin (1977[i]) assigned 43 families with aggressive or withdrawn children (5–12 years) to three groups: father involved, father not involved, and waiting-list control. Parent training was carried out in five individual sessions and included an adjunct of conflict resolution skills training. There was a 6-month follow-up. Improvement was the same, irrespective of father's involvement. The value of the adjunct was not tested. However, the heterogeneity of the sample makes the findings difficult to interpret.

Marital therapy was offered as an adjunct to parent training in a number of relatively small-scale studies. Assigning 9 of 17 mothers of young noncompliant children to parent training plus adjunctive training, Griest et al. aimed to assess the additional value of addressing the mother's perceptions of her children's behavior, personal and marital adjustment, and extrafamiliar relationships as part of parent training (Griest et al., 1982[ii]). Greater changes in child compliance and child deviant behavior were observed in the combined group at 2-month follow-up. Consumer satisfaction was also greater in the group that received additional treatment.

In a small study by Pfiffner et al., which balanced for the amount of therapist contact, 11 single-parent mothers were randomly assigned to either intensive parent training (IPT) or parent training plus training in social problem-solving skills (PTPS) (Pfiffner, Jouriles, Brown, Etscheidt, & Kelly, 1990[i]). Both groups improved relative to baseline (there was no control group), but mothers in the PTPS group reported significantly greater decreases of externalizing child behaviors, suggesting that single-parent families benefit more from parent training when nonchildrearing difficulties are also addressed in treatment.

In a study of 29 clinic-referred mothers of children with CD (mean age = 7.5), Wahler et al. (Wahler, Cartor, Fleischman, & Lambert, 1993[i]) compared parent training with an approach to social problem solving that integrates behavior management techniques within a structured curriculum, called synthesis training. This strategy aims to enhance traditional parent training interventions by facilitating a parent's discrimination between stressful stimuli emanating from child care and from other arenas. The therapist and parent discuss the parent's child care experiences and any other experiences that have some influence on child care, with the purpose of accentuating the differences between these two sets of experiences. There were three treatment conditions: parent management training (PMT), PMT + synthesis training, and PMT + synthesis training + friendship liaison. In friendship liaison, the mother brought a friend of her choice to the synthesis teaching session. There were no differences between the last two groups, and these were combined. There were significant benefits from parent training at the symptomatic (aversive behaviors) and transactional (indiscriminate reactions) levels but not at other levels. Synthesis training, however, enhanced the effect of parent training in reducing indiscriminate parenting, and the children demonstrated behavioral improvements. In contrast, neither the mothers nor the children in the PMT-only group demonstrated behavioral improvements. The small size of the sample ($n = 7$ per group) limits generalizability, however.

In an experimental study of 12 maritally discordant and 12 maritally nondiscordant families with a child with CD, Dadds, Schwartz and Sanders (1987[i]) randomly assigned 6 of each group to either basic parent training or parent training with partner support training. A strong feature of the study was that, unusually, the amount of therapist contact was consistent across the conditions. Measures of spousal support, marital satisfaction, and child deviance were collected at termination and 6-month follow-up. There was an interaction between the two conditions, with the adjunctive treatment improving maintenance of treatment effects for the discordant families assigned to this condition. In general, the most valued enhancements appeared to incorporate helpful discussions about other ongoing issues, such as marital conflict, distortion of perception of the child, and the parents' extra-familiar relationships (Prinz & Miller, 1994[i]).

In a controlled study of 42 intact Caucasian families with an alcoholic father and a child aged between 3 and 6, Nye et al. offered a 10-month (28-session) parent training and marital problem-solving program (Nye, Zucker, & Fitzgerald, 1995[v]). The data from the 23 families in an untreated control group were not included in the report. The program had limited success relative to baseline and control group. Of the 22 families in which both parents were involved, only 12 completed the treatment (55%), compared with 85% of the 20 families in which only the mothers were involved. Treatment effects were a function of maternal involvement. The group with high overall involvement (16 mothers who completed the program and were invested in the treatment) benefited from the child's negative behaviors decreasing and positive behaviors increasing. Moderate- (completers but uninvested) and low-involvement (terminated before 9 sessions) mothers ($n = 26$) reported no significant changes in the child's behavior. As maternal report of children's behavior was the main outcome variable, the internal validity of the study must be considered suspect.

Dadds and McHugh (1992[ii]) compared PMT for 22 preschool children with ODD or CD who had single parents. Mothers were randomly assigned to PMT or PMT with an adjunctive ally support training (AST). AST consisted of training an ally, recruited by the mother, to provide social support. Parent training lasted 6 weeks. Both groups showed significant improvement in terms of a reduction of disruptive and depressive symptoms, as well as an increase in positive parent–child interaction. The adjunctive AST, however, did not seem to generate extra benefit. Yet, treatment responders were more likely to report receiving social support from friends. Unfocused social support may reduce the rate of attrition in very high risk groups.

Strayhorn and Weidman (1989[ii]) reported a unique study that attempted to provide culturally sensitive parent training to multistressed low-income mother–child dyads. There were 89 predominantly African American parents (including 6 fathers) and 96 preschool children (ages 2½–6). Children had oppositional problems but no ODD diagnosis. Subjects were randomized between a minimal treatment control group of two IVM sessions and a parent training condition consisting of 10 2-hour sessions involving instruction and interactive play sessions with the children. The treatment was delivered by African American paraprofessionals recruited from the community. The interactive part was tailored to the child's developmental stage (e.g., reading, dramatic play, conversation). The PMT group was more successful in changing internalizing behaviors and attention deficit (mothers' ratings) and in an analog interaction task. In terms of oppositional behaviors (mothers' ratings), both groups improved.

Ducharme et al. reported an important and innovative modification of usual

PMT procedures for children with ODD from violent families (Ducharme, Atkinson, & Poulton, 2000[i]). Consequence procedures normally included in PMT packages can lead to confrontation between the parent and the oppositional child, potentially provoking more serious aversive interactions in parents prone to child abuse (Lutzker, 1996[vi]). "Errorless" compliance training, however, offers an alternative to the use of physical consequences for noncompliance. Following extended observation of parent–child interaction, compliance requests are categorized into four levels according to probability of compliance. In a hierarchy, easiest compliance requests are implemented first with ample rewards for compliance. Succeeding probability levels are faded in gradually. In a multiple baseline design across-group study, 15 children from 9 severely deprived families with a history of severe domestic violence against the mother, and in the majority of cases also against the child, were offered the treatment. The control in this design is maintained by experimentally delaying the initiation of the treatment for particular children. A complex observational procedure combined with parental recording was used to provide sessional information on compliance. Percentage of compliance increased by 50% at the most demanding level and remained high (in excess of 80%) for a follow-up period of 3 months. The study is an important demonstration of a new technique for adapting PMT procedures to families functioning in particularly difficult circumstances.

Cunningham, Bremner, and Boyle (1995[i]) carried out a large-group community-based parent training program and contrasted it with individual clinic-based parent training as well as a waiting-list control condition. The curriculum of the program included problem-solving skills, attending to and rewarding prosocial behavior, transitional strategies, when–then strategies for encouraging compliance, prompting the child to plan, time-out, and so on (Cunningham, 1990[vi]; Cunningham, Davis, Bremner, Rzasa, & Dunn, 1993[i]). The program used videotapes, role plays, and homework, but also had some systemic interventions to enhance problem solving, shared management responsibilities, and supportive communication. The study was particularly well controlled, with extensive effort to balance the samples and achieve treatment integrity. As enrollment was a dependent variable, inevitable differences between the groups arose. For example, as the community and control groups had somewhat higher numbers of severe problems, groups that were balanced for demographic and clinical characteristics were created. Forty-eight families participated in the community group, 46 in the clinic, and 56 in the control. There was 24% attrition by 6-month follow-up, and complete outcome data were available for only about one-third of the randomized sample. Take-up rates were higher in the community-based group for immigrant families and parents of children with severe behavioral problems. Surprisingly, parents in the community groups reported greater improvement at a symptom level in the child and in their own sense of competence at follow-up. The study, unusually, assesses the cost of the treatment, which was more than six times more cost-effective in the community than in the clinic. Although most of the children were not clinically diagnosable, this trial suggests a useful strategy for high-risk groups.

A similar study identifying children in kindergarten for high levels of aggression and hyperactive–impulsive/inattentive behaviors was reported by Shelton et al. (Barkley et al., 2000; Shelton et al., 1998, 2000[i]). Children were screened for ODD and ADHD symptoms, and those with scores of 1.5 SD or above were approached and 170 accepted (59%). Participants were randomly assigned to parent training, special treatment classroom, combined treatment, or no-treatment control. A comprehensive range of measures were implemented, including parent rating, teacher rating, psychological testing, and clinical observations. At posttreatment, the special classroom intervention appeared to produce improvements in aspects of classroom functioning, such as aggression, social skills, self-control, and so on. However, the impact on home functioning was minimal. The benefits of the parent training program were not evident posttreatment. The initial posttreatment gains for the special-classroom-treated group, however, disappeared over a 2-year follow-up period. No lasting benefits accrued to these children from an intensive, full-day, multimethod classroom intervention spanning their entire kindergarten year. Although treated children showed improvements over the study period, so did the controls, and all children remained abnormal relative to standardized measures. Posttreatment differences in the classroom should be treated with caution because neither observers nor teachers providing these measures were blind to the intervention.

Work in the United Kingdom yielded results that were different from those gained in this Canadian study. Harrington et al. (2000b[i]) randomized 141 subjects into community- or hospital-based treatment, both of which included parent training with either videotape modeling or parallel child groups. Approximately 50% of the community group and 60% of the hospital group completed more than 50% of the sessions. At 1-year follow-up there was no statistically significant difference between the two groups. The observed effects on the children in the sample were limited, however. The most marked changes associated with the intervention appeared in parental self-reports of depression. Teachers' reports of the child's behavior problems changed little, and even parental reports of the intensity of the child's behavior problems decreased only marginally. Thus, although the study was well controlled, the treatment may not have been of sufficient effectiveness in either setting for differences to emerge.

Sheeber and Johnson (1994[i]) describe a parent training program focused specifically on problems of temperament in preschoolers. The parent training program is based on one developed by Turecki (1985). It includes 9 weeks of 2-hour sessions of a principally psychoeducational nature. The program includes some skill-based components, teaching parents to recognize the way temperament characteristics contribute to the child's behavior and helping them to adjust their demands to the child's temperament characteristics. In addition, the program includes training in behavior management techniques. The program was tested on a sample recruited by advertisements. Twenty families were randomized to treatment and a waiting-list control group. All the children, ages 3–7, met criteria for being extreme on at least three of seven temperament characteristics. Comprehensive assessment revealed increases in satisfaction in the parent–child relationship, increased parental competence, and reduction in mother-rated child behavior problems. The effect was maintained at 2-month follow-up. However, the group was largely middle class and well educated.

Bradley et al. recently reported one of the briefest community-based programs of parent training (Bradley et al., 1999[ii]). Through school advertisements aimed at parents of children with problem behaviors, 222 primary caregivers were recruited. They were randomly allocated to waiting-list control or immediate intervention. Three once-weekly group psychoeducational sessions and a 1-month booster were offered, focused on supporting effective parental discipline and reducing parent–child conflict. Parenting practices and child problem behavior were assessed through parent reports. Substantial benefits were associated with this brief program, again underscoring the value of relatively low-dose early interventions for this group. Attrition rate is also reported to have been low, and user satisfaction was high.

MODERATORS OF OUTCOME

Our review has identified more than 50 studies and reveals important moderators to the effectiveness of parent training, substantiated by a number of investigations using somewhat different treatment approaches. To summarize, more severe and more chronic antisocial behavior and comorbidity with other diagnoses predict reduced responsiveness to treatment (Kazdin, 1995a[v]; Ruma, Burke, & Thompson, 1996[v]), including dropouts and negative outcomes (Patterson & Forgatch, 1995[vi]; Ruma et al., 1996[v]; Strain, Steele, Ellis, & Timm, 1982[v]; Webster-Stratton, 1996b[vi]). Extremely high levels of parental negativity toward the child also reduce responsiveness to the program (McMahon et al., 1981[ii]; Webster-Stratton, 1996b[vi]). Low SES is associated with more limited outcomes (Holden, Lavigne, & Cameron, 1990[v]; Kazdin, Siegel, & Bass, 1992[i]; McMahon et al., 1981[ii]) in particular if it occurs in combination with social insularity in the family (Dumas & Wahler, 1983[v]; Routh, Hill, Steele, Elliott, & Dewey, 1995[v]). Maternal psychopathology, particularly depression, and negative life events, also reduced the effectiveness of parent training (Dumas & Albin, 1986[v]; Kazdin et al., 1992[i]; McMahon et al., 1981[ii]; Webster-Stratton, 1996b[vi]). Single-parent status (Dumas & Albin, 1986[v]), marital disharmony (Dadds et al., 1987[i]), and maternal insecurity of attachment (Routh et al., 1995[v]) may undermine progress, but these associations are not sufficiently consistent across studies. Families with children in the preadolescent age group are more likely to drop out of treatment (Dishion & Patterson, 1992[v]).

SUMMARY

Observed abnormalities in families' interaction patterns, associated with externalizing problems, are an important empirically observable argument for parent training. Evidence that changing these patterns has the power to alter the child's behavior is very strong. Accumulating evidence shows that parent training programs may be applied to a wide range of conduct problems and effectively delivered in various settings. Aspects of service delivery that enhance its potency have been identified. On average, about two-thirds of children under 10 whose parents participate in parent training improve. Larger effects (fewer dropouts, greater gains, and better maintenance) also tend to be found for parent training when the children are younger, there is less comorbidity, the disturbance of conduct is less severe, there is less socioeconomic disadvantage in the family, the parents are together, parental discord and stress are low, social support is high, and there is no parental history of antisocial behavior. Failure to benefit from the program may be associated with parental disadvantage, lack of parental perception of a need for intervention, psychiatric difficulties (drug and alcohol problems, depression, personality difficulties), and comorbidity in the child (unmedicated hyperactivity, language disorders, mental retardation).

Helping the Noncompliant Child (Forehand & McMahon, 1981[vi]) is a program well supported by studies that show long-term improvements in behaviors, both targeted and untargeted by the program, although the studies that demonstrated this cannot exclude the possibility of spontaneous remission. However, evidence for generalization of gains from the home to school settings is poor. Adjuncts to this parent training program, addressing self-control problems in the child and mother, strengthen the maintenance of the program. The superiority of this program to systemic family therapy has not been demonstrated.

Videotape modeling group discussion (GDVM) (Webster-Stratton, 1996a[vi]) has been subjected to quite stringent tests of effectiveness and has been found to be more useful in the long-term than other therapist-assisted group discussions or videotape watching without the group discussion. Self-administered videotape monitoring is effective for relatively less severe, predominantly middle-class families. The treatment dose can be increased by including a child-oriented component and an additional parent-oriented component that facilitates children's problem-solving abilities and changes parental interpersonal skills; this appears to enhance treatment response and maintenance and increases the likelihood of clinically significant changes in the short term. Extending the process to a school setting has been partially successful, less evidently in the school than in the home. The approach so far is limited to younger children with limited adversity in their families, and a significant minority of those who participate request further help.

The *Oregon Social Learning Center program* (Patterson & Forgatch, 1995[vi]) is theoretically the most coherent approach. It has been extensively and successively applied in a wide range of contexts, with a range of adjuncts and modifications. It is effective for a somewhat wider age range than other parent training programs. It has been shown to be superior to alternative treatment (i.e. systemic family therapy), but the results of this study were not fully available to this review.

Parent–Child Interaction Therapy (Eyberg et al., 1995[ii]) is the version of parent training that most clearly follows up on general qualities of the parent–child relationship. Initial findings from the treatment of young children with ODD are quite promising, with some indication of generalization to outside the school setting. However, the approach has not been shown to be effective in older children (8–12), and it requires a clinic setting.

Adjunctive treatments such as social problem-solving skills training for single parents, partner support training for families with marital discord, and community-based treatment for high-risk and immigrant families, generally facilitate parent training.

Although parent training appears to be a powerful intervention in a number of its forms, it makes substantial demands on the families, including reviewing educational material, systematically observing the child, implementing reinforcement procedures, maintaining telephone contact with the therapist, and attending clinic sessions. These requirements may overwhelm some families, who may either fail to take up or prematurely discontinue treatment. Parent training is also culturally highly sensitive. Methods of child control are strongly culture bound. Although ethnicity has not been shown to influence outcome in all studies, parent training may not have generalized beyond the United States, partly because of the cultural specificity of many of its implicit assumptions. Evidence for the long-term maintenance of treatment gains is limited. Studies that show this most clearly are also those requiring highest therapeutic input and greatest client commitment. Dropouts can be as high as 30% in high-risk samples. The effects of parent training appear to decrease with age, and families characterized by the highest levels of disadvantage, psychopathology, and marital difficulties are least likely to benefit.

Although the literature on the effectiveness of parent management is large, and the effectiveness of this training relative to no treatment and other treatment procedures is considerable, the clinical significance of its effect is considered only in more recent studies. Generalizability beyond the home to other settings (to school, with teachers or peers) is insufficiently well demonstrated. These studies have neglected many outcome domains, including peer relations, social competence, academic functioning, and participation in activities. Although some studies show that gains from parent training can be maintained over extensive periods, less is known about whether the approach helps to prevent conditions developmentally linked to ODD, such as criminal activity and substance use in adolescents. Further long-term follow-up studies are needed to address these issues. Several reviewers note that training opportunities for professionals aiming to become competent in the parent training approach are limited.

Although the parent training approach is promising, it does not have the status of a panacea, and substantial subgroups of families with troubled children are likely neither to be suitable for nor to persist with the treatment. Families at greatest risk often respond to treatment, but the magnitude of these effects is attenuated by these risk factors.

IMPLICATIONS

All services for children under 8 should have some kind of parent training program. The evidence for the Webster-Stratton videotape modeling group discussion (GDVM program), which is also most cost-effective, is strongest. Training for staff in parent training techniques is not generally accessible and should become more widely available and affordable. Community-based treatments are cheaper and more effective than clinic-based ones, and therefore the integration of parent training programs with local activities should be explored.

More difficult children and children above the age of 8 require adjunctive treatment to parent training, to handle problems in the family, or, with older children, to address the cognitive (particularly problem-solving) deficits in the child. Some families will not be accessible and will need alternative treatments.

Child-Oriented Interventions

PSYCHODYNAMIC THERAPY

Besides a somewhat isolated study, psychodynamic treatments for disturbance of conduct in children under 10 have not been subjected to rigorous evaluation. In this study, Fonagy and Target (1994[iv]) report an uncontrolled retrospective open trial of 135 children with a range of disturbances of conduct. These children responded poorly to psychodynamic therapy, relative to a matched group of 135 children with emotional disorder. The treatments were long (2 years on average) and intensive (modal number of sessions = 4–5 sessions a week). One-third of the disturbance of conduct sample and 53% of the emotional disorder sample were no longer diagnosable at posttreatment, and 46% and 73% (respectively) showed clinically reliable improvements. These figures included a significant number of premature terminators (31%). At the end of at least 1 year's treatment, 69% of 93 cases of disruptive behavior-disordered children no longer warranted any diagnosis. Psychodynamic therapy seemed to be more effective for younger children than for adolescents, for children with ODD rather than CD diagnoses, and the additional diagnosis of anxiety disorder was found to predict persistence in treatment and good outcome. Treatment length and high intensity of treatment (4–5 versus 1–2 sessions per week) predicted greater improvements. Improvement rates compare unfavorably with those obtained with other approaches (e.g., parent training), but it should be noted that the assessment of improvement in this study aimed to encompass all contexts of the child's functioning, whereas in most other studies reported in this review, outcomes are based on either the home or school context (rather than both). In the absence of comparative studies, we cannot comment on relative effectiveness. However, the duration and intensity of psychodynamic treatment suggests unfavorable comparisons in terms of cost-effectiveness.

Moretti et al. (Moretti, Holland, & Peterson, 1994[v]) have developed an unusual therapy for CD based on attachment theory (Holland, Moretti, Verlaan, & Peterson, 1993[v]). The therapy starts with a residential program of 30 days, during which a multidisciplinary team works with the young person and the community to come to a formulation of his or her developmental and family history, the nature of the child's problem, and the functioning of the immediate family and the wider social community. During the third week the community is invited to join the team and the young person to develop a care plan. Discussion focuses on attachment issues in the family, including transgenerational attachment patterns and the functioning of the young person in that context. The outcome of the meeting is the development of a care plan covering (1) lifestyle issues (attachment issues related to vocational development, peer relations, personal hygiene, mental health, and sexuality), (2) home life issues (attachment issues related to the home settings, relationships with caregivers, significant others, and home responsibilities), and (3) school issues (attachment issues related to academic placement and educational goals, relationships with peers, and relationships with teachers). Under each of these headings the personal and family dynamics related to family issues are discussed, followed by management strategies. Recommendations from the care plan describe attachment issues rather than allocating treatment resources (e.g., the care plan may note that the youth would benefit from an adult role model and from developing vocational interests and skills—it is left to the community to decide how to implement these recommendations). From this point, community workers, the multidisciplinary team, and outreach workers work to reengage the young person with the community. The program's commitment extends to age 19. Respite care (e.g., from foster placements) may be requested at any time for 2 weeks at a time.

Data from 391 children (ages 10–17) are available at 6-, 12-, and 18-month follow-ups from this complex package of interventions. Only 32% of the sample lived with their natural parents. The caregivers reported improvements sooner than the children. At 6 months, the youths reported feeling more anxious, worrying about the past and the future. The caregivers reported a reduction in disturbance of conduct behavior on standardized scales. By 18 months, parents still reported reduction in disturbance of conduct behavior and the youths also reported lower levels of antisocial behavior and less anxiety. However, no control group was included in this study. Moreover, no official reports of conviction rates were reported to confirm the self-report measures of disturbance of conduct. The number of youths lost to follow-up threatens internal validity.

A relatively new psychodynamic approach claimed to be based on attachment theory, has been advanced at the Attachment Center at Evergreen, Colorado (Levy & Orlans, 1995). In a 2-week intensive intervention the entire family is offered 30 hours of therapy, during which cognitive restructuring, psychodramatic reenactment, inner-child metaphor, and therapeutic holding are used as the central intervention methods. In addition, the child is offered care by a "therapeutic foster mother" and has limited supervised contact with the parent. Therapeutic holding is designed to imitate the infant-nurturing position on a couch. The child lies across the therapist's lap with his or her head resting on a pillow. This allows for close proximity, eye contact, and physical restriction. There is a significant cathartic component in this intensive treatment. In a preliminary quasi-experimental evaluation, 12 treated and 11 comparison subjects evaluated before and 6 weeks after the 2-week intervention (30 hours of treatment delivered in 10 consecutive working-day sessions). Parent reports of disruptive behavior decreased in the treated group but not in the comparison group, which showed a slight increase. The measure used (CBCL) is not particularly sensitive to rapidly occurring symptomatic changes. Given that the parents are so intensively involved in the treatment, their ability to offer objective data must be treated with suspicion. A follow-up after an interval of 6 weeks also seems inadequate. The assignment to groups appears to have been driven by practical considerations, and it is unclear whether the children met diagnostic criteria for conduct problems. No follow-up was reported. This interesting and novel method of treatment is in great need of evaluation.

SOCIAL SKILLS AND ANGER COPING SKILLS TRAINING

The increasing prominence of models of conduct disturbance that emphasize social information processing deficits (Coie & Dodge, 1998; Kendall & MacDonald, 1993[vi]) has generated a range of treatment approaches that focus on the distorted appraisals of social events by children with conduct problems. The programs focus on modifying and expanding the child's interpersonal appraisal processes so that the child develops a more sophisticated understanding of beliefs and desires in others, as well as improving the child's capacity to regulate his or her own emotional responses.

A substantial body of evidence illustrates the deficits in the capacity of children with CD and ODD to establish adequate social relationships (Bierman & Welsh, 1997[vi]). Up to 40% of rejected children are aggressive. Children who are both aggressive and rejected have been shown to be at highest risk of developing antisocial behavior in adolescence (Coie, Underwood, & Lochman, 1991). Social rejection resulting from aggression may aggravate the child's violent tendencies (Fonagy, Moran, & Target, 1993). Social rejection may be an important cause of delinquent peer affiliation, which contributes significantly to adolescent criminality (Farrington, 1995[vi]). There is a good rationale, therefore, for the use of social skills training in the treatment of children with conduct problems.

A well-designed randomized controlled study compared the effect of social skills training, interpersonal problem-solving training, and a nondirective counseling control (Michelson, Mannarino, Marchione, Stern, Figueroa, & Beck, 1983[ii]). Sixty-one boys ages 8–12 years were assessed using parent, teacher, and self-report ratings, as well as peer sociometric ratings, at pre- and posttreatment and at 1-year follow-up. Only the social skills group reported significant gains, which slightly increased during the follow-up period. The other two groups declined significantly from posttreatment to follow-up.

Another group of investigators (Bierman, 1989[vi]; Bierman, Miller, & Stabb, 1987[i]) identified boys in grades 1–3 who were rejected by their peers because of their aggressive behavior. The intervention aimed at enhancing the social skills of these boys. It included coaching and shaping of social skills in the context of enjoyable activities. The program was brief (10 sessions), but according to independent assessments, disturbance of conduct in the aggressive children was markedly reduced. This outcome, as well as improved peer acceptance, was maintained at 1-year follow-up. More recent cognitive-behavioral approaches to the treatment of conduct problems often incorporate a social skills training component into multimodal treatment packages. Although these early studies illustrate the wisdom of this strategy, it is unlikely that social skills training alone will meet the complex clinical needs of severely conduct-disordered children.

Another program that has been subjected to outcome evaluation is Lochman et al.'s Coping Power, a school-based intervention (Lochman & Wells, 1996[vi]). The program is administered during the school day to primary school children with conduct problems. It is a well-manualized, well-structured 33-session program; each session has specific goals, objectives, and practice exercises. Children review examples of social encounters and discuss social cues and possible motives in these situations. The program incorporates problem-solving components. Children learn to identify problems, generate solutions, and evaluate these solutions using prosocial judgment criteria. Specific skills to manage anger arousal are practiced, with anger control strategies and anger-reducing self-talk. The range of contexts includes family and sibling interaction as well as the school situation. The first controlled evaluation (Lochman, Burch, Curry, & Lampron, 1984[ii]) showed that the program was more effective than a behavioral program with goal setting, or a no-treatment condition, in reducing aggressive and disruptive behavior in the classroom. This sample was teacher-identified, and the severity in terms of clinical diagnoses is unclear. In a subsample of this study followed up 7 months posttreatment, high levels of on-task behavior were maintained but the reductions in disruptive behavior were not (Lochman & Lampron, 1988[v]). Teacher consultation as an adjunct to the treatment appeared not to lead to significant improvements in a randomized controlled trial of 32 students (9–13 years), although both active treatment conditions were superior to the control condition (no treatment) (Lochman, Lampron, Gemmer, & Harris, 1989[ii]). A 3-year follow-up (Lochman, 1992[ii]) showed a reduction in substance use and alcohol use relative to untreated boys. Booster sessions significantly contributed to the maintenance of reduced off-task behavior. The study suggests that anger control and accurate interpersonal social understanding may be helpful to these children, but the evidence is not sufficient to suggest that anger coping skills training on its own is adequate for the treatment of ODD or CD.

A meta-analysis of self-statement modification studies (Dush, Hirt, & Schroeder, 1989) identified 48 controlled studies in which this cognitive-behavioral technique was used with children in a variety of settings (inpatient, outpatient, school, etc.) with a variety of disorders (anxiety, delinquency, hyperactivity, impulsivity). The ES for self-statement modification for disruption and aggression was small (ES = .18). The small ES reflects the commingling of disruptive and aggressive categories in the analysis, and the collapsing of data from school and clinical settings. The authors describe the range of students treated as those "vaguely identified as disruptive . . . to those . . . with extensive records of physical aggression and lack of rudimentary self-control" (p. 99). A more recent meta-analysis of school-based studies (Robinson, Smith, Miller, & Brownell, 1999[ib]) identified 6 investigations in which aggression was the primary focus of intervention and a further 6 in which hyperactivity–impulsivity and aggression were jointly addressed. The average ES across the 12 studies was 0.64. Only 6 of the 12 studies had follow-up data, and only 6 had a control group other than no treatment. Only 1 study that had both a control treatment and a follow-up produced significant ESs (Dubow, Huesmann, & Eron, 1987[ii]). On balance, then, the evidence base for the use of cognitive-behavioral methods designed to achieve increased self-control (such as verbal self-instruction) is as yet quite limited.

PROBLEM-SOLVING SKILLS TRAINING

Another well-investigated form of psychosocial treatment aimed at interpersonal cognitions is problem-solving skills training (PSST). PSST is derived from the work of Spivak and Shure (1974, 1976, 1978). It has been repeatedly shown that individuals with conduct problems are poor at generating alternative solutions to interpersonal problems and at means-to-ends thinking, fail to make appropriate attributions about the motivations of others, and fail to see the consequences of their own actions. PSST helps the young person develop interpersonal, cognitive problem-solving skills. It is an individual treatment, normally carried out in 20 sessions. The therapist explores the child's habitual ways of addressing interpersonal situations from a cognitive perspective, and encourages a step-by-step approach to solve such problems and to engage in self-talk that directs the child's attention to aspects of the problem that are likely to lead to an effective solution. Modeling and direct reinforcement foster prosocial behaviors. The treatment utilizes structured tasks, anchored to real-life situations of relevance to the young person. Other treatment components include practice, feedback, homework assignments, role-playing, and sometimes reinforcement schedules including mild punishment. Children with conduct problems receive *in vivo* practice and then learn to apply the skills to academic tasks, impersonal and interpersonal problems. Problem-solving skills training has become a component of a number of parent training programs (e.g., parent training developed by Webster-Stratton and some interpersonal skills training packages).

In one study, 56 children ages 7–13, who were inpatients on a psychiatric unit, were randomly assigned to PSST, relationship therapy or an attention placebo control condition (Kazdin et al., 1987b[i]). Behavioral ratings were collected from parents and teachers at pre- and posttreatment and at 1-year follow-up. PSST was clearly superior to the other conditions on all ratings at both posttreatment and follow-up. The PSST group moved closer to the normal range on the CBCL, but the majority of children remained in the clinical range for externalizing problems, according to both parents' and teachers' ratings.

The same investigators reported an early attempt to combine parent management training with PSST in 40 inpatient children (ages 7–12 years) (Kazdin, Esveldt-Dawson, French, & Unis, 1987a[i]). The combination treatment was contrasted with a minimal intervention control group in which the child's treatment was discussed over a comparable time period. The combined condition was highly effective: A reduction in aggression was reported both at home and at school in the combined condition but not in the contact control group. Prosocial behavior and overall adjustment were also superior in children in the combined condition.

In a further study, Kazdin et al. (Kazdin, Bass, Siegel, & Thomas, 1989[i]) contrasted PSST with (1) PSST and *in vivo* practice outside the treatment setting and (2) relationship therapy. Outcomes were assessed at symptomatic, transactional, and consumer satisfaction levels at 1 month and 1 year after the end of treatment. Children treated with relationship therapy were unchanged, but both problem-solving skills groups showed significant reductions in deviant behaviors at 1-year follow-up. Children who received client-centered relationship therapy failed to improve. The sample in this case was a mixed inpatient and outpatient group. PSST produced improvements with the milder or moderate severity outpatient group, as well as the inpatient group. Children with more severe disturbance of conduct (in terms of either frequency or intensity) were more likely to drop out or to have negative outcomes (Kazdin, Mazurick, & Siegel, 1994[v]).

In a later study (Kazdin et al., 1992[i]), these workers combined parent management training with PSST. All children participating in this exemplary study were within the clinical range of the CBCL for externalizing behavior. Sixty-four percent of the children who received PSST and whose parents received PMT were within the normal range on parent rating. When either of the treatments was administered on its own, only about one-third achieved this level of improvement. The level of stress reported in parents was also markedly reduced in the combined group. Both these effects were maintained at 1-year follow-up. Teachers' ratings of the children's behavior, however, showed smaller differences, signaling either a possible problem of generalization or, more likely, a reduced degree of sensitivity in teachers to changes in the behavior of their students. It should also be noted that the combined treatment group received more treatment than either of the other groups, raising the possibility that doubling the dose of each treatment on its own might have achieved similar outcomes. Nevertheless, the studies of PSST taken together effectively demonstrate the efficacy of a cognitive approach to pervasive conduct problems. The impact of the treatment was felt in the psychiatric unit in which the child was treated, by the parents, and by the child's teacher. These impressions of change also appeared to be unaffected by changes in the child's circumstances in the year following treatment. There is some indication from the findings that ethnic minority status may be associated with relatively poorer outcomes (Kazdin, 1996b[vi]). In general, children with comorbid diagnosis, academic dysfunction, and high levels of family impairment tend to respond more poorly (Kazdin & Crowley, 1997[v]). However, this limitation applies equally to many other treatments. The evidence for PSST, taken together with other combined treatment studies (Webster-Stratton, 1996a[vi]) is strong. It appears to be the best-supported approach currently available for the treatment of this group of children.

A challenge to the general applicability of this combination treatment is the relatively large percentage of families who discontinue treatment prematurely (approximately 40–60%; see Kazdin, 1996d[ib]). A large-scale study explored the reasons for dropping out of PSST and/or PMT treatment (Kazdin et al., 1997[v]). Of 242 children aged 3–14 years (mean age 81/2) who had been referred to a specialist outpatient unit, 39.9% dropped out. These individuals were more likely to be from minority groups, from single-parent families, on public assistance, to be from families with adverse child-rearing practices, of low SES, and with a child with a history of antisocial behavior. In addition, a specially designed Barriers to Treatment measure (Armbruster & Kazdin, 1994[vi]; Kazdin, Holland, & Breton, 1991) identified specific issues associated with dropping out, which were likely to be the immediate causes.

Families who dropped out had higher levels of stressors and obstacles that competed with treatment, including conflict with a significant other about coming to treatment, problems with other children and treatment being seen as adding to other stressors. Those terminating early also perceived the treatment as less relevant to the child's problems and appeared to have poorer relationships with the therapist. They liked the therapist less, perceived less support from him or her, and were more reluctant to disclose private information. Two further important findings emerged. First, the perceived demands of the therapy as rated by the parent (confusing, too long, costly, difficult, demanding) did not predict dropping out, although the clinician's judgment concerning this dimension did so. Moreover, low Barriers to Treatment scores served to protect these individuals whose family and child characteristics appeared to place them at high risk of dropping out. In general, it appears that social and clinical factors, as well as experiential and attitudinal ones, contributed to premature termination of treatments. Although the former factors, to some degree, may mediate the latter, they also appear to moderate them, raising the possibility of specific interventions with high dropout risk cases aimed at ensuring a reduction of treatment barriers scores before commencing the administration of the program. This is analogous to the model currently adopted in studies of psychotherapy process in adults (Safran & Muran, 2000).

These conclusions were supported by an uncontrolled study of 250 children and families treated with PSST and PMT (Kazdin & Wasser, 2000). The combination of these treatments administered to children referred to a community-based university clinic, diagnosed with ODD (33.3%), CD (38.2%), ADHD (6.0%), or major depressive disorder (MDD) (6%), was found to be quite effective in causing change over an average of 22 weeks of treatment (20–25 sessions of PSST and 16 sessions of PMT). Pre- to posttreatment effects were large in terms of child behavior change (ES = 1.25), small to medium in terms of change in parental symptoms and stress (ES = .34), and small for changes in family relationships and systemic family changes (ES = .23). Marital satisfaction did not change significantly. The changes across these domains were moderately correlated but predicted by slightly different combinations of variables assessed at referral. The greater the severity of the child's dysfunction and the higher the perceived barriers, the smaller the observed changes in the child's problems associated with treatment. The greater the barriers, the smaller the change in parental problems. Greater social disadvantage predicted less change in the domain of family function. These findings emphasize that in comparing treatments, the impact on the target problem alone may not be sufficient, and that adequate comparisons between treatments may entail comparisons in the domains of parental adjustment and family function as well.

In the Montreal Parent Training Prevention Trial, a sample of boys identified as aggressive or disruptive in kindergarten were selected from the Montreal low SES group. In second and third grade, these boys and their families were assigned to a parent training, cognitive problem-solving skills training and social skills training intervention. Annual assessments were conducted from 10th to 15th grade (Tremblay, Masse, Pagani, & Vitaro, 1996[v]; Tremblay, Pagani-Kurtz, Masse, Vitaro, & Pihl, 1995[i]; Tremblay et al., 1992). Up to age 12, the boys in the intervention condition (*n* = 46) were rated as having fewer problems, were more likely to have a positive peer group (Vitaro & Tremblay, 1994), and were performing better at school (McCord, Tremblay, Vitaro, & Desmarais-Gervais, 1994[v]) than those in the control condition (n = 58). Overall, 22% of the treated group manifested serious difficulties in school adjustment, as compared with 44% of controls. Teachers reported that boys in the treatment group were less likely to be involved in fights and that their school achievement was better. They were also less likely to be engaged in covert disturbance of conduct (stealing and trespassing). The results were more mixed at age 15, but positive outcomes in terms of substance use, friends arrested, and gang involvement were still evident (Tremblay et al., 1995[i]). There was no difference in crime record, but there was a difference in self-reported delinquency; the overall rate of 8% should be considered as low. Interestingly, there was no difference in the boys' perception of either punishment or supervision by the parents by age 15. Earlier effects on school adjustment were not maintained into adolescence.

INTEGRATED COGNITIVE THERAPY

The approaches considered earlier use a single treatment focus in their approach to the child's problems. A number of outcome studies have reported attempts at a broader treatment program, which combines a number of treatment components in a more complex package. In a meta-anlysis of cognitive-behavioral therapy (CBT) interventions for children with antisocial behavior (Bennett & Gibbons, 2000[ib]), the range of treatment components was as follows: (1) perception of social situation, (2) response generation, (3) response evaluation, (4) assertiveness training, (5) relaxation training, (6) generalizability component, and (7) self-instruction. The meta-analysis identified 30 studies. Overall, the effect on antisocial behavior was small to moderate (ES = .23). There was a trend suggesting that older children were more likely to benefit from CBT. As important aspect is that study quality was negatively correlated with ES, indicating that better studies had, in general, smaller effects. There appeared to be very large differences between the reported effectiveness of the interventions, suggesting that each of the specific CBT packages must be considered independently of the value of the general approach.

Kendall and his co-workers (Kendall & Braswell, 1985[vi], 1993) have integrated a number of elements of previously discussed programs in a 20-session CBT program for impulsive children. The treatment is well manualized and takes place over 20 sessions. In one study, 6- to 13-year-old children with DSM diagnoses of CD were randomly assigned to CBT or to supportive, insight-oriented therapy in a crossover design (Kendall, Reber, McLeer, Epps, & Ronan, 1990[i]). CBT was superior to the comparison treatment on teacher rating of self-control and prosocial behavior as well as on self-reports of social competence. Significantly more children moved out of the clinical range in the CBT treatment. A number of behavioral measures, however, showed no improvement for either of the groups. Children with lower levels of rated hostility and an internalized style of interpersonal attributions had significantly better outcomes in the treated group.

Another integrated cognitive model is the Peer Coping Skills (PCS) training program, which incorporates many important components found in the literature on risk factors for conduct problems (Blechman, Prinz, & Dumas, 1995[vi]). The program is school based and is designed to support prosocial coping by integrating low- and high-risk groups in a group information exchange, in which children are encouraged to share information about controllable and uncontrollable challenges in their lives. The focus is on sharing thoughts and feelings and engendering collaboration in the discussion of coping mechanisms (Blechman, Dumas, & Prinz, 1994[vi]). The program has undergone one evaluation (Prinz, Blechman, & Dumas, 1994[ii]). Two groups of children (6–9 years) were compared. Both samples were large (n = 60 and n=96) and included approximately 50% of children with and 50% without significant conduct disturbance. The group receiving PCS had 22 sessions. The comparison group received only a minimal classroom-based intervention. The groups were followed up at 6 months. Children both with and without disturbance of conduct benefited from PCS in terms of improved prosocial coping and social skills. Children who entered the training with significant conduct problems further benefited in terms of a reduction in teacher-rated aggression. However, this reduction did not take them out of the clinical range. Importantly, there was no evidence of behavioral contagion to the children who entered the program without disturbance of conduct. However, peer ratings of social acceptance were unchanged by the process. This implies that at least one risk factor, peer rejection, continues to be present at the end of the treatment. The research is promising, but in view of the iatrogenic effects observed in other group treatment studies, it should be implemented with caution.

Fire setting, although associated with a diagnosis of CD, is generally accepted as a particularly extreme, complex, and potentially highly dangerous problem. In the United States the Federal Emergency Management Agency (FEMA) offers a specific multicomponent program of fire safety education for fire setters. Adler, Nunn, Northam, Lebnan, and Ross (1994[v]) have shown this to be no more effective than simple distribution of educational material. Kolko (1996[v]) reported preliminary findings from a multicomponent skills training cognitive-behavioral program for fire setters. The study was based on a randomized allocation of 19 children to psychosocial treatment and 15 to fire safety education; a third group, of those who refused random allocation, were referred for a home visit by a firefighter (minimal treatment control group). The children were all male, 5–13 years of age, and had a documented child fire-setting episode in the previous 2 months in which property was burned and damaged. Children with major stressors or crises (e.g., recent physical or sexual abuse) were excluded. Psychosocial treatment consisted of cognitive-behavioral procedures designed to modify characteristics and correlates of fire setting. Children were taught generalized self-control, and therapy aimed to establish environmental conditions that encouraged behavior other than fire setting. The treatment program focused on the child's social and cognitive skills and the functional context in which they occurred (e.g., problem-solving skills, assertion skills, generating alternatives, choosing solutions, as well as creating a contingency management system). Parents also received parent management training with a particular focus on improving child monitoring. The treatment lasted for eight weekly sessions. Outcomes were available only for the presence and severity of fire setting. Initial analyses showed significant reductions in the child's and parents' report of fire involvement in the CBT group as compared with the group who had had fire safety education. These observations are preliminary and only posttreatment. As with all brief treatments, the critical question is the effectiveness of the treatment over the follow-up period.

Integrated cognitive programs are clearly well justified, both theoretically (given the wide range of problems manifested by children with CD) and empirically (given that a wide range of approaches appear to be only partially effective). The danger with the integrated approach to treatment, at least from the point of view of effectiveness research, is obscuring or even diluting genuinely effective treatment components with inert or iatrogenic ones. From a practical standpoint, multicomponent packages may be harder to translate into effective theoretical interventions in clinical settings, because they frequently require training in a number of distinct treatment approaches. Rather than ad hoc integration of various treatment components, Kazdin and Webster-Stratton's approach of systematically examining the added value of specific treatment components approaches in controlled experimental investigations is more desirable.

However, as most of the singular approaches considered are relatively complex and entail a considerable number of therapeutic components, the distinction between integrated and singular approaches may be far less clear-cut than it appears at first sight. Rather than further obscuring this picture by attempting to enhance effectiveness through integration, it may be preferable to initiate further decomposition studies that aim to identify uniquely therapeutic components of treatment procedures of known efficacy (such as PSST).

SUMMARY

Psychodynamic treatments have not been shown to be effective for children with conduct problems relative to an untreated or alternative treatment control group. Rates of clinically significant improvement appear to be lower in psychodynamic therapy than in other treatments, whereas treatment length and number of sessions are greater. Mild conduct problems are ameliorated with the help of social skills and anger management coping skills training, but there is no evidence for the use of these approaches on their own with more chronic and severe cases. Problem-solving skills training is the most rigorously investigated singular approach to the cognitive-behavioral treatment of conduct problems. Its effectiveness in combination with parent training has been demonstrated by two independent studies and it seems to be the treatment of choice for conduct problems in school-age children (8–12). Approaches that integrate social cognitive-behavioral strategies have not been shown to be superior, in terms of adaptability or effectiveness, to singular approaches, although they may be particularly relevant to some treatment-resistant individuals. The Barriers to Treatment measure offers potential for devising specific interventions aimed at the therapeutic engagement of those families at highest risk of premature treatment termination.

School-Based Interventions

Classroom-based treatments of conduct problems have not received as much attention as interventions for conduct problems in the home. Classroom intervention programs, recently reviewed by Little and Hudson (1998[ib]), are diverse; many lack empirical support, and others are not consistent with intervention strategies used in the home setting. A recent literature review (Papatheodorou, 2000[iv]) identified four approaches in current use: (1) the psychoeducational approach rooted in a psychodynamic/medical approach offering individual intervention (counseling, individual and group therapy) to the child with behavioral problems; (2) the behavioral approach applying behavior enhancement or reduction strategies in the classroom environment; (3) the cognitive approach bringing a range of skill-enhancement techniques that have emerged from developmental and social psychology, such as affective education and self-control curriculums; (4) the ecosystemic approach that sees disruptive behavior in the classroom as the function of the dynamic interactions between personal and environmental variables, rather than attributing it to either an internal or an environmental cause.

A number of attempts to tackle conduct problems have taken the school as their primary context for intervention. The rationale for such treatments is compelling (Rutter et al., 1998[ib]): (1) Children spend a high proportion of their time in schools. (2) There are major variations among schools in terms of the prevalence of disturbance of conduct, which are not accounted for by case mix. (3) Children who migrate between schools worsen or improve their behavior in the direction of the trends prevailing in the school they move to. (4) The prevalence of the level of disturbance in a school is systematically related to organizational characteristics (Maughan, 1994; Mortimore, 1995[vi]). In general, strong positive leadership; high pupil expectations; close monitoring of pupils; good opportunities to engage in school life and take on responsibility; well-functioning incentive, reward, and punishment systems; high levels of parental involvement; an academic emphasis; and a focus on learning are factors associated with schools with lower levels of problem behavior (Mortimore, 1995[vi]; Reynolds, Sammons, Stoll, Barber, & Hillman, 1996).

MODIFYING TEACHER BEHAVIOR

Psychosocial treatments of disruptive conduct in the classroom have a long history that is independent, at least to some degree, of the history of mental health interventions. Consequently, few studies include psychiatric assessments that would permit the diagnosis of ODD or CD. Nevertheless, the behaviors addressed by many school-based behavior modification programs, many of which have been carefully evaluated, are manifestations of these conditions and are therefore relevant for consideration here.

It has been argued that as teachers normally pay relatively little attention to prosocial behaviors, the amount of reinforcement offered by teachers is not sufficient to maintain the prosocial classroom behavior of children with disturbance of conduct (Martens & Hiralall, 1997[v]). Simply instructing teachers to offer more praise is unlikely to succeed, not only because teachers assume that they already praise the children adequately, but also because praise alone may have negative effects on children with severe aggressive behavior (Walker, Colvin, & Ramsey, 1995[vi]). Studies have demonstrated that changing the social behavior of the teacher on its own is unlikely to be effective for children who meet criteria for ODD or CD (Little & Hudson, 1998[ib]).

CONTINGENCY MANAGEMENT IN THE CLASSROOM

Behavioral interventions tried in the classroom initially focused on token systems (Abramowitz & O'Leary, 1991[ib]; Pigott & Heggie, 1986[ib]). One of the most effective procedures is the Good Behavior Game, in which groups within the class compete for reinforcement. Thus, the contingency is the behavior of a team rather than of an individual (e.g., Deitz, 1985). As with other token systems, the problem is maintaining treatment effects after the contingencies have been removed. For example, there is no evidence that the effect of these programs can travel across academic years (Walker, Hops, & Johnson, 1975[v]).

To strengthen the effect of contingency management, Hops, Walker, and colleagues (Hops & Walker, 1988; Walker, Hops, & Greenwood, 1981) designed a range of classroom contingency management programs. These programs are based on social learning principles, some with an emphasis on decreasing disruptive behavior (CLASS) and others on reducing aggression with peers (RECESS). The CLASS program for disruptive behavior has been evaluated with 119 children in both urban and rural settings (Walker, Hops, & Greenwood, 1984[iv]). There is evidence for both these effects being maintained at 1-year follow-up. Disruptive children participating in the program are more likely to be able to continue in mainstream schooling 2–3 years after the end of treatment. RECESS, the classroom-based program focusing on aggression with peers, is more intensive, requiring more than 40 hours of consultation time per child over a 3-month period. Data are available indicating that the program has a powerful effect while it is in place (Walker et al., 1995[vi]), but as yet there is no evidence concerning its generalizability over time. Nor have these studies examined the impact of adaptive changes on children's academic achievements and other aspects of their social adjustment. Further, the behavior of the children outside the classroom is not known. Narrow definitions of outcome such as those used in these behavioral studies may have social validity, principally for the teacher, but far less so for the child and his or her family.

A number of studies have examined the effectiveness of contingency management strategies in reducing stealing in elementary school classrooms. These studies all use response cost for stealing combined with positive reinforcement for periods when no stealing occurs (Brooks & Snow, 1972[v]; Rosen & Rosen, 1983[v]; Switzer, Deal, & Bailey, 1977[iv]). None of these studies, however, offer evidence beyond the anecdotal that interventions generalize to other settings even within the school (e.g., the cafeteria), let alone the home or other settings (e.g., stores). Further, no evidence is offered that these improvements are maintained after the unannounced theft probes (Switzer et al., 1977[iv]) or systematic searches (Rosen & Rosen, 1983[v]) have come to an end.

With the increasing burden on teachers to meet tough educational objectives, it is probably less realistic now than it was in the 1970s and the 1980s to train teachers to implement complex social-learning-theory-based programs. Given that the number of "difficult children" is limited within each class, teachers are more likely to opt for alternatives that are easier to implement than the programs themselves. One such approach pioneered by Ayllon, Garber, and Pisor (1975[v]) is home-based reinforcement. Within this system, parents administer the reinforcers and the teacher notes the child's achievement of prearranged targets.

Several outcome studies have demonstrated the value of the approach, which has the further advantage of being relatively acceptable to the parents (e.g., Rosen, Gabardi, Miller, & Miller, 1990[i]). A similar rationale underlies interventions for homework problems, whereby parents are taught to help the child divide homework into small, specific goals and to establish a time limit for completion (Kahle & Kelley, 1994[ii]). This program can also be taught relatively easily, via videotape instructions if need be (Forgatch & Ramsey, 1994[i]). For both these programs, the shared contingency management approach increases parental involvement in the child's school life, which is known to protect children from disturbance of conduct. The long-term outcome of these interventions is unknown, but their relatively low cost recommends them as part of preventive interventions.

A large-scale randomized controlled study contrasted the impact of parent training, multiple behavioral interventions in a special classroom, and combined treatment with an untreated control group (Barkley et al., 2000[i]). A large group of kindergarten children were screened for disruptive behavior with the use of a parent report form, and 158 were identified for randomization into four groups. Fifty-seven percent of the sample met criteria for ODD, 12% for CD, and more than 50% of the sample met criteria for ADHD. The classroom intervention included a token system, a response cost, overcorrection and time-out from reinforcement, group cognitive-behavioral self-control training, group social skills training, group anger control training, and a daily report card for home based reinforcement. A parent training program was offered to parents in a group format over 10 weekly sessions and monthly booster sessions for the rest of the school year. The program was based broadly on the Oregon model. A comprehensive set of outcome measures were used pre- and posttreatment by parents and teachers, as well as psychological testing and clinic behavioral observation. Children who received the classroom intervention were reported by their teachers to be superior in their behavior and social skills (Social Skills Rating Scale), to show less aggression and attention problems (CBCL-Teacher Report Form), to show less externalizing behavior (CBCL—Direct Observation Form), and to score higher on the Normative Adaptive Behavior Checklist as rated by parents. There were no benefits from parent training. There were no effects on any of the laboratory or psychological test measures. This well-conducted study is important because it highlights the limited value of parent training when applied to groups of parents who did not themselves seek treatment, yet whose children are relatively disruptive. School based treatments appear to be effective, but the generalizability of these effects to the home setting are suggestive rather than compelling. No follow-up of the sample has been reported so far.

APPLICATIONS OF THE ECOSYSTEMIC APPROACH

At a theoretical level, the ecosystemic approach appears to be promising in dealing with behavior disorder at school, but many have suggested that the approach is resistant to the quantitative methods used in the field (Carpenter & Apter, 1988).

Several attempts have been made to tackle disturbance of conduct in schools by modifying the school atmosphere. These initiatives have taken bullying as their focus. Bullying has surprisingly high prevalence in both the United States and Europe (e.g., Farrington, 1993). The interventions increase awareness of bullying throughout the school, promote antibullying attitudes by highlighting the dangers of bullying, encourage both victims and bystanders to seek adult assistance, and include peer mentors who observe the bullying and report it to teachers. On balance, these interventions are system oriented rather than person oriented, although the extent of person orientation varies somewhat between implementations.

The approach originated in Norway in the work of Dan Olweus (1996[v]). A nationwide antibullying campaign was undertaken and evaluated, including 2,500 students from 4th to 7th grade in Bergen schools (Olweus, 1991[v]). The design was quasi-experimental, permitting time-lagged comparisons between children in the trial and others of the same age who had not yet received the intervention. The principal outcome data were self-reports by the students. The program succeeded in substantially reducing bully–victim problems after 8 months of intervention, an improvement that was maintained at 20 months. School atmosphere also improved, and there were reductions in truancy, vandalism, and theft (Olweus, 1992[v]; Olweus, 1993[v]). The causal influence of the intervention is further supported by the finding of a dose–response relationship between the success of implementing the program and the size of the reduction in bullying. An important feature of the program is the inclusion of difficult-to-treat preadolescents in the sample. It may be argued on the basis of the prevalence rates of serious offenses in the two countries, however, that Norwegian preadolescents reflect risks of delinquency comparable with much younger children in the United States.

Smith and his colleagues administered a somewhat modified program in a replication study in 23 U.K. schools (Smith & Sharp, 1994a[vi], 1994b[vi]). The U.K. program was also quasi-experimental in design and incorporated an antiracial harassment component. It too reported substantial success in terms of a reduction in the level of aggression and intimidation in participating schools. However, these effects were most evident in elementary schools and there was substantial variation between the schools in terms of the degree of change effected.

A similar program in Canada was somewhat less successful (Pepler et al., 1993[vi]; Pepler, Craig, Ziegler, & Charach, 1994[v]). The program was implemented in four Toronto schools over an 18-month period. There were student-reported improvements in terms of personal experience of bullying as well as changes of atmosphere at the school level. Teachers also reported an increased level of interventions with bullying problems. However, victims' reports of racial bullying increased over the same period. This may have been the consequence of the greater awareness of violence created by the program. Perhaps critically, parent involvement, although a goal in this program, was not fully achieved. Similarly, Boulton and Flemington (Boulton & Flemington, 1996[ii]) found no substantial changes in secondary school students' attitudes after a single antibullying video session.

A Flemish study (Stevens, Van Oost, & de Bourdeaudhuij, 2000[i]) randomly assigned 24 primary and secondary schools to an experimental control condition from a pool of 50. The program was in place for 1 year, and posttests were obtained at the end of the school year and at the end of the subsequent year. The primary outcome measure was a questionnaire based on Olweus's instrument measuring students' attitudes toward bullying and involvement in solving bully–victim problems. One hundred thirty children from the experimental group and 193 from the control group completed the measure. The instrument yielded relatively small treatment effects for primary school children, indicating smaller decreases in rates of intervening for pupils in the experimental condition as compared with the control condition. In the secondary school children there were more substantial differences in attitudes and behavior at the end of treatment, but these disappeared in the year after the treatment was completed. The major limitation of the study is the lack of demonstrated validity for the key outcome measure.

A pilot program in the United States introduced by Twemlow in (Twemlow, Fonagy, & Sacco, 2001; Twemlow, Sacco, Giess, Ewbank, & Fonagy, 2001[iii]) Topeka, Kansas, used a quasi-experimental design to contrast two elementary schools, one with a schoolwide antibullying program, the other with an individual-focused antiviolence program supported by mental health consultation. The systemwide implementation included a 2-week martial arts training for all the children. Over a 2-year period, substantial improvements associated with the schoolwide implementation were observed. Disciplinary referrals to the principal for aggression and violence were reduced. There was also an almost 15% improvement in Standardized Achievement Test scores.

School-systemwide nonviolent programs show promise. Their effectiveness in reducing conduct problems is unknown. None of these studies report the number of clinical referrals for ODD and CD as variables. The precise characteristics of the program administered may be critical to its effectiveness. As with any systemwide implementation, experimental controls have been difficult to implement, and therefore the variability of outcomes may be explained by partial or even poor implementations. Experimental, in particular randomized, control studies, contrasting antibullying programs with best available alternative treatments, are urgently needed.

Conflict resolution training programs are quite widespread in the United States. *Resolving Conflicts Creatively* (RCC) operates in at least 350 schools nationwide and provides conflict resolution training for teachers, administrators, and parents, along with classroom instruction for students and peer mediation to resolve disputes between students. A comprehensive evaluation found that students in classrooms where teachers taught many RCC lessons (an average of 25 per year) showed far less aggressive behavior and better academic achievement than children who were not exposed to the program (Aber, Brown, & Henrich, 1999[ii]). *Peacebuilders*, which operates in some 400 schools, does not offer a classroom curriculum but focuses on improving the school climate by teaching and reinforcing five schoolwide principles: (1) Praise people, (2) avoid put-downs, (3) seek wise people as advisors and friends, (4) notice and correct the hurts one causes, (5) right wrongs (Flannery, 1997). This program is currently being evaluated as part of a 6-year federal program. Preliminary findings suggest teacher-rated increases in social competence and declines in aggressive behavior. Participating schools experienced reductions in visits to the nurse's office for the treatment of injuries. A multicomponent social development program in Seattle offered schoolchildren 6 years of social competence training, parenting skills training and training, for teachers in classroom management and interactive instructional techniques. The program followed the students to age 18 and found that, as compared with the control group, the participants committed fewer violent acts, drank less heavily, were less likely to have multiple sexual partners, misbehaved less in school, and were more committed and attached to school (Catalano, Berglund, Ryan, Lonczac, & Hawkins, 1999[ii]).

SUMMARY AND IMPLICATIONS

The modification of teachers' behavior is unlikely by itself to cause clinically significant outcomes in individuals with severe conduct problems. Classroom contingency management methods are demonstrated to be effective in controlling the behavior of children with conduct problems in that setting, but they have not yet been shown to generalize beyond the classroom situation or beyond the termination of the programs. The primary goal of teachers is to deliver an educational service. Complex programs may be seen as compromising this goal, yet disruptive children may prevent effective learning for the silent majority over the long term. Parent-administered reinforcements may enhance classroom contingency management in universal or selective prevention programs. Where children have behavior problems in the classroom, the addition of contingency behavior management programs in the classroom should be considered, in addition to family-based treatments. All schools should consider the implementation of antibullying, antiviolence programs.

Psychosocial Treatment Interventions for Adolescents

Meta-Analytic Findings and Reviews

Meta-analyses of treatment approaches to juvenile delinquency have produced relatively clear-cut findings (Andrews et al., 1990[ib]; Lipsey, 1995[ib]; Lipsey & Wilson, 1998[ib]; Lösel, 1995a[ib], 1995b[ib]). In his 1995 meta-analytic review, Lipsey attempted to address the broad question of whether treatments for delinquency work, by considering together the results of nearly 400 published control or comparison group studies from English-speaking countries, yielded by searching the literature since 1950. He found an overall reduction of 10% in reoffending rates in treatment groups as compared with untreated or "treatment as usual" groups. Lipsey reports considerable variation in results across studies. Part of this variance is accounted for by the associations of ESs with a range of alternative available outcome measures (categorized by Lipsey as psychological outcome, interpersonal adjustment, school participation, academic and vocational performance). ES also varied with client characteristics and different treatment approaches.

Lipsey found that older juvenile offenders with longer histories of offending were slightly more likely to benefit from treatment. He suggests that this unexpected finding may be due to the fact that there is more room for improvement with these individuals. He divided treatments into juvenile justice treatments (treatments provided in addition to supervision within the juvenile justice system) and non-juvenile justice treatments. Of the former, employment and multimodal, behavioral, and skill-oriented treatments produced a 20% or greater improvement in reoffending rates as compared with the control group. Of the latter, skill-oriented, multimodal, and behavioral treatments and group counseling produced comparable improvements. Lipsey commented that there was little information in the original reports regarding details of the treatment process, making it more difficult to use the meta-analysis for recommending treatment strategies for clinical settings.

Broadly speaking, the largest reported effects among the domains of outcome organized by Lipsey emerge within those categories least associated with a reduction in reoffending rates, an intriguing finding that he does not discuss. For example, there is most improvement on measures of psychological outcome (28%), followed by academic performance (14%), interpersonal adjustment and school participation (both at 12%), and vocational accomplishment (< 10%). On the other hand, reduced recidivism is most highly associated with school participation, followed by vocational accomplishment, interpersonal adjustment, psychological measures of outcome, and academic performance. There are a number of possibilities: (1) Many interventions may be focusing on the wrong mediators of offending behavior (mental health professionals, for example, persist with the notion that psychological health is the most significant causal mediator of delinquent behavior in the face of the evidence); (2) reduction of recidivism may not always be the most important aim in the treatment of adolescent offenders; (3) treatments may sometimes be focused on one aspect of a young person's difficulties but end up producing change in another. Most likely, all these possibilities apply to many studies to varying degrees.

The meta-analytic results of these studies in both juvenile justice and non-juvenile justice settings, which include many studies of various punishment and custodial care alternatives beyond the scope of the present review, appear to point to clear conclusions. Highest ESs within both settings derive from behavioral, skills-oriented, and multimodal methods. This conclusion is consistent with the U.K. Home Office Research Study Report (Vennard, Sugg, & Hedderman, 1997[ib]), which concluded that cognitive-behavioral methods have greatest promise in reducing antisocial behavior in adolescents. More specifically, they observed that treatment approaches that were active, participatory, and problem solving, were aimed at the genesis of the offending behavior, were of sufficient intensity and duration, and were rigorously administered were most likely to be successful. Kazdin (1997c[vi]) offered a set of further stipulations. He suggested that treatments based on a clear and evidence-based model of the cause of CD were most likely to be effective, that independent measurement of the mechanisms implied by the causal model was possible, and that there was evidence that the treatment changed these intervening mechanisms.

However, it should be noted that systemic, psychodynamic, and integrative eclectic approaches are underrepresented. Further, although ESs suggest significant change, these are substantially smaller than the ESs normally obtained for psychosocial interventions. It seems that the effectiveness of interventions aimed at the reduction of adolescent antisocial behavior is only about half that of comparable interventions aimed at addressing educational or other mental health problems (Lipsey & Wilson, 1993[vi]). Nevertheless, the limited effectiveness of "traditional" methods of intervention, based on the principle of deterrence, justifies interest in mental health interventions in delinquency.

Lipsey reported interesting results for traditional deterrent approaches to juvenile crime (shock incarceration, boot camps, transfer to criminal court). Deterrent approaches, presumably based on the negative reinforcement of offending behavior, constituted one of only two treatment categories that produced a negative effect, calculated as a 25% increase in reoffending rates; the other was "vocational counseling," which produced a less marked negative effect. Lipsey qualified this result by explaining that the number of studies measuring the effect of deterrence on reoffending was quite small.

However, Bishop et al.'s study of the effects on reoffending rates of transferring young offenders from the juvenile justice system to criminal court in the state of Florida between 1985 and 1987 impressively backs up Lipsey's summary of the negative outcome of punitive approaches (Bishop, Frazier, Lanza-Kaduce, & Winner, 1996[iv]). Bishop et al. used a case-control design; 2,738 young offenders transferred to criminal court within this time period were matched on a case-by-case basis with young offenders retained within the juvenile justice system, based on the number and seriousness of transfer offenses, the number and seriousness of prior offenses, and sociodemographic characteristics (age, gender, and race). Their outcome measures were individual and group rates of rearrest, the severity of the charge leading to rearrest, and the time that elapsed before rearrest. They took into account the possibility of a misleadingly positive outcome as a result of transferred juveniles being locked up and therefore unable to reoffend during the 2-year follow-up period, by excluding from the sample those subjects who remained locked up and being explicit about a standard estimate of 3 months for the average time of imprisonment, because this information was not available. Bishop et al. found that within their matched pair comparisons, juveniles in the rearrested transfer group were significantly more likely to reoffend across all but the lowest of seven levels of severity of offense. Group levels of rearrest were 30% in the transfer group, compared with 19% in the nontransfer group, after an average of 135 days since release for the former and 227 days for the latter. Overall, 93% of the rearrested transfer group were charged with felony offenses, compared with 85% of the nontransfer group—a small but telling difference.

In the conclusion to a definitive volume reviewing the effectiveness of efforts at reducing reoffending, McGuire and Priestley (1995[vi]) identified six principles that could guide effective programs. These were that (1) the intensity of the program should be in line with the size of the risk represented by the individual, (2) active participatory methods for working should be used that are neither didactic nor experiential and unstructured, (3) there needs to be a close integration with the community from which the youth originates, (4) programs should seek to target several problems, using a predominantly behavioral and cognitive-behavioral approach, (5) the program should have high integrity, with aims and methods tightly integrated, high level of staff training, and a close monitoring of treatment delivery, and (6) the focus needs to be on factors that are closely rather than distantly related to offending behavior. These factors include antisocial attitudes, feelings, peer associations, the promotion of family affection and communication, family monitoring and supervision of the adolescent, identification and association with anticriminal role models, increasing self-control, self-management, and problem-solving skills, reducing chemical dependencies, shifting the balance of rewards and costs from criminal to noncriminal activities across a range of settings, changing life circumstances in the direction of reducing risk, helping clients to recognize risky situations and providing them with well-rehearsed plans to deal with them (Andrews & Bonton, 1994). Unpromising targets are enhancement of self-esteem, increasing the cohesiveness of antisocial peer groups, increasing conventional ambition in the areas of school and work without assistance to the means to realize these ambitions.

These are logical and reasonable conclusions from the literature, but are not, strictly speaking, evidence based, insofar as they have not formed the basis of independent experimental outcome investigations. General conclusions such as the ones mentioned earlier may point to quite large groups of interventions, only some of which may be efficacious.

Innovative Methods of Service Delivery

Historically, juvenile justice policy has tended to oscillate between rehabilitative and punitive approaches to managing juvenile delinquency. In the 1970s and early 1980s policy and practice in the United States and Europe mostly emphasized individual treatment for young offenders in nonsecure, community-based programs. A perceived increase in violent youth crime during the late 1980s and early 1990s renewed interest in punishing delinquent youths. Mapping such fluctuations in policy to overall crime rates does not reveal any clear relationship (Jenson & Howard, 1998). Although it is beyond the scope of this chapter, it is important to note that various psychosocial models of CD/delinquency have been integrated with juvenile justice delivery systems in both the United Kingdom and the United States.

The Audit Commission (1996[vi]) describes a range of interesting and innovative service responses to the problem of youth crime in the United Kingdom, Europe, and North America. Some of these have not been evaluated. For example, the NCH Action for Children Project is particularly comprehensive, offering young offenders the opportunity to explore the causes of their criminal activity, as well as offering training in basic educational and social skills, job searches (for those ages

17 and above), and information on drug abuse; yet this program has not been evaluated and is vastly underused. It appears that either writers of presentence reports have recommended lower levels of intervention to the courts or the courts have ruled in favor of custodial sentences. Full evaluation of the program may persuade probation officers that a multilevel approach tackles reoffending among juveniles more effectively in less severe cases.

The innovative projects that have been evaluated have produced impressive results. The South Carolina Department of Mental Health program for juvenile offenders revealed that 50–70% of youths within the juvenile justice system had diagnosable psychiatric disorders (Cuffe, Hall, & Rogers, 1999[v]). In the first 3 years of the program, which offers highly intensive and long-term treatment, only 28 of 224 juveniles have reoffended. In Orange County, California, an intensive intervention program was initiated in 1994 specifically for youths ages 15 or younger at first offense who displayed multiple risk factors for recidivism (e.g., school failure, family discord, substance abuse, and predelinquent behavior)—thought to be 8% of delinquent youths. The program was aimed at intervening with the 8% of youths who become chronic juvenile offenders (Schumacher & Kurz, 2000). The pilot results indicate that 49% of extreme risk offenders were adjudicated, compared with the historic rate of 93%. More recently, Orange County has randomly assigned extreme risk youths either to the 8% *program* or to usual probation services. After 1 year, 20% of the treatment group had been arrested two or more times, compared with 43% of those receiving usual services. In general, there is ample evidence that diversion away from detention prior to trial helps in reducing recidivism by 50% (Shelden, 1999[ii]) and that keeping youths out of the adult penal system also decreases the risk of reoffending (Mendel, 2000[iii]). Despite high recidivism rates, there will always be a need for locked facilities for young people, but the degree to which these encourage reoffending appears to vary considerably depending on structural and programmatic factors. For example, the Florida Environmental Institute, also knows as the Last Chance Ranch, serves some of Florida's most serious juvenile offenders (average of 18 prior offenses). The program has a low offender-to-staff ratio and uses a three-step rehabilitative process: (1) a work and education phase, (2) an intermediate phase, in which youths participate in paid work projects to help make restitution payments, and (3) an intensive aftercare phase. The 1-year recidivism rate of this facility has ranged from 15–29%, which is far below that of most correctional programs (Associated Marine Institutes, 1999[v]).

The Dalston Youth Project in the London Borough of Hackney (United Kingdom), which provides a range of activities as well as local volunteer mentors, led to a 61% drop in reoffending among the users of the project in comparison with the rate the year before they joined. The project, however, also reported high rates of noncompliance. The Northamptonshire Diversion Unit, which combines individually tailored programs to prevent reoffending with reparation for victims, resulted in significantly lower than normal reoffending rates and large measures of satisfaction in victims. The HALT scheme, which is based in Rotterdam and involves reparation and education, led to 40% rates of reoffending, compared to 80% rates in young offenders who were prosecuted in the usual way (Audit Commission, 1996[vi])

A variety of "restorative justice programs" are under way in the United States. These include family group conferencing, peacemaking circles, juvenile drug courts, teen courts, and youth aid panels. There are limited evaluation data on these initiatives, although the trend is encouraging. In Philadelphia, 80% of young people participating in youth aid panels complete their contracts success-fully and recidivism rates are reported to be only 22% (DiIulio & Palubinsky, 1997[v]).

These evaluations are comparatively wide ranging in terms of the outcome measures used. They not only examine reoffending rates but also assess rates of inte-gration into mainstream schooling and employment. Generalizing from these and many similar projects is also particularly difficult because of their complex structure and necessarily idiosyncratic character, which is comprehensively adapted to par-ticular service contexts. Moreover, they are rarely driven by comprehensive theo-ries of the causes of delinquency (Kazdin, 1997c[vi]). They are mentioned here only to indicate the largely untapped potential for improvements in service delivery in reducing reoffending rates. In particular, there appears to be support for the integra-tion of efficacious psychosocial treatment strategies with juvenile justice service provision.

Family-Based Interventions

Family-based interventions for adolescent conduct disorders are commonly recom-mended (e.g., Lebow & Gurman, 1995[vi]), inasmuch as family factors are clearly associated with adolescent behavior problems (e.g., Kumpfer & Szapocznik, 1998). Families of adolescents with conduct problems tend to show less warmth, affection, and emotional support for the adolescent, more negative communication, and less participation in joint family activities (e.g., Steinberg, Darling, Fletcher, Brown, & Dornbush, 1995). Studies of parent training are abundant, but relatively few out-come investigations specifically focus on adolescents with conduct problems. A re-view by Chamberlain and Rozicky (1995[vi]) identified only seven studies between 1988 and 1994. In the 3–10 year age group the kind of parental influences encour-aged in this treatment model (for example, the delivery of praise, attention, and privileges) are likely to have quite a significant impact on the child's behavior. As the child enters adolescence, however, the importance of parents appears to de-crease and peers acquire a more central role, particularly in terms of the promotion and maintenance of antisocial behavior (Allen & Land, 1999[vi]; Elliott, Huizinga, & Menard, 1988[vi]). This may be one reason that adolescents appear less respon-sive to parent training. An alternative account is offered by the severity of symp-toms. In general, youths referred in adolescence for conduct problems suffer from a more chronic and more severe disorder (Kazdin, 1997b[ib]). Another explanation may be that the treatment needs to be modified to achieve greater age appropriate-ness.

MODIFICATION OF THE OREGON MODEL

The Oregon model was modified to address conduct disturbances in adolescents that were considerably more severe than those in the younger group (Bank et al., 1991[i]; Forgatch & Patterson, 1989[vi]; Patterson & Forgatch, 1987[vi]). The extension of the program involved targeting risk behaviors for delinquency (such as poor class attendance, affiliation with antisocial peers, drug use, etc.), general enhancement of parental monitoring, and replacement of the time-out procedure with more radical punishments (e.g., restriction of free time and restitution of stolen property). Parents are asked to report the child's offending behavior to the juvenile authorities and then act as advocates in court. The adolescent is actively engaged in setting up behavioral contracts.

The effectiveness of this procedure appears limited. In one study (Bank et al., 1991[i]), 55 boys (mean age 14) with an average of eight previous offenses were randomly assigned to modified parent training or treatment as usual, which in this case normally included services available to the court through local agencies (group counseling focused on drug use, behavioral family systems therapy, etc.). The primary outcome measure was court-documented offenses. In addition, home observation and parent daily report forms were completed, but only in the parent training condition. Treatment duration was 45 hours, but approximately 50% of these sessions were over the telephone. Posttreatment booster sessions were included for about half of the families. Each control group family received treatment estimated at more than 50 hours on average. During the treatment there was a reduction in offense rates in the experimental group. At 1-year follow-up and 3-year follow-up, both groups showed reduced rates of offending. However, the amount of time in institutions during treatment and during the first 2 years of the follow-up period was significantly reduced for the experimental group. The differences disappeared by the third year. On the whole, the effects, including the impact on family interaction patterns, were small and consisted mostly of a more rapid rather than a larger change. The Oregon program seems to be more effective with a younger, less severe group.

In a more successful but smaller-scale study including 28 families of children ages 5–14, the referral problem was specifically stealing (Reid, Hinojosa Rivera, & Lorber, 1980[ii]). The treatment was a modification of the Oregon model with increased emphasis on the identification of stealing, including suspicion that the child had stolen. A mild negative contingency was attached to such an event. The treatment lasted 32 hours, and at posttreatment and 6-month follow-up parent-reported stealing was significantly reduced. A waiting-list control showed no changes over the treatment period. A complication is presented by the finding that children referred for stealing, a number of whom do not complete treatment, are more likely to be labeled as delinquent years after the referral (Moore, Chamberlain, & Mukai, 1979[ii]). Seymour and Epston (1989[v]) implemented a similar program with 45 consecutive cases; in this study there was no control group. The reduction from pre- to posttreatment was substantial, with more than half reporting no stealing at 2-month follow-up and the overall frequency of stealing markedly reduced for the whole sample. At 1-year follow-up, 62% of the sample reported no stealing and 90% reported substantial reduction. However, none of these studies explored generalization across settings, and the parents' reports on which these findings were based are particularly suspect because of the relatively low parental involvement with the adolescents in this group.

The Oregon model was tested most stringently by a study that compared it with an approach focused on the 10- to 14-year-olds themselves (Dishion, Patterson, & Kavanagh, 1992[vi]). Dishion and Andrews (1995[i]) studied 158 families with adolescents ages 10–14 randomly assigned to one of five groups: parent training (n = 26), an adolescent group for self-regulation enhancement (n = 32), combined parent and adolescent treatment (n = 31), a self-directed change control group (n = 29) and a quasi-experimental placebo control with no intervention (n = 39). An attempt was made to balance girls and boys across groups. The sample was only in part clinical, with a number of families identified through newspaper advertisements and community flyers. The adolescents participating were mostly within the clinical range on the CBCL. There was a 1-year follow-up. The parent training followed the Oregon 12 group session model. The adolescent-focused treatment approach concentrated on self-monitoring and tracking, prosocial goal setting, peer relationships, communication skills, and problem-solving skills. Teenagers defined their own behavior change goals (in this study, 75% selected improved school performance). The adolescent-focused cognitive-behavioral treatments also took place in group settings. The self-directed change condition did not involve weekly group meetings or therapist contact. Members of this group received the intervention materials that accompanied the other interventions (six newsletters and five brief videotapes). The quasi-intervention group received no intervention and were contacted only for assessment purposes. Attrition was high: 30% in the three intervention conditions and 53% in the self-directed change control group.

The results were disappointing. According to mothers' reports, significant decreases in externalizing behaviors occurred in all groups (including both control groups) by termination, but this was not maintained at 1-year follow-up. The adolescent-only condition and the parent and adolescent condition were comparable to the control groups. According to teacher report at termination, adolescents assigned to the parent-focused group showed significantly lower rates of externalizing behavior relative to control, mainly accounted for by a steep increase in externalizing behavior in the control group over this period. Thus, the parent training program appeared to arrest an underlying tendency toward deterioration. At follow-up, the control groups were below baseline level, but the adolescent-only group and combined groups deteriorated relative to posttreatment. The externalizing ratings for the adolescent-only CBT groups were significantly above the control group levels. A similar pattern was reflected by tobacco use as an outcome variable. The study suggests that group treatment of adolescents with behavioral problems may have iatrogenic effects. The parent training model was only marginally superior, probably due to the negative effects of the group setting in which the adolescents were treated.

The available evidence suggests that parent training is not a particularly effective intervention for adolescents. Studies showing high levels of effectiveness with this approach tend to have predominantly younger children with ODD diagnoses. Severe and chronic CD appears to require more intrusive treatment approaches. It seems that behavior patterns are too well established by adolescence for the young person to respond to changes in the management or behavior contingencies deployed by parents alone. Moreover, the systems established within the families of conduct-disordered adolescents over years of transactional interaction may be too deeply rooted in the parents' behavior to be shifted by a relatively brief intervention.

FUNCTIONAL FAMILY THERAPY APPROACHES

The functional family therapy (FFT) approach advocated by Alexander and Parsons (1973[v], 1982) assumes that an adolescent's problem behavior is serving a necessary function, such as regulation of support and intimacy or regulation of distance between family members, and the treatment focus extends to interactional aspects of the family processes as well as behavioral and cognitive dysfunctions. The goal of treatment, therefore, is the achievement of a change in patterns of interaction and communication, in a manner that engenders adaptive family functioning. Highly conflicted family interactions are a primary target of family interventions with youths who have behavior problem. An initial goal of therapy involves disrupting negative interactions to facilitate a treatment atmosphere conducive to enhancing adaptive family functioning, by reframing conflicted interactions in a manner that is benign and nonblaming and disrupts the family's normal negative style of interactions. The therapist's goal is not to change underlying beliefs or feelings, but rather to disrupt or alter negative family interactions. The formulation is based on social learning concepts, with a focus on specific stimuli and responses that have the power to produce change. Like multisystemic therapy (MST) (see the discussion following) FFT works with youths in their homes and targets both the family and the individual behavior of the youth.

The treatment approach effectively integrates behavioral perspectives with family systems principles and cognitive and emotional processing perspectives (Alexander, Jameson, Newell, & Gunderson, 1996[vi]). The current FFT approach consists of several treatment components (Alexander, Waldron, Newberry, & Liddle, 1988[vi]). Initially, the blaming attributions prevalent in the families of delinquent adolescents are identified. The behavioral, cognitive, and emotional expectations, inappropriate attributions, and systemic processes in need of change are pinpointed and addressed, using predominantly cognitive methods. For example, negative labels assigned to specific family members are reframed in a positive light. The therapist points out interdependences and contingencies in the day-to-day functioning of family members in the context of the child's behavioral problems. The cognitive aspects of the program are followed by behavioral components, including communications skills training, behavioral contracting, and contingency management. The treatment encourages reciprocity and positive reinforcement among family members. There is emphasis on clear communication, both in the expression of interpersonal needs and in the constructive process of negotiation to arrive at a solution to interpersonal problems. Family members reciprocally identify desirable behaviors in others, and these are integrated into a reinforcement system aiming to promote adaptive behavior. The focus is on family communication patterns as these are observed in the consulting room. The therapist provides social reinforcement throughout.

Alexander and Parsons (1982[i]) contrasted FFT with client-centered and psychodynamic family interventions, as well as with attention placebo and no-treatment control groups. The latter treatments were provided as part of community services. FFT was superior to the other treatments on measures of family interaction and recidivism rates over the next 2 years. The recidivism rate was 26% for the FFT condition, 50% in the no-treatment group, 47% in client-centered counseling, and 73% in psychodynamic counseling. Particularly encouraging was the offending rate of siblings over the 3-year posttreatment period (Klein, Alexander, & Parsons, 1977): 20% of the siblings of adolescents involved in FFT, compared with 40%, 59%, and 63% for the no-treatment, client-centered and psychodynamic counseling groups, respectively. Although these findings are encouraging, the relatively small size of the groups and the relative lack of gravity of the offending behavior detract from their significance.

Unusually for child treatment outcome studies, this group explored the role of therapist factors in outcome (Alexander, Barton, Schiavo, & Parsons, 1976[v]). The graduate student therapists delivering the program were rated in terms of their capacity to build relationships (warmth, affect–behavior integration, humor) and their capacity to structure the therapy (directiveness, self-confidence). The former dimension accounted for almost half of the variability in predicting outcome, and the latter, more treatment-specific, dimension accounted for a further 15% of the variability. Further process work by this group showed that reframing statements were associated with positive within-session attitudes in the adolescents but less so for the parents (Robbins, Alexander, Newell, & Turner, 1996[v]).

More recently, a strengthened version of the program including remedial education and job training has been applied to families of multiply offending, previously incarcerated delinquents (Barton, Alexander, Waldron, Turner, & Warburton, 1985[ii]). The comparison group was made up of adolescents placed in group homes. The primary outcome criterion was offending in the 15 months following the treatment. Three-fifths (60%) of participants in FFT committed an offense in this period, compared with 93% of the comparison group. The number of offenses committed also differed significantly, with FFT subjects committing significantly fewer than those in the comparison treatment. The treated subjects were six times more likely to avoid arrest than members of the control group. This finding is impressive, although the control group may have been poorly chosen in that group homes may represent an iatrogenic rather than a therapeutic influence (Dishion & Andrews, 1995[i]).

A different team from the University of Utah replicated the findings in a rural context. Gordon et al. (Gordon, Arbuthnot, Gustafson, & McGreen, 1988[ii];

Gordon, Graves, & Arbuthnot, 1995[ii]) used a somewhat longer treatment period, based in the home, with a more extensively trained and supervised therapist. Twenty-seven adolescents with multiple offenses took part and were contrasted with a probation-only control group. The recidivism rates were 67% for the probation-only group, compared with 11% in the FFT group. The subjects were followed up in young adulthood, where recidivism was 9% in the FFT group and 41% in the comparison group. Recidivism was practically eliminated for the females in the sample. However, recidivism as a primary outcome variable is fraught with problems (Gordon & Arbuthnot, 1987[vi]). These studies also offered preliminary data on intersibling generalization, with reduced likelihood of subsequent court involvement among the siblings of the identified clients (Gordon & Arbuthnot, 1987[vi]).

FFT appears to have clinically significant and lasting effects on recidivism. In nine studies carried out on FFT between 1973 and 1997, improvement of 25–80% in recidivism, out-of-home placement, or future offending by siblings of the treated young people was found. The cost of the treatment has been estimated at $2,000 per person. In contrast to parent training, which traditionally does not involve the adolescent directly addressing the maladaptive cognitive and communication patterns in such families, using the framework of social behavior theory appears to empower the family to reduce delinquent behavior in these adolescents. The program of work using FFT is particularly noteworthy because at least tentative information is available on specifically effective treatment strategies. Effective delivery of this treatment requires considerable training and supervision. This may explain why, despite the relatively well-established manner of this treatment approach, the number of FFT practitioners is limited.

FFT is unusual among psychosocial therapies for children and adolescents in having a respectable body of research work on the therapeutic process supporting and extending the research on the outcome of this form of treatment. This work includes investigations of therapist variables (e.g., Mas, Alexander, & Barton, 1985) as well microanalytic studies of interaction processes (e.g., Robbins et al., 1996[v]). Recently, Robbins et al. (Robbins, Alexander, & Turner, 2000[iii]) studied the immediate impact of therapist reframing interventions. The results indicated that such interventions had a specific impact in reducing family members' defensive statements and generating favorable responses from the adolescents.

STRUCTURAL FAMILY THERAPY

There have been a number of studies of structural family therapy (Family Effectiveness Training, FET), for adolescents with conduct problems, advocated by Szapocznik et al. (Szapocznik & Kurtines, 1989[vi]; Szapocznik, Kurtines, Santisteban, & Rio, 1990[vi]; Szapocznik et al., 1989[ii]). In one study, Szapocznik et al. (1989[vi]) contrasted structural family therapy with individual dynamic therapy. The sample consisted of 69 Hispanic boys, of whom 26 were randomly assigned to structural family therapy, 26 to individual therapy, and 17 to recreational control. Different sets of analyses were carried out with and without covarying pretest differences between the groups. Families in the FET condition showed significantly greater improvement on independent measures of structural family functioning, on problem behaviors of the child as reported by the parent, and on a self-report measure of self-concept. On parent-report data, however, all groups showed significant improvement.

At 1-year follow-up, the adolescents in family therapy improved and those in child (individual) therapy deteriorated. There was no change in the recreational control. Adolescent self-report data indicated that all treatments led to improvements in child behavior and family functioning as well as in psychodynamic aspects of family functioning, which were maintained at 1-year follow-up. However, at 1-year follow-up, although child behavior remained improved for both treatment groups, family functioning had deteriorated for the individual therapy group but had continued to improve for the family therapy group. These findings underscore the importance of measuring transaction as well as symptomatic and adaptational measures. Treating only the child appears to sufficiently treat the symptom but neglects and increases risk for family functioning.

In a more recent study, structural family therapy was far more successful than group counseling for 12- to 18-year-old Hispanic adolescents with behavioral problems (Santiseban et al., in preparation[i]). In nearly half of the structural family therapy participants with severe conduct disorders, substantial improvements were observed, compared with only 5% of youths in group therapy. The youths in structural family therapy were also three times as likely to reduce their aggression (see Szapocznik & Williams, 2000[vi]).

There are other promising family-based approaches, similar in conception to FET, from the substance abuse field (see also Chapter 10). For example, multidimensional family therapy (Schmidt, Liddle, & Dakof, 1996[v]) led to improved parenting skills in 69% of the participating families. Moreover, 71% of participating youths significantly reduced acting-out behaviors and 79% significantly reduced substance use. In a further study, hard drug use was observed to decline from 53% of participating youths at the outset to 9% at the end of treatment and 3% at 1-year follow-up. A third study found that substance abuse declined in the treatment period. This was maintained at 12-months follow-up, whereas group therapy produced only a 37% decline and multifamily education yielded only 25%.

MULTISYSTEMIC THERAPY

Multisystemic therapy (MST) is arguably the most promising intervention for serious juvenile offenders. This approach fully recognizes the multidetermined nature of serious antisocial behavior (Hawkins et al., 1992[vi]; Offord et al., 1992[v]). The treatment uses multiple interventions in combinations indicated by the clinical picture. The constituent treatments include techniques from systemic and structural family therapy (e.g., joining, reframing, enactment, paradox, the assignment of specific tasks), parent training, marital therapy, supportive therapy related to interpersonal problems, social skills components, social perspective training, behavioral methods (e.g., contingency contracting), and cognitive therapy techniques (e.g., self-instructional training), as well as case management with the therapist acting as an advocate to outside agencies.

A family focus is key to the intervention. The overriding goals of MST are to give parents the skills and resources needed to independently address the inevitable difficulties of raising adolescents, and to empower adolescents to cope with familial and extrafamilial problems. Assessment and treatment explore the adolescent's role in various systems and consider the interrelationship between these systems. Specific attention is given to strengthening the various systems and an attempt is made to promote appropriate and responsible behavior amongst all family members. Medications are offered as part of the program when necessary.

Although MST includes a number of techniques from a range of approaches, it is far more than a mere amalgamation, and the focus on the interrelationship between systems is retained. Interventions are individualized and highly flexible but are documented in treatment manuals (Henggeler, Schoenwald, Borduin, Rowland, & Cunningham, 1998[vi]). Weekly group supervision meetings with a doctoral-level supervisor ensure treatment fidelity, and supervision meetings may also include a medical consultant. The entire team reviews goals weekly to ensure a multisystemic focus. The therapy is generally delivered by a master's-level therapist with a caseload of four to eight families. The MST therapist is a full-time generalist who directly provides most of the mental health interventions and directs access to services, coordinating these to monitor quality control. The therapist is available to the family 24 hours a day, 7 days a week, but input is adjusted according to need. The course of treatment generally lasts 3–5 months. Sessions are held in the family's home and in community locations (Henggeler et al., 1998[vi]).

There is evidence that the treatment impacts on processes critical to the generation of delinquent behavior (Mann, Borduin, Henggeler, & Blaske, 1990[vi]). For example, interactions between parents and teenagers improve in terms of levels of overt conflict and hostility, there is an increase in support among family members, and the amount of verbal communication between parents increases while conflict is reduced. Importantly, adolescent symptoms have been shown to decrease in association with increased supportiveness and decreased conflict between parents.

There have been a number of trials of MST (Henggeler et al., 1996a[vi]; Henggeler et al., 1992[i]; Henggeler et al., 1993[v]; Henggeler et al., 1986[ii]). Borduin (1999[vi]) provides a helpful review. Henggeler et al. (1986[ii]) evaluated the effectiveness of MST with delinquents who were repeat offenders ($n = 57$). The number of behavioral problems reported by parents decreased significantly with MST, compared with an alternative service provision condition ($n = 23$). Associations with deviant peers also decreased. Observations of family interaction indicated improvements relative to the control group during a discussion exercise.

A second study randomized a sample of 84 chronic (mean of 3.5 previous offenses) and/or violent offenders (mean age = 15.2) into MST or treatment-as-usual groups (Henggeler et al., 1992[i]). Youths in the usual service condition received court orders including one or more stipulations. Probation officers monitored adherence. Although youths were often referred to mental health services, few treatments were delivered. Youths whose families participated in MST were less likely to be arrested or incarcerated than youths in the comparison group. There were also improvements in terms of self-reports and parental reports of youths' behavior, and the families reported greater cohesion and reduced peer aggression. Neither demographic characteristics nor family functioning variables predicted outcome, but those youths who were able to create emotional bonds with peers appeared to have fewer rearrests (.87 versus 1.52) and were reincarcerated for shorter periods (5.8 weeks), as opposed to the control group (16.2 weeks). Costs of MST were $2,800 per adolescent. The costs encountered in the control group were in excess of $16,000 (mostly associated with the justice system). An important finding was that the severity of disturbance of conduct did not predict either dropping out of treatment or outcome, indicating that the treatment is useful for even the most severe cases. At 2½-year follow-up (Henggeler et al., 1993[v]) the MST group had fewer rearrests (61%) than the comparison group (80%).

These early trials demonstrated that MST using the family preservation model of service delivery could double the percentage of youths not arrested 2 years after treatment. However, the sample sizes of these studies were relatively small and lacked a comparison group with a roughly equivalent number of treatment hours. Further, the attrition from the research portion of the study was 23% for MST and 44% for usual services, and the loss appeared to selectively exclude the less functional families.

Borduin et al. (1995[i]) reported on the long-term effects of MST on the prevention of criminal activity in a sample of serious juvenile offenders. They assigned 176 families in which young people had multiple arrest records and were currently living with at least one parent, to MST or individual therapy. Individual therapy (IT) was supportive and was designed to address personal, family, and academic issues, including psychodynamic, client-centered, and behavioral components, all focusing on the adolescent rather than the system the adolescent was in. Treatment integrity for both therapies was independently assessed by therapist reports and videotaped sessions.

Differences in outcomes in the symptom realm were impressive. An average 4-year follow-up showed recidivism in the group who completed MST to be significantly reduced (22.1%) relative to the group who completed IT (71.4%). Even among those (26%) in the MST group who had been arrested, these arrests were generally for less serious crimes than the arrests for the 71% in the IT group who had been charged. The recidivism rate for MST noncompleters ($n = 15$) was 46.6%, as opposed to the IT noncompleters ($n = 21$), for whom the recidivism rate was 71.4%. Although there was no control group, 24 of the original 200 adolescents refused treatment, and the recidivism rate for this group was 87.5%. The reduction in arrests for violent crimes is of particular interest. Reductions in psychiatric symptomatology in both the parents and the adolescents were also of interest. MST produced significant improvements in mothers' and fathers' reports of psychiatric symptomotology and in mothers' reports of adolescents' behavior problems. The same measures showed deterioration in the IT group. Adolescents' own reports of their mental state are not included in the results, although they seem to have been measured. Not surprisingly, family functioning, both as measured by questionnaire and by direct observation, improved with MST and deteriorated with IT. The cost of the treatment has been estimated as $4,500, which is less than one-quarter the cost of an 8-months incarceration.

MST also appears promising in the treatment of substance-abusing or substance-dependent delinquents (Borduin, 1999[vi]). A particular strength of MST is the relatively low dropout rate, which is generally substantial in delinquent populations (Henggeler, Pickrel, Brondino, & Crouch, 1996b[i]). Henggeler et al. (1996b[i]) demonstrated that 98% of 58 families randomly assigned to home-based MST completed a full course of treatment, lasting an average of 138 days, in contrast to 78% of 60 families assigned to usual community services, who received no substance abuse or mental health services in the 5 months following referral, principally because they dropped out. The success of MST in eliminating dropouts echoes the finding of Szapocznik et al. (1988[i]). These authors reported that a strategic structural systems approach reduced the dropout rate from 58% to 7% and increased completion rates from 25% to 77% in 108 Hispanic families randomly assigned to the two conditions. When MST is implemented in a less rigorous manner—for example, without a weekly consultation with an expert in MST—the treatment is less effective and has a higher dropout rate (Henggeler, Melton, Brondino, Scherer, & Hanley, 1997[i]). In this latter community-based implementation (an effectiveness trial as opposed to an efficacy trial), treatment effects, although significant, were less strong, particularly where adherence to the treatment manual was somewhat weaker.

This study supports a radical rethinking of crime prevention services in the direction of emphasizing child-centered, family-focused, comprehensive, and ecologically valid services. The general approach has received substantial confirmation from independent studies of family preservation programs, in which the successful prevention of out-of-home placements was strongly related to the prevention of juvenile justice system involvement (Collier & Hill, 1993[vi]). Outcome studies on MST have provided preliminary data on the usefulness of this approach in addressing a range of problems related to disturbance of conduct, such as soft drug use (Henggeler et al., 1991[i]), drug-abuse-related arrests (Borduin et al., 1995[i]), and rearrests for sexual offenses (Borduin, Henggler, Blaske, & Stein, 1990[i]). The implications of these findings are limited by small sample sizes and relatively high dropout rates. Ongoing studies are investigating treatment processes and potential moderators of MST and the dissemination of MST in various community settings (Henggeler et al., 1997[i]). A 10-year follow-up of the major randomized trials of MST is under way (Borduin, 1999[vi]).

Although this approach has major strengths (see review by Borduin, 1999[vi]), a number of challenges remain. The combination of techniques required for effective practice has not been made clear. It is not clear which techniques are essential, and which are optional, or how the therapist may decide between the two categories. There is no unequivocal algorithm for the dosage required for the treatment to be clinically effective. Further, given the difficulties in delivering high-quality care even within a single modality, the challenge of combining these components, yet retaining treatment integrity, is considerable. The treatment program has not yet been shown to be effective by workers not involved in its development. Training is obviously crucial (Henggeler et al., 1997[i]), but training opportunities are not yet readily available.

Adolescent-Oriented Interventions

SOCIAL AND PROBLEM-SOLVING SKILLS TRAINING

Social skills training and problem-solving skills training are the two main derivatives of cognitive–behavioral therapy used to treat offending in young people (Tate, Reppucci, & Mulvey, 1995[vi]). Social skills deficits in adolescent delinquents have been repeatedly demonstrated. It has been suggested that given a deficit in socially acceptable ways of achieving goals within the social environment, delinquents will resort to socially inappropriate behaviors to achieve them.

An early trial of social skills training randomly assigned 76 adolescent male delinquents to a social skills training group, an attention placebo group, and a no-treatment control group (Spence & Marzillier, 1981[ii]). The training was relatively nonintensive (12 1-hour sessions for groups of four adolescents). The training package was comparable to other social skills interventions (discussion, role play, videotape modeling and feedback, social reinforcements, homework tasks, etc.) The program was individually tailored to the social skills needs of each adolescent. Improvements in social skills were assessed in analogue tests. Significant improvements were observed, which were maintained at 3-month follow-up. However, the program offered no evidence that these skills generalized beyond the treatment setting in terms of either observer ratings or staff ratings. Ratings by the social worker indicated no generalization to family, school, or social relationships. Nor was there an effect on officially recorded or self-reported delinquent behavior. Assertiveness training was also tested in a group of 48 8th- to 9th-grade African American children referred to school counseling for aggressive behavior (Huey & Rank, 1984[i]). The children met diagnostic criteria for CD; there was also a no-treatment control group. Teacher-reported aggression was significantly reduced following peer- and counselor-led assertiveness training groups. Learning assertiveness responses was associated with a reduction in aggressive behavior. The follow-up was too short (3 months) to demonstrate a durable effect, however.

The Viewpoints Training Program, described by Guerra and Slaby (1990[ii]), aims to change beliefs about the legitimacy of violence and to teach social problem-solving skills to replace aggressive responses. This 12-session cognitive mediation training program was assessed with 120 male and female adolescent incarcerated offenders with a history of aggression and violence. Subjects were randomly assigned to cognitive mediation training, an attention placebo control, or a no-treatment group. Staff rated the treatment group as less aggressive and impulsive than attention/control and no-treatment groups. Compared with subjects in the control groups, the treated group's skills in solving social problems increased and endorsement of beliefs supporting aggression and aggressive, impulsive, and inflexible behaviors decreased, as rated by staff. Most of these measures are too closely related to the intervention to be useful indicators of outcome. Posttest levels of aggression appeared to be directly related to change in cognitive factors (This analysis, however, was reported only across the whole sample. To ensure a demonstration of process and outcome, the two groups should have been analyzed separately). In terms of parole violations, there were no group differences 24 months after release.

Social skills-oriented training programs appear to improve the social functioning of delinquent adolescents. Training in social problem solving appears effective in reducing aggressive behavior. However, the long-term maintenance of these gains is limited. The widespread use of perspective taking programs outstrips the evidence base currently available to support them. In view of the far greater intensity of other programs that have proved to be effective for this group (e.g., MST), it is likely that social skills based approaches have not been administered in a sufficient dose to generate clinically significant outcomes.

ANGER MANAGEMENT

Feindler and colleagues have developed an anger management program based on the assumption that anger motivates aggressive behavior (Feindler, 1990[ib], 1995[vi]; Feindler & Guttman, 1994[vi]). The program (appropriately named "ChillOut") was evaluated in an inpatient psychiatric unit with adolescents who had been given a CD diagnosis. The treatment is offered in group settings and includes a stress inoculation component. Staff ratings of self-control differentiated the treated group from an untreated control. An analogue role-play test of behavior only partially differentiated the groups (33 out of 11 measures). There were no group differences at the end of treatment related to the key outcome variable, namely, the number of violations of the regimen for physical aggressions. No long-term follow-up data are available. An earlier study (Schlichter & Horan, 1981[i])2.1 showed that stress inoculation was effective in building anger and aggression management skills in 38 (13- to 28-year-old) institutionalized delinquents. However, the sample size was relatively small (there were three groups), and the outcome measures were highly reactive (anger inventory, imaginary provocations test, role-played provocation test, and irrational beliefs test), without adequate long-term follow-up.

The effectiveness of an anger control training program with stress inoculation was tested in a high school setting with 36 adolescents (ages 12.5–25 years) (Feindler, Marriott, & Iwata, 1984[i]). The sample was selected from 100 delinquents who had been multiply suspended because of high rates of disruption in the classroom or the community. They were randomly assigned to group anger control treatment or to a noncontact control condition. The treatment group included training in self-control strategies and strategies specific to controlling anger leading to disruptive and/or aggressive incidents. At posttest, subjects in the treatment group were found to have received fewer suspensions and expulsions. The interpretation of these findings is complicated by the presence of other ongoing behavior modification programs at the school (e.g., fines for disruptive behavior). Thus, the findings pertain to the effectiveness of anger control only as an adjunct to behavioral programs and not as a stand-alone intervention.

The generally acknowledged limitation of anger management skills training is the absence of demonstration of skills generalization and maintenance into contexts beyond that of the therapeutic session. A unique study randomized 50 adolescent inpatients who were identified by clinicians as potentially benefiting from this kind of intervention and who scored above the 75th percentile on the State–Trait Anger Expression Inventory (Snyder, Kymissis, & Kessler, 1999[ii]). Participants were assigned to a four-session group anger management training program or a placebo control condition. Attrition was minimal. Behavior ratings were carried out by teachers and nurses blind to group assignment. There was no analysis of data obtained from parents or guardians in the home environment. There was a significant reduction on the Minnesota Multiphasic Personality Inventory Anger Content Scale for the experimental group, but not for the control group. There was also a significant difference between experimental and control group in nursing staff and teacher rating, but this was significant only at the .05 level and was not adjusted for possible preintervention differences, which appeared not to be available for this measure. The study therefore has severe limitations, notwithstanding the reasonable quality of randomization, in showing significant benefit from anger management only on a self-report measure and providing no data on follow-up.

A physical exercise program has also been tested as a method of reducing disruptive behavior (Basile, Motta, & Allison, 1995[ii]). Physical exercise may be conceived of as an emotion-regulation, anger control strategy. Fifty-eight children (7–13 years) were randomly assigned to the "antecedent physical exercise" (APE) program, to a mastery task group, or to a no-treatment control group. There was a 4-week baseline observation period. Subjects in the APE group produced significantly less disruptive behavior than those in either of the other groups. There was no follow-up, and the hypothesis that the effects of exercise on disruptive behavior are mediated by changes in self-esteem was not supported.

Anger control training has high face validity, given the obvious problems of impulsiveness and aggression in this group. However, improvements in this capacity have not yet been shown to generalize to clinically significant behavioral problems. Given the popularity of this approach in clinical settings, the empirical weakness of the treatment is somewhat surprising. On the basis of the evidence available, we have to conclude that the effectiveness of anger control programs is not yet demonstrated. It is likely that anger, as a target for intervention, is not sufficiently central to problems of aggression for its control to be an appropriate goal on its own.

TRAINING IN MORAL REASONING

The immaturity of conduct-disordered and delinquent adolescents in moral reasoning and moral judgment tasks is well demonstrated (Chandler & Moran, 1990[vi]; Gregg, Gibbs, & Basinger, 1994[vi]; Nelson, Smith, & Dodd, 1990[ib]). An early study (Block, 1978[ii]) examined the effectiveness of a rational–emotive therapy approach in 40 11th- to 12th-grade Hispanic and African American high school students. Although this approach is not uniquely focused on moral reasoning, addressing inappropriate moral cognitions is an important component of the treatment. The treated group received five weekly sessions of rational–emotive therapy over a full semester. The rational–emotive therapy group obtained higher grade point averages, manifested lower incidences of disruptive behavior, and fewer absences from classes. The differences between those receiving rational–emotive therapy, client-centered therapy, and no-treatment (control group) were maintained over a 6-month follow-up period. Unfortunately, the treatment is not well described in this early report, and there have been no further investigations of this approach.

Arbuthnot and Gordon (1986[i]) evaluated the benefit of a moral dilemma discussion group for a behaviorally disordered group of adolescents. Forty-five-minute discussion groups were held once weekly for 16–20 weeks in the school. Significant benefits were associated with the program, including reduced disciplinary referrals, improved academic performance, and reduced police or court contacts. The differences between treated and untreated groups were maintained at 1-year follow-up, although neither group had a significant number of encounters with the police or the courts. Teacher ratings of adolescent behavior also failed to reflect differences, but this is well known to be a relatively insensitive parameter. However, the promising results of this study are not reflected by a number of other investigations (Gibbs, Arnold, Ahlborn, & Cheesman, 1984[ii]; Power, Higgins, & Kohlberg, 1989[vi]). As the programs offered differed in subtle ways, identifying the reasons for such discrepancies may be difficult at this stage. In general, although the programs succeed in improving moral reasoning in these youngsters, a reduction in conduct disturbance does not necessarily follow.

MULTICOMPONENT PACKAGES

None of the single-component or single-focus individual skills programs have generated unequivocal evidence of effectiveness, raising the question of whether they may be more effective in combination. Combination treatments are more likely to administer psychosocial treatments in a clinically effective dose, as well as simultaneously addressing the multiple causes of the severe behavioral problems of adolescence (Kazdin, 1996a[vi]).

There have been several attempts at addressing deficits in skills and cognitive functioning in delinquents at a number of levels within a single program, but few have been subjected to rigorous evaluation. One such program, Aggression Replacement Training (ART), which integrates social skills training, anger control, and moral reasoning training, has been used with institutionalized delinquent adolescents (Goldstein, Glick, Reiner, Zimmerman, & Coultry, 1986[vi]). The program is associated with skills improvements particularly when administered in a community setting. Young offenders who received ART showed significant increases in constructive, social behaviors and moral reasoning and decreases in impulsivity, compared to a no-treatment group (Goldstein & Glick, 1994). There is limited evidence for generalization, but preliminary data suggest reduction in 3-month rearrest rates and higher ratings on adjustment measures by social workers at 1-year follow-up. However, at that time, the adolescents did not differ significantly from controls in either the number or intensity of their acting-out behaviors.

A second multicomponent package (Equipping Youth to Help One Another, EQUIP) combines social skills training, anger management, moral reasoning training, and problem-solving skills training approaches administered in a group setting (Gibbs, Potter, Barriga, & Liau, 1996[v]). A controlled outcome study, with 15- to 18-year-old incarcerated male offenders, compared EQUIP with an attention placebo group and a no-treatment group (Leeman, Gibbs, & Fuller, 1993[i]). The experimental group had 20 subjects, the control groups 37. Assignment was random to the EQUIP group, a simple control group, or a motivational control group in which subjects were challenged to show "that they can have power and control over their lives." Despite a relatively small sample, the program generated promising results. Within the institutional setting's staff-filed incident reports, truancy and self-reported misconduct were reduced. At 1 year following release from the institution, the recidivism rate of participants was stable at 15%, whereas for the control groups it was 41% and climbing. Gains in moral judgment scores did not correlate with measures of conduct improvement, but gains in social skills did. Unfortunately, the design of this study does not allow the conclusion that the therapeutic effect is curriculum specific.

It is unfortunate that so few multicomponent packages have been the subject of systematic study. Given the complex problems presented by adolescent, delinquent, and conduct-disordered youths, it is most likely that a multicomponent program would be needed to adequately address the causes of their disorders. Evaluation of multicomponent treatments presents special difficulties. Parsimony and cost-effectiveness considerations dictate that the minimum number of components necessary for an effective treatment intervention should be used. Further, the sequencing and specific combination of components generate limitless permutations, only some of which may be clinically efficacious. The theoretical rationale of multicomponent approaches tends to be limited, with pragmatic rather than conceptual considerations guiding the selection of approaches. The contrast with alternative treatments is made more challenging by the relatively high doses in which multicomponent treatments are delivered. Treatment integrity should be separately assessed for each of the treatment components. Nevertheless, multicomponent treatments are more likely to be effective for serious and chronic disorders such as CD.

School-Based Interventions

The extensive literature on the link between delinquency and school performance, attitudes toward school, and school attendance (Farrington, 1992; Farrington, Loeber, Stouthamer-Loeber, Van Kammen, & Schmidt, 1996; Loeber, Stouthamer-Loeber, Van Kammen, & Farrington, 1991) makes the question of the efficacy of alternative education programs an especially interesting one. According to Cox et al., who published a meta-analysis of evaluations of these programs in 1995, alternative education is principally characterized by individualized assessment and instruction and low student–teacher ratios. Only 57 out of 241 studies yielded by computer searches of the literature from 1966 to 1993 met minimum research criteria (i.e., statistical assessment of one type of outcome that was adequate for the purposes of the meta-analysis, the presence of a separate curriculum, and location of the program outside conventional school). The researchers coded studies on four outcome variables: levels of delinquent activity, school performance, attitude to school, and self-esteem. Their surprising finding was that alternative education programs have small positive effects on school performance, attitude to school, and self-esteem, but none on delinquency. Cox suggests that the effects of the programs on their hypothesized mediators of delinquency (that is, the school-related variables and self-esteem) were not strong enough to produce a consequent effect on delinquent activity.

Gottfredson and Gottfredson (1992[vi]) contrasted the effectiveness in reducing delinquency of three secondary-school-based programs: Positive Action through Holistic Education (PATHE), Student Training through Urban Strategies (STATUS) and Peer Culture Development (PCD). The PATHE program involved strengthening the bond between students and schools through counseling, tutoring, and extracurricular activities. The STATUS program aimed to strengthen the adolescent's involvement with the school, as well as with community organizations, by providing a range of opportunities for active participation. The PCD program aimed to alter peer interaction and foster positive styles of behavior and social interaction. The key outcome variable was self-reported delinquency. PCD was superior to the other two programs. The PATHE and STATUS programs appeared to have little impact in reducing delinquency. Unfortunately, the implementation of a random allocation was unsuccessful in the PCD condition, and it is possible that its apparent superiority was due to a higher-functioning sample. The disappointing results from the other two programs, however, imply that enhancement of positive social features of a school may not be sufficient to reduce delinquency in adolescence.

By contrast, programs tackling gang involvement sometimes appear to have significant effects. Gang Resistance Education Training (GREAT) has been evaluated recently in a national study (Esbensen & Osgood, 1999[v]). The program entails uniformed law enforcement officers teaching a 9-week curriculum to middle-school students. The curriculum includes structured exercises and interactive approaches to learning aimed at spelling out the ramifications of gang violence. The curriculum includes extended activities aimed at teaching goal setting, resisting peer pressure, and peaceful conflict resolutions. More than 3,000 specially trained officers have implemented the program in over 1,300 communities. Results from a survey of nearly 6,000 8th-grade students suggest that the students participating in the program (45%) had lower levels of self-reported delinquency and gang involvement than the comparison group. They also exhibited more prosocial behaviors and attitudes, they were more attached to their parents and to school, and more of their friends were involved in nondelinquent activities. However, these results cover only the first postprogram year. A longer-term follow-up is awaited.

The literature exploring causal models for young people who break the law does not provide conclusive evidence that school-related variables are causally associated with juvenile delinquency. There are suggestions, for example, that performance at school is associated with delinquency but that both are primarily mediated by psychological difficulties, disorders of conduct in particular (Farrington, 1996). Given the support in the literature for multiple models of cause for offending behavior, a linear causal link between school-related variables and delinquency is a simplistic construct that excludes too many other important factors. Nevertheless, the school remains an important point of entry to a treatment program for adolescents with CD and delinquency. Many initiatives attempt to bring mental health services into the school setting. Unfortunately, these mental health programs tend to be relatively traditional implementations of the same treatments that were previously available in the community context. If a concerted effort were made to take advantage of school-based mental health resources for the systemwide modification of school environment in the direction of changing those characteristics associated with delinquency, there might be a substantial added benefit.

Community-Wide Programs

BROAD COMMUNITY-BASED PROGRAMS

Ultimately, outcome research aims to guide mental health services policy, and, ideally, the quality of interventions should be assessed in terms of their benefit to an entire community or geographical area. This kind of public health perspective is relatively rare in treatment research; trials tend to be restricted to a specific treatment program within a particular health care (usually university clinic) setting. The issue of generalization of findings beyond the specialist clinic has been a burning issue within psychosocial treatment research for some years. Surprisingly, community-wide programs, although frequently implemented, are rarely systematically evaluated, and controlled trial methodology is even less likely to be used.

A unique large-scale study, for disruptive behavior-disordered children living in certain counties of Tennessee, contrasts an integrated case management model (involving child welfare, mental health, education, and juvenile justice systems) with traditional methods of service delivery. Children treated within the integrated case management model were better off in terms of psychosocial functioning than those living in counties without the new system. The new system also appears to be associated with a reduction in residential and inpatient care (Glisson, 1994).

Evaluation of services to status offenders in the state of Florida examined the use of family therapy in family preservation or family unification programs over a 3-year period (Nugent, Carpenter, & Parks, 1993[vi]). Family preservation programs aim to keep adolescents at home. Family reunification programs aim to reunite adolescents, who have been placed out of home or who had run away, with their families. More than 8,000 families took part in preservation programs and more than 1,300 in reunification programs. Participation in family therapy, as well as the number of sessions of family therapy, were significant predictors of the success of these programs. No effect was observed for individual or group counseling, but families receiving five sessions of family therapy were twice as likely to remain together as those who received none. Families who had 10 sessions were 2.5 times more likely to remain together. In terms of family reunification, as the number of group counseling sessions increased, the probability of family unification decreased. Families receiving family therapy, however, were about 3.5 times more likely to reunite than those who received none. Positive effects of family therapy were seen in all 3 years of the evaluation. The findings indicate the value of family therapy, but data of this kind do not indicate why certain families took up this help while others did not. It is quite likely that the most dysfunctional family units could not accept family intervention, and the failure of unification is a further indication of their problems. However, it is possible (particularly in light of the success of other family-based interventions) that family therapy has a synergistic effect when used in the context of multitarget ecologically based interventions. The study unequivocally demonstrated that family therapy is, at least, not iatrogenic, and its effective implementation, population-wide, may be associated with important therapeutic gains.

Another comprehensive statewide program providing violent youths with appropriate mental health services has been less successful. The program is based on a case-management therapeutic approach whereby managers oversee the development and execution of treatment plans. Plans are individualized for all youths participating in the program. Normally, referral is made to existing community services in the least restrictive environment possible. The program evaluation failed to identify measurable relative gains for the program participants (Weisz, Walter, Weiss, Fernandez, & Mikow, 1990[v]).

Numerous other community-based programs aim to reinforce mental health provision within the criminal justice system. For example, in the New York-based Mobile Mental Health Teams program (Fagan, 1991[vi]), mental health professionals travel in mobile units to justice facilities at all levels of security. Unfortunately, although these programs are costly, as well as imaginative, they have not in general been evaluated in experimental trials. In particular, case-management approaches that simply funnel clients into existing services may fail because of the relative lack of effectiveness of these community-based programs (Weisz et al., 1995a[vi]).

The Yale Child Study Center has reported an extraordinary program of coordinated mental health care and policing that led to multiple changes in the delivery of both clinical and police services (Marans, Berkowitz, & Cohen, 1998[vi]). The program involves joint response by law enforcement and mental health services to the needs of children and families exposed to or involved in violence. Police officers receive training in child development and mental health issues, and child mental health professionals are on call to attend crime scenes that involve children as victims, perpetrators, or witnesses. The program's involvement with juvenile offenders has led to a coordinated response from the police, mental health professionals, and the juvenile justice system. Community surveys have confirmed substantial improvements in the sense of safety experienced by young people over the period of the program, and they report witnessing fewer violent incidents. Of course, it is hard to provide conclusive evidence that there is a causal relationship between the provision of the program and the reduction of reported violent crime. Nevertheless, the program has been widely adopted by police forces across a number of major cities in the United States.

The Iowa Strengthening Families Program includes a brief family-based intervention with seven consecutive weekly meetings, separate parent and child skills-building curricula, and a family curriculum (Kumpfer, Molgaard, & Spoth, 1996). A randomized trial including 22 public schools and 117 treatment and 208 control families provided preliminary data supporting the value of the intervention (Spoth, Redmond, & Shin, 2000[i]). On observer ratings and adolescent self-reports of aggressive and hostile behaviors, the family intervention was found to have statistically reliable effects 4 years after the original intervention. Although family member reports also favored the family intervention group, the difference was not significant. The ESs relative to the minimal contact control group were small, which is hardly surprising given the duration of the follow-up and the brief nature of the intervention. The outcome measure is of unknown clinical significance. However, the mere fact that the impact of a skills-oriented family intervention is detectable on adolescent behavior 4 years after the intervention, is a remarkable testament to the impact such relatively modest interventions can have on the lives of receptive families.

A truancy intervention program established a processing center to assist in dealing with truants as part of a community project to reduce youth crime (Thomas, Holzer, & Enriquez, 1999[v]). Truants violating a schoolday curfew are brought to the center by officers after a background check for outstanding warrants. The young person is interviewed, the school and parents are contacted, and referral is made to other resources for identified problems. Over 4 years of operation, 865 truancy incidents have been dealt with. The average monthly rate of truancy cases has dropped from 50 to 30. During the same period, youth crime and high school dropout rates have significantly declined. The absence of a comparison sample limits the study's generalizability, however.

A number of Positive Youth Development programs have successfully tackled problems of delinquency. In Ottawa, Canada, an afterschool recreational program targeting all children in a local public housing project led to a 75% drop in the number of arrests for youths residing in the project while the arrest rate in a neighboring project showed a 67% increase (see Howell, 1995). A Columbia University study compared public housing complexes with and without an on-site Boys and Girls Club. Clubs that also delivered a social skills training curriculum were associated with significantly less vandalism, drug trafficking, and juvenile crime (Schinke, Orlandi, & Cole, 1992[iii]). The Big Brothers/Big Sisters mentoring project showed that youths assigned a mentor were 46% less likely to take drugs, 27% less likely to drink alchohol, and 30% less likely to strike another person than controls who applied for mentors but ended up on a waiting list (Tierney, Grossman, & Resch, 1995[ii]). A study of the Quantum Opportunities Program (QOP) showed that high risk youths who participated in a 4-year intensive afterschool program of career preparation, life skills training, and academic enrichment were far more likely than a randomly assigned control group to graduate from high school, attend college, and delay parenting and were convicted of less then one-sixth of crimes, compared with control group youths (Hahn, Leavitt, & Aaron, 1994[ii]).

A large number of therapeutic and treatment programs are introduced in communities, particularly in North America, yet the findings of many studies are equivocal. There is an urgent need to evaluate these different treatment approaches. Too little is known about which community-wide initiatives work and what methods of implementing such programs are effective. It is unlikely that a program developed for one community easily translates to other, sometimes quite different, social environments. Issues of generalizability are substantial, and protocols for cross-site transfer are rarely available and even less often demonstrated. The communities that are most successful at reducing crime rates are those that have focused comprehensively and engaged key leaders from multiple sectors. With a steep rise in juvenile and young adult violence in the late 1980s, Boston suffered 152 homicides in 1990, after experiencing fewer than 10 per year in the 1980s. A major source of the violence was youth gangs struggling for control territory and crack distribution. Guns acquired for this purpose were used in murders unrelated to drugs. In 1998, Boston suffered only 35 murders (a 78% decrease). The city's success was due to the comprehensive approach adopted by all agencies and leaders in various sectors, followed by an organized, coordinated, customized antiviolence campaign. Some elements focused on law enforcement; the police department convened a youth violence task force (45 officers working alongside 15 officials from other agencies) that concentrated on the highest-crime neighborhoods and maintained a database on gang leaders and dangerous ex-offenders in the community. A specific project for tracing the guns used and identifying those who profited from gun trafficking was developed. A zero-tolerance policy for gun violence was established, and all those carrying guns were turned over to the more severe federal courts. In addition, the city strengthened its efforts in the juvenile justice system and delinquency prevention. The probation department and the police started joint and coordinated activities—for example, visiting the homes of high-risk probationers together. Those out after curfew were warned at the first instance and then returned to court and sometimes to jail (National Criminal Justice Reference Service, 1996[v]). In addition, an alternative-to-incarceration network was created, providing community-based supervision and positive support to less malignant offenders. The program also included an outreach element whereby local counselors and street workers worked hand in hand with local police officers to send the message that gunplay would not be tolerated. Boston is not an isolated example. The key to the success of these initiatives is the comprehensive nature of the approach adopted. Sadly, these are expensive and complex programs that depend on broad-based adoption by a community; this is often not forthcoming, particularly in less receptive social and cultural contexts. The concept of community collaboration appears surprisingly difficult to adopt. Harsh punishment regimes send a simpler message, to which many communities are receptive, even in the absence of a reasonable evidence base.

TEACHING-FAMILY MODEL

The Teaching-Family Model (TFM), also known as the Achievement Place Model, was developed in the 1960s and is now widely used in group homes across the

United States. There are probably more than 250 group homes in the United States for aggressive and delinquent adolescents organized according to TFM principles (Fixsen & Blase, 1993[vi]; Wolf, Kirigin, Fixsen, Blase, & Braukmann, 1995[vi]). Each group home is run by a married couple with at least 1 year's training in TFM principles, certified by the Teaching-Family Association (Kirigin, 1996). Each group home has between five and eight adolescents. The treatment components of TFM include a multilevel points system, self-government procedures (including conferences and a peer manager), social skills training, academic tutoring, and a reinforcement system for monitoring school behavior. Early publications emphasized learning theory based motivational procedures and behavioral skills training. More recently, the establishment of positive relationships, both within the peer group and between the teaching parents and the adolescents, has also become a focus. A strong feature of the program is the high level of quality control, which includes evaluators, community boards, and judges (Wolf et al., 1995[vi]).

An early evaluation of the program compared 13 TFM group homes with 9 traditional community-based residential programs (Kirigin, Braukmann, Atwater, & Wolf, 1982[ib]). The primary outcome variables were court and police records. The groups were comparable in terms of their records prior to treatment. During the treatment TFM participants had significantly fewer recorded offenses, but there was no difference between the two treatment conditions during the year following treatment. Measures of consumer satisfaction, taken from schools as well as the participants, favored the TFM group homes.

A larger-scale study (Weinrott, Jones, & Howard, 1982[ib]) considered 26 TFM group homes and 25 comparable programs, the majority of which were also group homes. The sample size was 354 in the TFM group and 363 in the comparison group. The primary outcome variable was cost, measured at intake, during treatment, and annually for 3 years following the end of treatment. There was a saving of 22% in a cost-per-youth calculation and 7% in a cost-per-day calculation. Four composite indices were used to compare the program's effectiveness: (1) deviant behavior was assessed on the basis of self-reports of delinquent behavior and court records; (2) education was assessed as a composite of average grade points and courses passed; (3) occupation was assessed in terms of positions achieved after leaving the home; and (4) various social and personality measures were taken. There was surprisingly little difference between the two groups in terms of effectiveness, although there was evidence that the educational element of the program slowed the decline of grade point averages. Because of the lower cost of the TFM program, it was favored in effectiveness by cost ratios. A strong feature of this study, besides the unusually thorough examination of costs, is the independence of the investigators. However, all group home programs are expensive and less than half of those participating in these programs complete the treatment. Two to 3 years after the end of treatment, there appeared to be few differences between treatment completers and dropouts.

A third study considered a broader range of comparison groups and a wider range of measures of effectiveness, looking at self-reports and reports from staff members, as well as official records (Wolf, Braukmann, & Ramp, 1987[vi]). The treatment was effective in terms of officially recorded delinquency rates, social skills levels, educational attainment, and consumer (youth) satisfaction. As in previous studies, the effects dissipated once the youths left the program.

The failure to generate long-term benefit from such programs underscores the importance of a continuum of services for young people with severe disturbance of conduct. The possibility of integrating the group homes approach with a treatment foster care program has been suggested (Chamberlain, 1994[vi]; Hudson, Nutter, & Galaway, 1994[ib]). The results also echo the more general finding that the effects of behavioral interventions do not readily generalize to other settings.

TREATMENT OR THERAPEUTIC FOSTER CARE

Treatment foster care (TFC) is an intervention model that offers an alternative to group residential care for serious chronic juvenile offenders. TFC is an extension of parent-mediated treatments developed by the Oregon Social Learning Center that have previously been shown to be effective in working with children with aggression and antisocial behavioral problems. In TFC, community families are recruited and trained to provide placements for children as an alternative to group homes (Chamberlain & Moore, 1998a[ii]). Therapeutic foster care for children with chronic delinquency has been shown to be relatively effective in reducing the recidivism rate. The program uses carefully selected foster parents in conjunction with individual therapy and case management. There has been a substantial increase in the number of adolescents who are displaced or removed from their family homes in the United States. In many of these cases institutional care would be an added risk factor (Rutter et al., 1998[ib]). Group homes, like any effort to bring together deviant youngsters, must be questionable because involvement with deviant peers in adolescence predicts the exacerbation of disturbance of conduct and enhances a deviant identity (Dishion & Andrews, 1995[i]; Dishion, Patterson, Stoolmiller, & Skinner, 1991[v]).

The therapeutic foster care approach has received support from a meta-analysis of 40 studies (Reddy & Pfeiffer, 1997[ib]). Across more than 12,000 subjects substantial ESs were shown for lengthening the placement of hard-to-place adolescents and increasing their social skills. ESs for the reduction of behavior problems were moderate, as was improvement in psychological adjustment. There was considerable variability between the studies. One of the most effective approaches was that of Chamberlain and her colleagues (Chamberlain, 1994[vi]; Chamberlain & Reid, 1994[vi]). The approach, which is strongly influenced by the Oregon Social Learning Center model, offers preservice training for foster parents and further support through individual consultations, group meetings and 24-hour crisis management. Foster parents are also supported with training in school advocacy skills. Family therapy is offered to the biological parents to facilitate transfer to the home as appropriate. Individual therapy is also offered to the child, specifically problem-solving skills training and anger management.

Chamberlain (1990[iii]) provided 2-year follow-up data on 16 young people with chronic delinquency who were provided with specialized foster care services, contrasted with a matched group of 16 who received community treatment as usual. Although 94% of the comparison group were reincarcerated, only 50% of the experimental group experienced this outcome. The number of days' incarceration was reduced from 160 days in the comparison group to 86 days in the foster care group in the first year, and 67 days versus 44 days at follow-up. The follow-up lasted 2 years.

In a second study (Chamberlain & Reid, 1991[i]), hospitalization rates for 19 children and adolescents who had spent the year before referral in state mental hospitals were examined for therapeutic foster care and treatment-as-usual placements. Children in therapeutic foster care were placed somewhat earlier and once placed in the community spent somewhat less time in the hospital, but the difference was not statistically reliable. The therapeutic foster care group showed a reduction in problem behaviors of, ore than 50%, compared with no significant decrease in the comparison group.

In a third study (Chamberlain, Moreland, & Reid, 1992[ii]), these workers explored whether the extra support and training or the extra payment that accompanied this was responsible for the superior performance of the children who received therapy with foster care. The therapeutic group participated in weekly foster parents' meetings and received daily telephone consultations. The results showed that in those foster homes where parents received enhanced training and support, there was greater stability; fewer changes of foster homes; reduction of behavior problems; and fewer instances of running away, juvenile detention, residential care, or other restrictive setting placements. Furthermore, fewer foster parents dropped out of providing foster care.

Chamberlain and Reid (1994[vi]) report interesting gender differences in the effectiveness of therapeutic foster care. Girls appear to respond more poorly to therapeutic foster care than boys. Although boys' behavior improves, the behavior of girls deteriorates slightly. Girls also show less improvement in terms of arrests, particularly for property crimes. The authors speculate that because of the past history of family sexual abuse of a far greater number of girls than boys (almost five times as many), the choice of therapeutic foster care may be less appropriate for girls.

Chamberlain (1996[i]) and Chamberlain and Moore (1998b[i]) described preliminary findings of a randomized, controlled comparison of 79 12- to 18-year-old boys placed either in therapeutic foster care or in residential group care. All the boys were at risk for commitment to a state training school. In this study, therapeutic foster care appears to be associated with a reduction of problem behaviors, a reduction in self-reported delinquency, and an indication of better relationships between the carers and the adolescents. Preliminary data on 68 subjects who completed a 6-month follow-up showed substantial and significant benefits in the therapeutic foster care group in incarceration rates, frequency of running away, and self-reported delinquent behavior arrests. The foster care group spent more time with adults and less time with delinquent peers. At 1 year (Chamberlain & Reid, 1998[ii]), running away in the TFC group, was 31% versus 58% in the control group. Incarceration rate was also substantially lower (53 days versus 129 days). Program completion was 73% in the TFC group, compared with 36% in the control group. There was a significant reduction in official criminal referrals. Detailed analysis of the data suggested that association with delinquent peers was the best predictor of continued offending, and this in turn appeared to depend on the quality and quantity of discipline and supervision the youngsters received from their adult carers. Independently, the relationship with adult carers appeared to be a protective factor that buffered youths from delinquent peers and, in turn, from subsequent arrests (Chamberlain, 1998[vi]).

These results suggest that the integration of case management and consultation is a powerful therapeutic tool. The treatment program is individualized and flexible, responsive to a wide range of clinical problems and shifting community needs, thus posing major challenges for evaluators who wish to identify components that are specifically efficacious. The program is costly, but nevertheless may be cost-effective, because alternatives (group homes, institutionalization) are at least as, if not more, costly. Programs may require that a child and adolescent psychiatrist is an integral part of the regime rather than just a consultant (Fine, 1993).

There have been other attempts at assessing assistance to children in foster care, but none has been assessed as extensively as Chamberlain's program. Most of these studies principally reorganize existing mental health services, rather than providing qualitatively different interventions. For example, one study (Clark et al., 1994[i]) randomly allocated 132 children to the Fostering Individualized Assistance Program (FIAP) or to standard practice foster care. This program involves strength-based assessments, life domain planning, clinical case management, and follow-along support services. Children in the FIAP placements had moderately better outcomes, based on caregivers' CBCL ratings, interviews, and foster care and school records. Their social adaptation ratings were higher, and there were fewer episodes of running away, official records of criminal acts, incarceration, and placement changes. However, the input received by the families of these children was also substantially greater, better organized, and more costly. Further, the treatment was not manualized as a package.

The limited effectiveness of other assisted foster care approaches supports the specific efficacy of Chamberlain's program rooted in the Oregon Social Learning Center model. Foster parents may be useful therapeutic agents. They have excellent access to the adolescent in their care and have not yet established the kinds of negative interaction pattern with the young person that the biological parents have. Given sufficient support and direction, the change of home environment can clearly be used to substantial therapeutic advantage.

PARTIAL HOSPITALIZATION PROGRAMS

Interestingly, there are no controlled studies of the effects of hospitalization on conduct problems. A follow-up study of inpatient treatment (Sourander, Helenius, & Piha, 1996[v]) showed that although children hospitalized for emotional or mixed antisocial and emotional problems continue to improve in the year after discharge, antisocial problems ameliorated during inpatient stay tend to reappear during the follow-up period. A study of a 10- to 12-week residential behavior modification (token economy) program in Dartmouth, Canada, also reported limited successes with male adolescents with conduct problems (Al Ansari, Gouthro, Ahmad, & Steele, 1996). Day treatment programs for preadolescents with severe disturbance of conduct are offered with the aim of keeping these young people in the community. Most studies of day hospital treatment are descriptive in character, report clinical impressions, and have heterogeneous samples, and the duration and type of treatment are not standardized. In a 1-year follow-up of 114 patients, Kiser, Millsap, and Hickerson (1996[v]) found that children's behavior scores, as assessed by the CBCL, fell from 70 to 63, the majority still remaining in the clinical range. The number of school suspensions decreased, and peer and family relations improved. The study had a somewhat heterogeneous sample that included a majority of youths with disturbance of conduct, but there was no control group. In a long-term (8-year) follow-up study of 88 5- to 14-year-olds, Tissue and Korz (1993[v]) demonstrated that 61% of the sample made a successful transition from adolescence to adult life. However, this study lacked a control group and standardized measures.

We identified one effectiveness study with a relatively homogenous CD sample (Grizenko, Papineau, & Sayegh, 1993[ii]). Thirty children were assigned to either day treatment or a waiting-list control group. They were compared on measures of disruptive behavior, self-perception, academic performance, peer relations, and family functioning. Children participating in the intensive day hospital treatment program showed greater benefit in terms of parental behavioral ratings and self-esteem, both at discharge and at 6-month follow-up. Academic functioning was comparable in the intensive day hospital group and a comparison outpatients/waiting-list group. The day treatment takes place after school and on Saturdays and includes a range of models, such as skills training, parent training, and school consultation. A follow-up of 33 children (80% of the original sample) who completed the day treatment program (Grizenko, 1997[iii]) showed that improvement was maintained at 5-year follow-up. Only 9% of the children needed further psychiatric treatment after discharge, and 18% required further social service intervention, including temporary placement. Parental cooperation was the most significant predictor of success, accounting for more than 50% of the explained variability in outcome.

Rey et al. evaluated an Australian multimodal partial hospitalization program at 3-year follow-up (Rey, Denshire, Wever, & Apollonov, 1998[ii]). Parents and children were interviewed separately. Those adolescents who attended the program ($n = 38$), many with diagnoses of CD and CD/ADHD, functioned better overall and were more satisfied with the treatment than the controls ($n = 35$). The groups were matched on delinquency and aggressivity scores as well as age and gender. However, the study yielded poor outcome for both the treated and the treatment-as-usual control groups. Initial diagnosis of CD and high delinquency and total problem scores predicted poor outcome.

An Ontario-based study (Olds, Nixon, & Votta, 1999[v]) reported on a group anger management program as part of a partial hospitalization program. Forty-three adolescents completed the treatment (dropout rate was 19%). A significant treatment effect is reported in terms of youth self-report on the State–Trait Anger Expression Inventory. Consumer satisfaction ratings were also positive. No behavioral observations or postdischarge follow-up was reported.

A similar Canadian study from Ottawa (Kotsopoulos, Walker, Beggs, & Jones, 1996[v]) reported on 46 children (39 males, 7 females) who attended a day treatment program for a school year (average 9 months). Overall, 80% of the sample had conduct problems, 28% with ADHD. The program included classroom contingency management, social skills training, and stimulant medication, as well as specialist help for language and speech and visual–motor problems. Behavior improvement on the CBCL was reported by parents, but not by the teachers, and no long-term outcomes were reported. Although there was academic gain in terms of grade levels, the pre–post differences on reading, spelling, and mathematics were not significant in terms of percentile measures. There was no control or comparison group.

The current evidence for partial hospitalization is equivocal. Some studies suggest that partial hospitalization may be helpful, but the treatments are not specified clearly enough to permit replication. In particular, the observation that poor parental cooperation and greater symptom severity are associated with worse outcome suggests that this may not be the most suitable approach for the treatment-resistant families who need such interventions most. The optimal partial hospitalization approach remains to be specified.

"WRAPAROUND SERVICES"

Wraparound services emerged in the United States in the 1980s with the aim of reducing out-of-home, and especially out-of-state, placement of troubled youths. They are designed to "wrap" individualized services and supports around the individual rather than forcing the young person into a predetermined program. Each young person is assigned a care coordinator, who provides mentoring support and leads a process to assess the needs of the young person, work with his or her family, identify and coordinate needed services, and maintain close supervision. Wraparound Milwaukee is a $27 million project serving 600 young people each year. The program is demonstrating powerful results with a difficult population (69% of court-ordered participants were delinquent offenders and 72% were diagnosed with CD or ODD). It is reported (Mendel, 2000[iii], p. 18) that not only did arrest rates fall dramatically, but also clinical problems were reduced in their severity. Although 45% of participants committed two or more offenses in the year prior to enrollment, only 11% committed two or more offenses in the year of treatment. Among 54 youths with 1-year follow-up data, the average number of arrests declined by 85%. Hooper et al. (Hooper, Murphy, Devaney, & Hultman, 2000[iii]) provided cross-sectional follow-up data on 111 adolescents in a reeducation residential facility with a strong emphasis on community involvement, specifically community/family-oriented wraparound services, starting while the student was still in residence. The most stringent of the outcome criteria (involving improvement in legal, school, and level of care domains) indicated successful outcomes for nearly 60% of the adolescents. Improvement was inversely correlated with length of follow-up and was greater for girls than boys. Eighty percent of the adolescents did not engage in criminal activity in the 2-year follow-up period, but only less than half the sample had legal involvement prior to admission.

Summary

By the time young people with CD reach adolescence, many of the behaviors encompassed by CD involve breaking the law, although the juvenile justice system will not deal with all such adolescents. Interventions based on the traditional principles of punishment and deterrence have not been adequately tested, but effectiveness studies indicate that there is a possibility of adverse outcomes from these interventions. There is evidence that psychosocial treatment strategies can be effectively integrated with juvenile justice provision.

Meta-analytic reviews indicate that reoffending rates are most likely to be reduced by multimodal, behavioral, skills-oriented treatment programs, but the largest ESs are normally observed in outcome measures that are not closely related to reoffending rates (e.g., academic performance). In general, the strongest evidence is for those multilevel, relatively intensive, community-based, highly structured and well-integrated programs focusing on goals proximal to offending behavior (for example, family monitoring and supervision of the adolescent). FFT has been shown to be effective in reducing recidivism in adolescents who have multiply offended. This promising treatment has not yet been widely applied. Several studies have shown that integrating a training program for carefully selected foster parents with problem-solving skills and anger management skills training for delinquent adolescents is a powerful approach, reducing behavior problems as well as recidivism. MST is the most effective treatment for delinquent adolescents in reducing recidivism and ameliorating individual and family problems. It is substantially more effective than individual treatment, even for quite troubled and disorganized families. MST shares a particular strength with other systemic family approaches in reducing attrition rates in this highly volatile group. A number of treatment packages combining a range of individual skills-oriented techniques appear promising, but the most effective combination of specific techniques has not yet been identified and results on long-term outcomes are equivocal. A selective cost-effectiveness of successful crime prevention program models undertaken by the Washington State Institute for Public Policy found that FFT saved taxpayers $6.85 for every $1.00 spent in justice system costs alone. MST saved taxpayers $8.38 for every $1.00, and multidimensional treatment foster care saved $14.07 for each $1.00 spent (Aos, Phipps, Barnoski, & Lieb, 1999[iii]).

Numerous other approaches have been tried, but none of these are as effective as multisystemic therapy. The effectiveness of parent training has been assessed in adolescents; although trials show statistically significant gains associated with these programs, these gains are of low clinical significance. Group treatments of conduct-disordered adolescents appear to carry a risk of worsening rather than improving the individual's behavior problems. Social skills and social problem solving approaches lead to desirable short-term changes, but do not generalize well across settings or engender lasting improvements. Anger management is a promising treatment approach, but the evidence for its efficacy is quite limited. School-based approaches have considerable potential, but studies to date have failed to demonstrate powerful effects on delinquency. The evidence for community-wide implementation of psychosocial treatment programs is inadequate and the results are mixed, although family preservation and systemic family therapy implementations appear most promising. Group homes run according to behavioral principles are less costly and perhaps more effective at reducing criminal behavior during the program than ordinary group homes, but the superior effects dissipate once youths leave the programs.

Day hospitalization represents a promising approach to severe CD and delinquency, as it preserves the community and family contexts of the adolescent while removing him or her from the context within which the problem behaviors originated. Available evidence only partially fulfills the promise of this approach, with most studies reporting either equivocal findings or basing conclusions on rather heterogeneous samples.

Implications

Conduct disturbances are difficult problems to treat. A specialist set of services, well integrated with the juvenile justice and educational systems, is needed to provide interventions for conduct-disordered and offending youths. Multisystemic treatment has the strongest evidence for effectiveness, but this expensive and complex treatment requires lengthy special training. Individual treatment approaches appear to be less effective than family-based approaches, but if individual approaches are implemented, they should focus on proximal causes for delinquent behavior rather than more distal underlying problems. The programs for adolescents with CD should be skills oriented wherever possible, identifying the skills deficits. Current priorities for research in this area include a need for more precise indications for titrating and combining treatment modalities; effective extensions of the program to community settings; and the development of effective dissemination strategies, as inadequate implementations appear to have poorer outcomes.

Physical Therapies for Children and Adolescents

In the last 20 years there has been increasing interest in identifying appropriate medication for disturbance of conduct, particularly problems associated with high levels of aggression (i.e., overt and destructive disturbance of conduct). No single drug has emerged that may be unequivocally considered as an agent of choice in the management of aggression, but a range of preparations have now been evaluated in controlled research for their potential antiaggressive properties (Vitiello & Stoff, 1997[vi]). These studies mostly use inpatient settings for trials of medication, which is not the context in which most treatments are normally offered. Hospital admission may entail additional parameters that can mediate the effects of medication. In a study of 44 subjects with CD (9–17 years) admitted to a hospital for aggression, 48% were found to respond in 2 weeks to the hospital milieu with reduced levels of aggression (Malone et al., 1997[i]). The study raises the obvious possibility that if medication is commenced during the initial phase of inpatient treatment, improvements associated with hospitalization may be inaccurately attributed to pharmacotherapy, resulting in the unnecessary medication of children. Another study investigating the effect of diphenhydramine (an antihistamine) found that although active medication was no more effective than placebo, either diphenhydramine or placebo was more effective when administered as intramuscular injections than when administered orally (Vitiello et al., 1991[i]). This suggests that an accurate assessment of the value of medication may well be obtained if an "active" (credible) placebo is used in a randomized controlled trial.

Combined pharmacotherapy (CPT) is relatively common in the United States. In one study, 40% of 131 inpatients receiving neuroleptics were also prescribed two or more strongly anticholinergic agents (Zito, Craig, & Wanderling, 1994). In another study that assessed child psychiatrists' outpatient prescribing practices, CPT was found in 11–22% (Kaplan, Simms, & Busner, 1994[iv]). In a survey of 65 young people with ODD or CD diagnoses, the 3-month CPT prevalence rate was 18.5% (Stoewe, Kruesi, & Lelio, 1995[vi]). In 83 consecutive admissions to an inpatient child and adolescent center, a history of CPT was found in more than 60% and was specifically associated with aggression (Connor et al., 1997b[iv]). In this latter study only 10% of the children had never been on medication. The high prevalence of CPT is surprising in light of expert advice that it should be used only in treatment-resistant, complex presentations (Spencer et al., 1995b[vi]; Walkup, 1995[vi]). A study of incarcerated female delinquents showed that more than 50% were skeptical about the benefits of pharmacotherapy, despite their prior experience with medication (Williams, Hollis, & Benoit, 1998[vi]). These findings underscore the importance of establishing the evidence base for pharmacological treatments in order to avoid the unnecessary prescription of agents with significant side effects and known implications for neural development.

Psychostimulants

The effectiveness of methylphenidate and dexamphetamine in the treatment of ADHD are reviewed elsewhere in this volume. The rate of comorbidity between ADHD and disturbance of conduct raised the question of the potential specific effects of stimulant medication on disordered conduct. Studies by Hinshaw et al. (Hinshaw, Buhrmester, & Heller, 1989a[ii]; Hinshaw, Henker, Whalen, Erhardt, & Dunnington, 1989b[i]) demonstrated that in children with a diagnosis of ADHD, .6 mg per kg methylphenidate reduced retaliatory aggression during verbal taunting from peers in a laboratory simulation. Further, both the same dose and half this dose of methylphenidate could reduce noncompliance and aggression in classroom and playground settings. Similar findings were reported in nonresearch settings in 11 aggressive/hyperactive boys where the dependent variable was aggression toward peers (Gadow, Nolan, Sverd, Sprafkin, & Paolicelli, 1990[i]). A further randomized controlled trial (RCT) of nine boys (ages 13–16), comorbid for ADHD and aggressive conduct disorder, found that methyphenidate reduced verbal and physical aggressive symptoms (Kaplan, Busner, Kupietz, Wassermann, & Segal, 1990[i]). A double-blind placebo trial of methylphenidate was carried out with 18 6- to 12-year-olds diagnosed with ADHD and attending a summer treatment program for youths with disruptive behavior disorders (Bukstein & Kolko, 1998[i]). Based on staff ratings, children showed significant improvements both in ADHD and aggressive behavior with both low- and high-dose methylphenidate. However, at home, few significant differences were reported in either the low- or high-dose condition. In a unique study of 22 boys with ADHD (10 comorbid for ODD and 4 for CD), methylphenidate was found to be effective in reducing stealing and property destruction in a laboratory setting (Hinshaw, Heller, & McHale, 1992[ii]). However, there was a significant increase in cheating. On balance, there is consistent evidence to support the use of methylphenidate in children with a comorbid ADHD and ODD/CD diagnosis.

Studies of the effect of stimulant medication on children referred for a primary diagnosis of CD are fewer and troubled by the problems of comorbidity and intercurrent treatments. In one study, although marked reductions of disturbance of conduct were observed, all but a few subjects had a comorbid diagnosis of ADHD (Abikoff, Klein, Klass, & Ganeles, 1987, October). A more recent study compared the effectiveness of Ritalin (methylphenidate) and Adderall (a 75:25 ratio of dextro and levo amphetamine) in 25 children diagnosed with ADHD of whom 21 were comorbid for either ODD or CD (Pelham et al., 1999a[i]). Two doses of each agent administered morning and noon were compared (10 mg and 17.5 mg of Ritalin and 7.5 mg and 12.5 mg of Adderall) with placebo. Measures were taken at lunchtime and 5 P.M. Adderall, which has a longer half-life than Ritalin, was more effective in the doses administered on a number of measures, but comparable in terms of side effects. The lower dose of Adderall was comparable in terms of effectiveness to the higher dose of Ritalin. The study supports the use of Adderall in the treatment of symptoms of conduct disturbance. However, the study was carried out in the context of an ongoing behavioral program. Thus, although a quarter of the children were judged to be nonresponders to the medication, this may have been because the incremental benefit from medication was small relative to the concurrent behavioral intervention.

Another study contrasted methylphenidate with lithium and placebo in children with a primary diagnosis of CD, treated on an outpatient basis (Klein, Abikoff, Klass, Shah, & Seese, 1994[i]). In the 80 children and adolescents in the trial, methylphenidate produced improvement in conduct problems whereas lithium did not. A well-designed randomized placebo-controlled trial by the same team tested methylphenidate for 5 weeks in 84 children with CD, two-thirds of whom also met ADHD criteria (Klein et al., 1997[ii]). Behavioral ratings were taken from parents, teachers, and clinicians, and direct classroom observations were also used. The children's ages ranged from 6 to 16. Contrary to expectations, ratings of antisocial behaviors specific to CD were significantly reduced by methylphenidate. This was also true when clinically significant change was used as a criterion. Controlling for the effects of the severity of the ADHD did not alter the significant superiority of methylphenidate on CD ratings specifically. This study suggests that methylphenidate is as relevant to the treatment of conduct problems as it is to problems more specifically associated with ADHD. Expert opinions tend to recommend a trial of stimulants in combination with intensive psychosocial treatment in all cases of disorders of conduct and behavior (e.g., Kruesi & Lelio, 1996[vi]; Werry, 1994[vi]). Despite problems of comorbidity in these studies, it appears that children and adolescents with a primary diagnosis of conduct disturbance are likely to respond to stimulant treatment.

Combination treatments of psychosocial and stimulant treatments have also been assessed in experimental studies. A unique prospective study demonstrated that delinquency consequent to disruptive behavior was more likely to be prevented by a multimodal treatment (MMT), including psychosocial intervention with child and parent and stimulant medication ($n = 50$), than by a treatment with stimulant medication alone ($n = 80$) (Satterfield et al., 1987[iii]). The two groups had been reasonably matched on pretreatment variables, and both were hyperactive with conduct problems, including antisocial behavior. The subjects were about 17 years old at follow-up. Official teenage arrests and institutional rates were significantly lower in the MMT group. The study highlights the importance of long-term follow-up in assessing the value of multimodal treatments.

A small double-blind study by Carlson et al. (Carlson, Pelham, Milich, & Dixon, 1992a[ii]) also found that stimulant medication alone had limited or negative effects on behavioral symptoms. In an experimental single-case study, Blum et al. (Blum, Mauk, McComas, & Mace, 1996[iib]) contrasted methylphenidate with behavioral management in three individuals with severe to profound mental retardation. Two of the three children benefited from drug treatment, and all three benefited from behavioral interventions. In this study there was no evidence of additive effects, but this may be accounted for by ceiling effects on the measures used. Kolko and colleagues (Kolko, Bukstein, & Barron, 1999[i]) conducted a randomized placebo-controlled study of the separate and incremental effects of two doses of methylphenidate and behavior modification. There were 22 children with ADHD and comorbid CD in the trial. Only 72% of the subjects completed the trial. Both treatments appeared to benefit the child and the treatments in combination led to incremental improvements. For example, methylphenidate treatment was associated with positive mood and behavior, whereas behavior modification was associated with a reduction of negative behaviors. The study suggests that multiple dimensions of behavior in multiple settings must be assessed in outcome trials of ADHD/CD treatments and that the combination of behavioral and psychostimulant treatments is justified in cases of comorbid disorders.

Thus, evidence on combination treatments is equivocal. Although long-term follow-ups suggest that the effect of psychosocial treatments may be amplified and made more durable by stimulant medication, other studies find no evidence for additive or interactive effects, and yet others indicate that psychosocial and pharmacological treatments may act on different response systems. At present there is no clear indication as to which stimulant may be most effective for a particular child (Stoewe et al., 1995[vi]), although those with longer half-lives may require lower doses.

Lithium

It is suggested that the feature of CD most likely to respond to psychopharmacological intervention is aggression (affective subtype) (Campbell & Cueva, 1995b[ib]). Recommendations for the use of lithium in the treatment of affective aggression are based on the work of Campbell and her co-workers, who carried out double-blind placebo-controlled studies of inpatient children with a formal diagnosis of CD and major problems with explosive behavior and aggression. In one study (Campbell et al., 1984[ii]), 61 5- to 12-year-olds with a diagnosis of CD were given lithium, haloperidol, or placebo. The trial lasted 4 weeks. Outcome measures included the Children's Psychiatric Rating Scale (CPRS) and a clinical global impression instrument (CGI). There were significant changes with both types of active medication on the aggression, hostility, and hyperactivity cluster of the CPRS. Lithium was superior to haloperidol, both in terms of the size of the effect and the relative infrequency of adverse side effects. The authors make the clinical observation that although lithium reduces explosiveness and thus permits other positive changes, haloperidol merely makes children more manageable, making the children feel "slowed down" rather than helping them control themselves. There was some evidence of a reduction in aggressive behavior on a number of independent measures. However, the lithium treatment had some untoward side effects, including increased confusion and bewilderment and increased tension and anxiety, perhaps accounted for by the relatively high upper end of the range of serum lithium levels (up to 1.79 mEq/l).

Campbell et al.'s double-blind placebo-controlled study of lithium with conduct disordered children deserves special mention (Campbell et al., 1995[i]). This more recent study included children who had been hospitalized for treatment-resistant severe aggressiveness and explosiveness, and who had been diagnosed with CD. The double-blind placebo controlled trial of lithium lasted 6 weeks and was completed by 50 children. Lithium was superior to placebo, although on some measures this was a more modest gain than the previous study found.

Some studies have not found lithium to be beneficial in the treatment of aggression in CD. For example, 33 adolescent conduct-disordered inpatients were administered lithium in a double-blind, placebo-controlled study (Rifkin et al., 1997[i]). Three patients out of 14 improved on lithium, compared with 1 of 12 in the placebo group. This may be due to the inadequate length of treatment, which was only 2 weeks. Other studies, with the same treatment duration, demonstrated only limited effects (Lavin & Rifkin, 1993[vi]; Rifkin, Doddi, & Dicker, 1989). In still other studies (Abikoff & Klein, 1992[vi]; Klein, 1991; Klein et al., 1994[i]), the severity and subtype of the aggression appeared to be the critical determinant of effectiveness. In the Klein study, 80 outpatients participated, but only a few children manifested the kind of aggressive, explosive, dangerous behavior that was an indication for lithium in the Campbell trials. In one of these trials, a single long-term controlled study of 11 patients, equal improvement was observed in the treated and the placebo groups (Campbell et al., 1995[i]). A more recent study (Malone, Delaney, Luebbert, Cater, & Campbell, 2000[i]) found that the affective subtype of aggression predicted treatment response to lithium in 28 aggressive conduct-disordered children. However, this group also responded more markedly in the placebo condition. Large placebo effects are not surprising in view of the demanding nature of the treatment protocol. The same workers conducted a large randomized 6-week double-blind placebo-controlled study of lithium in inpatients with conduct disorder, hospitalized because of severe aggression (Malone et al., 2000[i]). Of 86 patients who enrolled, 40 entered and completed the treatment phase of the trial. In the lithium group, 16 of 20 subjects were responders on the consensus ratings versus 6 of 20 in the placebo group. More than 50% of the participants in the lithium group experienced nausea, vomiting, and urinary frequency, which not only threatened the blindness but indicates the complexity of this treatment protocol. The subjects in this study were somewhat older than those in the original Campbell et al. trials, but doses were broadly the same.

On balance, the findings suggest that lithium may be appropriate for the pharmacological treatment of explosive, severe, aggressive manifestations of CD. Evidence is available from a follow-along study of 196 adolescents treated for 1 to 10 years that long-term lithium therapy can be safely undertaken in clinical settings (DeLong & Aldershof, 1987). An appropriate treatment protocol (Campbell, Gonzalez, & Silva, 1992[vi]) should include baseline laboratory investigations (complete blood count with differentials, electrolytes, blood uria nitrogen, creatinine, and liver function tests, thyroid function tests, and electrocardiography). Blood lithium levels need twice-weekly checks until stabilized, followed by monthly essays. Side effects are common. Sixty percent of children aged 6 years or younger manifested various side effects during the initiation of lithium treatment (Hagino et al., 1995[vi]). In view of the dangers associated with the use of lithium, the significant side effects such as weight gain and tremor, and the need for regular monitoring of blood levels, expert opinion suggests that lithium should be considered only with very cooperative families where other treatments for the child's explosive aggressive behavior have failed (Werry, 1994[vi]).

Clonidine

A relatively small number of studies support the use of clonidine in the treatment of destructive and aggressive manifestations of conduct disturbance. Clonidine, an antihypertensive agent sometimes used in adult psychiatry in disorders of arousal, has been investigated in an open study of 17 outpatients ages 5–15 who presented with treatment-resistant conduct problems, including destructiveness and cruel behavior (Kemph, DeVane, Levin, Jarecke, & Miller, 1993[ii]). Fifteen patients showed improvement with clonidine. The most troubling side effect was drowsiness. In a small-scale double-blind placebo-controlled trial of 10 boys with ADHD (Hunt, Minderaa, & Cohen, 1986[i]), clonidine over 8 weeks was found to reduce explosive aggression, according to teachers' reports. The reports also indicated that the children tended to be more readily accepted by peers. Further double-blind controlled studies will be required before an evidence base for the use of clonidine is established.

Carbamazepine and Other Anticonvulsants

The use of carbamazepine is based on the speculation that the aggressive outbursts common in CD may in some cases be due to abnormal electrical activity in the temporal lobe. Anticonvulsant medication may be expected to control such neural overactivity. Carbamazepine was used in a pilot study of 10 conduct-disordered children (Kafantaris et al., 1992[ii]). They were inpatients with severe aggressivity and explosiveness and were reported to have fewer of these symptoms with carbamazepine. There was, however, a high incidence of side effects. Carbamazepine, in some respects, has similar clinical effects to lithium but is free of extrapyramidal side effects (see Kowatch & Bucci, 1998). Two further open trials suggested positive effects (Mattes, 1990[ii]; Vincent, Unis, & Hardy, 1990[ii]). The study by Mattes (1990[ii]) of 80 patients, ages 16 years and older, compared propranolol and carbamazepine for the treatment of rage outbursts. Although propranolol was more effective for patients with comorbid ADHD, carbamazepine was superior for patients with intermittent explosive disorder.

Trials with better controls yielded less promising outcomes. In a double-blind placebo-controlled trial over 6 weeks, Cueva et al. (1996[i]) did not find carbamazepine superior to placebo in reducing aggression in 12 hospitalized conduct-disordered children (ages 5–12), contrasted with 11 controls. Carbamazepine had a significant number of side effects, even at optimal doses, including moderate and marked leucopenia, rash, dizziness, and diplopia, which disappeared only with tapering and discontinuation of the drug. However, the sample size was rather small and the elimination of placebo responders in the trial reduced the likelihood of identifying significant group differences.

Sodium valproate is another anticonvulsant with beneficial effects on temper outbursts. Donovan et al. (1997[ii]) conducted an open trial of 10 adolescents with chronic temper outbursts and mood lability over a 5-week period. All subjects showed clear improvements at 5 weeks. Those who continued on medication maintained their improvements. Five of the 6 who discontinued relapsed and recovered when they continued medication once again. In a randomized double-blind replication (Donovan et al., 2000[i]), the authors administered sodium valproate to 20 outpatient children and adolescents with ODD and CD diagnoses, who met criteria for explosive temper and mood lability. Treatment lasted 6 weeks, with doses of the drug increased over 2 weeks to 10 mg/lb/day. The main dependent variable was the Modified Overt Aggression Scale. The drug was well tolerated, with only four subjects developing mild side effects (increased appetite). There were significant differences between the placebo and active treatment groups after 6 weeks. After crossover, six of the eight responders to medication began relapsing on placebo. The results support the use of anticonvulsants in the treatment of explosive temper and mood lability. Although this study yielded promising results, the small sample size and the crossover design suggest caution in interpreting the findings.

In summary, anticonvulsants have not been adequately assessed. Pilot studies showing promising results are undermined by the indifferent results from better-controlled trials.

Beta-Blockers and Minor Tranquilizers

Beta-adrenergic receptors of both beta-1 and beta-2 types are involved in the fight-or-flight response. Connor et al. (Connor, Ozbayrak, Benjamin, Ma, & Fletcher, 1997a[ii]) conducted an open trial of 12 subjects (mean age 13.8 years) who were placed on nadolol (mean dose 109 mg, representing .6–5.8 mg/kg). Length of baseline varied, and outcome was evaluated in weekly observational assessments. Entry to the trial was on the basis of clinically significant aggression or significant inattention to an activity. Most subjects had either autism or mild or moderate mental retardation. Five subjects were on other concurrent medication, including anticonvulsants, anticholinergics, neuroleptics, or lithium. Overall, 83% of the subjects showed clinical improvement. The improvement was most marked on the observer aggression scales.

Minor tranquilizers have not been used extensively because of the risk of disinhibition or aggressive dyscontrol, which has been identified in about 1% of child and adolescent patients (Dietch & Jennings, 1988[vi]). Buspirone has shown promise in reducing aggression in a number of case studies (Quiason, Ward, & Kitchen, 1991[iib]; Ratey, Sovner, Parks, & Rogentine, 1991[ii]). One case report, however, showed children undergoing a psychotic reaction with this agent (Soni & Weintraub, 1992[vi]). An open-label study of buspirone in 25 prepubertal psychiatric inpatients presenting with anxiety symptoms and moderately aggressive behavior reported limited but significant therapeutic effects on aggression, anxiety, and depression (Pfeffer, Jiang, & Domeshek, 1997[ii]). However, buspirone had been discontinued with over 25% of the sample, with four developing increased aggression and agitation and two, euphoric mania.

Neuroleptics

Neuroleptics are powerful sedatives. It would not be surprising if they had anti-aggressive effects. Controlled studies showed that neuroleptics resulted in decreased aggression (Greenhill, Solomon, Pleak, & Ambrosini, 1985[i]). The investigators showed that both molindone and thioridazine reduced aggression somewhat, but raters were not blind to active treatment and blind teachers noticed no differences. In a study by Campbell and her team (Campbell et al., 1984[ii]), cited earlier, neuroleptics were found to be inferior to lithium, in terms of both outcome and side effects. Neuroleptics, though effective in reducing aggressiveness, are frequently excessively sedative, thus interfering with learning and performance (Campbell & Cueva, 1995b[ib]; Findling, Schulz, Reed, & Blumer, 1998[vi]). The other side effects of neuroleptics can also be very severe (leucopenia, tremor, dystonic reactions, tardive dyskinesia, neuroleptic malignant syndrome) and potentially irreversible (Campbell & Gonzalez, 1996[vi]). Case reports of tardive dyskinesia observed in children are accumulating (e.g., Demb & Nguyen, 1999[v]; Lyons, 2000[v]).

One of the atypical antipsychotics (clozapine) was tested in an open trial with 36 psychotic adolescents (Remshmidt, Schulze, & Martin, 1994[v]). Aggression was measured directly, but results were comparable with those of a previous study

(Schmidt, Trott, & Blanz, 1990[v]) that found that paranoid hallucinatory symptoms, states of excitement, and aggressive behavior responded to clozapine. An open clinical study of risperidone in a clinically heterogeneous group of 11 children ages 5–16 showed moderate to marked improvement in 7 children (Schreier, 1998[v]). A similar open-label study (Buitelaar, 2000[ii]) of 26 subjects with borderline or mild mental retardation and aggressive behavior reported that 14 of the subjects manifested a marked reduction in aggression, and a further 10 a moderate reduction. The dose range was 0.5 to 4.0 mg/day over periods of 2 to 12 months. Seven children experienced tiredness and sedation, necessitating dose reduction, and 2 had marked weight gain. Similar observations on a similar sample have been reported by Holford et al. (Holford, Van der Walt, & Peter, 2000[ii]). Further clinical reports suggest that risperidone has a place in the treatment of aggression in nonpsychotic children and adolescents (e.g., Fras & Major, 1995[v]).

A study of 118 mentally retarded 5- to 12-year-olds with CD compared risperidone (0.02–0.06 mg/kg/day) with placebo over a 6-week period in a randomized trial (Aman, Findling, & Derivan, 1999[i]; Brecher, 1999[i]). On clinician's rating, risperidone was more effective than placebo and appeared to be well tolerated, apart from increased sedation (51%), headache (29%), and weight gain (15%) in some children. There were no detected effects on attention or short-term memory. However, because the sample was comorbid with mental retardation, it is unclear how far the findings are generalizable to CD. A study of 20 aggressive youths with CD ages 6–14 (Findling et al., 2000[i]) compared risperidone (up to 1.5 or 3.0 mg/day according to weight) with placebo in a randomized controlled trial. Six subjects assigned to risperidone and 3 to placebo completed the 10-week protocol. The subjects were free of significant comorbidity. Findings indicated that risperidone was well tolerated, but side effects included increased appetite, sedation, headache, insomnia, restlessness, and irritability. No subject experienced parkinsonian symptoms. Risperidone was superior to placebo in ameliorating aggressive symptoms on clinician ratings, although significant differences were not found on all measures, which is hardly surprising given the limitations of the study. The very small size of the sample suggests caution in interpreting the results. Atypical antipsychotics may have improved tolerability and greater ability to reduce some target symptoms (Findling et al., 1998[vi]), but as the receptor-binding profile of the atypical agents is not the same, it should not be assumed that what is demonstrated for one of these agents also applies to the others. Furthermore, reports are accumulating that the atypical antipsychotics are not as free of side effects as initially hoped. For example, hyperprolactinemia (elevated levels of prolactin in the blood) may be a concern for youths on atypical antipsychotics, which could potentially cause amenorrhea and irregular periods, sexual dysfunction, breast engorgement and lactation, and gynecomastia (Cohen & Biederman, 2000; David, Taylor, Kinon, & Breier, 2000; Dickson & Glazer, 1999; Frazier & Matthes, 1975[v]; Kleinberg, Davis, de Coster, Van Baelen, & Brecher, 1999; McConville et al., 2000; Nicolson, 2000; Sallee et al., 2000; Wudarsky et al., 1999). Other reports suggest that clozapine may be associated with myocarditis and cardiomyopathy (Kilian, Kerr, & Lawrence, 1999).

Tricyclic Antidepressants and Selective Serotonin Reuptake Inhibitors

Clinical reports have suggested that disturbances of conduct were reduced in boys who were comorbid for depression and conduct disorder, upon administration of imipramine (Puig-Antich et al., 1987[i]). In an open trial of 75 mg trazodone with three children, significant decreases of aggression were observed (Ghaziuddin & Alessi, 1992[v]). In a further open trial of the same drug in hospitalized children, disruptive behavior problems decreased (Zubieta & Alessi, 1992[v]). Another open-label trial of 13 nondepressed adolescent inpatients with comorbid CD, ADHD, and substance abuse, found that a 5-week treatment of 300 mg bupropion resulted in significant decreases of hyperactivity, daydream inattention score, and CGI/S (Clinical Global Impression of Severity) (Riggs, Leon, Mikulich, & Pottle, 1998[v]). The study was uncontrolled.

There is evidence of reduced concentration of the neurotransmitter serotonin and its 5-HIAA metabolite in the central nervous system in association with increased aggressive behavior in animals and humans. Controlled clinical trials of serotonin agonists in depressed adults have suggested that aggressive behavior is less likely during treatment with selective serotonin reuptake inhibitors (SSRIs) than with placebo. There is, however, no evidence for the effectiveness of SSRIs in the treatment of children with CD or oppositional defiant disorder (ODD) (DeVane & Sallee, 1996[ib]). Only a small number of double-blind controlled studies and 16 open-label trials are available, and very few of these concern aggressiveness. Only sparse evidence, mostly anecdotal, exists for the effectiveness of SSRIs for conditions other than depression and obsessive–compulsive (OCD). An open study of 19 inpatient adolescents who were receiving fluoxetine, paroxetine, or sertraline for a minimum of 5 weeks did not show overall improvement in levels of aggressive behavior (Constantino, Liberman, & Kincaid, 1997[ii]). There was, in fact, an increase in some ratings of aggression. In another study of 24 children receiving fluoxetine, 50% of the children experienced side effects of restlessness, hypokinetic behavior, insomnia, and excitation (Riddle, King, Hardin, & Scahill, 1990/91[v]). The reported modest side effects of behavioral disturbances limited recommendations and warranted caution for widespread use.

Summary and Implications

There is survey evidence for the significant use of polypharmacy in the treatment of children with ODD/CD in the United States and of substantial active placebo effects with these disorders, at least in inpatient settings.

Psychostimulants have been shown to be effective in reducing antisocial behaviors in children and adolescents with comorbid ADHD–ADD/CD diagnoses, independent of the effect of these medications on attention deficit and hyperactivity symptoms. Combinations of psychosocial and stimulant treatments have been tried, and there are some indications that the two in combination may have broader and longer-lasting effects than either alone. There is suggestive evidence of somewhat clearer gains from psychostimulants with longer half-lives.

Lithium is likely to be less effective than methylphenidate in the treatment of antisocial behavior. Lithium may be appropriate for the pharmacological treatment of explosive, severe aggressive manifestations of CD, but in view of the complexities of the treatment protocol, substantial side effects, and limited advantage over placebo, this treatment should be restricted to very cooperative families where other treatments for explosive aggressive behavior have failed.

Clonidine has been shown in small-scale open trials to improve destructive and aggressive behavior, but evidence at the moment is suggestive rather than compelling. Anticonvulsants have been tried and found useful in the treatment of impulsive behavior in open trials, but better-controlled investigations have reported more equivocal findings, including substantial side effects. Traditional neuroleptics appear to be effective in reducing aggressiveness, but these effects are associated with sedation and interference with learning as well as more severe side effects. Atypical antipsychotics show promise in the reduction of aggressiveness and are less likely to be associated with unwanted effects, although weight gain may prove to be a problem. There is no strong evidence to support the use of either beta-blockers or minor tranquilizers in the treatment of ODD/CD. Antidepressants have not yet been demonstrated to be helpful in the treatment of ODD/CD symptoms.

Medication cannot be justified as the first line of treatment for conduct problems. A diagnosis-based approach, which defines primary or comorbid psychiatric disorders associated with aggression, should guide the pharmacological treatment of CD.

6

Attention-Deficit/ Hyperactivity Disorder

In this chapter and the next we discuss attention-deficit/hyperactivity disorder (ADHD) or hyperkinesis, and Tourette's disorder. These are seen as neuropsychiatric disorders because of the frequent association with central nervous system manifestations. Neurological signs and symptoms are part of the definition of Tourette's syndrome. It is also frequently associated with hyperkinesis and learning difficulties. The situation with the attention deficit disorders is more varied, depending on the definitions used, but there is a frequent association with learning difficulties. There is other evidence of brain involvement, such as epilepsy, clumsiness, language delay, and a variety of syndromes (e.g., fragile X, fetal alcohol syndrome). This chapter reviews the clinical presentation of ADHD and then summarizes the literature review on treatment. We will refer to only the more robust studies from the vast literature on the attention deficit disorders in this chapter.

DEFINITION

The characteristics of ADHD are reduced levels of concentration or attention, impulsivity, and overactivity or restlessness. There is no clear demarcation between extremes of normality and truly abnormal degrees of these behaviors. ADHD has been variously named minimal brain dysfunction, hyperkinesis, attention deficit disorder (ADD), attention deficit disorder with hyperactivity (ADD-H), and attention-deficit/hyperactivity disorder (ADHD) at different times and in different locations. Opinions differ about the interchangeability of these names. In America and Australia, DSM-IV refers to the diagnosis of attention-deficit/hyperactivity disorder. In Europe, the ICD-10 (World Health Organization) classification system refers to hyperkinetic disorder. In practical terms, *hyperkinetic disorder* is a narrower term describing a subgroup of ADHD. European experts have argued that the diagnostic category of ADHD corresponds largely to the conduct disorder diagnosis of ICD-10 (Prendergast et al., 1988; Sandberg, 1982), because inattention is a required diagnostic criterion for the hyperkinetic diagnosis but not for ADHD. Pervasiveness of the problems and an absence of clinically significant anxiety are also criteria for diagnosis of hyperkinetic disorder. Children so diagnosed also tend to have other neurodevelopmental delays (Taylor, Sandberg, Thorley, & Giles, 1991).

Work of the last two decades has indicated at least two, and probably three, subtypes of attention deficit disorder. DSM-III-R gave a polythetic definition of ADHD consisting of 14 symptoms covering the problems of inattention, hyperactivity, and impulsiveness. Any 8 of these could constitute the full syndrome; hence, there could be great heterogeneity among those receiving the diagnosis of ADHD. It failed to take into account the findings from several factor-analytic studies, such as the study by Lahey and Carlson (1992), that there appear to be two separate dimensions: the impulsive hyperactive, and the inattentive disorganized dimension. DSM-IV describes three types of ADHD: predominantly inattentive, predominantly hyperactive, and combined (both sets of symptoms). Six or more symptoms are required for each symptom group. Some symptoms must have been present before the age of 7 years and must have persisted for longer than 6 months. ICD-10 requires age of onset before the age of 6, whereas DSM-IV requires onset before 7 years.

The difficulty caused by cross-cultural variations in perceptions of hyperactivity are highlighted by a recent study (Mann et al., 1992), which asked 37 health professionals from China, Japan, Indonesia, and the United States to rate four video vignettes of 8-year-old boys. Chinese and Indonesian clinicians gave significantly higher ratings of hyperactive and disruptive behaviors despite the use of standardized rating scales. This confirms the concern about comparing prevalence rates across cultures, although much of the difference may be attributed to the criteria set by the two classification systems. Prendergast et al. (1988) found that if diagnosis was based on the respective criteria of the two systems, there was agreement on caseness. In other words, clinicians on either side of the Atlantic could be taught to use the opposite side's criteria, after training.

The significance of the differences in diagnostic criteria for attention deficit disorders needs further evaluation. However, because far more of the relevant literature on attention deficit problems comes from the United States rather than Europe, in this chapter we will use the term ADHD, as defined in DSM-III-R and DSM-IV, to describe attention deficit disorders.

PREVALENCE

Suspected hyperkinesis or ADHD is now the most frequent reason for referral to child and adolescent mental health services in the United States. A similar situation is beginning to develop in the United Kingdom. Prevalence rates vary according to the diagnostic system and criteria used. The American Psychiatric Association (1994) estimates the rate in school-age children at between 3% and 5%.

Taylor et al. (1991) found that 1.7% of 7-year-old boys in a London population sur- vey fulfilled criteria for the more restricted hyperkinetic disorder diagnosis. The authors commented that this probably overestimated the true prevalence of hyperkinetic disorder in the general population, as it is commoner in boys and in urban areas, and 7 is the peak age for recognition of the disorder. They suggested that a prevalence of at least 0.5% in the general population may be more accurate. As this figure applies to the extreme end of problems with hyperactivity, it can be seen that a significant number of children are affected by the disorder. Studies of the prevalence of the less restricted diagnosis of ADD-H or ADHD have found a prevalence in children in the range of 4.2% to 12% (August, Ostrander, & Bloomquist, 1992; Bergeron, Valla, & Breton, 1992). The prevalence of ADHD in adolescents is in the range of 1.5% to 5% (Bergeron et al., 1992; Lewinsohn et al., 1993).

ADHD is thought to occur much more frequently in males. There is no consis- tently reported prevalence ratio between males and females. The American Psychi- atric Association (1987) reports a male–female ratio in clinic-referred samples ranging from 9:1 to 6:1. This contrasts with a ratio of 3:1 from population-based studies (Szatmari, Offord, & Boyle, 1989).

CLINICAL PRESENTATION

Children with ADHD and, to a greater extent, hyperkinesis show impaired func- tioning in most areas of their lives, including home and school settings. Their impulsivity and inattention leads to frequent criticism from relatives, peers, and teachers. Their hyperactive and often aggressive behavior leads to peer rejection.

The peak age of referral for ADHD or hyperkinesis is between 7 and 9 years, but peak age of onset appears to be in the preschool period at around 3 years. Onset of the more restricted hyperkinetic disorder is probably earlier, at 2 or 3 years, be- cause of the associated neurodevelopmental problems (Thorley, 1984). Sandberg, Rutter, and Taylor (1978) reported that the more pervasive the hyperkinesis, the earlier the onset. Children with attention problems without hyperactivity have later onset at about 6 years (Green, Loeber, & Lahey, 1991).

A recent meta-analysis of 18 studies describing gender differences based on rel- evant variables highlights gender differences in presentation (Gaub & Carlson, 1997). Clinic-referred girls with ADHD showed lower levels of hyperactivity and fewer externalizing behavior problems, but greater intellectual problems than boys. The sexes did not differ in terms of impairment due to inattention, internalizing behavior, peer aggression and disliking. Among the nonreferred children, however, boys with ADHD were more likely to be impaired by inattention, internalizing behavior problems, and peer relationship difficulties. These findings suggest that many of the gender differences may be attributable to referral bias; there may be a different threshold for referral of boys than for referral of girls. Boys are more likely to be referred for treatment than girls because of the increased rate of disruptive externalizing behavior problems in boys. This could mean that although boys with

ADHD are generally more severely impaired than girls with ADHD, studies of clinic samples fail to detect these inequalities because only the most severely affected girls are referred. The ratio of boys to girls who attend treatment clinics is between 6:1 and 9:1, despite the ratio of boys with ADHD to girls with ADHD in the community being lower, at 3:1 (Brown, Madan-Swain, & Baldwin, 1991). Further research is needed to determine whether boys and girls with ADHD are receiving appropriate services.

The behaviors causing impairment in ADHD are difficult to measure. Although there is an understanding of the necessary behaviors required to make the diagnosis, recognizing the point at which the behaviors in question become abnormal can be problematic, especially in very young children. Hyperkinesis or ADHD often has its onset in the second or third year, but because children of this age are normally active and have a short attention span, certainty about a diagnosis is even more problematic with these children than with older children. The varying presentations of ADHD or hyperkinesis also add to the difficulty of accurate diagnoses.

At assessment parents and child should be interviewed; interviews should include an inquiry about possible comorbidity and environmental causes of the problems. It is also important to ask about the home situation (e.g., parental conflict, financial hardship, parental mental disorder) and about the child's educational progress. This information can be obtained by way of standardized rating scales and an open report from the school. Classroom observations are also informative. A variety of questionnaires are available; the best validated are the Child Behavior Checklist (CBCL) (Achenbach, 1991a; Achenbach & Edelbrock, 1983b), which includes a teacher report form, and the Conners parent and teacher rating scales (Goyette, Conners, & Ulrich, 1978). Children should be medically examined, and a comprehensive assessment of their learning abilities, including reading and writing, should be made.

The etiology for the primary problems of inattention and hyperactivity is heterogeneous. Multiple secondary factors, such as parental disharmony, bullying, and additional learning difficulties, in many cases produce the behavior problems that lead to referral.

Comorbidity

Biederman, Newcorn, and Sprich (1991) have recently reviewed the literature and reported that the comorbidity of ADHD is high: 30–50% of children with this disorder have comorbid conduct or oppositional disorders, 15–75% have a mood disorder, and 25% an anxiety disorder. The type of comorbid problem seems to vary in the two subtypes. Those with hyperactivity are more likely to have a comorbid conduct disorder. Those without hyperactivity are more at risk of internalizing symptoms such as anxiety and depression (Barkley, DuPaul, & McMurray, 1990a; Cantwell & Baker, 1992). Little is known about the differences in response to medication or outcome. Further research is clearly required in this area.

Several authors have reported that 50% of children with ADD have speech or language impairments (Love & Thompson, 1988). Similar numbers of children go on to have reading and writing difficulties. Visuomotor problems and clumsiness are also common (Losse et al., 1991; Taylor et al., 1991). Hallgren, Gillberg, Gillberg, and Enerskog (1993) found that visuomotor problems persisted into adolescence, placing the young person at higher risk of accidents than the control group. Taylor et al. (1991) similarly report a higher rate of accidents in pervasively hyperactive youngsters. Richters et al. (1995) report that 10–25% of children with ADHD have comorbid learning disorders.

In a study of 7-year-old children in Sweden, Gillberg et al. (Gillberg, Rasmussen, Carlstrom, Svenson, & Waldenstrom, 1982) reported that 1–2% of the sample had a combination of severe pervasive hyperactivity and impaired motor control and perception (DAMP). This combination of problems is often seen clinically but is not included in either classification system. Many (50%) children with severe DAMP have also been found to have autistic features (Gillberg & Gillberg, 1989). In an attempt to clarify the problems of social relationships often associated with ADHD, Clark et al. (Clark, Feehan, Tinline, & Vostanis, 1999) have reported a retrospective case study in which 49 cases of ADHD were examined; 65–80% of subjects reported significant difficulties in social interaction (particularly in empathy and peer relationships) and communication (maintaining conversations, imagination, and nonverbal behavior).

Natural History

There have been few follow-up studies of preschoolers, in whom until recently hyperkinesis and ADHD were rarely diagnosed. In a study of a 3-year follow-up of "problem" 3-year-olds, Campbell, Ewing, Breaux, and Szumowski (1986) reported that 33% met criteria for ADD at follow-up. Fifty percent showed some of the features of the disorder, such as being inattentive and impulsive and/or aggressive at follow-up. Children rated as more hyperactive at age 3, with more externalizing behavior problems generally, were more likely to have persistent problems at age 6, but at age 3 the future hyperactive children could not be distinguished from those who would be oppositional or conduct disordered.

McGee, Partridge, Williams, and Silva (1991) reported a 12-year follow-up of 21 hyperactive preschoolers. They were compared with a "difficult to manage group," and a 'developmental control group', selected because the hyperactive group showed poor language skills. At follow-up the hyperactive group had poorer language development, lower verbal and performance intelligence scores, and poorer reading ability in primary school. Children in the matched developmental control group were similar to those in the hyperactive group in these areas, suggesting that the problems at outcome in this group were due to the presence of delayed language development in the hyperactive preschoolers, rather than hyperactivity per se. However, the reading ability of the hyperactive preschoolers at age 15 was lower than that of the developmentally delayed group, suggesting that hyperactivity does affect academic outcome. At follow-up the hyperactive group showed a higher level of psychiatric disorder, particularly ADD, than the developmentally delayed group or the normal controls. Seventy-five percent of the hyperactive preschoolers had some form of behavior disorder at age 15. A similar number of the difficult-to-manage group had behavior problems at age 15, but they were less pervasive.

Many authors have reported the high risk of continuity of behavior problems in hyperactive children. Fischer, Barkley, Fletcher, and Smallish (1993b) reported the findings of a prospective 8-year follow-up study comparing 158 hyperactive children with 81 well-matched controls. They used standardized assessment tools to measure the degree of behavioral disturbance. At follow-up, on all measures the hyperactive subjects were significantly worse than the controls, although their behavior problems had improved over time.

Barkley, Fischer, Edelbrock, and Smallish (1991[i]) reported an 8-year follow-up study comparing outcome from childhood into adolescence in 100 hyperactive children and 60 controls. At follow-up the hyperactive children still had conduct and learning problems and were more hyperactive, inattentive, and impulsive than controls. Mothers of hyperactive children reported more frequent family conflicts and higher levels of distress in adolescence as compared with controls. These authors found that lower childhood verbal intelligence and greater pervasiveness of behavior problems in the home predicted greater conflict at follow-up. These variables and the rate of maternal commands in free play accounted for a large amount of the variance in predicting the presence of conduct problems at follow-up. Aggressive behavior is more predictive of long-term outcome than inattention or hyperactivity.

Fischer, Barkley, Fletcher, and Smallish (1993a) used multiple linear and logistical regression equations to relate childhood predictor variables to adolescent outcome. Academic success in adolescence was predicted by higher intelligence in childhood and a reduced need for special education. These two variables explained more than 21% of the variance of adolescent outcome.

Biederman, Wilens, Mick, Spencer, and Faraone (1999) have reported an important study on the risk of substance abuse in adolescence. They followed up male subjects diagnosed with ADHD who were older than 15 at the time of the study. The study compared the rate of substance abuse in ADHD subjects who had received medication (mean duration of treatment 1.7–7.1 years) with those who had not. None of those treated with medication were receiving treatment at follow-up. The authors found that the untreated ADHD subjects were at significantly increased risk for substance misuse at follow-up, compared with non-ADHD controls. Medicated ADHD subjects had a significantly lower risk of substance misuse than the nonmedicated ADHD group. Stimulant medication reduced the risk for substance misuse even in the ADHD subjects with a comorbid conduct disorder.

Up to 80% of school-age children will have the same diagnosis of ADHD or hyperkinesis 5 years later or in adolescence. The disorder will persist into adulthood in up to 65% of these individuals (Weiss & Hechtman, 1993). At least one-third will continue with a conduct disorder and will have increased rates of substance abuse in adolescence, with problems persisting into adulthood in the form of trouble with the police and personality disorder. The factors most highly predictive of poor outcome include family history of ADHD or hyperkinesis, psychosocial adversity, and comorbidity with conduct, mood and anxiety disorders (Biederman et al., 1996).

TREATMENT

Physical Therapies

Psychostimulants

Stimulants are the most frequently prescribed drugs for children with ADHD and have been shown to be effective in the control of hyperactive and aggressive behavior in these children. There are two available stimulants: methylphenidate and dexamphetamine. They are both fast-acting drugs. They are rapidly absorbed after oral ingestion and have an onset of action within the first hour. The duration of effect is no more than 4 hours. Several authors (Wilens & Biederman, 1992[ib]) have reported that the serum blood level and onset of action have a similar time course with methylphenidate, with a half-life for both of approximately 3 hours. On the other hand, the blood level of dexamphetamine does not peak until 4 hours.

Methylphenidate is the most frequently used psychostimulant (Swanson, Lerner, & Williams, 1995a[vi]), despite the fact that there is little evidence for its superiority over other stimulant preparations. Methylphenidate has a short half-life, which often necessitates several doses throughout the day. Another problem is that as many as 40% of children with ADHD do not respond to methylphenidate, although they may respond to other stimulants; there is, however, no way of predicting which child will respond to which stimulant preparation. Greenhill et al. (1996) confirmed that methylphenidate and dextroamphetamine (also known as dexamphetamine) were similarly efficacious in a meta-analysis of five studies comparing the two drugs. Thirty-eight percent of 141 subjects responded equally well to either stimulant, 35% responded best to dexamphetamine, and 26% responded best to methylphenidate.

Methylphenidate is also available in long-acting form or extended-release tablets (known as Ritalin-SR), but the time course has been found to be too variable (Pelham et al., 1990b[i]). Attempts have been made, therefore, to develop a more reliable treatment. With this in mind, a long-acting presentation of methylphenidate (Concerta) designed to provide cover for 12 hours has been tested in structured and unstructured settings in 70 children between the ages of 6 and 12 years over a trial period of 3 years (Pelham, Burrows-Maclean, & Gnagy, 1999b[i]; Pelham, Gnagy, Burrows-Maclean, Williams, & Fabiano, 1999c[i]). The study found that there were no significant differences in responses to the two drug preparations, apart from a significantly better parental report of their child's behavior in the evening with the long-acting preparation, as compared with the immediate-release preparation. There were no significant side effects from either preparation. Further studies are required, but based on these findings Concerta may be beneficial when children need to be medicated in the evening and compliance is poor.

A long-acting amphetamine compound (Adderall) has been developed, and so far results from trials appear to be hopeful. Adderall is a 75:25 ratio of dextro- and levoamphetamine. It has been shown to have a longer half-life than methylphenidate (Swanson et al., 1998[i]), which could be advantageous in reducing the frequency with which the drug needs to be taken during the day.

Two randomized controlled studies have compared the response to Adderall and methylphenidate. The first to be published is by Pelham et al. (1999a[i]). These authors compared the response of 25 children with diagnoses of ADHD when taking 10 mg methlyphenidate, 17.5 mg methylphenidate, 7.5 mg Adderall, 12.5 mg Adderall, and placebo. Both drugs led to significant improvements, but the two doses of Adderall produced significantly higher effect sizes (ESs) than the methylphenidate, particularly at midday and at 5 P.M. The side effect profile was similar for both drugs. The authors also found that the 7.5 mg Adderall dose was equivalent to the 17.5 mg methylphenidate dose and that there was no advantage from a higher Adderall dose. However, the children in this study were taking part in an intensive behavioral program, which could have led to an additive effect on the medication response. The results therefore may not be generalizable to all settings. The authors also emphasize the need to explore adjustment of dose to the child's weight in future studies. Pelham et al. (1999a) recommend prescribing Adderall in preference to methylphenidate when the latter wears off midmorning or midafternoon and compliance or the school setting prevents the use of extra methylphenidate doses.

Pliszka, Browne, Olvera, and Wynne (2000[i]) have also compared Adderall and methylphenidate. These authors compared the two drugs in a sample of 53 children who were not also engaged in a behavioral program, hence assessing the generalizability of the findings of Pelham's study. The children were randomly allocated to either methylphenidate, placebo, or Adderall for a 3-week trial. The dose was varied according to the child's weight. Those weighing less than 60 pounds were treated with 5 mg and those heavier than 60 pounds received 10 mg initially. A psychiatrist blind to the drug status adjusted the dose, depending on response and side effects. Both stimulants led to significant improvement, with significantly more responders in the Adderall group. None of the Adderall group required a midday dose; however, some of the methylphenidate group also managed without a second dose. The authors concluded that the behavioral improvements with Adderall treatment persist for longer during the day than occurs with methylphenidate. Manos, Short, and Findling (1999[i]) have confirmed this finding.

There appears to be a reasonable consensus among experts on both sides of the Atlantic (Greenhill, 1992[ib]; Swanson, McBurnett, & Wiwal, 1993[ib]; Taylor, 1994[ib]) about the procedure for stimulant treatment. Stimulants should commence with a suboptimal dose (5 mg methylphenidate and 2.5 mg dexamphetamine in school-age children) in order to reduce the risk of side effects. There is great individual variation in responsiveness. The dose should be increased gradually while monitoring for effectiveness and any adverse reactions. The recommended average daily dose of methylphenidate is 10–40 mg per day, divided into between two and six doses. The maximum dose is 60 mg. An adequate trial is between 4 and 8 weeks.

Overall, 20–25% of patients who respond poorly to one treatment will respond well to another (Dulcan, 1990[ib]). Side effects are common and dose related, but rarely serious. Probably the most severe side effect is precipitation of a psychosis (Bloom, Russell, Weisskopf, & Blackerby, 1988), but this is rare. Possible adverse reactions include appetite suppression, insomnia, irritability, mood changes, nausea and vomiting, growth suppression and an increase in heart rate and/or blood pressure. Height and weight should be monitored regularly. Pulse and blood pressure should be monitored after an increase in dose. Some children may have a behavioral rebound 5 hours after the last dose. Adding clonidine may be necessary for a severe rebound. Alternatively, a small dose of stimulant in the late afternoon may reduce the rebound effect.

Klein, Landa, Mattes, and Klein (1988[iii]) investigated the effect of methylphenidate on height using data from 58 hyperactive children (mean age 10 years 2 months). Subjects were either taken off medication for the summer vacation or continued on medication during two consecutive summers. There was no difference after one summer, but after two summers subjects who had been taken off medication were significantly taller. These findings support the practice of having annual drug holidays.

Interestingly, Barkley et al. (1990a[i]) reported a high (>50%) placebo rate of side effects. Some of these, such as anxiety and sadness, were decreased with stimulant treatment.

Recommendations regarding dosage are difficult to make, as there is considerable individual variation in response. Several studies have questioned whether there is an ideal dosage. For example, Brown, Wynne, and Slimmer (1984[iii]) reported a study in which they examined which dose (0.15, 0.3, 0.6 mg/kg) or a placebo dose of methylphenidate produced the optimal effect. They found that a dose of 0.3 mg/kg produced optimal performance in concentration and impulse control. Varley and Trupin (1983[i]) also evaluated the optimal dose in a 3-week double-blind study of 85 boys and 13 girls ages 5–15 years. Of those who had not previously been on medication, 74% improved. Nineteen of the 24 who had previously been on medication also improved. Low doses produced optimal effects in learning. The authors suggest that side effects are not the best guide to dosage. Despite the obvious appeal, only two authors so far have reported using individual placebo-controlled trials (Kent, Camfield, & Camfield, 1999[i]; McBride, 1988[i]). Kent et al. demonstrated in a 3-week double-blind, placebo-controlled trial that comparing individual children's responses to placebo capsules and methylphenidate in the clinical setting helped the family decide whether to use methylphenidate long-term.

On the issue of monitoring, Taylor (1999[vi]) suggests that "intense and frequent monitoring of response with clear guidelines about actions to be taken is likely to be the key to improving results" (p. 1097). A multimodal treatment study of children with ADHD (The MTA Cooperative Group, 1999a[i], 1999b[i]) showed that the response to medication at a research center was significantly better than at a community treatment center. As the children were randomized to the community treatment site, this result was not due to case selection. However, it is not known whether intensive monitoring is required for all affected children, and, if not, which features indicate the requirement. Taylor suggests that this is an important area for further research.

Another important recent paper is that by Jensen et al. (1999[iib]), which reported findings from the Methods for the Epidemiology of Child and Adolescent Mental Health Disorders (MECA) study. The study sought to determine what proportion of children with ADHD were treated, how they were treated, and whether children without ADHD were prescribed stimulants. The authors found that only 12% of the children with ADHD were receiving stimulants. Approximately 25% were receiving extra input in school, and 33% were receiving behavioral or psychotherapeutic help. Fifty percent of children receiving stimulants did not meet criteria for a diagnosis of ADHD, although they had high levels of certain ADHD symptoms. The authors suggest that over- and underprescribing occur and that further studies with more detailed measurements of these treatment patterns are required.

EFFECT ON THE PRIMARY SYMPTOMS

The beneficial effects of the stimulants for the primary symptoms of inattention, hyperactivity, and impulsivity have been confirmed by more than 100 trials of medication. Some of the better known include those by Porrino, Rapoport, Behar, Ismond, and Bunny (1983[i]); Abikoff and Gittelman (1985[i]); Taylor et al. (1987[i]); Pelham et al. (1990a[i]); Hinshaw (1991[i]); DuPaul and Rapport (1993[i]); and Wilkison, Kircher, McMahon, and Sloane (1995[i]). In addition, there have been several helpful recent reviews (AACAP Official Action, 1997[ib]; Barkley, 1990[ib]; Greenhill, 1992[ib]; Jacobvitz, Sroufe, Stewart, & Leffert, 1990[ib]; Simeon & Wiggins, 1993[ib]; Swanson, McBurnett, Christian, & Wigal, 1995b[ib]; Taylor, 1986[ib], 1994[ib]; Wilens & Biederman, 1992[ib]). In the recent National Institute of Clinical Excellence (NICE) (United Kingdom) review of the evidence for methylphenidate treatment, the Institute concluded that methylphenidate is recommended for children with a diagnosis of severe ADHD or hyperkinetic disorder (NICE, 2000). The review also recommended that "in some cases treatment may be appropriate for children and adolescents who do not fit the diagnostic criteria for Hyperkinetic Disorder but are experiencing severe problems due to inattention or hyperactivity/impulsiveness" (p.17). There is no doubt that stimulant medication relieves the primary symptoms, at least in the short term. There is less certainty, however, regarding the extent of the benefit. Swanson et al. (1993[ib]) have helpfully undertaken a review of the literature. They found that there is a fairly good consensus that the ES of stimulant treatment on the primary symptoms of ADHD or hyperkinetic disorder is 0.8 and that 70% of treated children respond. In contrast, the ES on academic performance is approximately 0.4. The placebo response rate appears to be approximately 30%.

As observed in the classroom, stimulants have been shown to improve the primary behavior problems of ADHD to the level of normal controls in 75% of treated children. Abikoff and Gittelman (1985[i]) reported a randomized controlled study in which 28 hyperactive boys ages 6–12 years were treated with methylphenidate for 8 weeks to examine the effects on behavior. After the treatment the subjects were indistinguishable from the controls in terms of interference with peers, time spent off the chair, noncompliance, minor and gross motor movement, and aggression. DuPaul and Rapport (1993[i]) similarly found that 75% responded to the point of being indistinguishable from their peer controls. The remaining 25% failed to achieve normalized levels of classroom performance and required additional input such as a classroom aide. It is difficult to predict which children will fail to respond.

In addition to assessments of the response to medication as observed in the classroom, more recent studies have looked at laboratory measures of the symptoms of ADHD, such as impulsivity. Two types of impulsivity have been described in the literature. *Behavioral impulsivity* refers to a disregard for the consequences of an action and a lack of tolerance for any delay in gratification. *Cognitive impulsivity* refers to a tendency to give answers without adequate consideration as to their accuracy. The Matching Familiar Figures Test was developed to assess cognitive impulsivity. Unfortunately, it is unclear whether inaccuracy alone or a fast inaccurate response is characteristic of children with ADHD. Other tests, such as the Continuous Performance Test and the Porteus Maze Test, have been developed, but are thought not to be specific to impulsivity.

Using the Matching Familiar Figures Test, several authors have reported a decrease in errors when the child is treated with a stimulant. Some of these authors have shown an increase in response time, and others have reported no change. Similar approaches have used other test paradigms such as a word-matching test (Malone & Swanson, 1993[i]), and it has been reported that the control children made fewer impulsive errors than the children with ADHD on placebo. The children with ADHD on medication performed nearly as well as the nonaffected control group and significantly better than untreated children with ADHD.

THE INFLUENCE OF AGE AND COMORBIDITY ON THE RESPONSE TO STIMULANT TREATMENT

Stimulant Use in Adolescents. The response of adolescents to stimulant medication has also been assessed in three open and three double-blind, placebo-controlled studies: 75% showed a good response (Evans & Pelham, 1991[i]). In one of the largest studies of stimulant use in this age group, Klorman, Brumaghim, Fitzpatrick, and Borgstedt (1990[i]) reported findings from a study of 48 adolescents with ADHD ages 12–18 years who had not previously received stimulant therapy. They used a randomized controlled trial design with 3 weeks of medication and placebo. Methylphenidate significantly reduced teacher and parent ratings of hyperactivity, inattention, and oppositionality, although parents were more likely to report improvement than teachers. Thirty-seven percent of adolescents failed to benefit from the methylphenidate treatment, which is higher than the nonresponse rate in younger children (20–25%).

How stimulants are of benefit in any age group is not fully understood, but one small study suggests that stimulants have a positive effect on the underlying mechanisms in addition to the primary symptoms in this age group, as well as in younger children. Coons, Klorman, and Borgstedt (1987[i]) reported a significant improvement in information processing in 19 adolescents ages 12–19 years, compared to placebo.

There have been concerns that stimulants may be abused in adolescence, but studies have found no evidence for this (Hechtman, 1985[i]; Loney, 1988). In fact, Hechtman reviewed eight outcome studies comprising 580 adolescents and found no increase in substance abuse in those who had received stimulants. In Hechtman's own prospective study of 25 subjects (mean age of 22), who had all received stimulants for a minimum of 3 years at the time of follow-up, the treated subjects had fewer car accidents, later onset of delinquency (prognostically better than earlier onset), better social skills, higher self-esteem, and more positive memories of childhood than the untreated comparison group. It therefore seems likely that appropriate stimulant treatment may protect against the development of substance abuse, because of the improvement in self-esteem and frustration tolerance.

For those interested in further reading, there are some helpful reviews of stimulant treatment in adolescence by Wilens and Biederman (1992[ib]), Greenhill and Setterberg (1992[ib]), and Spencer et al. (1996[ib]).

Stimulant Use in Preschoolers. Five randomized controlled studies have assessed the response of preschoolers to medication (Barkley, 1988[i]; Barkley, Karlsson, Strzelecki, & Murphy, 1984[i]; Mayes, Crites, Bixler, Humphrey, & Mattison, 1994[i]; Musten, Firestone, Pisterman, Bennett, & Mercer, 1997[i]; Schleifer et al., 1975[i]). They show that children of this age respond to stimulant medication. On the whole, these studies did not find a higher rate of side effects in preschoolers as compared with school-age children. Improvement was observed in structured tasks, in addition to mother–child interaction. The authors reported that generally the response is less predictable in preschoolers and suggest that medication should be used in this age group only when parent training and behavioral interventions have failed. Musten et al.'s study found that stimulant medication in 31 children with ADHD ages 4–6 years produced an improvement in cognitive measures of attention, in addition to parent-reported benefits. More than 80% of children showed some improvement on the parent rating scales. Side effects were not severe.

In summary, therefore, regardless of age, 75% of children with ADHD show normalization of inattention, hyperactivity, and impulsivity when treated with stimulants. It is not possible to predict reliably which children will show a good response. In addition, 70% of children with ADHD with comorbid aggression will show significant improvement in aggressive behaviors to the level of controls. However, prosocial behaviors do not improve and it has, in fact, proved difficult to improve them by treatment generally.

Stimulant Use with Comorbid Internalizing Disorders. Spencer et al. (1996[ib]) reviewed the findings from 11 studies that examined the interaction of internalizing symptoms on the response of children with ADHD to stimulant medication. Most of these studies reported that the presence of a comorbid internalizing disorder such as anxiety or depression reduces the response to stimulant medication (DuPaul,

Barkley, & McMurray, 1994[i]; Plizka, 1989[i]; Taylor et al., 1987[i]). In a well-designed trial, DuPaul found that in a sample of 40 children with ADHD and varying degrees of internalizing symptoms, significantly fewer of the children in the high internalizing group exhibited a positive response to methylphenidate than subjects with fewer internalizing symptoms. Fifty percent of the children with significant comorbid internalizing symptoms either failed to respond or had an adverse reaction to methylphenidate. Twenty-five percent of the children with a comorbid internalizing disorder showed deterioration in behavior with stimulant use, compared with 9% in the groups with few internalizing disorder symptoms. It should be noted that this deterioration was based on teacher reports of classroom behavior.

There have been three notable exceptions to the aforementioned studies. The first was that of Tannock, Ickowicz, and Schachar (1995a[i]), who reported a study in which 22 nonanxious children were compared with 18 anxious subjects. Although methylphenidate failed to improve the working memory of the anxious group, it improved motor activity equally in the two groups.

Second, Diamond, Tannock, and Schachar (1999[i]) reported findings from their randomized controlled study in which the presence of comorbid anxiety did not reduce the behavioral response to methylphenidate. Nor did it predict an increased number of adverse reactions to methylphenidate. Although the anxious group had a higher rate of somatic complaints and conduct disorder symptoms prior to the initiation of the treatment, there are some concerns about the reliability of the anxiety diagnoses in this study. The third study that failed to find an impact of comorbid anxiety on stimulant responsiveness is the large Multimodal Treatment Study for Children with Attention-Deficit Hyperactivity Disorder (MTA) (March et al., 2000[i]), described later in the section on multimodal therapies.

In summary, when ADHD is comorbid with depression and/or anxiety, until recently it was observed that only 50% of the children significantly benefited from stimulant treatment. In addition, there was presumed to be an increased risk of adverse reactions and deterioration in the mental state. The findings from three recent studies have led us to conclude that, at least in the case of anxiety, this may not be the case. The findings from the MTA study also suggest that when ADHD occurs in the presence of comorbid internalizing disorders, additional behavioral interventions may be appropriate and more beneficial than when ADHD occurs on its own.

Stimulant Use with Comorbid Conduct Disorder and Aggression. Spencer et al. (1996[ib]) report 17 controlled studies of stimulant treatment in ADHD. They conclude from their review of these studies that stimulants produce a significant improvement in ADHD symptoms in children with comorbid aggression. They also found that stimulants reduce both verbal and physical aggression in these subjects. This concurs with the findings of an earlier review of the subject by Hinshaw (1991[i]).

In a randomized controlled trial of 83 children that initially set out to assess the response of children with CD in the absence of ADHD, Klein et al. (1997[i]) similarly reported that the presence of comorbid CD did not affect responses to stimulant medication. They also found that the symptoms of CD responded to stimulant medication at least in the short term and the response was independent of the severity of ADHD symptoms. This is an important finding, as to date stimulant medication has not been recommended for the first-line management of CD. The only behavior that did not significantly improve was socialized aggression (severe delinquent behavior such as gang membership). Further studies are required with a longer period of follow-up before these findings can be seen as conclusive.

In summary, 70% of children with ADHD who have comorbid aggression will show significant improvement of aggressive behaviors to the level of controls when treated with stimulants. Prosocial behaviors do not improve, however.

Stimulant Use with Comorbid Learning Disability. ADHD and hyperkinesis are approximately four times more prevalent in children with learning disability than in those with normal intelligence (Biederman et al., 1991). There is no consistent view in the literature regarding the efficacy of medication in children with ADHD who have comorbid learning disabilities because most studies have excluded such children from their samples. Those few that have included learning-disabled subjects have tended to contain only those with mild deficits. Earlier studies had reported stimulants to be ineffective in this group (Barkley et al., 1990a[i]). More recent studies, however, by Payton, Burkhart, Hersen, and Helsen (1989[i]), Aman, Marks, Turbott, Wilsher, and Merry (1993b[i]) and Handen, McAuliffe, Janosky, Breaux, and Feldman (1995[i]) have reported a response rate averaging 65%, which is useful, although lower than the rate of 70–80% reported in the literature for non-learning-disabled school-age children. Handen et al. (1999[i]) have also reported a small (11 subjects) randomized controlled study confirming that preschool children with learning disabilities respond to methylphenidate at a similar rate to school-age children, although there is a suggestion that there is a higher rate of side effects in the younger age group. Aman and colleagues (Aman, Kern, McGee, & Arnold, 1993a[i], 1993b[i]; Aman et al., 1991[i]) reported that children with higher IQs and better overall functioning showed better responses than those whose IQs were lower. More severely mentally retarded children are more difficult to treat; these children appear more likely to develop adverse reactions and are less likely to show behavioral improvement than their nonretarded peers.

Mayes et al. (1994[i]) report a small study in which 19 children with a learning disability (an IQ less than 80) and ADHD, and 44 children with ADHD only, were blindly allocated to methylphenidate. Conners rating scales were used to assess response. Side effects were monitored. The response rate for the learning-disabled group was 68.4% and was not significantly different from the non-learning-disabled group. The rate of side effects did not differ between the two groups.

An important subgroup of children with ADHD are those with fragile X, because most of these children have ADHD or hyperkinesis. Hagerman, Murphy, and Wittenberg (1988[i]) have reported a crossover double-blind study of a small sample (n = 15) of children with ADHD with fragile X who were treated with methylphenidate, dexamphetamine, or placebo. The authors found that these children showed significant behavioral improvement in response to stimulant medication.

Stimulants, therefore, are often beneficial in the presence of a comorbid learning disability; the more severe the learning disability, however, the poorer the response.

Stimulant Use with Comorbid Specific Learning Disabilities. Many children with ADHD or hyperkinesis have a comorbid specific learning disability such as a specific reading retardation, although the estimated prevalence of these two disorders occurring together varies between 10% and 92% (Biederman et al., 1991). One study (Kupietz, Winsberg, Richardson, Maitinsky, & Mendell, 1988[i]) has shown that children with ADHD who have a comorbid specific learning disability respond as well to stimulant treatment as children with ADHD without a comorbid learning disability. A second placebo-controlled study demonstrated that behavioral improvement in class was associated with increases in reading scores (Richardson, Kupietz, Winsberg, Maitinsky, & Mendell, 1988[i]). In summary, in the presence of ADHD and a specific learning disability, stimulant therapy facilitates improvements in the learning disability.

Stimulant Use with Comorbid Pervasive Developmental Disorders. Early studies suggested that stimulants should not be used when ADHD was comorbid with a pervasive developmental disorder because of the risk of increasing stereotypic behavior (Aman, 1982[vi]). However, a more recent open study (Birmaher et al., 1988[ii]) of methylphenidate in nine autistic children reported significant behavioral improvement without a worsening of stereotypic behaviors. Further studies are required in this area.

Stimulant Use with Comorbid Seizure Disorders. Until recently, stimulants were avoided in children with ADHD who had comorbid seizures because they were thought to lower the seizure threshold. Some clinicians would prescribe dexamphetamine but not methylphenidate, because it was thought that dexamphetamine raised the seizure threshold. One double-blind study (Feldman, Crumrine, Handen, Alvin, & Teodori, 1989[i]) of stimulant treatment of ADHD in 10 children with a comorbid seizure disorder has shown that stimulants did not affect the seizure threshold and did not lead to an increase in seizures. The authors concluded that if the seizure disorder is adequately treated, stimulants are safe to use. As there has been only one well-designed study addressing this question, however, stimulant treatment should be administered with caution in children with well-controlled epilepsy.

Stimulant Use with Comorbid Tics and Tourette's Disorder. This subject is discussed in Chapter 7, on Tourette's disorder.

ADAPTATION TO PSYCHOSOCIAL ENVIRONMENT

Social Relationships. Children with ADHD and hyperkinesis usually have serious social difficulties. They tend to respond impulsively and aggressively in the context of social relationships (Hinshaw, 1991[i]).

There have not been many studies of the effects of stimulants on social relationships, but those that have been done suggest a benefit in this area, showing that children who respond positively to stimulant medication receive increased warmth and decreased maternal criticism, with an increased frequency of maternal contact (Schachar, Taylor, Wieselberg, Thorley, & Rutter, 1987[i]; Whalen & Henker, 1991[vi]). Hinshaw, Henker, and Whalen (1984a[i]) assessed the effects of methylphenidate at doses of 10–40 mg on the social performance of 24 8- to 13-year-old hyperactive boys. Social interactions were directly observed and rated in classroom and playground settings. The authors found that medication and cognitive-behavioral treatment were optimal in terms of improving prosocial behaviors and self-control. Placebo plus reinforcement alone led to the worst outcome. However, other studies have found no advantage from the addition of cognitive-behavioral therapy to medication alone.

In support of the suggestion that medication alone improves social relationships, several authors have reported a decreased incidence of arguments and fighting in stimulant-treated boys with ADHD (Barkley, McMurray, Edelbrock, & Robbins, 1989[i]). Children also become more popular with their peers, but some social difficulties often remain (Gadow, Nolan, Sverd, Sprakin, & Paolicelli, 1990[i]; Whalen et al., 1989[i]). About 70% of children and adolescents treated with medication show a good response. Nevertheless, Swanson et al. (1993[ib]) concluded that although stimulants may reduce the negative behaviors, they do not increase the positive prosocial behaviors; other therapies are required if social relationships are to be fully normalized.

Academic Performance. Discussion in the literature of the benefits, if any, of stimulant medication on learning in children with ADHD is ongoing. In a meta-analysis of 135 studies, Kavale (1982[ib]) found moderate positive effects favoring the drug treatment. The results revealed a 15% increase in achievement for those treated with methylphenidate.

More recently, in a randomized controlled study, Rapport, Denney, DuPaul, and Gardner (1994[i]) evaluated the effects of methylphenidate on the classroom behavior and academic performance of 76 subjects ages 6–11 years. The measures included (1) observations of the children's attention, (2) percentage of assignments completed, and (3) teacher ratings of classroom behavior using the Abbreviated Conners Teacher Rating Scale. Standardized statistical assessments showed that medication significantly improved all three areas. This finding continued to apply when academic efficiency was divided into percent completed and percent correct. The methylphenidate accounted for a significant amount of the variance in attention (46%), academic efficiency (32%), and teacher ratings (41%). Doses of 10 mg or more significantly increased the performance in all three areas, as compared to placebo or a 5 mg dose.

Overall, 76% of the sample showed either improved or normalized attention (72% were normalized), with 24% showing no change; 53% showed improved or normalized academic efficiency (50% normalized); and 47% showed no change in academic efficiency. Increasing the dose of stimulant improved attention and classroom performance but not academic accuracy, which stabilized at the lower dose of

10 mg. In contrast, the numbers for normalized attention and classroom behavior increased as the dose of methylphenidate was raised toward 20 mg. Hence, for some children academic performance may not improve in line with changes in behavior. Moreover, the children who failed to show improvements in academic accuracy were less likely to have shown improvements in attention.

Several authors (Alto & Frankenberger, 1995[iii]; Carlson, Pelham, Swanson, & Wagner, 1991[i]) have suggested that mathematical skills are particularly sensitive to methylphenidate. However, Zentall and Ferkis (1993[i]) failed to support this finding in their study. Another question has been the dose effect on learning. This is an important question, as Swanson, Cantwell, Lerner, McBurnett, and Hanna (1991[ib]) have suggested that high doses of stimulant may produce such an overfocusing effect that it impedes learning. These authors suggest that higher dosage levels may optimize achievement in some tasks and lower dosages may maximize other tasks, such as those demanding greater cognitive effort.

Several studies have attempted to clarify the mechanism for improvement in academic performance. Richardson, Kupietz, Winsberg, Maitinsky, and Mendell (1988[i]) investigated the effects of methylphenidate and placebo on reading achievement in 42 7- to 13-year-olds with hyperactivity and reading disorder. Methylphenidate produced improvements in reading mediated through behavioral control after 12 weekly reading sessions. A specific effect of methylphenidate on word recognition involving verbal retrieval, as opposed to phonic skills, was also found. Similarly, in an attempt to delineate the mechanism of improved performance, Balthazor, Wagner, and Pelham (1991[i]) examined performance in a classroom reading comprehension test in 19 boys treated with methylphenidate (Posner Letter-Matching task). The improvement with methylphenidate was attributed to nonspecific aspects of information processing, as opposed to specific aspects. The responses in the methylphenidate condition were faster and of greater accuracy than they were with placebo. A third study by Forness, Cantwell, Swanson, Hanna, and Youpa (1991[i]) confirmed a significant improvement in reading comprehension but not reading recognition, in stimulant-treated children with ADHD.

However, longer-term follow-up studies have often failed to confirm the beneficial effects of stimulants on academic performance. Weber, Frankenberger, and Heilman (1992[i]) used a group achievement test to assess the response to methylphenidate versus control before and after 1–2 years of treatment of 22 subjects with ADHD. They concluded that methylphenidate did not improve achievement.

Alto and Frankenberger (1995[iii]) reported a study of 17 subjects with ADHD aged 7–8 years. Each of these children was matched with a control child according to age, gender, and cognitive abilities. The authors found that even when subjects were matched on verbal cognitive scores, they showed significantly lower achievement in the areas of word analysis and reading. The performance of subjects with ADHD in math approached a significant increase in rate of learning as compared with the control group. Listening skills were more likely than vocabulary skills to respond to medication. Increase in dosage further increased listening but had an opposite effect on vocabulary. The authors concluded that although the children with ADHD were behind their normal peers in most areas of learning at onset, once they were placed on methylphenidate their learning rate was equal to that of the controls so that they did not fall further behind, although they did remain behind in reading skills. Because the study lasted a year, it was not possible to assign children to a placebo treatment, as parents and teachers were reluctant to consent to this.

In practice, medication alone is unlikely to be an adequate intervention for optimal academic achievement. Studies such as that by Pelham, Milich, and Walker (1986[i]) have found that when behavioral approaches incorporating a reward system were combined with methylphenidate, performance was maximized.

Therefore, although attention and output during academic tasks improve by 70% with stimulant medication, efficiency and accuracy show only approximately 50% improvement. In the long term, subjects with ADHD treated with stimulants do not achieve as much as nonaffected control individuals, probably because there is too much to catch up. Further studies are required to verify this as the cause of poorer long-term academic progress.

UNDERLYING MECHANISMS

Working Memory. Working memory involves the ability to hold a small amount of information in mind while carrying out further activities, such as remembering an address while purchasing a birthday card.

Working memory is required for many areas of learning and classroom functioning. It is highly correlated with performance on several academic and language-related tasks, such as vocabulary, reading comprehension, arithmetic, and problem solving (Swanson et al., 1995b[ib]). In a recent well-designed double-blind trial by Tannock et al. (1995a[i]), the authors compared the response of working memory to stimulant medication in children with ADHD both with and without comorbid anxiety. The authors chose this design because of the hypothesis that the presence of anxiety preempts some processing and storage resources of the working memory system.

In this study the authors used a serial addition task—the Children's Paced Auditory Serial Addition Task (CHIPASAT) (Dyche & Johnson, 1991)—to assess working memory. The CHIPASAT consists of tape-recorded single-digit numbers; children are required to add each new number to the immediately preceding number. Methylphenidate significantly improved working memory as compared with placebo in 22 children with ADHD without comorbid anxiety, but not in the 18 children with ADHD with comorbid anxiety. Interestingly, there was no difference in the response of the two groups in terms of the children's motor activity. The finding of a difference of effect on working memory demonstrates why outcome should, where possible, be measured in terms of the underlying mechanisms or cognitive and emotional capacities that are thought to underpin symptomatology and adaptation.

Cognitive Flexibility. Cognitive flexibility refers to the ability to shift freely from one concept to another or change a course of action or thought according to the demands of the new situation (Tannock, Schachar, & Logan, 1995[i]). Several studies have found that children with ADHD show deficits in response inhibition (Schachar, Tannock, & Logan, 1993[i]; Tannock, Schachar, & Logan, 1995b[i]). In a study of 28 children with ADHD, Tannock et al. (1995b[i] entered a placebo-controlled trial in which the children received 0.3 mg/kg, 0.6 mg/kg, or 0.9 mg/kg of methylphenidate or placebo. The study assessed response inhibition by way of a stop signal paradigm, which tests the subjects' ability to modify their responses to different stimuli. Methylphenidate was found to enhance cognitive flexibility, although the lower doses were better than the higher doses in enhancing response inhibition. Dose response curves for response reengagement were linear but, for response inhibition, were an inverted U-shape. None of the doses impaired either aspect of cognitive flexibility. Rather, methylphenidate accelerated both so that children were faster to stop their ongoing actions and faster to replace them with alternative actions. The results on dosage suggest that the optimal benefit overall will be obtained by using a medium dose.

Response Inhibition and State Regulation. These concepts are based on the hypothesis that the rate of presentation of stimuli affects the activation state of subjects (Sanders, 1983). The term "activation state" as used here relates to the subject's readiness to initiate motor action. It is suggested that a fast presentation of stimuli leads to a rapid inaccurate response and a slow presentation leads to a slow and inaccurate response. The theory goes on to suggest that when stimuli are rapidly presented, subjects are required to inhibit activation (response inhibition). When stimuli are presented slowly, subjects have to increase activation. A test paradigm known as the GO–NO GO measure has been developed (Van der Meere, Stemerdink, & Gunning, 1995[i]). Children with ADHD appear to be poor at modulating their activation states and make many errors in the fast and slow presentations. In the medium condition, however, the number of errors is equivalent to the number made by normal controls (Van der Meere, Gunning, & Stemerdink, 1996[i]). In learning-disabled children the error rate is independent of the speed of presentation of the stimuli. Using a randomized controlled trial, Van der Meere, Gunning, and Stemerdink (1999[i]) tested whether methylphenidate or clonidine had any effect on response inhibition and state regulation, but the treatments showed no advantage as compared with placebo. The authors concluded that these problems appear resistant to the medications tried and that they are not the underlying mechanisms of the improvements observed in the drug treatment of ADHD. Similarly, Kempton et al. (1999[i]) reported that the general measure of executive function is impaired in ADHD but returns to normal levels with methylphenidate treatment.

SUMMARY: PSYCHOSTIMULANTS

Seventy-five percent of children with ADHD show normalization of inattention, hyperactivity, and impulsivity when treated with stimulants. It is not possible to predict with certainty who will show a good response. Attention and output during academic tasks improve by 70% with stimulant medication, and efficiency and accuracy show approximately 50% improvement. Prosocial behaviors do not improve.

The outcome of ADHD is still uncertain. However, it appears that treatment is preferable to no treatment, although subjects with ADHD treated with stimulants do not achieve as much as nonaffected individuals long-term, probably because there is too much to catch up. Nevertheless, young adults who were treated for ADHD with stimulants in childhood and adolescence have fewer accidents, improved social skills, and happier childhood memories as compared with untreated individuals with ADHD.

Depending on the type of comorbid problem, stimulant medication is beneficial to varying levels. In the case of CD, 70% of children with ADHD will show significant improvement of aggressive behaviors as well as ADHD behaviors when treated with stimulants. In contrast, when ADHD is comorbid with depression and/or anxiety, until recently it was observed that only 50% of the children significantly benefited from stimulant treatment. In addition, there was presumed to be an increased risk of adverse reactions and deterioration in mental state. The findings from three recent studies have led us to conclude that, at least in the case of anxiety, this is not so.

Stimulants are also often beneficial in the presence of a comorbid generalized learning disability; however, the more severe the learning disability, the poorer the response. They also lead to improvements in the learning problems of specific learning disabilities. Children with a pervasive developmental disorder and ADHD have recently been found to benefit from stimulant therapy without showing an increase in stereotypies. Stimulants are safe to use in the presence of epilepsy as long as the underlying seizure disorder is appropriately treated.

Tricyclic Antidepressants

The tricyclics are the most frequently used alternatives to stimulants. Spencer et al. (1996[ib]) have reviewed the literature on their use in ADHD or hyperkinesis. These authors reported that 92% of the 26 studies of tricyclic antidepressant treatment of ADHD in latency-aged children reported significant behavioral improvement as compared with placebo. Twelve studies evaluated the response to imipramine, nine evaluated desipramine, three amitriptyline, four nortriptyline, and one clomipramine. Recent studies have tended to use higher dosages, and they report a better outcome than the earlier studies (Biederman, Gastfriend, & Jellinek, 1986[i]; Gastfriend, Biederman, & Jellinek, 1985[i]; Wilens, Biederman, Geist, Steingard, & Spencer, 1993[iv]). However, ECGs should be performed regularly and with each significant increase in dose, because of the risk of arrhythmias. Several children receiving tricyclic medication have suddenly died, although the rate may be no higher than the sudden death rate in the general population. Both parents and teachers have reported that behavioral symptoms improve as well with tricyclics as with stimulants. Four studies, including two controlled trials, have included preschool children and have shown significant improvements. Similarly, eight studies included adolescents (Gastfriend et al., 1985[i]; Wilens et al., 1993[iv]), and these reported a similar degree of benefit.

The possible benefits of the tricyclics, as compared with stimulants, are longer duration of action and improved response in children with comorbid anxiety and depression (McClellan et al., 1990). Other advantages include the use of a single daily dose, a reduced risk of medication abuse, and a reduced risk of an afternoon rebound in hyperactive behavior.

Baseline blood pressure, pulse, and ECG, to rule out any preexisting conduction anomalies, should be recorded before tricyclics are prescribed. Pulse, blood pressure, and ECG should also be obtained regularly during treatment, and with each subsequent dose increase.

Biederman et al. (Biederman, Baldessarini, Wright, Knee, & Harmatz, 1989[i]) have reported one of the largest randomized controlled studies, of desipramine in 62 children ages 6–17 years. Forty-three of these children had responded poorly to stimulants. Treatment included 6 weeks of either desipramine or placebo. Significant behavioral improvements occurred at an average dose of 4.6 ± 0.2 mg/kg. Sixty-eight percent of desipramine-treated subjects were considered very much or much improved, as compared with only 10 % when treated with placebo.

In a second paper, these authors reported that this improvement occurred even in those cases with comorbid CD, depression, or anxiety. Cases with "pure ADHD" showed a trend toward a lesser placebo response and a greater desipramine/placebo difference (Biederman et al., 1993a[i]).

In summary, tricyclic antidepressants have been shown to be beneficial in the treatment of the primary symptoms of ADHD in 70% of children of all ages. Although children with "pure" ADHD are likely to show the most improvement with stimulant treatment, those with comorbid depression, anxiety, or aggression also respond. When comorbid anxiety and/or depression worsens with stimulant therapy, it may be preferable to use a tricyclic antidepressant. Tricyclics may also be indicated when there is a severe rebound with stimulant treatment.

Nontricyclic Antidepressants

Spencer et al. (1996[ib]) report that there have been six studies of the use of nontricyclic antidepressants in the treatment of attention deficit. An open-label trial of fluoxetine use in children and adolescents with ADHD has been reported (Barrickman, Noyes, Kuperman, Schumacher, & Verda, 1991[ii]). In this trial 60% improved moderately, and there were few adverse reactions.

An earlier study by Zametkin, Rapaport, Murphy, Linnoila, and Ismond (1985[i] was the first to consider the use of the monoamine oxidase inhibitor (MAOI) group of antidepressants. This 12-week double-blind crossover study evaluated the effects of an MAOI as compared with dexamphetamine in a sample of 14 boys with ADHD ages 7.7–10.7 years. Tranylcypromine sulphate or clorgyline was given twice a day in 5 mg doses. Dexamphetamine was given as 10 mg in the morning and 5 mg at lunchtime. The Conners Questionnaire and a Parent Questionnaire were used, as was a Continuous Performance Test while subjects were on placebo and in treatment week 4. Low tyramine diets were required, and blood pressure was measured weekly. There were no significant adverse reactions. The MAOIs and dexamphetamine improved disruptive behavior, as rated by both teacher and parent to an equivalent degree. Attention also improved with both types of drug. There were no significant differences between them. The main difficulty with the MAOIs is the need for a low tyramine diet because of the risk of a hypertensive crisis. This was a small study of good design and suggests that the newer, more selective MAOIs may provide a promising alternative to stimulant treatment.

A recent German paper (Trott, Friese, Menzel, & Nissen, 1991[ii]) reported a trial of a selective MAOI, moclobemide, in children with ADHD who had failed to benefit from stimulants. The authors reported that there was some improvement in attention and concentration span. There was less improvement in behavior.

Barrickman et al. (1995[i]) have reported a double-blind crossover study contrasting the effectiveness of bupropion and methylphenidate in 15 subjects with ADHD ages 7–17 years. Bupropion is an antidepressant whose pharmacological profile is similar to the stimulants'. The Conners Questionnaire, the Continuous Performance Test, and the Matching Familiar Figures Test were used to monitor response to treatment. According to the parents' reports, methylphenidate was significantly more successful in improving attention than bupropion. The two treatments did not differ significantly in relation to improvement of conduct. Both treatments significantly improved conduct above the baseline behavior.

Casat, Pleasants, and Van Wyck Fleet (1987[i]) reported a double-blind study in which 30 children were treated with bupropion and placebo. The bupropion was superior to placebo in terms of improvement of hyperactivity. A study by Clay, Gualtieri, Evans, and Guillion (1988[i]) similarly reported benefits of bupropion in 28 subjects with ADHD.

Side effects of bupropion include skin reactions, which abate after stopping the drug. Bupropion lowers the seizure threshold at a similar frequency to the tricyclic drugs. As it is a weak dopamine agent, there is a small risk of its precipitating a psychotic illness. Four such cases have been reported in the literature.

The scarcity of studies of treatment with nontricyclic antidepressants in ADHD makes it impossible to advise about their use at this stage, other than to comment that they are worth consideration if stimulants and tricyclic antidepressants are contraindicated.

Clonidine

Clonidine has been used in treating the symptoms of agitation and hyperarousal in Tourette's disorder for the last 15 years. Spencer et al. (1996[ib]) report two controlled trials of clonidine treatment for ADHD alone; These are Hunt, Minderaa, and Cohen (1985[ii]) and Gunning (1992[i]). Based on parents' and teachers' reports, Hunt et al.'s double-blind placebo crossover study of the use of clonidine in children with ADHD found clonidine as effective as methylphenidate and more effective than placebo in reducing motor activity, and in increasing compliance as well as reducing the level of irritability. In a review of the use of clonidine in ADHD with comorbid tics, Hunt, Capper, and O'Donnell (1990[ib]) suggest that it is useful in those with comorbid tic disorders, extreme overactivity and hyperarousal, oppositional or conduct symptoms, and poor response to stimulants.

Four other controlled studies have reported significant improvements in ADHD symptoms in the presence of comorbid disorders with the use of clonidine. Two of these were for ADHD comorbid with tics or Tourette's disorder (Leckman et al., 1991[i]; Singer et al., 1995[i]). The two other studies reported on the response of ADHD with comorbid autism (Fankhauser, Karumanchi, German, Yates, & Karumanchi, 1992[i]; Jaselskis, Cook, Fletcher, & Leventhal, 1992[i]). These four studies are discussed in Chapter 7, on Tourette's disorder, and Chapter 9, in the section on autism. However, it is important to mention them here, as Connor et al. (1999[ib]) have recently reported a meta-analysis of the findings from these studies and three further open studies (Hunt, 1987[iii]; Schvela, Mandoki, & Sumner, 1994[iii]; Steingard, Biederman, Spencer, & Gonzalez, 1993[iii]).

The meta-analysis found that clonidine had an overall ES of .58, based on the results from studies rated as more methodologically sound by the authors: This means that the chance of a clonidine-treated subject showing a better response than a placebo-treated one is 66%. Connor et al. (1999[ib]) compared this result with their own meta-analysis of the controlled trials of tricyclic use, in which they obtained an ES of .44. These findings support the impression from clinical experience that they are less effective than stimulants (which have an ES of .82; see Swanson et al., 1995b[ib]). Another important finding is that clonidine was significantly more effective in the children with ADHD alone than in those with a comorbid tic disorder. There were no other significant differences between groups, but the authors suggest that this could be attributed to the small sample sizes.

It is important to note that meta-analysis confirmed a high rate of side effects with clonidine use. Nine out of 10 studies reported sedation and 6 out of 10 reported irritability. The skin patches were associated with localized skin reactions such as redness, rash, and irritation. No cardiovascular system side effects were described, although Connor et al. reported electrocardiographic changes in the sample in their own study (in press).

Hunt (1987[iii]) had recommended the combination of clonidine and stimulants for those children who did not respond to either drug alone, commenting that as many of the side effects of clonidine are the opposite of those caused by stimulants, combining the two treatments often keeps the side effects to a minimum. Simeon and Wiggins (1993[ib]) have supported this recommendation for combined use of stimulants and clonidine and suggest that the indications for combining these drugs include partial response to stimulants alone, rebound effects, insomnia, impulsiveness, and emotional lability. However, Swanson et al. (1995a[vi]) suggested that as there have been no randomized controlled studies of the combination of stimulant and clonidine medication, the practice of combining them should be avoided until more is known. Connor, Fletcher, and Swanson (1999[ib]) reiterate the concerns about using these drugs in combination.

In summary, although there have been only two studies of the use of clonidine in ADHD alone, it appears to be as beneficial as the tricyclics in the treatment of ADHD symptoms and should be a second-line treatment for those unable to use stimulants, for whatever reason. Until recently it was recommended that an ECG was required prior to treatment and at regular intervals during treatment, but a recent statement from a committee of pediatric cardiologists, accepted by the American Heart Association, states that electrocardiograms are not required (Gutgesell et al., 1999). The risk of a hypertensive rebound means that this treatment must not be stopped suddenly. Two children treated with methylphenidate and clonidine in the United States and one in Australia have died; sudden cessation of clonidine may have been the cause, although this is unproven. Clonidine also frequently causes drowsiness. Although no definite recommendations can be made about the combination of clonidine and stimulant medication until there is more scientific information regarding the safety of their combined use, the rate of prescribing of clonidine, both separately and in combination with methylphenidate, has greatly increased in recent years (Swanson et al., 1995a[vi]). Until more is known about the safety of this drug combination, an ECG should be obtained at the start of treatment and with each dose change.

A drug related to clonidine is guanfacine, which has a longer half-life and is less sedating. It is also more selective in its binding with the alpha receptors and does not bind with the alpha-1 receptors. Hunt, Arnstein, and Asbell (1995[ii]) have reported an open-label study of guanfacine in 13 children with ADHD. Parents rated hyperactivity and inattention as significantly improved when their child was receiving guanfacine. The authors are in the process of completing a double-blind trial.

Carbamazepine

Silva, Dinohra, Munoz, and Alpert (1996[ib]) have conducted a meta-analysis of carbamazepine use in ADHD. They found reports of seven open studies involving a total of 189 patients and three double-blind studies including a total of 53 patients. Overall, 71% of those treated with carbamazepine in the controlled studies showed significant improvement, compared with 26% of those treated with placebo. There was an ES of 1.01 for the drug–placebo comparison in the double-blind studies. Meta-analysis confirmed that carbamazepine was significantly more effective than placebo at controlling ADHD symptoms. A similar response rate was found in the open studies. In terms of side effects, monitoring of the leucocyte count is required because of the risk of leucopenia. Liver function tests should also be checked regularly because of the risk of liver damage. Other side effects include rashes, ataxia, and drowsiness.

Antipsychotics

Antipsychotic drugs should be resorted to only if all of the aforementioned groups of drugs have been tried and the child is extremely disturbed. The child should be reassessed first to ensure that the diagnosis of ADHD is correct. This group of drugs must be used only in the short term and at low dosage because of the risk of side effects. On the whole, the risks are so great that the antipsychotics should probably be avoided in ADHD, although no good studies have evaluated the risks and benefits of this class of drugs.

Combination of Stimulant and Tricyclic Antidepressant

Children with ADHD and a comorbid mood disorder have been treated with the combination of a stimulant and an antidepressant. This practice seems to be more prevalent in the United States than in the United Kingdom. There is no good evidence to support the practice of this type of drug combination.

Exclusion Diets

For some time there has been a suggestion that certain food additives increase behavioral problems in normal and hyperactive children (Mattes & Gittleman, 1981). One of the best-known examples of such additives is tartrazine (Rowe & Rowe, 1994). Where parents have observed a deterioration in their child's behavior following exposure to a particular additive or food, withdrawing this substance may be effective in reducing problems of hyperactivity in an unknown but relatively small number of children (Carter et al., 1993; Egger, Carter, Graham, Gumley, & Soothill, 1985; Kaplan, McNicol, Conte, & Moghadam, 1989; Wender, 1986). However, there is no good evidence for more rigorous exclusion diets despite one earlier study suggesting that about 5% of hyperactive children show behavioral and cognitive benefits with an additive-free or Feingold diet (Feingold, 1975[ii]). Such dietary approaches may be appealing, but are difficult to sustain because they are so restrictive and time-demanding for the family. Contrary to popular belief, there is no evidence for the benefits of large doses of vitamins or herbal remedies.

Psychosocial Therapies

Behavioral Therapies

A variety of behavioral approaches are used in the management of children with ADHD. Progress in this area is summarized in the AACAP review (American Academy of Child and Adolescent Psychiatry, 1997[ib]). Although behavioral approaches are less effective than medication in reducing the primary symptoms of ADHD, they have been shown to improve the targeted behaviors to a degree, in addition to improving social skills and academic performance. The study by Carlson, Pelham, Milich, and Dixon (1992b[ii]) illustrates this well. These authors reported a trial of the single and combined effects of methylphenidate and behavior therapy on the classroom performance of children with ADHD. Twenty-four boys ages 6–12 years participated in an 8-week treatment program. Two doses of methylphenidate were crossed with two classroom settings, which were (1) behavior modification with token economy, time-out, daily home report card and (2) a classroom setting not using these procedures. Both methylphenidate and behavior therapy alone significantly improved subjects' classroom behavior, but only methylphenidate improved academic productivity and accuracy. Singly, behavior therapy and 0.3 mg methylphenidate produced roughly equivalent improvements in classroom behavior. However, the combination of behavior therapy and 0.3 mg methylphenidate resulted in maximal behavior modification, which was nearly identical to 0.6 mg methylphenidate alone.

A study by Pelham et al. (1993[i]) confirmed Carlson et al.'s (1992b[ii]) finding that behavioral management training is beneficial, although less so than medication. These authors evaluated the separate and combined effects of behavior modification and two doses of methylphenidate (0.3 and 0.6 mg/kg), compared with a baseline of no behavior modification and placebo medication. They examined the classroom behavior and academic performance of 31 boys with ADHD attending a summer training camp. Results demonstrated significant benefits of both interventions with a mean ES of medication being more than twice that of behavior modification. Relatively small additional benefit was obtained with the higher dose of medication or with the addition of behavior modification, compared with the effects of low dose medication. The addition of either dose of medication resulted in improvements beyond the effects of behavior modification alone. Comorbid CD did not affect the response to the interventions.

Several authors have compared a variety of behavioral interventions aimed at improving attention, accuracy, and work output in the classroom. The approaches reported have included positive reinforcement, response-cost, and group contingencies. Pfiffner and O'Leary (1987[vi]) have suggested that positive reinforcement alone is insufficient and needs to be combined with mild punishment for optimal behavioral and academic performance. Several authors have suggested that response-cost is the best approach (Abramowitz, 1994[vi]; DuPaul, Guevremont, & Barkley, 1992[vi]; Pfiffner & Barkley, 1990[vi]). The response-cost approach has been refined into an Attention Training System, a battery-operated feedback system that is placed on the child's desk. It displays accumulated points earned at a fixed interval; for each minute the child remains on-task, a point is added. When the teacher observes that the child is off-task, a small remote control button is pressed, which activates a red light on the child's module, signaling the loss of a point from the total. At the end of the lesson the points accumulated are exchanged for free time or small toys. So far this approach has been used with children in small classroom settings. It is not known whether it can be generalized to a mainstream setting where the majority of children with ADHD are taught. The provision of a classroom aide would facilitate its use.

As summarized in the AACAP review (1997[ib]), the main shortcomings of behavioral management in ADHD are the tendency for improvements in behavior not to be sustained over time and the poor generalization of behavioral improvements to situations other than those in which the training occurred. Booster sessions, and training in the setting where the behavioral improvement is required, should help to remedy these problems.

In summary, then, behavior therapy alone is less effective than stimulant medication. Combining behavior therapy with a lower dose of stimulants, however, may lead to sufficient behavioral improvement that a higher dose of medication is not required. Behavioral therapy is most likely to lead to improvements in on-task behavior and a reduction in disruptive and rule-breaking behavior. Improvements in academic performance usually require medication. The main shortcomings of current behavioral management programs are the failure of behavioral improvements to generalize across settings and to be sustained over time.

COGNITIVE-BEHAVIORAL THERAPIES

Cognitive-behavioral treatment combines the techniques of behavioral management with training in problem solving and self-monitoring. Several studies have evaluated the efficacy of cognitive-behavioral therapy (CBT) in children with ADHD, but, unfortunately, all used small samples. The most promising studies were those by Hinshaw, Henker, and Whalen (1984a[i], 1984b[i]), who reported two studies of cognitive-behavioral interventions. The first reported on a sample of 21 boys ages 8–13 years, who had been taking methylphenidate regularly for at least 3 months. Consecutively recruited boys were formed into groups of three. For 3 weeks, the groups met twice a week for 2 hours. All sessions were manualized. The curriculum consisted of problem-solving strategies, which were initially applied to cognitive tasks; in the later sessions, interpersonal problem solving was introduced. Subjects were randomly allocated to a medication or medication-free status for the 3 weeks. For the testing of outcome, subjects were told that they would be teased and had to practice the strategies they had learned. The responses were recorded on video and rated by two blind observers who had good interrater reliability.

Methylphenidate significantly reduced the intensity of the boys' hyperactive behavior, as measured by the vigor and forcefulness of behavior and the likelihood of moving away from a tormentor. However, methylphenidate had no effect on self-control, whereas the cognitive-behavioral treatment, using rehearsal of specific strategies, led to greater levels of self-control and a reduced tendency to vocalize, show verbal retaliation, or fidget. There was strong evidence that the children were mastering appropriate alternative strategies ($p < .001$).

In their second study, Hinshaw et al. (1984b[i]) reported findings from a 5-week summer camp for 24 boys ages 8–13, who had been receiving stimulant medication for at least 3 months. In addition to classroom and playground activities, the boys participated in cognitive therapy training groups with a focus on self-control. The intervention was manualized. A control group did not receive training in cue recognition or specific strategy training and rehearsal. Medication was taken as usual and was randomly replaced by placebo. Methylphenidate significantly reduced the intensity of reactions. However, boys trained in the cognitive-behavioral strategies used a significantly greater proportion of purposeful coping skills during provocation.

In contrast, several recent studies have failed to confirm benefits from CBT. Brown, Wynne, and Slimmer (1985[i]) report a study in which 30 boys ages 6–12 years with a diagnosis of ADD with hyperactivity were randomly assigned to one of three treatment groups: (1) methylphenidate therapy, (2) cognitive training, and (3) methylphenidate combined with cognitive training. There was a no-treatment control group of 10 children on the waiting list (nonrandomly assigned). The treatment lasted 12 weeks and was provided as two hourly sessions a week (24 sessions in total).

The methylphenidate group improved significantly, compared with the cognitive training or no-treatment groups. With the exception of the Durrell Subtest of Listening Comprehension, there was no significant improvement on academic measures. Combining methylphenidate and CBT had no significant advantages over methylphenidate treatment alone. CBT alone produced some improvement in attention, but the benefits were not as large as with methylphenidate.

Abikoff et al. (1988[iii]) evaluated the effectiveness of a 16-week intensive cognitive training course using 33 methylphenidate-treated academically deficient males with ADHD ages 7.4–12.3 years. Eleven subjects received medication plus cognitive training focused on academic skills and self-control. There was no evidence that academically based cognitive training improved performance and achievement. It did not enhance self-esteem or attributional perceptions of academic performance.

As with behavioral therapy, there is a problem with teaching children to generalize any problem-solving strategies they master to different settings and in getting them to use them spontaneously. The current view of experts in the field (AACAP Official Action, 1997[ib]; Abikoff, 1991[ib]) is that CBT is only occasionally beneficial in children with ADHD, and even then is less efficacious than medication.

In summary, CBT appears to be less effective than medication in treating the primary symptoms of ADHD; however, it must also be said that the majority of studies in the field so far have been limited in design. This approach has no advantages over behavioral therapy in relation to academic performance, medication appearing to be required in preference to these psychological approaches. CBT may improve self-control, although most studies to date have failed to confirm this.

PARENT TRAINING

Anastopoulos, DuPaul, and Barkley (1991[ib]) have helpfully reviewed parent training for children with ADHD. They emphasize the need to share with the parents the objective "not to cure or eliminate [the child's] ADHD problem, but to learn methods of coping with and compensating for this ongoing learning and behavioral disability" (p. 214).

A course of parent training would consist of 6 to 12 sessions and is best carried out when the children are prepubertal. Children with more severe behavioral problems will require medication first. Booster sessions are usually necessary. Pisterman et al. (1989[i]) used the nine-step parent training course designed by Anastopoulos (Anastopoulos, DuPaul, & Barkley, 1991[ib]). They reported a well-designed controlled study of parent training with preschoolers with ADHD, comprising 23 children in the treatment group with the same number of controls. Using the group parent training therapy described by Anastopoulos and based on treatment programs of Barkley (1981) and Forehand and McMahon (1981), Pisterman et al. found a significant reduction in noncompliance from pretreatment to 3 months posttreatment. There were no significant changes in the control group. In a second study (Pisterman et al., 1992[i]) these workers looked at the response of other outcome variables in addition to noncompliance. The treatment included a 12-session extension to the course referred to in the first study. The authors reported both a significant increase in compliance and a decrease in the time required to complete tasks.

However, the authors reported a higher dropout rate among the less educated parents and suggest that there must be greater efforts to involve this needy group of parents as further parent training courses are developed. On a more positive note, the majority of parents did complete the treatment and were observed to improve their style of parenting with an increase in appropriate commands and positive feedback for compliant behavior.

Anastopoulos, Shelton, DuPaul, and Guevremont (1993[ii]) examined the changes in parent functioning following participation in a nine-session parent training course specifically designed for children with hyperactivity. The children were ages 5 years 3 months–10 years 3 months. Relative to 15 waiting-list controls, the 19 mothers who completed the course showed significant posttreatment gains maintained 2 months after treatment. Both child and parent functioning improved. On measures of the ADHD rating scale, Parenting Sense of Competence Scale (PSCS), and Parenting Stress Index (PSI), 26–64% of the parent training subjects displayed reliable change and/or normalization, compared with 0–27% of the waiting-list controls. There were reductions in parenting stress and increases in parental self-esteem, which accompanied parental reports of a reduction in severity of the children's symptoms.

Although there have been a limited number of studies, the evidence so far is that parent training increases child compliance and reduces the time for task completion. It also appears to improve parental self-esteem and reduces parental stress.

SOCIAL SKILLS TRAINING

There is no questioning the fact that children with ADHD show social deficits, but the basis of these difficulties is not yet fully understood. Whalen and Henker (1985) have shown that these children struggle to modulate their behavior to changing demands. This applies particularly to social interactions. Hinshaw (1992b) has shown that the strongest predictor of whether children would be rejected in a summer camp was their level of aggressive behavior. Milich and Dodge (1984) have shown that children with ADHD and aggressive behavior are prone to negatively distorting their perceptions of social interactions.

These social deficits are nearly always impairing for the child. Attempts have been made to correct them by social skills training (reviewed by Cousins & Weiss, 1993[ib]), which combines many of the behavioral and cognitive-behavioral approaches discussed earlier. Unfortunately, several studies have shown that despite improvements in behavior as observed by parents, teachers, and researchers, these improvements are often not perceived by peers, leading several authors to suggest involving peers in social skills treatment programs. This is an important area for further research, as impaired social skills appear to be the most disabling and persistent deficit in children with ADHD (Hechtman, Weiss, & Perlman, 1984).

Humanistic and Counseling Approaches

Families with one or more child affected by ADHD or hyperkinetic disorder often require social support. Examples of such support are child care relief, additional help in the home, and assistance with parenting by way of family aides. However, studies are required to evaluate the benefits of these interventions.

Multimodal Interventions

Recent years have seen increasing interest in multimodal therapies for ADHD, because treatments of any kind rarely produce a complete "cure" with generalization of behavioral improvements to all settings (Pelham & Murphy, 1986[ib]). There have been few well-designed studies in this area, and the conclusions have been mixed. One of the best-designed studies, by Horn et al. (1991[i]), reported a controlled trial of high (0.8 mg/kg) and low dose (0.4 mg/kg) doses of methylphenidate alone and in combination with behavioral parent training and child self-control training. Each intervention group receiving the parent training and self-control therapy met for 12 90-minute sessions. There were 96 subjects and 21 controls, and the children were ages 7–11 years. There were no advantages to the combined treatments as compared with the methylphenidate alone, although there was some limited evidence that the effects of a high dose of medication could be achieved by a low dose with a behavioral intervention. However, as the authors pointed out, these findings were based on a single teacher rating.

The authors argue that the failure to demonstrate the supremacy of the combined interventions may be attributed to the limitations of the behavioral interventions used (in particular, their failure to be generalized to settings outside the laboratory) as well as ceiling effects. None of the interventions had any benefit on spelling or arithmetic attainment scores. This finding indicates the need for remedial instruction specific to the cognitive and/or academic disability of the child with ADHD.

Abikoff and Hechtman (1996[ib]) have reported a multimodal intervention for children with ADHD, incorporating methylphenidate, academic study skills training, remedial tutoring as required, individual psychotherapy, social skills training, parent management training, and strategies to provide home-based reinforcements for school behaviors and performance. The authors describe advantages to the combined treatments as compared with attention training or medication alone.

A major problem with all of these studies is that they followed the children for short periods only. One long-term follow-up study of a large sample of boys, which was, unfortunately, uncontrolled (Satterfield, Satterfield, & Cantwell, 1981[ii];

Satterfield et al., 1987[iii]), found that combined treatments were more efficacious than medication alone at follow-up when the child was 14–21 years old. The treatments included parent training, group therapy, psychotherapy, and educational interventions. The combination of treatments depended on the needs of the child and family, very much as happens in clinical practice. The sample, consisting of boys ages 6–12, was divided into two groups, drug treatment only and the multimodal therapy described earlier.

The children who continued with multimodal therapy for 2 to 3 years did best, with significantly lower levels of delinquency than the medication-only group. These findings support the use of multimodal therapy and long-term treatments for this group of children. However, the allocation to therapy was not randomized and the treatments were not standardized. Although the complexity and variation of cases means that this is often the reality of case management in clinical practice, these results must be interpreted with caution.

THE MTA STUDY

The MTA study is a 5-year multimodal treatment study set up by the National Institute of Mental Health. Richters et al. (1995) initially reported the background; since then the results have been eagerly awaited. This study aims to address unanswered questions about the disorder and the possible benefits of multimodal treatments for ADHD as compared with medication alone. At this time, at least seven preliminary reports of the findings at 14 months into the study have been produced. As there has been, according to several of the study investigators, a lot of confusion about the results, there have also been several papers explaining the results. The first official report of the findings (The MTA Cooperative Group, 1999a[i]) describes a sample of 539 children with ADHD. The children were randomly allocated to 14 months of treatment in one of four possible groups: (1) medication, (2) intensive behavioral management with the parents, child, and school, (3) the two combined, or (4) standard care provided by a community team.

The parent training component (Wells et al., 2000[i]) was based on programs developed by Barkley (1987) and Forehand and MacMahon (1981). There were 27 groups with six families per group and eight individual sessions per family. The therapist also provided consultation to the school. The child-focused behavioral work was a summer treatment program developed by Pelham and Hoza as a summer camp (Pelham et al., 2000[i]; Pelham & Hoza, 1996a). The same therapist who provided the parenting and school consultation supervised the child-focused behavioral work, which was provided in a group format. The school-based intervention consisted of a part-time behaviorally trained classroom assistant working directly with the child in the classroom, using methods suggested by Swanson (1992), and fortnightly consultation with the teacher targeting classroom behavioral management strategies, as described by Pelham and Waschbusch (1999[i]).

Medication was optimal for parents' and teachers' ratings of inattention, and teachers' ratings of hyperactivity–impulsivity. There were no other differences between medication and behavioral management. The combined intervention was also superior to behavioral intervention alone on the aforementioned parameters and, moreover, was significantly better than behavioral intervention in three particular areas: (1) parent-rated oppositional/aggressive behaviors, (2) internalizing symptoms, and (3) reading achievement scores. The authors concluded that combined behavioral intervention and stimulant medication—multimodal treatment, the current criterion standard for ADHD interventions—yielded no significantly greater benefits than medication management for core ADHD symptoms. However, the combined treatment was more favorable than community treatment for internalizing symptoms, oppositional behaviors, peer relationships, and parent–child interactions. The authors point out that the evidence is that long-term stimulant medication (14 months) is beneficial and safe and that "carefully monitored" drug treatment may make intensive behavioral interventions unnecessary.

The second MTA paper (The MTA Cooperative Group, 1999b[i]) describes interesting findings on the moderators of treatment response. The main finding is that in the presence of comorbid anxiety (present in 34% of the sample), there was a trend toward a better response to the combined treatment than to medication on its own, and behavioral intervention alone was better than the standard community care; the presence of comorbid anxiety reduced the relative advantage of medication over the other treatments, but it did not reduce the rate of response to medication. The presence of comorbid oppositional or conduct problems had no impact on the response rate. The authors conclude that improvements in ADHD symptoms resulting from medication can lead to a reduction in anxiety symptoms and, therefore, that some of the anxiety present in ADHD-affected children may be generated by their distress about the ADHD problems.

In the first commentary on the responses to the findings, Jensen (1999) suggests that the findings do not mean that behavioral treatment is ineffective. Pelham (1999) makes a similar argument. Firstly, he notes that it had a large ES improvement (.9 to 1.3) from baseline to endpoint across all measures. Second, he points out that the MTA medical management did not differ from withdrawn behavioral treatment (faded out several months before the 14-month review) for most of the measures. Third, there was no difference between the behavioral treatment and community treatment for all of the measures. Therefore, behavioral treatment is nearly as effective as the ongoing MTA medical management.

Pelham points out the relevance of this finding for parents, who often prefer the combined or behavioral approaches. Another important finding, supported by previous studies, was that the combined approach required a 20% lower dose of medication than when the medication was used on its own. The fact that the beneficial effects of the behavioral treatment appeared to remain several months after the treatment had ceased supports the notion that combining treatments may allow earlier discontinuation of medication. Longer-term follow-up reports will, it is hoped, be able to clarify this point.

Systemic Therapies

There have been very few outcome studies of family therapy in this group of children. The only study to systematically examine the response is reported by Barkley et al. (1992[ii]). This study randomly allocated 61 adolescents with ADHD to one of three therapies: behavior management training, problem-solving and communication training, and structural family therapy. Unfortunately, the authors do not say how many children were also on medication, but it is clear that some were. Only 5–30% of the sample showed significant improvements. The improvement rate was the same for all three treatments. Family therapy per se may not be the most efficacious treatment for this disorder, but a systemic approach to the impact of this disorder on family and school functioning is important (Bernier & Siegel, 1994).

Psychodynamic Therapies

There have been no trials of the use of psychotherapy in children and adolescents with ADHD, but the relatively poor insight of these children (Pelham et al., 1993[i]) suggests that it is unlikely to be particularly beneficial.

CONSULTATION AND TRAINING

Consultation with schools and teachers by mental health professionals is crucial. Social workers also need an opportunity to discuss the children with whom they are involved. There is a need for clinical practice guidelines regarding the management of these children, as the problem is so highly prevalent and professionals from various backgrounds, especially pediatricians and primary care physicians, become involved in managing these cases.

SUMMARY

ADHD is probably a disorder along a continuum that has heterogenous etiology, whose severity relates to long-term outcome. Depending on the definition, its prevalence is 1–5% of school-age children. There are often high rates of comorbid CD, attachment disorder, mood disorder, and specific learning disabilities. Diagnosing and treating ADDs early improves the prognosis. ADDs are particularly persistent in the presence of a family history, psychosocial adversity, and comorbidity.

Stimulants have been shown to be effective with inattention, hyperactivity, and impulsivity in the classroom, irrespective of age and with any comorbid condition except anxiety and depression. There is no evidence of misuse of stimulant medication in adolescence by individuals with ADHD. The evidence is somewhat less compelling for the impact of stimulants on academic performance, and there is no evidence that prosocial behaviors increase with their use. There is no evidence as to who will respond well to stimulants and no evidence of serious, irreversible side effects. There is no evidence for the superior effectiveness of antipsychotics or tricyclic antidepressants in combination with stimulants. There is less compelling but still good evidence for the effectiveness of clonidine, tricyclics, MAOIs, and carbamazepine, but these drugs have more serious side effects.

There is no good evidence for the blanket exclusion of additives and colorings in the child's diet. Studies demonstrated that the exclusion of certain foods from the diet is effective in a selective group, but no particular foods are implicated.

Behavior therapy on its own is less effective than stimulant medication, but it can prevent a need for higher doses of medication. It improves task behavior and reduces disruptive behavior, but there is little evidence of generalization across settings so far. Multimodal treatments have not yet consistently demonstrated superiority, but a number of trials are in progress with promising results. There is no good evidence that CBT is effective on its own, and its effective component may be the behavioral one. Parent training is effective in improving compliance with instructions, but not all families are able to persist with the approach. There is no evidence that social skills intervention leads to an improvement in poor relationships. There is no evidence, either, for or against the effectiveness of systemic or psychodynamic therapy.

IMPLICATIONS

Service

The outcome of attention deficit problems is poor if untreated, but effective treatments exist. Intervention should be earlier rather than later, and thought needs to be given to early case identification services (child health surveillance or other measures). Services should be organized so that adequately trained staff can assess, treat, and monitor treatment over long periods, continuing throughout the school years. A service needs individuals with a range of skills to be involved at all these stages, which should include medical input from a child and adolescent psychiatrist. There needs to be monitoring by specialist clinics because of the large number of children affected and the need for specialist skills.

Clinical

Assessment needs to look beyond core symptoms of ADHD to include associated physical, educational, and social contexts. It is important to exclude other reasons for the problem behavior. If diagnostic criteria are met and the behavior problems are pervasive in at least two different types of setting, then a trial of medication is indicated as the first line of intervention. Medication can be given when there are comorbid problems such as conduct disorders, anxiety, or depression. As it is not possible to predict which dose is effective, dosage should be increased within safe limits until an effect is achieved. Effective monitoring of dose medication is needed to minimize adverse side effects of drug treatment. In the MTA study, this meant monthly monitoring appointments. Stimulants may impact on a range of symptoms. There is no evidence that the trial of other drugs during this phase is particularly helpful. If there is no or only partial resolution of symptoms, other medication should be considered, such as discontinuing the stimulants and replacing with tricyclics, clonidine, or selective serotonin reuptake inhibitor (SSRI) antidepressants. Some experts recommend adding clonidine to the stimulants, but there is no good evidence for or against this practice at present. If stimulants aggravate emotional problems (anxiety) or depression, then tricyclics should be considered instead. There should be annual trials of drug holidays to see whether the medication is still required.

If parents have noticed adverse reactions to specific foods, then evidence suggests that it would be worth considering a trial of exclusion. If parents have not noticed a specific allergic reaction, then the evidence does not warrant the effort involved in imposing a selective exclusion diet, which requires exceptionally strong parental commitment for effective implementation.

If there is unsatisfactory/insufficient response to physical treatment, then psychosocial treatments should be added. The most compelling evidence is for parent training and behavioral therapy with the child. There is evidence that further educational input is required to help children with delayed attainments to catch up, but there is no evidence for specific educational approaches.

Research

There needs to be more understanding of the optimal method of monitoring treatment with medication, as well as of the predictors of the requirement for more intensive monitoring. Given the significant proportion of children who are nonresponders to methylphenidate, further studies exploring combination treatments should be undertaken. Although we know that methylphenidate and other medications are effective, it is less clear as to how long treatment should continue. There is also a lack of long-term outcome studies. Given the evidence for better prognosis following early diagnosis and treatment, there should be studies of early detection and screening protocols. More research is needed on effective educational interventions that address the educational retardation of many children with this disorder.

7

Tourette's Disorder

Tourette's disorder is a common childhood-onset disorder with unknown neurobiological etiology (Comings & Comings, 1985). It presents with motor and vocal tics. It was initially reported in the French medical literature in 1825 (Robertson, 1989). It is thought that Tourette's disorder is the most severe form of chronic tic disorder. It appears that Tourette's and chronic tic disorder are different phenotypic expressions of the Tourette's disorder gene. Family genetic studies have demonstrated that the gene may be expressed as a transient tic disorder, chronic tic disorder, or Tourette's disorder in the same family (Park, Como, Cui, & Kurlan, 1993). Because tics do not necessarily cause impairment, only the problems of Tourette's disorder will be considered here.

There is reliable evidence of a strong genetic influence on the expression of the disorder (Comings, Comings, Devor, & Cloninger, 1984; Pauls, Raymond, Stevenson, & Leckman, 1991) Pauls et al. (Pauls, Towbin, Leckman, Zahner, & Cohen, 1986) have also reported a significantly high rate (26%) of obsessive–compulsive disorder (OCD) in the first-degree relatives of 13 subjects with Tourette's disorder without OCD. Similarly, Leonard et al. (1992) have confirmed the association of the two disorders in a follow-up study of 54 children presenting with OCD and suggested that an earlier age of onset of OCD predicted the development of Tourette's disorder. These findings have led to the suggestion that OCD may be an alternative phenotypic expression of the gene(s) responsible for Tourette's disorder. Further studies are required to clarify the relationship between the two disorders.

DEFINITION

A tic is a sudden repetitive motor or verbal movement and is usually of brief duration. Motor tics vary from simple movements such as blinking or shrugging to more complex movements such as facial expressions or gestures of the arms or legs

(Leckman & Cohen, 1994[vi]). When most severe, these movements can be self-injurious, such as biting. Vocal tics vary from throat clearing to use of obscene language (coprolalia). Young children are mostly unaware of their tics. Above the age of 10 years, however, individuals may be aware of urges to tic before the involuntary movement occurs and may be able to suppress some of these movements.

Tourette's disorder is characterized by the presence of both motor and one or more vocal tics (repetitive involuntary stereotyped movements) at some time during the illness. The tics occur many times a day (usually in bouts), nearly every day, or intermittently throughout a period of more than a year. The onset is usually in early childhood, with bouts of tics that come and go but eventually become more persistent. Vocal tics, if present, tend to develop 1–2 years following the onset of motor tics. Most often these consist of grunts, squeals, and throat clearing.

PREVALENCE

The prevalence of Tourette's disorder appears to be in the region of 3–6 per thousand children in the general population (Apter, Pauls, & Bleich, 1993a; Kurlan, Como, Deeley, McDermott, & McDermott, 1993[i]). The prevalence of tics insufficient to fulfill diagnostic criteria for Tourette's disorder is higher: as many as 0.5–2.0% of all children are affected at some time. There is often a strong family history of tics.

CLINICAL PRESENTATION

In an attempt to analyze the usual modes of presentation of this frequently underrecognized disorder, Comings and Comings (1985) reviewed the features of 250 consecutive cases seen over a period of 3 years at the City of Hope National Medical Center. The male/female sex ratio was 4:1. The average age of onset of tics or vocal noises was 6.9 years. The most frequent symptom was facial muscle tics, occurring in two-thirds of patients. The most common facial tic was eye blinking, followed by a variety of other movements, including nose twitching, stretching the mouth, and pursing the lips. Easily missed is the problem of frequent lip licking, which often leads to discoloration or sores around the mouth. One-third of patients presented with vocal noises, the most common of these being throat clearing. Nearly two-thirds of cases developed other nonfacial motor tics at some stage, the most common of these being what the authors refer to as the "hair-out-of-eyes tic." Thirteen percent had self-abusive tics such as hand, tongue, and cheek biting, self-hitting, and scratching sufficiently to form sores.

Comings and Comings (1985) reported a high rate of behavioral problems in their cases. Greater than 40% had "discipline problems" and poor anger control, and although these were more often present in children with comorbid hyperactivity, they did occur in a significant number of nonhyperactive cases. However, there was no normal control group for this case series, so the findings must be interpreted with some caution.

It is essential to establish the degree of impairment caused by the tics. The child and family's understanding of the symptoms must be ascertained. School performance also needs assessment, as many of these children have learning difficulties as a result of poor attention and obsessions or compulsions. In deciding whether treatment is required, the key question is whether the child can develop appropriately without treatment. None of the current treatments cure Tourette's disorder, and they all have some side effects. Leaving tics untreated is harmless as long as they are not impairing the child in some way.

Comorbidity

Tourette's disorder is usually associated with emotional and behavioral problems. A recent study by Spencer et al. (1995a) compared the phenomenology of Tourette's disorder and chronic tic disorders and found that, apart from the severity of the problem, they were identical, including comorbidity and cognitive impairment. Currently, it is unclear as to what extent the emotional and behavioral symptoms are part of Tourette's disorder or how much their occurrence indicates the presence of one or more comorbid disorders.

Tic disorders are sensitive to stress. Life events may exacerbate the signs and symptoms. Shapiro, Shapiro, Young, and Feinberg (1988) reported that such life events do not need to be negative to trigger deterioration. In a more recent study, Silva, Munoz, Barickman, and Friedhoff (1995) explored the effect of 29 environmental factors on symptomatology in Tourette's disorder and found that factors such as social gatherings and trauma, as well as anxiety-inducing situations, exacerbated the symptoms of the disorder. Reading for pleasure and talking to friends reduced symptoms. Several authors have suggested that the family's coping style is likely to influence the symptoms (Carter & Pauls, 1991; Leckman et al., 1990). In addition to the frequent presence of comorbid psychiatric disorders, it is consistently found that children with Tourette's disorder frequently have social problems and delayed acquisition of academic abilities (Leckman & Cohen, 1994[vi]; Wodrich, Benjamin, & Lachar, 1997).

Leckman and Cohen (1994[vi]), Bruun (1984), and Robertson (1989) provide three useful reviews on the subject of Tourette's disorder in children and adolescents. These and other authors consistently report frequent comorbidity with other psychiatric disorders, with at least 25% of children with this disorder having learning difficulty and 20% having a conduct disorder. Attention deficit disorders (ADD) are often present, with studies reporting rates as high as 90% (Sverd, Curley, Jandorf, & Volkersz, 1988), although two more rigorously designed recent studies (Park et al., 1993; Wodrich et al., 1997) reported a lower rate of 55%. A significant number of cases have OCD, with figures varying from 13% (Coffey, Frazier, & Chen, 1992) to 43% (Singer & Rosenberg, 1989). Anxiety and depression are also frequently present (Singer & Rosenberg, 1989). A study by Singer et al. (Singer, Schuerholz, & Denckla, 1995) reported a 5- to 20-fold increase in these comorbid disorders in Tourette's disorder, as compared with the general population.

Natural History

There have been few outcome studies (Bruun, 1988; Lees, 1985; Park et al., 1993) of Tourette's disorder; however, poor prognoses are particularly associated with the presence of comorbid disorders. In the absence of comorbid disorders, there is often complete resolution in late adolescence and early adulthood. Generally, as children and adolescents approach adulthood, their symptoms improve, although they may not completely resolve. It appears that at least half will improve in their late teens and early twenties. At least one-quarter will be able to stop their medication eventually (generally in early adulthood).

TREATMENT

Physical Therapies

The few clinical trials of medication in Tourette's disorder undertaken so far confirm that drug treatments reduce its severity in about 50% of patients (Cohen, Riddle, & Leckman, 1992[vi]; Dysken, Berecz, Samarza, & Davis, 1980[i]; Erenberg, 1992[vi]; Goetz et al., 1987[i]; Leckman et al., 1991[i]; McKeith, Williams, & Nicol, 1981[i]; Ross & Muldofsky, 1978[i]; Shapiro & Shapiro, 1984[i]; Shapiro et al., 1989[i]). However, all the medications (haloperidol, pimozide, clonidine) produce side effects and should be tried and continued only if benefit occurs. If the child or adolescent does not respond to one drug, an alternative should be found. Because of the risk of side effects, these children should be kept under regular medical review. Because at least 50% of patients will have other psychiatric diagnoses, these need to be looked for, diagnosed, and treated appropriately.

Treatment of Tourette's Disorder without Comorbid Disorders

NEUROLEPTICS

Haloperidol. Surveys of patients with Tourette's disorder show that haloperidol is the most frequently prescribed treatment (Bornstein, Stefl, & Hammond, 1990[vi]). The empirical evidence supporting the use of this drug, which commonly induces significant side effects, is limited. Although there have been 10 or more single- or double-blind case studies, there have been only two randomized controlled trials, using very small samples of children. In a double-blind crossover study, Ross and Moldofsky (1978[i]) showed that in a sample of nine patients with Tourette's disorder, haloperidol treatment led to a significant reduction in tics, but there was an increased risk of sedation. A more recent study by Shapiro et al. (1989[i]) compared the benefits of haloperidol and pimozide in 31 subjects. Haloperidol led to significant (38–51%) improvements in severity and a reduction in frequency of tics in approximately 70%.

Cohen et al. (1992[vi]) have recommended that haloperidol be commenced at a dose of 0.25 to 0.5 mg/day and increased gradually to a dose of 1 to 3 mg/day, in twice-daily dosages. The improvement is usually apparent within a few days of initiating treatment. Unfortunately, long-term, only 20–30% continue to benefit. Higher doses lead to side effects and are less effective (Shapiro & Shapiro, 1982a[i]; Shapiro et al., 1989[i]). Tardive dyskinesia has been reported in one child taking haloperidol for treatment of Tourette's disorder (Riddle, Hardin, Towbin, Leckman, & Cohen, 1987[iib]). The significant side effects of haloperidol include tiredness, weight gain, lability of mood, neurological symptoms such as tremor and rigidity, restlessness (akathisia), dystonic reactions, and oculogyric crises (Cohen et al., 1992[vi]). A study of neuroleptic treatment in hospitalized children and adolescents found that 34% of the sample developed severe neurological symptoms (Richardson, Haugland, & Craig, 1991[i]). Antiparkinsonian drugs such as procyclidine can be prescribed for neurological side effects in the short term, but they will not reduce the risk of developing tardive dyskinesia. There is no evidence to support their prophylactic use.

Pimozide. Three randomized controlled studies found that pimozide produces a significant reduction of tic severity (34–52%) in 70% of Tourette's disorder (Sandor, Musisi, Muldofsky, & Lang, 1990[i]; Shapiro & Shapiro, 1984[i]; Shapiro et al., 1989[i]). A recent double-blind, three-treatment crossover comparison study (Sallee, Nesbitt, Jackson, Sine, & Sethuraman, 1997[i]) compared the efficacy of pimozide (1 mg), haloperidol (1 mg), and placebo. Each treatment was given blind to a sample of 22 children with Tourette's disorder, with a 2-week placebo washout between treatments. The dose could be adjusted over 4 weeks by a maximum of 2 mg/week. At the end of each treatment, the authors undertook a standardized assessment of (1) tic severity, using the Tourette's Disorder Global Scale (Harcherik, Leckman, Detlor, & Cohen, 1984), the Clinical Global Impression tic severity scale (CGI; see Walkup, 1992) and the Tourette's Syndrome Symptom List (Leckman, Towbin, Ort, & Cohen, 1988); (2) behavior, using the Children's Global Assessment Scale (CGAS; Shaffer, Gould, & Brasic, 1983); and (3) side effects, using a semistructured interview and the Abnormal Involuntary Movement Scale (Guy, 1976) and the Extrapyramidal Symptoms Rating Scale (Chouinard, Annable, Ross-Chouinard, & Kropsky, 1979).

Sallee et al. (1997[i]) found that both active treatments reduced tics by 70% in 64% of cases, compared with a placebo response of 23%, which is a significant difference. At identical doses, pimozide was significantly more effective in reducing the primary symptoms of Tourette's disorder. Neither drug affected behavior significantly. The rate of extrapyramidal side effects was significantly higher with haloperidol in comparison with pimozide and placebo. Pimozide treatment led to the same incidence of side effects as placebo. There was no increase in cardiovascular system side effects with either drug and no significant electrocardiograph changes. Two patients receiving haloperidol had substantial impairment in school performance. Two patients on haloperidol developed depression, which resolved spontaneously during the placebo washout period.

Sallee, Sethuraman, and Rock (1994[i]) have also attempted to clarify the effect of pimozide and haloperidol on cognition, especially in the subgroup with comorbid attention-deficit/hyperactivity disorder (ADHD). They randomly allocated a sample of 65 children with Tourette's disorder (mean age 10.5 years) to haloperidol, pimozide, or placebo. Computerized assessments of memory and vigilance (Continuous Performance Test, by Lindgren & Lyons, 1984) were completed. The mean doses of medication required for a 70% reduction in the severity of primary Tourette's disorder symptoms were 0.05 mg/kg/day for haloperidol and 0.14 mg/kg/day for pimozide. At this dose, pimozide treatment led to significantly fewer errors of commission than haloperidol in those with comorbid ADHD, but there were no differences between the treatments for the rest of the sample. In contrast, haloperidol was associated with significantly more errors of commission than placebo in the ADHD-comorbid group. The authors suggest that pimozide may offer effective treatment of Tourette's disorder with comorbid ADHD when stimulants exacerbate the tics.

Cohen et al. (1992[vi]) recommend a starting dose for pimozide of 1 mg/day, which is gradually increased to a maximum of 10 mg/day in children (0.2 mg/kg). It can usually be given once a day. Pimozide should not be given if there is an abnormal ECG (e.g., QT interval > 0.47 seconds). Side effects, if they occur, are similar to those of haloperidol, with an important additional risk of ECG changes that appear to occur in approximately 20% of children taking the treatment. Pimozide should be withdrawn if there is T wave inversion or the development of U waves, and the ECG should be checked before any increase in dose, as well as prior to initiating treatment and at regular intervals every few months.

Atypical Neuroleptics. This relatively new group of drugs is characterized by having relatively greater affinity for 5HT2 receptors than dopamine receptors, which makes them less likely to cause extrapyramidal neurological side effects than the so-called typical neuroleptics, such as haloperidol and pimozide. Four atypical neuroleptics have so far been tried in a small number of subjects with Tourette's disorder: risperidone, olanzapine, clozapine, and ziprasidone.

Lombroso et al. (1995[ii]) have reported an open-label trial including five children with Tourette's disorder who were treated with *risperidone*. The patients showed a significant reduction in tics following the gradual introduction of risperidone. The starting dose was 0.5 mg/day, increasing by 0.5 mg every 5 to 7 days. Most children showed improvement after 4 weeks of treatment on a dose of 1–2 mg/day. The most frequent side effect was weight gain. Bhadrinath (1998[iib]) has reported partial resolution of symptoms with *olanzapine* treatment in one case. Caine, Polinsky, Kartzinel, and Ebert (1979[i]) did not find any significant benefits from *clozapine*.

Ziprasidone has similar dopamine (D2) and serotonin (5HT2A) antagonistic action to risperidone but appears to have certain differences from risperidone (Seeger et al., 1995), which provides hope that it may lead to a lower rate of side effects as compared with the other treatments in use (Sallee, 1999). Sallee et al. (2000[i]) have given a preliminary report of very promising findings from ziprasidone treatment in 28 children aged 7–17 years. In this parallel design study the subjects were randomized to ziprasidone or placebo for 56 days. The starting dose was 5 mg/day, increased as required to a maximum of 40 mg/day. Ziprasidone was significantly more effective than placebo in reducing the frequency and severity of tics, based on observation and report. The tics reduced by 54%, compared with less than 1% with placebo. Mild tiredness was the only side effect.

Overall, the response to the atypical neuroleptics is very promising, but double-blind studies are required before definite conclusions can be drawn about their benefits and safety.

CLONIDINE

Clonidine is an alpha-2 agonist and has been shown in open and double-blind studies to be beneficial for treatment of tics in children with Tourette's disorder (Borison, Arg, & Hamilton, 1983[i]; Leckman et al., 1991[i]; McKeith et al., 1981[i]). However, not all studies have reported benefit (Dysken, Berecz, Samarza, & Davis, 1980[i]; Goetz et al., 1987[i]). In the most recent randomized controlled study of the subject, Leckman et al. (1991[i]) reported a double-blind trial of 40 subjects ages 7–48 years. Thirty-one subjects were younger than 18 years. Clonidine significantly reduced the number and severity of motor tics. Vocal tics did not improve. Clonidine also significantly reduced impulsivity and hyperactivity problems.

Clonidine is commenced at doses of 50 μg/day (3 to 5 micrograms per kilogram) and increased over several weeks to a maximum dose of 300 μg/day. The dose should be titrated against the response. Side effects are less severe than with the neuroleptics. The most frequent side effect is drowsiness. Until recently it was recommended that an ECG should be checked prior to initiating treatment, as well as at regular intervals during treatment, because it was thought that ECG changes such as prolongation of the P-R interval occurred. However, a recent statement from a committee of pediatric cardiologists, accepted by the American Heart Association, states that electrocardiograms are not required (Gutgesell et al., 1999). Parents should be warned about the risk of hypertension should clonidine suddenly be discontinued. Blood pressure monitoring is required at the higher dosages. Clonidine has a slower onset of action than the neuroleptics and usually takes 3 weeks to show any benefits. Parents should be warned that their child may be more irritable and tired for the first 6 weeks of clonidine treatment.

PERGOLIDE

Pergolide is another dopamine agonist. It activates a specific dopamine receptor known as the D2 autoreceptor, which in turn inhibits dopamine activity in the substantia nigra area of the brain. Gilbert et al. (Gilbert, Sethuraman, Sine, Peters, & Sallee, 2000[i]) have reported a randomized controlled trial with crossover design in 24 children aged 7–17 years with chronic tic disorder or Tourette's disorder. A well-validated scale of tic severity (Yale Global Tics Severity Scale) indicated that pergolide led to significant improvements without serious side effects. Further studies are required before any definite recommendations can be made about the use of pergolide.

COMBINED MEDICATIONS

In an attempt to reduce the effective dose of neuroleptic medication, an open-label trial (Saccomani, Rizzo, & Nobili, 2000[i]) has reported the combination of trazadone antidepressant and haloperidol. The authors reported that a lower dose of haloperidol was required than in common clinical practice. However, randomized controlled trials are required before recommendations about using combined treatments can be made.

Treatment of Comorbid Attention Deficit

Many children with Tourette's disorder are more impaired by their attention deficit symptoms than their tics, and most children with Tourette's disorder have comorbid attention deficit. Several groups of drugs have been tried for children with Tourette's disorder and ADD.

PSYCHOSTIMULANTS

There has been a great deal of disagreement about the administration of stimulants in children with Tourette's disorder and ADD. An exacerbation of tics has been reported by some (Robertson & Eapen, 1992[vi]); however, others (Gadow, Sverd, Sprafkin, Nolan, & Ezor, 1995[i]) have found no more than a transient increase in tics when stimulants were taken in conjunction with haloperidol by 42 subjects. Barkley et al. (1990b[i]) similarly found that tics were not exacerbated in 83 children treated with methylphenidate, in comparison with placebo treatment. Law and Schachar (1999[i]) replicated this finding. Higher doses of stimulant made tics slightly more likely to increase.

More recently, Nolan and Gadow (1997[i]) have reported a double-blind placebo-controlled study of methylphenidate use in 34 children with ADHD and tic disorder, in which all the children showed significant behavioral improvement with methylphenidate. A variety of measures failed to detect a significant increase in tic severity, although the frequency of motor tics tended to increase when methylphenidate was given at low dosage (0.1 mg/kg). A second double-blind placebo-controlled study by Castellanos et al. (1997[i]) reported a crossover trial of methylphenidate in 20 subjects. This sample was also followed up monthly over a 2-year period. Three had severe enough exacerbation of tics during the trial to require discontinuation of the treatment. Tic severity was worse with dexamphetamine as compared with methylphenidate and at higher doses of medication. Although continuing with methylphenidate led to a decrease in tic severity in the majority, during follow-up most patients required additional medication for the tics. Although this was a small sample, it suggests that some children with tics and ADHD respond well to stimulants, but careful monitoring for exacerbation of tics is always required.

Because of the possibility of stimulants aggravating tics and the uncertainty about the long-term effects of stimulants on the course of Tourette's disorder, other medications are often tried. The most frequently used alternatives to the stimulants that have been shown to be effective with attention deficit problems are clonidine, an alpha2-agonist and the tricyclic antidepressants.

CLONIDINE AND RELATED TREATMENTS

A double-blind study showed clonidine to be effective and superior to placebo in treating both tics and comorbid symptoms of ADHD (Leckman et al., 1991[i]). Unfortunately, children are often affected by sedation; in Leckman's study this occurred in 90% of subjects.

Guanfacine is a selective alpha 2-adrenergic agonist that is much less sedating than clonidine. Chappell et al. (1995[ii]) reported an open-label study of the use of this drug in 10 children ages 8–16 years with Tourette's disorder and ADHD. These authors reported a significant improvement in both tic severity and symptoms of ADHD without any serious adverse reactions, although drowsiness did occur in some (reported to be less severe than with clonidine). A double-blind study is required to confirm these findings.

TRICYCLIC ANTIDEPRESSANTS

There has been a case report of the use of imipramine in comorbid ADHD and Tourette's disorder (Dillon, Salzman, & Schulsinger, 1985[iib]). Riddle, Hardin, Cho, Woolston, and Leckman (1988a[iii]) have reported a case series of seven children treated with desipramine and found a 70% improvement of ADHD symptoms without deterioration in Tourette's disorder. Singer et al. (1995[i]) reported a placebo-controlled trial of desipramine and clonidine and found that desipramine was significantly more efficacious than placebo or clonidine. Spencer, Biederman, Wilens, Steingard, and Geist (1993[i]) reported an 80% improvement in ADHD and Tourette's disorder symptoms in 33 children with the comorbid disorders. This group has also reported a similar rate of improvement in 12 cases of the comorbid disorders treated with nortriptyline. There is, however, concern about the risk of sudden death in children treated with tricyclics, although there is little definite evidence to date that this is a major risk (Biederman, 1991[vi]; Biederman et al., 1993a[i]). Nevertheless, the possibility of sudden death being attributed to tricyclics warrants ECGs, prior to initiating treatment, at intervals throughout treatment, and prior to any increase in dose.

MONOAMINE OXIDASE INHIBITORS

Deprenyl is a selective monoamine oxidase-B inhibitor, and therefore does not necessitate the child's having a strict diet as with nonselective monoamine oxidase inhibitors (MAOIs). Jancovic (1993[ii]) reports an open study of deprenyl use in 29 children ages 6–18 years with Tourette's and attention deficit. The symptoms had not been controlled by conventional therapies such as stimulants, clonidine, imipramine, or dopamine receptor blockers such as haloperidol. The author found that 90% reported meaningful improvement with no serious adverse reactions. A randomized controlled trial is required to support these findings.

Treatment of Obsessive–Compulsive Disorder Comorbid with Tourette's Disorder

Several studies suggest that fluoxetine may be beneficial when used for the treatment of comorbid OCD and Tourette's disorder (Riddle, Hardin, & King, 1990[ii]; Riddle, Leckman, Hardin, Anderson, & Cohen, 1988[ii]). However, a controlled study (Kurlan et al., 1993[i]) of fluoxetine in nine boys with OCD and Tourette's disorder failed to confirm improvement of the OCD symptoms as a result of 4 months of treatment, as compared with placebo. As the drug has a long half-life, it is possible to take fluoxetine on alternative days, at least initially, in order to reduce unwanted side effects. There is now a liquid preparation available that allows the administration of smaller doses than the lowest dose possible by tablet. The symptoms of Tourette's disorder and OCD usually begin to show improvement in 2–4 weeks. If they do not, the dose can be gradually increased. The maximum adult dose is 80 mgs. Possible side effects are not serious and include hyperarousal such as sleep difficulties and hyperactivity, agitation, and drowsiness. They are dose dependent and usually resolve after the first few weeks of treatment.

There have been no trials of the use of clomipramine for children with comorbid OCD and Tourette's disorder. ECG monitoring is required, as discussed earlier.

Various combinations of medication have been tried, although currently no clinical evidence supports their use. Examples of the combinations tried are haloperidol and methylphenidate, and haloperidol and clomipramine (Cohen et al., 1992[vi]).

Behavioral Therapies

Behavioral treatments have been found to be beneficial with such interventions as habit reversal (performing a movement that is opposite to the tic in question) and relaxation (Azrin & Peterson, 1990[iib]). This approach requires approximately a year's course of monthly behavioral treatments, but it is not beneficial for all children with Tourette's disorder. Other techniques, such as massed negative practice, whereby the child performs the tic as quickly and forcefully as he or she can, have been attempted. The results have been uncertain (Azrin & Peterson, 1988[ii]). Leckman and Cohen (1994[vi]) found that families generally report only short-term benefits from these interventions. Nevertheless, Azrin and Peterson (1990[iib]) reported good results from a waiting-list control group comparison of 10 subjects. The treatment program lasted 10 months, and subjects were randomly assigned to an immediate treatment group or a 3-month waiting-list control group. The treatments consisted of awareness training, enabling the subject to identify the tic and the precursors of a tic both in themselves and in the environment; relaxation training, consisting of a variety of strategies including visual imagery and deep breathing muscular relaxation; and competing response training, consisting of tensing the muscles opposite to those used during the tic so that the tic cannot occur. The most frequent or disruptive tic was treated first. Parents were requested to praise efforts at home and to inform the child about any improvements they had observed in the tics. Two subjects dropped out of treatment. A mean of 20 sessions was attended, initially weekly and subsequently at least monthly. The reduction in tics in the treatment group was 93%. Further studies are required, but this treatment appears promising.

There is great need for more studies of promising behavioral approaches, especially as there are no ideal drug treatments. We also speculate that involving parents in a behavioral approach may be beneficial, but to date there does not appear to have been any evaluation of this approach.

Psychotherapy and Other Psychosocial Approaches

Leckman and Cohen (1994[vi]) report that psychotherapy may be useful in helping children and families cope with the distressing illness of Tourette's disorder, but there have been no controlled studies of its use. Similarly, although not clinically evaluated, studies have suggested that supportive interventions with the family and with the school are beneficial.

SUMMARY

The onset of Tourette's disorder is usually in early childhood, with bouts of tics that come and go but eventually become more persistent. Its prevalence appears to be in the region of 3–6 per 1,000 children in the general population. Its characteristic features include the presence of both motor and one or more vocal tics (repetitive involuntary stereotyped movements) at some time during the illness. The tics occur many times a day (usually in bouts), nearly every day, or intermittently throughout a period of more than a year. If the tics do not impair the child, leaving them untreated is safe. Functional impairment is usually caused by the impact of the tics on social relationships. There needs to be more understanding of the etiology of tics, such as the role of anxiety, but there is currently thought to be at least a degree of neurobiological influence in their development. Although there are likely to be neurobiological and emotional determinants, environmental risk factors strongly influence the presentation. Comorbid psychiatric problems are common in children with Tourette's disorder. Although the tics can lead to impairment during a bad phase, they are often less debilitating than the symptoms resulting from the comorbid disorder(s).

There is no one ideal drug treatment for Tourette's disorder either in isolation or in the presence of comorbid disorder(s). All the drugs in current accepted usage have a risk of side effects. The treatment of Tourette's disorder often requires a delicate balance between treating a comorbid disorder and treating the primary Tourette's disorder symptomatology. In the absence of comorbid problems the current treatments of choice are haloperidol and clonidine, with little to choose between them. There are significant side effects from haloperidol, including neurological symptoms such as rigidity and tremor. Clonidine must not be stopped suddenly and may induce drowsiness. A potential second-line treatment is pimozide, which is less sedating than haloperidol but has a greater risk of ECG abnormalities. If there are further studies confirming its safety, as the rate of neurological side effects is lower, pimozide may be preferable to haloperidol.

In the presence of comorbid ADD, methylphenidate, clonidine, and tricyclic antidepressants and pimozide have all been shown to be effective, albeit in only a very limited number of trials. Currently, clonidine is probably the first choice of drug, although methylphenidate is the least likely drug to lead to troublesome side effects. Early evidence that methylphenidate routinely exacerbated tics has not been confirmed. Tricyclic antidepressants may also lead to ECG changes, and there have been very occasional reports of sudden death associated with tricyclic use, although no definite proof that the deaths were due to the drugs.

Individual behavioral approaches and parent training approaches are promising but require further evaluation.

IMPLICATIONS

The psychosocial determinants of tics imply that there may be an important place for both psychoeducation and parenting/family work with the children's carers. Because of the relapsing nature of the condition, long-term involvement with the child and family is often necessary.

Comorbid psychiatric disorders are very frequently present, and therefore a comprehensive psychiatric assessment is essential in every case and multiple treatments may be needed. Drug treatments require regular monitoring, particularly as the treatment of the comorbid disorder may have an impact on the severity of the tics and most of the recommended drugs have a significant risk of side effects.

Further randomized controlled studies of medication for Tourette's disorder are urgently required, especially of the drugs with lower risks of side effects, such as the selective serotonin reuptake inhibitors (SSRIs), selective MAOIs and atypical neuroleptics.

Psychotic Disorders

The two main groups of psychotic disorders in children and adolescents are the schizophrenias and the bipolar disorders. Each of these will be discussed separately. Until fairly recently there was considerable debate in the literature as to whether adolescent mania occurred (Carlson, Davenport, & Jamieson, 1977). However, a number of studies have shown that bipolar disorder does arise in this age group, but it is frequently misdiagnosed as schizophrenia (Carlson, 1990). Carlson and Strober (1978) reviewed the records of six late adolescents who were clearly bipolar by that stage and found that they had all initially been wrongly diagnosed as schizophrenic, usually because the affective episodes were psychotic. This finding suggests that adolescents with bipolar disorders are predisposed to developing psychotic symptoms. Several authors suggest this may be the case (Ballenger, Reus, & Post, 1982; Joyce, 1984; Rosen, Rosenthal, Van Dusen, Dunner, & Fieve, 1983). The propensity to present with psychotic rather than affective symptoms may have led to misleading prevalence rates, outcome figures, and estimates of treatment response for both bipolar disorder and schizophrenic disorders. As the diagnoses of these two disorders become increasingly refined, facilitated by the development of reliable diagnostic tools (i.e., Schedule for Affective Disorders and Schizophrenia for School-Age Children (K-SADS), Chambers et al., 1985; Diagnostic Interview Schedule for Children (DISC), Costello, Edelbrock, & Dulcan, 1984), these errors should become less of a problem.

SCHIZOPHRENIA

Definition

The schizophrenic disorders comprise characteristic distortions of thinking and perception and an inappropriate affect. Intellectual ability is usually maintained, although certain cognitive deficits may appear over time. It is useful to divide the symptoms into groups, which often occur together. These include *abnormalities of thoughts*—for example, thought echo, thought insertion, withdrawal, and broadcasting; *abnormal beliefs*, either about the self (e.g., delusions of control, influence, and passivity) or beliefs relating to religious or political identity or to superhuman powers and abilities (e.g., being in communication with aliens); and *abnormal experiences*, such as hallucinatory voices giving a running commentary on the patient's behavior. In addition to these "positive" symptoms, there are often negative symptoms, such as apathy, reduction of speech, and incongruity of emotional responses, which lead to social withdrawal. The ability to achieve at school, to maintain social relationships, and to self-care is markedly reduced.

Symptoms should have been present for 1 month in ICD-10 (World Health Organization, 1993) and 6 months in DSM-IV (American Psychiatric Association, 1994), although the patient is unlikely to have been floridly psychotic for the whole of this time. In the first instance a diagnosis of acute schizophrenia-like psychotic disorder should be made and reclassified as schizophrenia only if symptoms persist for longer periods. It is important to rule out drug-induced psychosis and any other possible organic cause prior to making the diagnosis. If there is a history of pervasive developmental disorder, the additional diagnosis of schizophrenia is made only if delusions and/or hallucinations are also present.

Prevalence

No studies specifically examine the epidemiology of schizophrenia during childhood. Torrey (1987) has reviewed the prevalence of adult schizophrenia. Unfortunately, because of inconsistency in diagnostic practices, it is difficult to be certain about prevalence rates (Werry & Taylor, 1994). Nevertheless, the accepted prevalence for schizophrenia in adults is about 1% with an incidence of 0.1% per year (Torrey, 1987).

In an attempt to assess the prevalence in children and adolescents, Zigler and Levine (1981) have assessed the age of first hospitalization for schizophrenia and reported an increase in the incidence in adolescents, with peak incidence in males occurring between the ages of 15 and 25 years. The peak incidence in females was higher, at 25–35 years. However, schizophrenia did occur during adolescence in some females. Eaton et al. (1992a, 1992b) have described a study on the rehospitalization of patients with a diagnosis of schizophrenia following their initial discharge, which was completed using data from psychiatric case registers in Australia, the United States, Denmark, and England. Approximately 10% of the schizophrenic subjects in each of the four countries had onset during late childhood and adolescence.

The prevalence in younger children is thought to be much lower than the 1 case per 1,000 thought to be the rate in adolescents. Spencer and Campbell (1994) suggest that the prevalence rate is 2 per 10,000 children under the age of 12 years. These authors and others have concluded that childhood schizophrenia is identical to adolescent- or adult-onset schizophrenia. These prevalence rates are supported by the findings of Von Knorring, Andersson, and Magnusson (1987), who reported the incidence and prevalence of various psychiatric disorders arising in Swedish subjects from birth to 24 years of age. The information was obtained from the hospital registers of child guidance clinics and drug abuse clinics. Unfortunately, schizophrenia was not diagnosed separately but was included under the label "schizophrenic disorders and other nonaffective psychoses." The incidence was approximately 1 per 1,000 9- to 19-year-olds. The 5-year period prevalence of schizophrenic disorders and other nonaffective psychoses was approximately 1.5 per 1,000 for males and females in the 10- to 24-year-age group.

It is essential that other studies using up-to-date diagnostic criteria are undertaken as soon as possible, to establish how many adolescents are affected by this disabling disorder.

Clinical Presentation

Schizophrenia typically has its onset in adolescence or early adulthood, although there have been occasional reports of onset in early childhood, with the youngest case reported to date being a child of 3 years (Russell, Bott, & Sammons, 1989). Schizophrenia in children this young is extremely uncommon, but incidence increases significantly at 11–12 years of age (Eggers, 1978; Werry, McLellan, & Chard, 1991). Schizophrenia is both debilitating and chronic, although its course varies across individuals and at different times within the same individual (Carpenter & Kirkpatrick, 1988). These factors make the disorder costly to health services. Sharfstein and Clark (1978) report that schizophrenia is a major contributor to the cost of the psychiatric services in most countries.

Prior to the 1970s, childhood schizophrenia was included with other childhood psychotic disorders; hence, few studies use ICD or DSM criteria. Probably the best-designed study of the natural history of schizophrenia that does use reliable diagnostic criteria is the study by McClellan, Werry, and Ham (1993). In this study, the medical records of all children with psychotic disorders, either at intake or discharge at the Child Study and Treatment Center in Tacoma, Washington, were reviewed. The length of these admissions averaged 4–6 months. Once subjects were identified, they were interviewed using the Structured Clinical Interview for DSM-III-R (parent version) (Spitzer, Williams, & Gibbon, 1987), the Schedule for Positive Symptoms and the Schedule for Negative Symptoms (Andreasen, 1982), and the Brief Psychiatric Rating Scale (BPRS) (Overall & Gorman, 1962). Subjects were interviewed where possible; otherwise, relatives and any other relevant sources were contacted for information. Interrater reliability for assessments was satisfactory. The authors divided schizophrenia in childhood and adolescence into "very early onset schizophrenia" (VEOS), which refers to those cases with onset before 12 years, and "early onset schizophrenia" (EOS), which refers to cases with onset after the age of 12 years but before the age of 18 years. The study assigned diagnostic categories by the symptoms at follow-up, rather than at onset, which increases the reliability of assigned diagnoses.

The outcome at follow-up, with a mean interval between treatment and follow-up of 3.9 years, was particularly poor in the schizophrenic group. Only 4% were classified as "recovered" with no further episodes of illness, 79% had experienced two or more episodes of illness, and a worrying 46% had required six or more readmissions during the follow-up period. Only 13% had a full-time occupation at follow-up. The authors remark on the high attrition rate in this study (59%), noting that among the subjects lost to follow-up were a higher number of children with very early onset schizophrenia. This means that the children who were not followed up had a more severe disorder. In addition, the study was retrospective, and hence recall of actual events was likely to be inaccurate. Nevertheless, these results suggest a poor outcome for schizophrenic disorder.

Other studies suggest a slightly more favorable outcome. Eggers (1989) reports on 57 patients diagnosed as schizophrenic prior to age 14 who were followed up 6–40 years later (mean 16 years). Just over half the sample were either in remission (27%) or with only slight defect (24%). More recently, Cawthron, James, Dell, and Seagroatt (1994) reported on the outcome of a cohort of 58 young people admitted to inpatient care with psychotic disorders as compared with nonpsychotic inpatients. Only 36% of the matched pairs were traced at follow-up, 11 years after admission. The schizophrenic group had the poorest outcome, with seven of the nine continuously ill. As Asarnow (1994) points out, cross-national differences may affect outcome. The McClellan, Eggers, and Cawthron studies are all from different countries, which may account for some of the differences.

Werry and McClellan (1992) assessed the predictors of outcome in schizophrenic and bipolar disorders. They assessed 59 patients, 30 with schizophrenia and 23 with bipolar disorder diagnosed according to DSM-III-R criteria. The mean age at presentation was 13.9 years, and follow-up occurred 5 years later when the mean age was 19 years. Fifty percent of the variance in outcome was predictable using stepwise multiple correlation. The most reliable predictors of outcome in schizophrenia were premorbid adjustment and personality. In bipolar illness the most reliable predictors of outcome were premorbid adjustment and intelligence. The authors emphasize the fact that the number of variables evaluated was small—for example, expressed emotion (Falloon & Pederson, 1985; Leff, Kuipers, Berkowitz, & Sturgeon, 1985) was not assessed—and the sample size was small. In a recent paper Falloon et al. (1998) point out that the patient variables associated with a better prognosis are the same as the characteristics that are most likely to lead to earlier detection and treatment.

Similarly, Eaton et al. (1992a, 1992b) reported a longitudinal prospective follow-up study of admissions for schizophrenia. This study examines the risk for rehospitalization following initial diagnosis of schizophrenia in four centers in Australia, the United States, Denmark, and England. In all these centers the follow-up was for at least 10 years. All those with onset between the ages of 10 and 19 years required at least one further rehospitalization in each of the centers. The finding that the readmission rate was lower in the patients with later onset of schizophrenia confirms the greater severity of early onset schizophrenia.

Treatment

The management of childhood and adolescent schizophrenia has been reviewed recently on both sides of the Atlantic, and authoritative recommendations have been made (Clark & Lewis, 1998[vi]; McClellan & Werry, 1997[vi]). Both reviews highlight the lack of clear empirical evidence on which to base treatment decisions for children and young people, comment on the similarities and continuities between childhood, adolescent, and adult schizophrenia, and extrapolate from the extensive adult literature to formulate guidance.

Assessment

Schizophrenia can be reliably diagnosed from middle childhood onward, using the same criteria as for adults (Asarnow, 1994). However, thorough assessment is essential for the application of diagnostic criteria and an accurate diagnosis. This should always include a full and accurate history of recent changes in mental state and functioning, premorbid developmental details about the index patient and other family members, and family history of psychiatric disorder. Information from others involved with the child, especially at school, should be sought. Neuropsychological assessment may assist both diagnosis and subsequent management. A full mental state examination is essential, as is physical examination and appropriate further physical investigation (Clark & Lewis, 1998[vi]). Assessment and investigation can be carried out on an outpatient basis, but many centers recommend a period of inpatient observation as part of the ongoing assessment process. This affords opportunities to assess the child in a number of different settings and engaging in a variety of activities, and is generally accepted to be very useful in complex cases.

Accurate diagnosis is complex, and assessment may take some time, given the difficulty in distinguishing between genuine psychotic symptomatology and apparent distortions of thinking and perception due to developmental status. Deciding whether impaired communication is related to the formal thought disorder of schizophrenia or to cognitive and language problems associated with speech and language disorders is particularly difficult. Caplan (1994) argues that such distinctions can be made, but are complex and time-consuming in routine practice using existing measures. Accessing the inner world of children is always difficult, and children with hallucinations and delusions may be reluctant to discuss them and, because of their developmental status, may have difficulty in accurately describing internal processes. Several interviews may be necessary, particularly with younger children (Volkmar, 1996a).

Differential diagnosis can include most mental health problems in young people, but of particular relevance are organic disorders, major affective disorders, pervasive developmental disorders and autism, severe obsessive–compulsive disorders, and substance abuse. Asarnow (1994) provides a useful list of standardized rating instruments that may assist the assessment and diagnosis of schizophrenia. Although many organic medical conditions may present with psychotic symptomatology, Adams, Kutcher, Antoniw, and Bird (1996) suggest that extensive routine endocrine and neuroimaging screening tests are not diagnostically useful. Instead, such investigations should be targeted specifically at children and young people whose history and physical examination suggest organic disorder.

McClellan and Werry (1997[vi]) describe the hesitancy of some clinicians in diagnosing schizophrenia early because of the associated stigma. They indicate that the overlap between symptoms of affective disorder, schizophrenia, and other diagnoses means that even when diagnostic criteria are met the initial diagnosis may be inaccurate. However, they suggest that although this is understandable, it denies children and families access to potentially beneficial treatments. Instead, they suggest educating patients and families about the diagnostic uncertainties of schizophrenia and carrying out regular reassessments to ensure accurate diagnosis. Schizophrenia is an episodic condition, and although some people experience only one episode, regular reassessment of the situation is essential.

General Approaches to Treatment

The consensus is that treatment of schizophrenia should be multimodal and should include specific treatments targeted at specific symptoms as well as more generic treatments relating to the psychosocial and educational needs of the child and family. However, much of the evidence for this approach is based on the similarities between childhood and adult schizophrenia and extrapolation from adult research. Once treatment of the acute, psychotic symptomatology has been addressed, most young people, and their families, will require interventions and extensive social support to deal with the associated psychosocial sequelae of having a chronic and deteriorating psychiatric condition. Although little formal evidence supports one treatment location over another, there is general consensus that a period of inpatient treatment is usually needed, at least in the early stages of treatment. This should be in a specialist child or adolescent psychiatric unit staffed by a multidisciplinary team including educational staff. However, Tolbert (1996[vi]) suggests that some young people may be managed successfully in the community even in the acute phase if there are low levels of behavioral disturbance and high levels of cooperation with treatment.

Informed consent must be obtained before treatment can commence. Treatment has risks as well as potential benefits, but the risks of nontreatment are also significant. Different countries have different approaches to dealing with issues of informed consent and refusal to participate in treatment. It is usually wise to try to enlist cooperation and consent from both the young person and his or her parents or legal guardians. If consent is not forthcoming, practitioners need to be familiar with relevant child care and mental health legislation and use this where indicated to ensure that treatment is given appropriately.

Physical Treatments

NEUROLEPTIC MEDICATION

Antipsychotic (neuroleptic) medication is usually the mainstay of treatment for schizophrenia in the acute phase. Controlled trials of treatment are, however, very rare, and most of the evidence comes from adult studies in which numerous randomized, controlled, double-blind studies have been reported, and in which the consensus as to treatment is reasonably clear (Frances, Docherty, & Kahn, 1996[vi]).

The studies of young people that do exist are often open trials or descriptions of case series; these studies tend to be more recent and to attempt evaluation of the "newer" antipsychotics. Gadow (1992[vi]), in a review of pediatric psychopharmacology, describes schizophrenia as "one of the least researched disorders in children and adolescents" (p. 172).

"TRADITIONAL" NEUROLEPTIC MEDICATION

Pool, Bloom, Mielke, Roniger, and Gallant (1976[i]) describe a double-blind, randomized evaluation of loxapine, haloperidol, and placebo in 75 children with schizophrenia. The sample comprised young people with consecutive admissions to an adolescent unit with an "undisputed diagnosis of schizophrenia" and who met the inclusion criteria of ages 13–18 and absence of organic disorder and/or significant developmental delay. Because of the timing of this study, formal diagnostic criteria were not used, but each participant had to be diagnosed unequivocally as having schizophrenia by two psychiatrists. Medication was given for 4 weeks after an initial 5-day drug-free period. Dosage started with one capsule per day and increased daily at the discretion of the clinical team, but with a maximum of eight capsules daily. Average daily dosage was 87.5 mg (3.5 × 25-mg capsules) for loxapine, 9.8 mg (4.9 × 2-mg capsules) for haloperidol, and 5.4 capsules of placebo.

The BPRS (Brief Psychiatric Rating Scale), the Nurses Observation Scale for Inpatient Evaluation (NOSIE), and the Clinical Global Ratings of Improvement (CGI) were completed at baseline, 2 weeks, and 4 weeks. All three groups showed improvements over the 4 weeks, but the authors report significant improvements for both drug groups over placebo, although no raw data are provided. Side effects, mainly sleepiness and extrapyramidal symptoms, were reported significantly more in the two drug groups.

Spencer, Kafantaris, Padron-Gayol, Rosenberg, and Campbell (1992[i]) report preliminary findings from a study of 12 children ages 5–12 years diagnosed with schizophrenia using DSM-III-R criteria. Exclusion criteria included systemic illness, seizure disorder, mental retardation, tardive dyskinesia, or psychoactive medication in the preceding 4 weeks. There are no details about the origins or representativeness of the subjects. Following a 2-week placebo baseline period, subjects were randomized to an 8-week crossover, double-blind treatment regime—either 4 weeks of placebo followed by 4 weeks of haloperidol or vice versa. Dosage was in three divided daily doses and was titrated against clinical response and level of side effects for each individual patient.

A battery of standardized instruments was administered at baseline and at the end of 4 and 8 weeks. Consensus Global Clinical Judgment of all ward staff indicated that all 12 children on haloperidol improved (marked in 9, moderate in 2, and mild improvement in 1), whereas only 2 children improved on placebo (moderate in 1, mild in 1). Statistically significant haloperidol treatment effects were obtained on Global Clinical Judgments, Clinical Global Impressions for severity, schizophrenia-related items of the Children's Psychiatric Rating Scale, and the "total pathology" score of the BPRS for Children. Side effects related to haloperidol

(commonly drowsiness, dizziness, or extrapyramidal) resolved on dosage maintenance or reduction. All 12 children were discharged on haloperidol following the
trial because of clinical improvements.

Side effects with traditional antipsychotics are a cause for serious concern. The
primary concerns in children are acute dystonic reactions, parkinsonian symptoms,
akathisia, neuroleptic malignant syndrome, and tardive dyskinesia (Gadow, 1992[vi]).
Richardson et al. (1991) suggest that parkinsonian symptoms in children on
antipsychotics are more common than in adults and less amenable to treatment.
They note a clear association between length of neuroleptic treatment and the
presence of parkinsonian symptoms. Tardive dyskinesia was less common than in
adult studies and unrelated to lifetime measures of neuroleptic treatment. There
was an association between tardive dyskinesia and a family history of psychiatric
hospitalization.

Less serious side effects may, nevertheless, have a significant influence on determining pharmacotherapy. Realmuto, Erickson, Yellin, Hopwod, and Greenberg
(1984[i]) carried out a single-blind comparison of thiothixene and thioridazine.
Subjects were 21 adolescent inpatients (11–18 years) who met DSM-III criteria for
schizophrenia, had IQs of greater than 70, were not on other medication or chemi-
cally dependent, and did not have physical illness. Subjects were randomly allocated to 4–6 weeks treatment with one of the two drugs. The drugs were equally effective in controlling symptoms (BPRS, Clinical Global Impressions Scale), but the
prevalence of drowsiness as a side effect necessitated dose reduction, which limited
therapeutic effectiveness. The importance of sedation as a side effect in children
leads the authors to suggest that higher-potency antipsychotics with lower rates of
sedative side effects may be the drugs of choice in childhood schizophrenia.

"ATYPICAL" NEUROLEPTIC MEDICATION

More recently, Kumra et al. (1996[i]) conducted a randomized double-blind, controlled trial of clozapine for children with refractory schizophrenia. Clozapine is a
newer, "atypical," antipsychotic with markedly reduced extrapyramidal side effects.
Twenty-one volunteers, ages 6–18 years, with a DSM-III-R diagnosis of schizophrenia with symptoms before age 12 and intolerance or nonresponse to at least two different neuroleptic medications, were recruited. Children with an IQ of less than 70
or with physical disease were excluded. On admission, all drugs were tapered off,
followed by a 4-week drug-free period. The 21 patients were randomly assigned to a
6-week course of haloperidol (up to 27 mg/day) plus prophylactic benztropine, or
clozapine (up to 525 mg/day) plus placebo. The BPRS and the Bunney-Hamburg
Psychosis Rating Scale were administered weekly, and other rating scales fortnightly, during the drug-free period and the trial. Adverse side effects were monitored weekly. Analysis of results was on an "intention to treat" basis. The
haloperidol group had an open trial of clozapine with similar measurements after
completing the controlled trial.

This was a severely disturbed group with baseline scores on the BPRS higher
than previously reported scores for adults. Clozapine gave statistically significant

improvements over haloperidol for all of the overall indices of improvement despite the small numbers of subjects. Clozapine also significantly decreased both positive and negative symptoms.

Adverse effect reporting was similar in both groups, with clozapine producing more drowsiness and haloperidol more insomnia. It should be noted that patients administered haloperidol were routinely given benztropine. However, more serious adverse effects were noted. Five patients given clozapine had neutropenia, 3 of whom resolved spontaneously. Two patients given clozapine experienced seizures. A further 3 in the open trial received prophylactic anticonvulsants after EEG abnormalities were noted in conjunction with clinical deterioration. Two patients experienced a sinus tachycardia, and 1 a clinically significant elevation of liver enzymes. One patient given haloperidol showed early signs of neuroleptic malignant syndrome. Significant weight gain with clozapine was also commonly reported. If clozapine is prescribed, patients must be closely monitored for evidence of these potential serious side effects. However, these concerns have to be balanced against the claimed reduction of risk of tardive dyskinesia, as compared with more traditional neuroleptic medication.

Only minimal information is given about longer-term follow-up. The research team attempted to stay in telephone contact with the subjects, and they report that adverse side effects remained a problem but that 13 patients continued to take clozapine for an additional mean 30 months. They conclude that despite serious concerns about adverse effects, clozapine has considerable clinical value and for most children improved positive and negative symptoms of schizophrenia, improved interpersonal functioning, and allowed a return to a less restrictive setting.

The results of this controlled trial are supported by a number of case reports (Birmaher, Baker, & Kapur, 1992[vi]; Gonzales & Michanie, 1992[vi]; MacEwan & Morton, 1996[vi]; Mozes et al., 1994[vi]) and open trials (Frazier, Gordon, & McKenna, 1994[vi]; Siefen & Remschmidt, 1986[vi]) of clozapine in children and young people with schizophrenia, emphasizing the usefulness of clozapine in cases where onset is early and/or where other treatments have failed. The reduced risk of tardive dyskinesia is also commonly mentioned.

Because the potential value of clozapine is compromised by its side effects, a new generation of "atypical" antipsychotics has been developed, characterized by their ability to be an antagonist at 5-HT_{2A} receptors as well as at the more traditional D_2 receptor. These drugs are as effective as haloperidol in adults (Thomas & Lewis, 1998) but have much reduced extrapyramidal side effects. As yet there are few studies of these new drugs in younger age groups.

Armenteros, Whitaler, Welikson, Stedge, and Gorman (1997[iv]) report an open trial of risperidone, which has a similar pharmacological profile to clozapine but without its serious side effects. Ten subjects ages 12–18 years with a DSM-IV diagnosis of schizophrenia were recruited. After a 2-week drug-free period, each subject started a 6-week trial of risperidone starting at 1 mg/day and increasing to a maximum of 10 mg/day according to response. The Positive and Negative Symptom Scale for Schizophrenia, the BPRS and the Clinical Global Impressions scale were administered weekly, as was a standardized screen for side effects. The mean dose of risperidone was 6.6 mg/day, and four subjects required concomitant benztropine for extrapyramidal side effects. Clinically and statistically significant improvements were found on all clinical measures in comparing baseline and end-point measurements. Adverse effects were minor, with somnolence common but no serious side effects. Clinical effects were noted early, with significant improvements in the first week of treatment. Sikich et al. (1999[i]) report the early findings of a randomized double-blind treatment with one of three agents, haloperidol, risperidone, and olanzapine. Subjects were 23 youths ages 9–19 with active psychosis (DSM diagnosis not specified). All agents reduced psychotic symptoms (measured on standardized scales), with haloperidol being least effective and olanzapine most effective. Olanzapine produced least side effects and was taken longer by subjects. Details of this study are minimal but worth describing here, as so few double-blind evaluations of atypical antipsychotic medications have been reported.

ELECTROCONVULSIVE THERAPY

Electroconvulsive therapy (ECT) is only rarely used in children and adolescents, and there are no adequate controlled trials. Its use tends to be considered when all other treatment approaches have failed and in the presence of severe and disabling symptomatology. The literature comprises case reports and is reviewed by Bertagnoli and Borchardt (1990[vi]). In their summary of published case reports, ECT was effective in only 11 out of 18 reported cases of schizophrenia. They conclude that there is inadequate information to make a judgment about the use of ECT in schizophrenia.

Psychosocial Treatments

There are very few evaluations of psychosocial treatments for children and young people with schizophrenia and only one small controlled trial (Rund et al., 1994[ii]). In this study, 12 young people ages 13–18 years with DSM-III-R schizophrenia (in fact, 9 with schizophrenia, 1 with schizophreniform disorder, 1 with schizotypal personality disorder, and 1 with schizoaffective disorder) were matched on age, sex, and psychosocial functioning with 12 other young people (9 with schizophrenia, 3 with schizophreniform disorder). The experimental group received a psychoeducational intervention comprising educational parent seminars for 1 whole day two to three times a year and structured problem-solving sessions for patient and family every 2 weeks during hospitalization, monthly during rehabilitation, and every 2 months thereafter. The intervention lasted 2 years and included a ward milieu designed to reduce expressed emotion and training and support for school staff and other key people in the family's social network. This was not a randomized trial; the subjects were compared with a matched control group comprising young people who had been through the unit's standard treatment program before the development of this structured psychoeducational approach. The authors claim that treatment was similar for both groups except for the psychoeducational program. Young people in the experimental group had significantly fewer episodes of relapse in the 2 years following first admission if they were receiving the psychoeducational program. However, there were no significant differences in psychosocial functioning as measured by the Global Assessment Scale 2 years after initial treatment. All families were rated as high expressed emotion (EE) families on the Camberwell Family Interview at the time treatment started. The authors note that in the experimental group 7 of the 12 families had changed to low EE status by the time treatment finished. None of the control group families changed their EE status. Overall treatment costs for the psychoeducational program subjects were less than for the control group because of the reduced rate of relapse and readmission.

Penn and Mueser (1996[vi]) review psychosocial treatments in adult schizophrenia. They conclude that there is considerable evidence for the effectiveness of social skills training and a variety of family interventions aimed at reducing expressed emotion and, thereby, relapse. Drury, Birchwood, Cochrane, and MacMillan (1996a[i]; 1996b[i]) in a controlled trial of cognitive therapy suggest that cognitive therapy can also reduce positive symptoms and improve recovery time. As with pharmacological treatments, this research has been extrapolated to guide the management of schizophrenia in children and young people. Practitioner reviews emphasize the need for a range of psychosocial interventions: clear, accurate, and developmentally appropriate information to be made available to patients and their families; psychological interventions for the patient aimed at improving social skills, self-care, and problem solving; and family-based interventions to improve family functioning and coping skills (Clark & Lewis, 1998[vi]; McClellan & Werry, 1997[vi]). However, there is little empirical evidence for these approaches and some suggestion that extrapolation from studies of adults is not always justified. Asarnow et al. (1994) did not find high levels of EE in the families of children with schizophrenia, suggesting interventions aimed at reducing EE may not be justified.

Nevertheless, it is difficult to argue against the need for information and support for children with schizophrenia and their families along with pharmacological treatments. Psychosocial interventions should deal not just with the psychosocial sequelae of illness but with the resulting deviations in development as well. One aim of treatment must be to allow young people to continue to engage with developmental tasks, which will almost inevitably involve close liaison with educational services. Children and young people with schizophrenia may need to be provided with special educational and additional support to reenter schooling. Continuity of care and a flexible approach to the individual's changing developmental needs are essential. Most services will need access to a flexible range of places in day hospitals and units and inpatient units, as well as outpatient and community services to meet all the therapeutic requirements of children with schizophrenia.

SCHIZOAFFECTIVE DISORDERS

A diagnosis of schizoaffective disorder is given only when schizophrenic and affective symptoms are simultaneously present. Some patients have recurrent schizoaffective episodes, which may be of the manic or depressive type or a mixture of the two. The prognosis for schizoaffective disorder in adults is more favorable than that for schizophrenia, but worse than that for affective disorders (Kendler & Tsuang, 1988). A study by Eggers (1989) followed up 16 children and adolescents with schizoaffective disorder over a period of 16 years. The 16 children were part of a sample of 57 children initially diagnosed with schizophrenia. The diagnosis of schizoaffective disorder was made according to ICD-9 criteria. The authors found that an acute recurrent course predominated, although 5 of the 16 patients were in complete remission. This finding suggests that, as with adults, the prognosis of schizoaffective disorder is more favorable than schizophrenia. Similarly, Freeman, Grossman, Pozanski, and Grossman (1985) reported the outcome of four prepubertal children with the disorder. These children were ages 6–12 years and were treated with antidepressants, neuroleptics, and psychotherapy. At follow-up a year later, two had recovered, one was psychotic, and one was depressed. Further longitudinal studies of the outcome of this disorder are required.

There are no outcome studies evaluating interventions for schizoaffective disorders that are of sufficient methodological rigor to allow clear treatment guidance to be given.

MANIA AND BIPOLAR DISORDERS

Definition

Bipolar Disorder

DSM-IV and ICD-10 give very similar definitions of bipolar disorder and bipolar affective disorder. Both classify bipolar disorders according to the current episode. DSM-IV distinguishes between bipolar I disorder and bipolar II disorder. In the latter, there are recurrent major depressive episodes but only hypomanic, not manic, episodes. For a diagnosis of bipolar affective disorder there must have been at least two episodes in which the patient's mood and activity levels are significantly disturbed, one of which must have been hypomanic or manic in nature. Typically, there is complete recovery between episodes. The first episode may occur at any time from late childhood onward. Each episode can be described as primarily either manic or depressive. Sometimes there is a mixed episode in which the mood changes rapidly.

ICD-10 describes three degrees of severity of mania, whereas DSM-IV describes only two (hypomanic and manic episodes). The ICD categories are described in the following paragraphs.

Hypomania

Hypomania is a lesser degree of mania in which mood and behavioral abnormalities occur but are not accompanied by delusions and hallucinations. There is a constant, mildly elevated mood for several days, accompanied by increased energy and activity and usually strong feelings of heightened mental and physical well-being. There may also be evidence of increased sociability, overtalkativeness, over-familiarity, increased sexual energy, and a reduced need for sleep. Concentration and attention may be impaired. To meet the diagnosis, several of these features should be present continuously for at least several days. The ability to take part in school or social activity is likely to be reduced. If this inability is severe or complete, mania should be diagnosed.

Mania without Psychotic Symptoms

In mania without psychotic symptoms, the mood is elevated out of keeping with the individual's situation and may present as uncontrollable excitement. Elation is accompanied by increased energy, resulting in overactivity, pressure of speech, and a decreased need for sleep. There is marked disinhibition, attention cannot be sustained, and there is often extreme distractibility. In some manic episodes the mood is irritable and suspicious rather than elated. The first attack occurs most commonly between the ages of 15 and 30 years but may occur at any age, sometimes in late childhood. To meet the diagnosis, the episode should be present for at least a week and should be severe enough to disrupt ordinary school and social activities more or less completely.

Mania with Psychotic Symptoms

In mania with psychotic symptoms, the clinical picture is that of a more severe form of mania as described earlier. Inflated ideas may develop into delusions, and irritability and suspiciousness into delusions of persecution. In severe cases delusions of identity or role may occur, and flight of ideas and pressure of speech may result in the individuals becoming incomprehensible.

Prevalence

There are very few epidemiological studies of the childhood psychoses. Lewinsohn et al. (1993) conducted a longitudinal study of 14- to 18-year-old adolescents in west central Oregon, using the standardized K-SADS interview. The incidence of current and follow-up episodes of bipolar disorder occurring a year later was approximately 0.3%, with a lifetime prevalence of approximately 0.6%. However, the authors interviewed adolescents but not teachers and parents. Although it has been reported that adolescents are usually the most reliable informants regarding their mental health, as insight is often impaired in bipolar disorder it is possible that they were underreporting problems in this study.

Costello et al. (1988) examined the prevalence of psychiatric disorder in 789 7- to 11-year-old children visiting their primary care pediatrician for a wide range of reasons. One-year prevalence (assessed using the DISC) of DSM-III bipolar disorder was 0.2%, similar to that found in the Lewinsohn et al. (1993) study.

Clinical Presentation

The presentation of children and adolescents with depressive disorders is described in Chapter 4. Presentation of mania is covered in the section "Definition" earlier in this chapter. Frequently children and adolescents present with a bipolar illness following treatment of a depressive illness with antidepressants (Bowring & Kovacs, 1992). It is therefore important to consider this diagnosis as a possibility in children being treated for a depressive illness. No studies have specifically described the disorders likely to be comorbid with bipolar disorder.

Because of a lack of diagnostic rigor until recently, there are very few adequate follow-up studies of bipolar disorders in young people. Strober and Carlson (1982) reported a study of 60 adolescents hospitalized for major depression who were prospectively followed up to assess the prevalence of bipolar disorder and the predictors of this being an outcome. Bipolar disorder occurred in 20% of the cohort. The subjects were 56 consecutive admissions to the adolescent unit of the UCLA Neuropsychiatric Institute, Los Angeles, who satisfied research diagnostic criteria (Spitzer, Endicott, & Robins, 1978) for depression and had received an adequate trial of antidepressant medication for the initial depressive episode. Two subjects refused treatment, and in another two cases medication was discontinued because of an allergic reaction. A trial of amitriptyline or imipramine was deemed adequate if the dose was 150 mg for at least 2 weeks. Follow-up contacts were made at 6-monthly intervals dating from discharge. At follow-up 20% had developed mania. The average point of development of the manic illness was 28 weeks. Unfortunately, there were no other outcome measures from this study.

Carlson et al. (1977) reported a comparison of 20 subjects meeting a diagnosis of bipolar illness with onset before 20 years of age, and 20 subjects in whom the onset of the disorder was after 45 years of age. The age range for onset in the younger age group was 8 to 19 years with a mean onset age of 15.9 years. The mean episode frequency was 0.40 per year, which is the same as that found in adults with bipolar disorder. At follow-up 20% were significantly impaired but functioning, and a further 20% were chronically incapacitated. There were two suicides in the late-onset group and one in the early-onset group.

Treatment

As with schizophrenia, the management of bipolar disorder has been comprehensively reviewed in recent years (Alessi, Naylor, Ghaziuddin, & Zubieta, 1994[vi]; Botteron & Geller, 1995[vi]; Geller & Luby, 1997[vi]; Hechtman & Greenfield, 1997[vi]; Kafantaris, 1995[vi]; McClellan & Werry, 1997[vi]). If anything, there are even fewer adequately controlled trials of physical or psychosocial treatments in children and young people with bipolar disorder than there are for schizophrenia.

Assessment

Diagnosis in children uses the same diagnostic criteria as used for adults. As always, there is no substitute for a comprehensive history from the child, family, and other adults involved with the young person, and repeated mental state examination. Physical examination and appropriate investigation are essential. Diagnosis is complicated by the fact that a mixed presentation with features of depression and mania is common in younger people. Presenting symptoms often fluctuate, and mood can be labile. The presence of psychotic features, and the atypical presentation of other psychotic disorders in childhood, add to the difficulty. Comorbid conditions are not uncommon, and a further problem is the likelihood that age-related restrictions on children will modify the "reckless" and "disinhibited" behavior typically seen in adults. Instead, such behaviors may be more akin to typical conduct disturbance. A longitudinal perspective can be helpful in assessment, and the presence of risk factors such as a positive family history or past depressive episodes in the index patient is important. Assessment can be managed on an outpatient basis, but as with other complex conditions in young people, a period of day patient or inpatient observation may aid diagnosis by affording opportunities to assess child functioning in a number of settings. The differential diagnosis includes schizophrenia, schizoaffective disorders, depressive disorders, posttraumatic stress disorders, and disruptive conduct disorders, as well as organic disorders and substance abuse.

General Approaches to Treatment

Research on the management of children with bipolar disorder is limited. Existing practice guidelines draw heavily on extrapolations from adult literature and from case reports of treatment of children and young people. These extrapolations should be treated with caution especially with affective disorders, as there is clear evidence that children and young people do not necessarily respond in the same way to antidepressants as adults (Harrington, 1992). If this is also the case for bipolar disorders, extrapolation from adult data may be misleading.

There is consensus that the severity and likely time course of the illness means that treatment must be multimodal and aimed at bringing about a decrease in acute symptomatology and associated psychosocial problems, preventing relapse, and promoting normal development. Affected young people and their families are likely to require extensive support. Maintenance of education and social relationships between episodes is an important priority. Informed consent is required before treatment can commence, but the nature of the condition and the possibility of psychotic symptoms require an assessment as to whether informed consent is possible. As with schizophrenia, cooperation and consent should be sought from both the young person and his or her parents or legal guardians. If consent is not forthcoming, practitioners need to be familiar with relevant child care and mental health legislation and use this where indicated to ensure that treatment is given appropriately.

With relatively low levels of behavioral disturbance and good cooperation, treatment can take place on an outpatient basis, but most guidelines suggest that inpatient treatment in the early acute phase is necessary.

Physical Treatments

A recent paper by Kowatch et al. (2000[ii]) compares the effect sizes (ESs) of three of the more commonly used mood-stabilizing drugs in bipolar disorder in an open, but randomized, trial of lithium, carbamazepine, and divalproex sodium. Participants were 42 young people (mean age 11.4 years) meeting DSM-IV criteria for bipolar I or bipolar II disorder during a mixed or manic episode. Subjects had to be free of medical illness requiring medication, of normal intelligence, and with no history of schizophrenia, obsessive–compulsive disorder, autism, substance misuse, or organic brain disease. Standardized measures were used with the Bipolar Clinical Global Impression Improvement subscale (CGI-BP) and the Young Mania Rating Scale (Y-MRS) as the main outcome measures.

Assignation to treatment group was random, using the minimization method, and treatment continued for 6 weeks. Dose and serum levels for each drug were monitored at 1, 2, and 4 weeks. Using a change in Y-MRS of 50% or more from baseline to exit as the response, the ES was 1.63 for divalproex sodium, 1.06 for lithium, and 1.00 for carbamazepine. All subjects tolerated the medications well with few significant side effects. This study suggests that all three agents show clinically significant ESs in an open trial. Within the report there is useful information about dosage regimes, cumulative times to response, and patterns of response. Further studies are needed to validate these findings, preferably with no-treatment comparison groups and raters blind to treatment status.

LITHIUM

There is clear evidence of lithium's efficacy in adults, both for treatment of the acute phase and as a prophylactic to prevent relapse (Roth & Fonagy, 1996[vi]). Consensus is for a similar approach in children, though good evidence for this is lacking. What little evidence there is supports the use of lithium as the treatment of first choice, although in clinical practice other agents are often used. There have been a number of reviews of lithium carbonate use in the management of children and young people. Youngerman and Canino (1978[vi]) were unable to report on any controlled trials, but summarized the treatment of 190 children treated with lithium for a variety of reasons. These were all case series and case reports, with about 30 children seeming to meet criteria for manic–depressive illness. More recent reviews describing the literature in some detail have not been able to report a large increase in the number of controlled trials in this area (Alessi et al., 1994[vi]; Botteron & Geller, 1995[vi]; Kafantaris, 1995[vi]; McClellan & Werry, 1997[vi]). The more important studies are summarized briefly later.

DeLong and Aldershof (1987[vi]) report a large open trial of lithium over a period of years on a group of children with a variety of diagnoses. Diagnosis of bipolar disorder was made retrospectively. Of the 59 children (mean age 10.9 years, range 3.1–20 years) with a diagnosis of bipolar disorder, 45 (74%) were felt to have benefited from lithium treatment at the time of treatment. On retrospective review and incorporating what follow-up data was available, 59 (66%) were felt to have benefited in the long run. There were no significant differences in outcome for those over and under 14 years of age at the time of initial treatment. Strober et al. (1988[vi]) describe a group of 50 young people (ages 13–17 years) treated with lithium for DSM-III bipolar I disorder. This was as part of a study looking at family history, but the outcome of treatment is reported briefly. Lithium dosage was titrated against clinical response and side effects to achieve plasma lithium levels in the 0.9–1.5 mEq/l range. Other psychoactive drugs were prescribed as well as lithium, but there is little detail about this. These authors report that the response of children with onset before 12 years was significantly poorer than in those with later onset. Resistance to treatment with lithium has been noted in a few other case series. Himmelhoch and Garfinkel (1986[vi]) reported a series of 46 lithium-resistant patients with bipolar disorder (DSM-III), 23 of whom were adolescents (ages 12–19 years). They suggest an association between "mixed mania" (defined as simultaneous Hamilton Depression score of greater than 16 and Kupfer–Detre System score of greater than 12), neuropsychiatric disorders (usually seizure disorders and substance abuse), and lithium resistance. Hsu (1986a[iv]) describes seven adolescents (ages 15–17 years) with first episodes of DSM-III bipolar disorder. Three of the seven responded poorly to lithium.

There are very few controlled trials of the use of lithium in young people. McKnew et al. (1981[i]) describe six children ages 9–12 selected because of "incapacitating" psychopathology and a lithium-responding parent or (in one case) grandparent. The children had a variety of diagnoses based on DSM-III. Only two were diagnosed as having a bipolar disorder, two more had major affective disorders, and one had a cyclothymic disorder. None of the children had received psychoactive medication in the preceding year. Other diagnoses were common. The study used a double-blind, crossover design with two periods of lithium and two periods of placebo. There was random allocation to the starting condition of either lithium or placebo. Lithium was maintained at plasma levels of 0.8–1.2 mEq/l. Only the children meeting DSM-III criteria for bipolar disorder responded to lithium. DeLong and Nieman (1983[i]) report on a cohort of 16 children (mean age 10.3 years, range 6.3–13.5 years) with clinical symptoms "suggestive of manic–depressive illness." Inclusion criteria were clinical symptoms for a manic episode as defined in DSM-III for at least 2 years, a family history of affective disorder, IQ greater than 80, and a history of a positive response to lithium in the past. Exclusion criteria were neurological signs, substance abuse, and evidence of schizophrenia. The trial used a double-blind, crossover methodology, with 3 weeks of lithium and 3 weeks of placebo, and took place on an outpatient basis. Order of presentation was by random allocation. Each child received the lithium dose that had previously been shown to produce a good response (mean plasma lithium levels were 0.6mEq/l during the trial). Ratings were made by parents, using a 20-item questionnaire adapted for the study. Parents were not suffering from symptoms of affective disorder or taking medication for affective disorder during the trial. Subjects improved significantly on a range of mood and behavioral measures with lithium and deteriorated when on placebo.

More recently, Geller et al. (1998[i]) published results of a double-blind, placebo-controlled, random allocation trial of lithium for adolescents with bipolar disorder and temporally secondary substance dependency. Subjects were 25 young people ages 12–18 years recruited from newspaper advertisements and contacts with other clinicians. Subjects had to meet DSM-III-R criteria for substance dependency disorder (SDD) and bipolar disorder (BPD), except for the substance abuse exclusion criterion. Bipolar disorder needed to have preceded SDD by at least 2 weeks and could take the form of bipolar I, bipolar II, mania, or major affective disorder with one of the adolescent predictors of BPD. Neurological problems and an IQ of less than 75 were exclusion criteria. Subjects were randomly assigned to lithium or placebo. Lithium levels were maintained in the range of 0.9–1.3 mEq/l by regular and random serum lithium levels and subsequent dosage adjustment. Subjects and those responsible for outcome measurements were blind to this process, with subjects receiving identical capsules irrespective of the dosage of lithium. Subjects were not expected to refrain from use of "substances" during the trial, which took place on an outpatient basis with two contacts per week, one scheduled and one random. Pre- and posttreatment measures included the K-SADS (present episode and lifetime version), the Children's Global Assessment Scale (CGAS), and a semistructured interview addressing the nine DSM-III-R items relating to SDD. Regular urine assays for substance abuse were also made. Data were analyzed on intention-to-treat and completion-of-treatment methods; four of the 25 subjects failed to complete. There were significant improvements on the percentage of positive drug assays and on CGAS scores, but not on K-SADS mood items or on SDD items. This important contribution still has many of the problems of the two earlier studies, with small numbers of an unrepresentative sample and no follow-up data.

Lithium is also likely to be effective for patients with psychotic symptoms associated with bipolar I disorder. Horowitz (1977[vi]) describes a series of eight cases, with adolescents ages 15–18 years with manic–depressive illness with psychotic features (all had either hallucinations and/or delusions). All subjects were treated with lithium and achieved remission of symptoms at serum levels of 0.5—1.2 mEq/l. Varanka, Weller, and Weller (1988[vi]) report on a series of ten children (mean age 9 years 6 months) who fulfilled DSM-III criteria for manic episode with psychotic features. Seven had visual hallucinations, five auditory hallucinations, seven persecutory delusions, and two grandiose delusions. All ten were treated with lithium carbonate alone in a daily dose designed to maintain plasma levels of 0.6–1.4 mEq/l. Optimum levels were achieved within 3–5 days on a mean dose of 1270 mg daily. All children improved rapidly (mean time for improvement 11 days), and all psychotic symptoms disappeared. Minor side effects such as fatigue, anorexia, nausea, abdominal discomfort, increased urination, and tremor were reported.

There have been no controlled studies of maintenance lithium therapy, but Strober, Morrell, and Burroughs (1990[vi]) describe the 18-month outcome of a cohort of 37 children (mean age 15.1 years) who met DSM-III and Research Diagnostic Criteria (RDC) criteria for bipolar I disorder. The subjects were treated as inpatients during the acute phase of their illness and discharged on maintenance lithium with a recommendation that this continue. Lithium levels following stabilization ranged from 0.7–1.4 mEq/l. Sixteen subjects received neuroleptic medication, and 4 carbamazepine in addition to lithium during the acute phase. Following discharge, all patients received adjunctive individual and family interventions of varying intensity and had lithium levels monitored every 4–6 weeks. Of the 37 children, 24 continued maintenance lithium therapy throughout the 18-month follow-up period. This group did not differ from the group that discontinued treatment on any measures of clinical or demographic features. Relapse occurred in 21 of the 37, but relapse rates were three times higher in the group that discontinued treatment. Strober et al. (1995) report on a prospective cohort of 54 consecutive admissions of adolescents with bipolar disorder but do not describe outcome in relation to treatment continuance.

Pharmacokinetics and Side Effects of Lithium. Lithium is an alkali metal that affects a number of neurochemical systems: ion channels; serotonin, dopamine, and norepinephrine transmitter systems; and second messenger systems such as phosphoinositides and adenylate cyclase (Alessi et al., 1994[vi]). It is usually administered orally in the form of a carbonate salt and is excreted by the kidneys. Blood levels peak 2.4 hours after administration of an oral dose of 300 mg (Vitiello, Behar, & Malone, 1988). In this study the elimination half-life was 17.9 hours, quicker than in adults and presumably due to the differing renal function of children. This study found serum to be a more reliable means than saliva for estimating levels of lithium. Recommended therapeutic serum levels of lithium are 0.6–1.2 mEq/l, which can usually be achieved within 4–5 days by a starting dose of about 900 mg/day (Alessi et al., 1994[vi]; McClellan & Werry, 1997[vi]). Serum lithium levels may need to be monitored weekly on commencement of therapy, but once stabilized, lithium levels, as well as renal and thyroid function, should be monitored every 3–6 months.

Children seem to tolerate lithium well, and few side effects are reported in the studies mentioned earlier. There are insufficient data to make predictions about longer-term side effects, but it seems safest to assume that children will be at least as much at risk as adults. Common side effects are nausea, vomiting, diarrhea, tremor, polyuria, weight gain, headache, and fatigue (Silva et al., 1992). Thyroid and renal changes are common. Lithium inhibits the action of antidiuretic hormone on the distal tubules leading to polyuria and polydipsia. Regular monitoring of renal function is therefore recommended. In lithium-induced hypothyroidism, levels of thyroid-stimulating hormone are high; therefore, this should also be regularly monitored. Rarer side effects can include arrythmias, leukocytosis, muscle weakness and exacerbation of skin conditions, and alteration of EEG patterns (Alessi et al., 1994[vi]; McClellan & Werry, 1997[vi]).

Repeated monitoring of mental state for children on lithium is obviously indicated, but careful notice should be taken of mood as children recover from the acute manic phase as periods of depression are common.

NEUROLEPTICS

There are no trials of neuroleptic medication for bipolar I disorder, although case reports indicate that neuroleptics are often used (Kafantaris, 1995[vi]; McClellan & Werry, 1997[vi]). Given the suggestion that lithium can effectively treat mania with psychotic symptoms in a relatively short time period (Horowitz, 1977[vi]; Varanka et al. 1988[vi]), and the potential adverse side effects of neuroleptics, this treatment is not generally recommended.

ANTICONVULSANTS

The anticonvulsants valproate and carbamazepine have been shown to be effective in adults with bipolar disorders (Roth & Fonagy, 1996[vi]). No controlled trials have been conducted in children or adolescents.

Papatheodorou and Kutcher (1993[vi]) report preliminary findings of an open trial of valproate with six older adolescent subjects (mean age 19 years, range 17–22 years). All met DSM-III-R criteria for bipolar affective disorder, manic or mixed manic subtype. Five of the six showed significant improvement on each of the three clinical rating scales used (Modified Mania Rating Scale, BPRS, and Global Assessment Scale) on a mean dose of 1,000 mg/day. Very few side effects were reported. All subjects also received adjunctive neuroleptic treatment. West, Keck, and McElroy (1994) added valproate to the treatment regimes of 11 patients ages 12–18 years whose DSM-III-R bipolar I disorder was not responding to antipsychotics alone (6) or in combination with lithium (5). Six showed a moderate improvement and 3 a marked improvement. Mean dosage was 1,068 mg/day.

There are fewer reports of carbamazepine use in young people with bipolar disorder. Himmelhoch and Garfinkel (1986[vi]) mention its use as an adjunct to lithium in lithium-resistant cases. Kafantaris (1995[vi]) cites Garfinkel, Garfinkel, Himmelhoch, and McHugh (1985) as describing the use of carbamazepine in 19 treatment-resistant bipolar adolescent patients. A combination of lithium and carbamazepine was said to bring about an excellent response.

BENZODIAZEPINES

Benzodiazepines have been used in adults (Kafantaris, 1995[vi]; McClellan & Werry, 1997[vi]), but there are no reports of their use in children.

ELECTROCONVULSIVE THERAPY

ECT is only rarely used in children and adolescents, and there are no adequate controlled trials. Its use tends to be considered when all other treatment approaches have failed and in the presence of severe and disabling symptomatology. The literature comprises case reports and is reviewed by Bertagnoli and Borchardt (1990[vi]). In their summary of published case reports, ECT was effective in cases of bipolar disorders with affective, manic, and rapid-cycling episodes.

Psychosocial Treatments

Comprehensive multimodal treatment programs that combine psychoeducation, supportive therapy for child and family, attention to comorbid conditions, and so on, are recommended by most authorities, but no research evidence supports these recommendations. Even with adults, little evidence supports particular psychosocial interventions for mania, although Miklowitz, Goldstein, Neuchterlein, Snyder, and Mintz (1988) report that family factors such as expressed emotion and affective style do predict relapse in adult manic bipolar patients, suggesting a possible way forward.

Given the levels of acute behavioral disturbance in the early stages of manic presentations, anything other than supportive interventions may be difficult to deliver, let alone evaluate. However, given the chronic, relapsing nature of the condition and the probable effectiveness of ongoing lithium maintenance therapy, education about the condition and its course and treatment seem to be an essential component of any treatment program. Current best practice suggests a variety of other psychosocial interventions aimed at reducing social disruption, enabling developmental tasks to be seen through, supporting education, and reducing distress (Kafantaris, 1995[vi]; McClellan & Werry, 1997[vi]).

RAPID-CYCLING BIPOLAR DISORDER

Rapid-cycling forms of bipolar disorder can occur in children and adolescents (Geller et al., 1995a). There are no studies indicating the best management for children, although Himmelhoch and Garfinkel (1986[vi]) suggest that anticonvulsants may have a role to play. This is similar to adult management, in which a combination of antimanic agents may be needed but antidepressants are best avoided (Prien & Potter, 1990).

SUMMARY

Schizophrenia

Childhood and adulthood schizophrenia can be reasonably well defined. The incidence of childhood schizophrenia is low, but the cost of providing services for the group with this disorder is high because of relatively high prevalence rates consequent on its lifetime morbidity. Little is known about factors affecting the long-term outcome of childhood schizophrenia, but early onset, poor premorbid adjustment, and withdrawn and isolated personality are associated with negative long-term outcome.

Although schizophrenia is a relatively common and very serious mental illness, there are remarkably few well-conducted trials of pharmacological treatment in childhood and adolescence and no such trials of psychosocial treatments. What studies there are use small numbers and not necessarily representative samples. Some older studies use no or outdated diagnostic criteria. Outcomes are reported almost exclusively in terms of symptom relief, and sometimes, psychosocial adaptation. Follow-up data are minimal or nonexistent.

The assessment of childhood schizophrenia is complex, and in most cases admission is required for a full assessment to exclude organic conditions or the effect of exposure to drugs. Traditional neuroleptic medication has been demonstrated to reduce acute positive symptoms, but there are relatively few trials for children. The side effects of neuroleptic medication can be serious and must be regularly monitored. As yet, there is little empirical evidence of the superiority of atypical over traditional neuroleptic medication for children with schizophrenia, and, again, there are concerns about their side effects. There is no systematic evidence for or against the use of ECT. Psychosocial treatments have promise on the basis of extrapolation from adult studies, but there is, as yet, insufficient evidence to make specific recommendations.

In the absence of empirical data, best practice guidelines are frequently based on extrapolation from adult studies and/or the consensus of child clinicians. Best practice advice includes admission as part of the assessment process; neuroleptic medications, with close monitoring (initially weekly) of side effects, which should continue well beyond the acute phase; and psychosocial interventions aimed at the reintegration of the young person into normal life. Attention should also be paid to any comorbid problems. Suggested dosage is usually 0.5–9.0 mg/kg daily of chlorpromazine equivalent, but the lack of research on children means that these recommendations need to be treated with caution. Haloperidol is often the drug of first choice and is usually started in doses of 1–2 mg daily up to a maximum of 10–15 mg daily in adolescents. Extrapyramidal side effects can be treated with antiparkinsonian agents, but some suggest that these side effects are an indication for transfer to an atypical antipsychotic. Dosage should be gradually increased and titrated against clinical response and level of side effects. If after 6–8 weeks there is no clear improvement, a second antipsychotic should be substituted. If there is no response to a second drug or if side effects are intolerable, consideration should be given to one of the atypical antipsychotics. If clozapine is used, there needs to be careful and regular monitoring for side effects. If a recovery is made following a first episode, consideration should be given to slowly withdrawing medication, as a small proportion of young people will not relapse. If problems persist or relapse occurs, medication may have to continue indefinitely.

Schizoaffective Disorders

The definition of schizoaffective disorders is clear and their prognosis is better than that of schizophrenia. There are few studies establishing the long-term course of the disorders. There is insufficient evidence to provide an empirically based guideline for the treatment of children and adolescents with this diagnosis.

Bipolar Disorder

Until recently, there was a lack of clear diagnostic criteria for bipolar disorder, and, consequently, evidence concerning its prevalence and natural history is poor. Retrospective studies of natural history indicate that high IQ and good premorbid adjustment indicate good prognosis.

There is some evidence supporting the use of lithium in the acute phase of the disorder, but there are no controlled studies of its long-term prophylactic use. There are no good studies supporting the use of neuroleptics, although best practice reviews suggest their use. Reviews of best practice suggest that medication is the treatment of choice in the acute phase, with lithium probably the drug of first choice, perhaps augmented by neuroleptics if response is poor. Maintenance lithium therapy should be considered for prevention of relapse. Anticonvulsants are used in adult patients to prevent recurrence and may be effective in the maintenance treatment of children and adolescents. There is no evidence to support the use of benzodiazepines or ECT in children with bipolar disorder. Support and education for families, liaison with schools, and integration back into as normal a life as possible are recommended, but there is little evidence to guide the choice of psychosocial intervention.

IMPLICATIONS

Because of the better prognosis of bipolar and schizoaffective disorders, it is important that all children and adolescents presenting with psychotic symptoms are comprehensively assessed and accurately diagnosed. There is a clear need for further research into schizophrenia and bipolar disorders in children and adolescents, with particular attention to the role of newer antipsychotic medications, anticonvulsants for bipolar disorders, and psychosocial treatments. Although some adult studies suggest that atypical antipsychotics should be used, there is as yet insufficient evidence in children and adolescents to suggest that they would be the treatment of choice. Given that most children and adolescents are living within families, it is particularly important to study the possible usefulness of family-based interventions.

9

Pervasive Developmental Disorders

The terms *pervasive developmental disorders* (PDD) and *social communication disorders* are sometimes used interchangeably because of the difficulty of telling which type of PDD is present. Improvements such as increased refinements of the *International Statistical Classification of Diseases and Related Health Problems* (ICD) (World Health Organization, 1992a) and the DSM (American Psychiatric Association, 1994) classification systems and development of research instruments (American Psychiatric Association, 1994; Le Couteur et al., 1989; Nordin, Gillberg, & Nyden, 1998; Wing, 1996) have helped, but the great variability in presentation still often makes it difficult to be certain what type of PDD is present. Much more work is required to improve our understanding of these disorders, especially on the question of whether atypical autism and Asperger's disorder are on the same continuum as classical autism, or whether they are separate entities. At the present time the various types are classified as childhood autism, atypical autism, Asperger's disorder, Rett's disorder, and childhood disintegrative disorder. We discuss each separately in this chapter.

CHILDHOOD AUTISM

The etiology of autism is unknown, but the associations with physical disorders such as congenital rubella (Chess, 1971), the MMR vaccine (Wakefield, Anthony, & Schepelmann, 1998), tuberous sclerosis (Hunt & Shepherd, 1993), fragile X (Bailey et al., 1993), and many others (Gillberg, 1990a[ib]) suggest a significant degree of underlying organic pathology. The significantly elevated risk of developing seizure disorders as compared with the normal population supports this view (Volkmar & Nelson, 1990). A few studies report microscopic abnormalities, including reduced cell numbers in the limbic system (Bauman, 1991), the cerebellum

(Courchesne, Yeung-Courchesne, Press, Hesselink, & Jernigan, 1988), and the brainstem (Gaffney, Kuperman, Tsai, & Minchin, 1988). It is uncertain whether the findings are specific to autism, as the majority of subjects in these studies also had learning difficulties. The findings of brain scans and EEGs have also been inconclusive (Bailey et al., 1993).

Although fragile X, a congenital abnormality of the X chromosome, may be present in a very small number of autistic individuals (Bailey et al., 1993), children with the fragile X disorder are generally more socially anxious than autistic individuals, although they are also more interested in making friends. Twin studies suggest a strong genetic influence in autism (Bailey et al., 1995; Bolton & Rutter, 1990). Currently, the risk of brothers or sisters of an affected individual having autism appears to be high, on the order of 4% (Folstein & Rutter, 1988; Piven et al., 1992).

Definition

Kanner (1943) first defined the condition of autism, having recognized that some young children presented by the age of 30 months with abnormal development of language and social relationships as well as ritualistic and obsessional behaviors. The definition covers problems in three main areas of functioning, with onset in the first 3 years of life: (1) qualitative impairments in social interactions that may be apparent as failure to comprehend that others have feelings, lack of interest in imitative or social play, and inability to seek friendships or comfort from others; (2) qualitative impairments in verbal and nonverbal communication, ranging from little or no use of language and gestures with avoidance of eye contact, to difficulty in engaging in conversation despite the presence of adequate speech; (3) restriction of interests and a resistance to change, which may be expressed as an insistence on certain routines or a desire to take part in only a narrow range of interests or activities. There may also be a variety of mannerisms or stereotypes, such as hand twisting, toe walking, head banging, and running in circles.

Prevalence

In their review of the literature, Gillberg, Steffenburg, and Schaumann (1991) concluded that there is international agreement that the prevalence of autism is 7 to 17 per 10,000 children in urban and rural areas alike. The highest reported prevalence is in school-age children, and is estimated as 12–20 per 10,000. Gillberg suggests that as autism is so difficult to diagnose in young preschool children, this latter figure is probably the most accurate population estimate. Another difficulty in assessing the reliability of prevalence estimates is ascertaining whether the figures describe rates for "nuclear autism," as defined by the classification systems, or for autistic-like conditions such as the "autistic continuum," or "autistic spectrum." Gillberg emphasizes that the apparent increase in prevalence rates reported over time is due to an improved detection rate rather than to a true increase in occurrence. The recently published practice parameters of the American Academy of Child and Adolescent Psychiatry (1999) suggest that the prevalence rate of 4.8 cases per 10,000 (Fombonne, 1998) should be accepted, as this is the median prevalence of 20 studies. However, a recent study by Bryson (1997) agreed with Gillberg in reporting a rate of 1 per 1,000.

Clinical Presentation

The age of onset of autism is at birth, although its presence frequently goes unrecognized before the second or third year of life, and in higher-functioning individuals, not until much later. Usually there is no period of normal development, but if there is, problems become apparent before the age of 3 years. Early recognition of autism is preferable because early intervention may reduce later morbidity (Simeonson, Olley, & Rosenthal, 1987), and the developmental level at age 5 predicts the final outcome (Lotter, 1978). There is often considerable delay between problems being reported by parents and diagnosis (Ornitz, Guthrie, & Farley, 1977; Siegel, Pliner, Eschler, & Elliott, 1988). Baron-Cohen, Allen, and Gillberg (1992) have recently developed a checklist for use by primary health care professionals to help alleviate this delay. The disorder occurs in boys three to four times more often than in girls. Learning difficulties are present in most cases. The severity of the disorder can vary greatly.

Usually the first problem to present is lack of sociability. Even autistic infants frequently show a lack of social reciprocity; they may dislike being held and avoid direct eye gaze. Older infants show less enjoyment in joint play than would be expected. Alternatively, some are clingy and indiscriminately affectionate (Le Couteur et al., 1989). They often do not reciprocate speech and play and may fail to imitate others. In the early childhood years the lack of social interest persists; children show unusual eye contact and a lack of interest in peers. They may fail to use their parents as a secure base and have little desire to be comforted or to offer comfort to others in distress. Not all these problems need to be present in every individual for the diagnosis to be made.

By the time the child is 3 years old, parents and/or health professionals become concerned about delayed language development and failure to make appropriate peer relationships. Parents and preschool teachers may find the severe tantrums and extreme desire for sameness very difficult to handle. Poor comprehension of social cues, as demonstrated by a lack of response to other people's emotions and/or a lack of modulation of behavior according to the social situation, leads to problems in interactions with peers. As a result, autistic children are frequently isolated and spend most of their time playing alone. Parents describe difficulties in taking their child outside the home because of how he or she responds in public.

Language delay and/or impairment is the second area of problems to emerge. About half of autistic individuals never speak. Those that can talk show unusual use of language, although often the ability to speak, from the phonological (making the correct sounds) and syntactical (putting words together) point of view, is equivalent to that of normal controls (Fay & Schular, 1980). Autistic individuals tend to show unusual intonation and stress when speaking, appearing to speak in a monotone. They are extremely literal in their expression and understanding, particularly when considering thoughts and emotions (Tager-Flusberg, 1981). In addition to these semantic difficulties, pragmatic difficulties are common: They may fail to observe conventions of speech such as turn taking, adapting the length of conversation to the listener, or introducing a subject where appropriate. It can be difficult to distinguish autism from a language disorder, particularly in individuals with high-functioning autism. Nevertheless, indicators include the pervasiveness of communication difficulties (nonverbal in addition to verbal), more profound social difficulties, and the large scatter of cognitive scores on psychometric testing (Cantwell, Baker, & Rutter, 1978; Cohen, Caparulo, & Shaywitz, 1976; Rutter, 1978a). Learning disability is the other differential diagnosis. Autistic features are often present where there is a generalized learning disability; in autism, however, the social dysfunction exceeds the level that the general cognitive abilities would predict (Rutter, 1978b).

Repetitive and restricted interests tend to become more apparent in the older preschool child, who may frequently become preoccupied with, for example, parts of toys such as spinning car wheels. Spontaneous imaginative play is rare; these children may enact the same scene repeatedly. Many autistic children show unusual interest in certain sensory properties of objects, such as taste or smell.

A significant but currently unknown proportion of autistic children have additional behavior problems, including hyperactivity, short attention span, aggressiveness, stereotypies, self-injurious behavior, and temper tantrums. Lainhart and Folstein (1994) looked for affective symptoms in 17 published case reports of autistic individuals. Affective symptoms were initially noticed in childhood in 6 cases. The authors emphasize that the possibility of mood disorder should be considered in the presence of a deterioration in performance in either behavior or cognition. Crying, decreased activity, and agitation are other features, as would be a sudden increase in self-injurious behavior. As the majority of autistic individuals have language delay and learning difficulties, it can be difficult to recognize the onset of affective disorder.

DeLong suggests that autism, in the absence of brain damage, is a "severe early-life phenotype of familial major affective disorder" (1999, p. 911). He bases this theory on the frequent finding of a strong family history of affective disorders in affected children, the clinical presentation of autism, and the response of affected children to antidepressant treatment. He supports his hypothesis further with the findings from a PET brain scan study of seven autistic boys, which showed reduced left hemisphere serotonin synthesis (Chugani, Chugani, Nimura, & Muzik, 1997). Reduced serotonin production in the brains of autistic children has been found in a second study. He also notes the relatively normal functioning of the right hemisphere in non-brain-damaged autistic children (Ehlers et al., 1997), leading often to the preservation of visual–spatial abilities, simple memory, and language and attention. Further studies with larger samples are clearly required, including findings from genetic studies.

Natural History

There have been few longitudinal studies of the progress of autistic children throughout childhood and adolescence. Gillberg (1991) reviewed the current literature on the outcome of autism; we will discuss this review as well as the current literature. It is useful to refer initially to two earlier papers by Lotter (1974, 1978). Lotter considered eight studies to be acceptable for the purposes of considering outcome. Four originated in the United Kingdom, three in the United States, and one in Belgium. They reviewed the outcome of 474 cases of autism, all diagnosed by criteria similar to Rutter et al.'s (1970b), although in Gillberg's (1991) opinion even in these studies there is considerable diagnostic variability. Only one reported on a community- or population-based series of autism cases. The outcome in the studies was variable, but the overall trend was toward a bad prognosis, with at least 313 of the 474 cases (66%) in the poor prognosis bracket (severe handicap, no independent social progress) or very poor prognosis bracket (unable to lead any kind of independent existence). In addition, 1.5% of the whole group died between the ages of 2 and 30 years. The mortality rate at this time in the general population was 0.5. Five of the eight studies reported a high rate of epilepsy: 11% at or after adolescence. Some cases were probably missed because the period of follow-up was not always sufficient, epilepsy tending to have onset in adolescence or beyond. Overall, 8% in these follow-up studies had jobs; one person was attending college.

At about the same time, Rutter et al. (1970b) similarly reported a follow-up study of 60 clinically referred cases of autism and other childhood psychoses. Rutter reported a figure of 12% for permanent deterioration. The findings regarding onset of epilepsy were similar to those of Gillberg (1991a) (discussed later). Generally, children with higher IQs had a better and less predictable outcome. Useful speech in childhood also predicted better outcome.

As the main problems with outcome studies have been variability in diagnostic criteria and a lack of standardized outcome measures, it is important to refer to studies in which autism has been diagnosed according to strict criteria, such as those of Rutter et al. (1970b), Wing (1989), Coleman and Gillberg (1985), or Le Couteur et al. (1989). Some studies have examined the general outcome of all severities of autism and others have tended to look at the outcome in high-functioning autistic cases only.

Gillberg (1991) reported a study in which children with autism were followed up at ages 16–23 years. The study concerned cases of population-based (nonclinic) children with autism diagnosed according to DSM-III criteria. The results were similar to Lotter's (1974, 1978). Of the combined group of children with autism and autistic-like conditions (described by the authors as "other childhood psychosis"), 59% did poorly or very poorly in late adolescence and early adult life. Only 4% were indistinguishable from normal, but 11%, although still showing very odd behaviors, had made "exceptional progress." Two percent of the whole group died. Almost a third (29%) of the autism group and 43% of the "other childhood psychosis" group developed epilepsy. Onset of epilepsy in puberty was common, with grand mal and psychomotor variants the most frequent. Overall, 30% showed a temporary worsening, and 22% a permanent worsening, of symptoms at adolescence, but there was no difference in outcome between the children with classic autism and those with the autistic-like conditions.

Deterioration in adolescence, manifested as hyperactivity, aggressiveness, self-destructiveness, and a return to the need for strict routines as seen in the preschool years, was often associated with the onset of epilepsy. The findings regarding epilepsy are similar to the results of Rutter et al.'s paper (1970b). However, they differ from the results of a population-based study by Olsson, Steffenberg, and Gillberg (1988) and one large-scale clinical referral study by Volkmar, Cohen, Hoshino, Rende, and Paul (1988), which both reported an increase of new epilepsy cases in early childhood rather than in adolescence.

Volkmar et al.'s (1988) study involved 165 children meeting Rutter's (1978a) criteria for autism, who were selected from referrals for assessment of possible autism. Every child completed a psychiatric and neurological examination, as well as neurological and psychological testing. The children were reviewed at ages 4.5 years to 25.5 years. At follow-up, 51.4% of individuals with early-onset (< 24 months) and 15.8% with late-onset (> 24 months) autism remained mute. In 17.6% cases of early-onset and 15.8% of late-onset autism, the subjects had developed epilepsy. Moreover, 38.2% of those with early onset and 47.4% with late-onset autism were in residential placements.

Venter, Lord, and Schopler (1992[v]) followed up 58 high-functioning autistic children over an 8-year period. They found that initial IQ, presence of communicative speech prior to 5 years, and the amount of deviant speech predicted good later adaptation. Initial verbal intelligence predicted 51% of the variance of this score. Early nonverbal intelligence and speech before 5 years significantly predicted academic attainment, including reading. Of those with an IQ greater than 70, 80% had a reading age of 8 years or more. This compared with a figure of 50% in the Bartak and Rutter study (1976). The authors suggest that improvements in the availability of educational resources for these individuals explain the different findings in the two studies.

Autism is on a spectrum of severity and is highly disabling, especially in terms of social relationships. It is one of the least prevalent conditions seen in child mental health services, but because of the degree of disability and the implications for the family, it often demands considerable resources. The outcome of autism is poor. There is deterioration in 50% of adolescents, some of which can be attributed to onset of seizures. However, 30% show some improvement in behavior and functioning. The outcome is best for the children with later onset of autism (> 24 months), those with higher general intelligence (IQ over 60), and intelligible speech by the age of 5 years.

Treatment

Treatment needs are best assessed by a multidisciplinary team. Assessment should include a detailed history of the neonatal period and early development. Descriptions of social and language difficulties, and of any repetitive or ritualistic behavior, need to be carefully recorded. Observation of the child with parents and siblings, engaged in both free and directed play, is required. A physical examination should be completed and should include a search for any features of tuberous sclerosis in addition to a neurological examination. Psychological testing of intellectual ability is essential. It is also important to gather information from other sources such as the nursery school teacher. Once the child's needs have been comprehensively assessed, a treatment plan should be devised. Gillberg (1990b[vi]) has suggested that three main areas should be included: a full diagnostic evaluation, provision of special educational, and a home-based treatment program including family support, behavioral management, and drug treatment where indicated. Rutter (1985b[vi]) suggested that treatment should be planned according to the child's needs in the following areas:

- *Promotion of normal development,* which necessitates focusing on cognitive, language, and social skills.
- *Reduction of rigidity/stereotypy.* Rutter emphasizes that it may not be possible to achieve a complete resolution of these behaviors. This reduction is more likely to be achieved by gradual adjustment.
- *Elimination of nonspecific maladaptive behaviors (e.g., overactivity, aggression, sleep disturbance).* This necessitates an understanding of the precipitants of such behaviors, which is best achieved by way of a functional analysis.
- *Alleviation of family distress,* which should include practical support in addition to teaching problem-solving skills.

Physical Therapies

Physical treatments have a relatively small part to play in the management of autism. There are no curative agents. Physical treatments are usually prescribed following attempts to rectify problems with behavioral approaches. Indications include aggressive outbursts/temper tantrums, overactivity, self-injurious behaviors, stereotypies, obsessive–compulsive behaviors, depression, and epilepsy. The problematic behavior is likely to vary with age, so that tantrums are frequent in the younger child but depression is more likely to occur in adolescent autistic individuals.

MEGAVITAMIN THERAPY

Several studies have found a small but insignificant, nonspecific benefit from megavitamin therapy, especially vitamin B_6. The mechanism of action is unknown (Gillberg, 1990b[vi]).

NEUROLEPTICS

Campbell et al. (1978[i]) were the first to report a double-blind trial demonstrating the beneficial effects of haloperidol on difficult behaviors in autism.

Anderson et al. (1984[i]) subsequently reported a placebo-controlled double-blind study of the use of haloperidol in 41 autistic children aged between 2.3 and 6.9 years. These authors found that haloperidol produced a significant decrease in unwanted behaviors, including hyperactivity, irritability, stereotypies, and preoccupations. These behaviors decreased in both the classroom and naturalistic settings. There was a trend toward an improvement in learning. There were no significant side effects at doses of 0.5–3 mg/day.

Locascio et al. (1991[i]) analyzed the data on 125 autistic children from the Anderson and Campbell studies to pinpoint the variables that predicted a positive response to haloperidol. This reanalysis confirmed the therapeutic effectiveness of haloperidol as compared with placebo. Higher intelligence predicted a better response, although it also predicted a positive placebo response. The older the child, the better the response to haloperidol. Haloperidol decreased both anger and noncompliance, as well as some of the primary autistic behaviors and language.

Campbell, Schopler, Cueva, and Hallin (1996[ib]) have reviewed the drug treatment of autistic children. Haloperidol is the only agent consistently reported to be effective, but it has major side effects such as tardive dyskinesia.

NALTREXONE

Naltrexone is a possible choice of medication in this group of children because of its relative safety, although it is difficult to administer because of its bitter taste. It is an opiate antagonist, and its effectiveness is thought to be mediated via the opiate system thought by some to underlie some of the maladaptive behaviors and cognitive deviances seen in children with autism. Campbell (1993[i]) reported an excellent double-blind placebo-controlled study of relatively large sample size for this group of children ($n = 41$). The children, ages 2.9–7.8 years, were all hospitalized for the trial. The authors found that naltrexone significantly decreased hyperactivity but did not reduce the core symptoms of autism. It had no effect on learning. Side effects were transient nausea and vomiting and drowsiness. There was no significant weight loss, although as the treatment period was only 3 weeks, it may have been too short to produce any detectable changes (Gonzalez et al., 1994[ii]). The authors did not observe a reduction in self-injurious behavior, in contrast to earlier studies, although they point out that these early studies were all of small sample size ($n = 1$–4). The authors used a dose of 1 mg/kg/day, which may be at the low end of the therapeutic range. Campbell, Anderson, Small, Locascio, Lynch, and Choroco (1990[ib]) reported that increasing age improved the efficacy of naltrexone relative to placebo.

Kolmen, Feldman, Handen, and Janosky (1995[i], 1997[i]) reported a randomized placebo-controlled double-blind study of the use of naltrexone in autistic children. Their sample ($n = 24$) showed a statistically significant behavioral response to naltrexone. The symptoms demonstrated to improve were hyperactivity and disruptive behavior. Of the 24 subjects, 11 showed this positive response, based on parent, teacher, and laboratory-standardized measures. As with the Campbell et al. study, no improvement in learning was associated with naltrexone use in the short term.

TRICYCLIC ANTIDEPRESSANTS

A study by Gordon, State, Nelson, Hamburger, and Rapoport (1993[i]) reported a 12-week double-blind comparison of desipramine, clomipramine, and placebo in autistic disorder. The total sample comprised 24 autistic children and adolescents. Twelve were compared with placebo and 12 were in a clomipramine/desipramine comparison. Clomipramine was superior to placebo in reducing autistic withdrawal and preoccupations, hyperactivity, and oppositionality. Desipramine was significantly less effective than clomipramine. The maximum dose of clomipramine given was 250 mg/day. We are unaware of any other studies of tricyclic antidepressant use with autistic individuals. Electrocardiographic monitoring is required. It is also important to ask about seizures and to warn parents that clomipramine lowers the seizure threshold. In the Gordon et al. study (1993[i]), one child had a seizure and clomipramine was withdrawn. Apart from the risk of seizures and arrhythmias, clomipramine is a safe treatment. Further studies are required to confirm its efficacy in the treatment of autism, however.

PSYCHOSTIMULANTS

For autistic children with comorbid hyperactivity and short attention span, the psychostimulants constitute a promising treatment (Quintana, Birmaher, & Stedge, 1995[i]), although to date there has only been one randomized controlled study with a sample of only 10 children. The children taking the stimulant medication showed a significant reduction of hyperactive behavior but no increase in stereotypies or other autistic behaviors. In addition, a fairly recent open study (Birmaher et al., 1988[ii]) of stimulant use in nine autistic children reported significant improvement in target behaviors without significant side effects. This finding contradicts earlier recommendations that psychostimulants should be avoided in these children because of the risk of increasing stereotypic behaviors (Aman, 1982[vi]).

FENFLURAMINE

Several studies have reported raised serum levels of serotonin in the blood of autistic individuals (Campbell et al., 1975; Ritvo et al., 1971[i]). Fenfluramine has antiserotonergic properties. It was first found to be beneficial in autistic individuals in 1983 (Ritvo, Freeman, Geller, & Yuwiler, 1983[i]). This study reported a placebo-controlled crossover trial in 14 autistic patients ages 2–18 years. However its authors then reported less favorable results in a multicenter study (Ritvo et al., 1986[i]). Other authors (Campbell et al., 1988[i]; Leventhal et al., 1993[i]; Stern, Walker, Sawyer, Oades, & Badcock, 1990[i]) failed to find a significant benefit of fenfluramine as compared with placebo. It is therefore not a recommended treatment for autism.

OTHER POSSIBILITIES

One randomized controlled study (Fankhauser et al., 1992[i]) of nine subjects, seven of whom were children, has reported that transdermal clonidine was significantly preferable to placebo in reducing hyperarousal responses such as noise hypersensitivity, angry outbursts, and repetitive behaviors. There was also reported to be an improvement in social relations. Unfortunately, a second randomized controlled study of the use of clonidine in eight boys (Jaselskis, Cook, Fletcher, & Leventhal, 1992[i]) failed to confirm any benefits over placebo. Moreover, medication with clonidine requires monitoring of the cardiovascular system. There have been a few reports of small samples of children given fluoxetine or lithium, but as there have been no double-blind studies, these should be given as a last resort.

AUDITORY INTEGRATION TRAINING

Auditory integration training as a treatment for autistic children has received a considerable amount of media coverage in the last decade. The treatment focuses on reducing the hypersensitivity to sound, which distresses possibly as many as 40% of autistic individuals. Rimland and Edelson (1995[i]) have reported their randomized controlled study of 17 autistic children ages 4–17 years. These children were paired and matched as closely as possible. After the degree of hypersensitivity was assessed, the treatment consisted of 10 hours of listening to electronically modulated music through the headphones of an Ears Education and Retraining System (EERS). The music was filtered, and the individual listened for two 30-minute sessions each day for 10 days. The experimental subjects significantly improved in terms of behavior and comprehension, despite a failure to reduce sound sensitivity. As this was a pilot study of a small sample, it is not possible at this time to draw conclusions apart from suggesting that there be further studies on larger samples.

SECRETIN

Recently there have been claims of "miracle cures" via a hormone called secretin. Secretin is a 27-amino-acid water-soluble peptide. It is not known how secretin accesses the brain, or whether it does, in fact, work at all. Indeed, to date the findings from studies have been disappointing. In addition, there have recently been reports of adverse reactions, including increased withdrawal and loss of skills. A recent suggestion (Connors & Crowell, 1999) is that cysteine hydrochloride, which is used to stabilize secretin, may be the component leading to behavioral improvement in a few cases. This is a sulphur-containing amino acid obtained from the diet. The authors suggest that one vial of secretin doubles the plasma concentration of cysteine in a preschool child. Cysteine is thought to have a narcotic-like action on brain opioid receptors. The authors recommend developing a cysteine-containing placebo for comparison with secretin.

SUMMARY

In summary, physical treatments are sometimes required if behavioral therapies are insufficient. However, only a small number of drugs have so far been found to be effective in double-blind studies. Psychostimulants are promising drugs for hyperactivity in children with pervasive developmental disorders, and there is an insignificant risk of serious adverse reactions. Haloperidol may reduce aggression, hyperactivity, and preoccupations, but there is a risk of tardive dyskinesias and other side effects. Naltrexone is a safe, bitter-tasting drug that has been reported in two controlled studies to improve hyperactivity and disruptive behavior, although there is no conclusive evidence that its use results in a reduction of self-injurious behavior, despite case studies supporting its use for this reason. In one controlled study, clomipramine was superior to placebo in reducing autistic withdrawal, preoccupations, hyperactivity, and oppositionality, and it was certainly more effective than desipramine. Many more studies of the use of medication in autism are required.

Behavioral Therapies

INDIVIDUAL

There is no cure for autism, or for the other PDDs. However, intensive, structured behavioral programs have had beneficial effects on some of the behavioral manifestations, such as tantrums, aggression, and sleep problems. The need for these interventions is likely to be long-term.

Thorough assessment of the antecedents and consequences of the child's problem behavior is required to plan a behavioral approach. Gillberg (1990b[vi]) comments that in most cases interventions should be personalized to the child's particular symptoms. He also emphasizes that families should be made aware that there is no cure for autism. Probably the most informative study of behavioral interventions with autistic children is that by Howlin and Rutter (1987[i]), which describes a detailed long-term case control study of the benefits of a home-based treatment program. This study compared the response to behavioral interventions of 16-high functioning autistic boys with a mean age of 6 years at commencement of treatment, to the outcome of 14 short-term and 16 long-term controls. The treatment consisted of behavioral modifications, encouragement of language skill development, and psychological support for the family. The authors showed that the treatment made a significant difference in the field of social competence, use of language, and behavior problems in the 6-month period of treatment, but less so by the 18-month follow-up. IQ was not affected. However, Gillberg (1990a[ib]) in his review, points out that these children were at the higher end of functioning in autistic children, with none of them having epilepsy or any other diagnosed medical condition. There were no significant sensory deficits and none of the children had an IQ of less than 60. In addition, most of the boys came from the higher social classes.

Wolfberg and Schuler (1993[iib]) have reported a study on the application of integrated play groups in a school setting and its impact on the play behavior of three children with autism. The treatment lasted 7 months, and a semistructured interview was conducted with the parent of each child and the special education teacher who facilitated the play groups to determine whether changes generalized to other settings such as the family home. Pre- and posttreatment samples of solitary play were videotaped for analysis of the proportion of diversity versus stereotyped play. Three separate play groups were established; each play group included two children with autism and two nondisabled children. From each play group, one male with autism with an average age of 7 years was targeted as the primary participant. The play groups were observed for half an hour, twice a week, and all sessions were videotaped. Interrater reliability was satisfactory, and the results showed that although during the baseline assessment all participants spent most of their time in stereotyped nonfunctional object manipulations, following the intervention the amount of functional and/or symbolic play doubled with all participants during all phases of treatment. In addition, although all participants spent approximately 50% of their time in isolated activities during the baseline assessment, their participation in common focused play more than doubled during the final treatment stage. The authors surmised that the integrated play groups were effective in enhancing play, though they were unable to say which aspect of the play groups achieved the benefit. This intervention has promise for improving the social skills of autistic children, but further studies are required to confirm these results.

Several authors have shown that behavioral treatment improves language and social skills while decreasing aggression (DeMyer et al., 1972[vi]; Newsom & Rincover, 1989; Rutter, 1985b[vi]). A randomized controlled trial by Lovaas (1987[i]) provided behavioral treatment to an experimental group of 19 children under 4 years of age with autism. The allocation was randomized, in that allocation to a treatment group was made for each of the alternating referrals to the unit. Treatment consisted of 40 hours or more per week of one-to-one behavioral treatment for 2 or more years, plus parent training. The control group also comprised 19 children, who received 10 hours a week of one-to-one behavioral treatment in their homes, in addition to a variety of other treatments such as parent training or special education classes. The children were followed up at a mean age of 7 years. It was found that subjects in the experimental group had gained an average of 20 IQ points and had progressed in their education. Nine of the 19 subjects were, in fact, in normal classes and had an average IQ. Only 1 control subject reached normal levels of IQ and educational functioning.

McEachin, Smith, and Lovaas (1993[i]) followed up the Lovaas sample at age 13 for the subjects and at age 10 for the controls. All children who had achieved normal functioning by the age of 7 years had ended treatment at that point. Outcome was assessed "blind" by a psychologist who was not associated with the study. At this later follow-up, the proportion of experimental subjects in regular classes was 47%, which was the same proportion as at age 7. In the control group, none of the 19 children was in a regular class, which again was unchanged from the position at age 7. The experimental group at follow-up had a significantly higher mean IQ than the control group ($p < .01$). In the experimental group, 58% obtained full-scale IQs of at least 80, as compared with only 17% in the control group.

In the McEachin study the experimental group consistently scored higher on the Vineland tests assessing communication, daily living, and socialization. The mean score in the treatment group was 72, compared with 48 in the control group and 100 in the general population. Maladaptive behavior was significantly higher in the control group ($p < .05$) than in the experimental group. This study showed that the children reported by Lovaas (1987 [i]) had maintained their level of intellectual functioning from their previous assessment at age 7 up to their current assessment at the mean age of 13. Their mean IQ was about 30 points higher than that of the control subjects; indeed, 42% of the experimental group made major and enduring gains in IQ, as compared with none of the control group subjects. In addition, the experimental subjects displayed significantly higher levels of functioning than controls on measures of adaptive behavior and personality. However, this study has been criticized because allocation to experimental or control groups was based on therapists' availability rather than the usual randomization techniques. Other authors have suggested that the technique used here was essentially randomized (Baer, 1993[vi]). What is clear is that the findings are extremely promising and require urgent replication, particularly as Rutter (1985b[vi]) found that only 1 of 64 autistic children improved without treatment.

The Lovaas and McEachin findings strongly suggest that behavioral treatments are beneficial, although longer-term outcome studies are required. It is also vital to know whether similar benefits can be obtained from a reduced amount of input. It is highly unlikely that resources would ever be sufficient to allow 40 hours input per week for any child seen in routine clinical practice. In an attempt to address this question, Anderson et al. (1987[i]) reported an open study of 14 children under the age of 5 years. The intervention comprised (1) 15–25 hours of individual training to address individually assessed deficits such as those of self-care, language, play, behavior, and socialization, and (2) parent training for 15–25 hours per week. This latter element meant that the parent joined the therapist during his or her input with the child for at least 50% of the time that the therapist was in the home, as well as receiving at least 10 hours of training at other times, some of which included general parenting skills. There was a statistically significant increase in the children's mental age and social maturity scores as measured by the Vineland scales. There was also a significant increase in the parents' abilities to "correctly use behavioral teaching techniques." Although the results were promising, there was less of an improvement than the Lovaas study reported, especially in terms of normalization of intelligence and the ability to be taught in a mainstream classroom. Whether this difference in response was due to the number of therapy hours or differences in sample selection is not clear at this stage. Unfortunately, there was no control group, so it is not possible to be certain that the improvements were due to the treatment package.

A community-based study by Birnbrauer and Leach (1993[ib]) also set out to replicate the Lovaas findings. The fact that this study was based in the community is a point in its favor. However, unfortunately, there were two serious methodological problems: The sample size was only 9 children and there was no statistical analysis permitting comparison between the treatment and control conditions.

Although further studies are required, there is fairly good evidence that behavioral interventions in the home and school setting lead to significant gains in autistic individuals. The studies have tended to focus on children under the age of 4 years at the time of commencing treatment. The improvements shown by these studies include persisting gains in IQ, daily living skills, communication, and the ability to socialize, as well as a reduction in behavior problems.

PARENT TRAINING

All the studies of behavioral interventions with autistic children have included a parent training approach. At this point, it is not possible to comment on the extent to which any improvement can be attributed to this intervention. Nevertheless, it is highly probable that the parent training component is a crucial part of the behavioral programs. Rutter (1985b[vi]) emphasized the importance of enlisting parents as co-therapists, helping them to learn problem-solving skills so that they are more able to deal appropriately with future as well as current behavioral problems.

SIBLING TRAINING

Several case reports (Celiberti & Harris, 1993[iib]) have described the successful training of siblings of autistic probands, enabling them to elicit play and speech by prompting their autistic sibling when there was no initial response and praising play behaviors. This is an interesting area for further research and could be incorporated into a behavioral parent training program.

SOCIAL SKILLS TRAINING

Despite a variety of approaches, there is no good evidence that individual social skills training significantly benefits autistic individuals (Campbell et al., 1996[ib]; Matson & Swiezy, 1994). More recent interventions have tried a group approach. One such group approach has been the use of integrated play groups (Wolfberg & Schuler, 1993[iib]). This study was described in the section on behavioral therapies. There were only three autistic subjects. Symbolic play increased and was accompanied by gains in language. Improvements in both these areas generalized to settings outside the play group. In a similar study, Kohler et al. (1995[iib]) obtained similar results with three autistic preschool children. This is a promising finding, but, obviously, further larger controlled studies are required before definite conclusions can be drawn.

This approach of integrating autistic children with nondisabled subjects has been extended to older subjects but with less impressive results. For example, Schleien, Mustonen, and Rynders (1995[iii]) reported the inclusion of 15 autistic students ages 4–11 years in an integrated art program. Nondisabled peers were taught ways of interacting with autistic subjects in order to involve them in a variety of activities. However, although the nondisabled peers increased the frequency of social approaches during the intervention, this was not reciprocated by the autistic subjects.

Another group approach that has been tried is teaching "theory of mind," which is the ability to infer the mental states of others. It has been reported that 80% of autistic children are unable to predict the beliefs of others (Baron-Cohen, Leslie, & Frith, 1986[vi]). A study by Ozonoff and Miller (1995[ii]) incorporated teaching theory of mind to nine autistic male adolescents with IQs above 70. Five received the treatment, and four became the no-treatment controls. The social skills group consisted of weekly 90-minute sessions. Although subjects were more likely to be more successful with false-belief tasks than controls, social competence as observed by teachers and parents did not improve significantly. It is possible that despite a well-designed methodology, the small sample size and relatively brief duration of therapy led to insufficient evidence of benefit. Nevertheless, at present there is insufficient empirical evidence to support the belief that social skills training is beneficial in autistic individuals.

Humanistic and Counseling Approaches

Rutter (1985b[vi]) emphasizes the importance of family support and counseling, especially the fostering of problem-solving skills. In addition, many parents find additional input from a parent support group useful. An autistic child places great strain on a family. The local social services special needs team should be involved to help support the family, including the provision of respite care, financial support for the care of the child, and so forth.

Although there have been no evaluative studies of various specialized treatments, several such treatments are currently available. One of the most controversial of these is holding therapy (Richer & Zappella, 1989[ii]; Wimpory & Cochrane, 1991[ii]). This approach consists of a course of approximately half-hour sessions, with the child being held regardless of whether it comforts or distresses the child. These treatments cannot be recommended at this point because of the lack of reliable data regarding their effectiveness.

Educational Approaches

Lord and Rutter (1994[ib]) have reviewed the school programs that have been used to encourage satisfactory vocational behaviors such as task completion and self-management. Mesibov (1986[vi]) and Dunlap, Koegel, Johnson, and O'Neill (1987[vi]) have described these. Lord and Rutter (1994) conclude that substantial improvements in education for autistic children and adolescents over the last half-century have resulted from the recognition that these individuals respond best to a well-structured environment where the individual needs of each child are considered (Harris, Handleman, Kristoff, Bass, & Gordon, 1990[vi]). In practice, this means that children with autism require special needs education. There is considerable debate on the possibility of incorporating the resources available in special schools into the mainstream setting, so that the child's needs are adequately understood and his or her potential maximized. It is important that the assessment, and hence the allocation, of appropriate educational resources is completed while the child is less than 5 years old so that he or she is not faced with the additional disadvantage of either no place or an inappropriate placement at the time of official school entry. Where possible, these extra resources should be made available in the nursery placement. The reason is that in addition to the obvious advantages of providing specialist input for the child, there is the benefit of the nursery school's providing useful information about the child's needs when planning the school placement.

Several case studies (Ingenmey & Van Houten, 1991[iib]; Matson, Sevin, Box, & Francis, 1993[iib]; Matson, Sevin, Fridley, & Love, 1990[iib]) have reported that spontaneous verbalizations can be increased using either time-delay or visual cue prompting—for example, through the use of colored cards. Another approach to further the development of autistic children involves using computers to improve reading and communication skills. A recent small, but interesting, study (Heimann, Nelson, Tjus, & Gillberg, 1995[iii]) compared autistic children ($n = 11$) with normal preschoolers and children with mixed disabilities. This study used a multimedia program known as Alpha Interactive Language Series, which involves the animation of nouns and verbs. In addition, the teacher provides a warm, responsive atmosphere aimed at guiding the child through the learning tasks. This program was previously reported to lead to improvement in reading abilities. The program consisted of 112 lessons. The authors reported that all three groups of children made progress. The children with autism increased their reading scores by 11% during the training period. They also showed significant improvements in language, with a 16% gain in phonological skills. However, these results should be interpreted with caution, as there was no control group and the sample was selected on the grounds of their willingness to learn. It is therefore impossible to comment on how the benefits reported here would generalize to less able autistic children.

Schopler, Mesibov, and Hearsey (1995[vi]) have described the TEACCH (Treatment and Education of Autistic and Related Communication Handicapped Children) system of education developed at the University of North Carolina. This system emphasizes the importance of parent–professional collaboration. Assessments involve the use of standardized instruments, leading to interventions aimed at improving both "individual skills" and "environmental adaptations to autism-related deficits." The interventions use cognitive and behavioral strategies developed for autism, and visual teaching tools are available to compensate for the difficulties with auditory processing. This approach requires further evaluation by way of double-blind studies.

NONAUTISTIC PERVASIVE DEVELOPMENTAL DISORDERS

Atypical Autism or Pervasive Developmental Disorder, Not Otherwise Specified

There has been little research into atypical autism or pervasive developmental disorder, not otherwise specified (PDD-NOS); consequently, it is poorly defined. It should refer to children with autistic features, but with better cognitive and communicative skills and some degree of relatedness.

The epidemiology of the nonautistic PDDs is less clear than that of autism (Klin & Volkmar, 1995). Ironically, it appears that the prevalence of atypical autism or PDD-NOS is higher than that of so-called typical autism. The treatments are as described for autism.

Asperger's Disorder

Asperger's disorder was first described by Hans Asperger (1944). There was not much awareness of this disorder until Wing's case series was published in 1981. For this reason, there is little information on effective treatments.

Definition

The same kind of qualitative abnormalities of reciprocal social interaction and stereotyped, repetitive repertoires of interests that typify autism characterize this condition. The essential difference is the history of appropriate development of language and cognition. Although most individuals are of normal intelligence, they are often markedly clumsy. The current use of the term *Asperger's disorder* varies considerably. The DSM-IV classification system makes it clear that the diagnosis should not be made if the child meets the criteria for autism. ICD-10, however, is less clear about the difference between the two disorders. Kugler (1998) sought to clarify the demarcation between Asperger's disorder and autism but concluded that "the paucity of reliable research findings allows few definitive conclusions to be drawn . . . a greater understanding of the behavioral heterogeneities within autistic spectrum or pervasive developmental disorders is crucial to improving clinical practice and research" (p. 11). Nearly all the studies comparing high-functioning autism and Asperger's disorder have been poorly controlled. The suggested differences between the two disorders require further clarification.

Prevalence

The prevalence of Asperger's disorder is probably similar to that of autism (Gillberg & Gillberg, 1989). Ehlers and Gillberg (1989) reported a study that was carried out in Göteborg, Sweden. The authors' population sample consisted of all children ages 7–16 years residing in a Göteborg borough. This target population consisted of 1,519 children. The questionnaire was developed between the authors and Wing of the MRC Social Psychiatry Unit of the Institute of Psychiatry in London. Test/retest reliability and interrater reliability were satisfactory. Teachers and parents were interviewed, and the children were directly observed. In addition, some children completed a neuropsychiatric examination. Final case selection based on clinical work showed a minimum prevalence of 3.6 per 1,000 with a male to female ratio of 4:1, including suspected and possible cases of Asperger's disorder. The prevalence rose to 7.1 per 1,000 children, and the male to female ratio dropped to 2.3:1; that is, 0.9% of all boys and 0.44% of all girls. ICD-10 criteria were used as much as possible, but the authors discuss the difficulty of adhering to this practice totally because it requires a retrospective history of onset of language delay in order to distinguish Asperger's disorder from both atypical and typical autism.

A methodologically less robust study by Gillberg and Gillberg (1989) concluded that the prevalence in 7- to 16-year-olds appears to be in the range of 8–11 per 10,000 children. Unfortunately, this study does not discuss the reliability or validity of the questionnaire used, and half of the children who may have had possible Asperger's disorder were not seen by a clinician, and the teachers and parents were not directly interviewed. The reliability of these results is therefore unknown. Further studies of the epidemiology of Asperger's disorder are required.

Clinical Presentation

Children and adolescents with Asperger's disorder present with normal intelligence but with social and behavioral characteristics that make it difficult for them to join in with their peers. The youngster and/or caregivers may complain about the child's motor delay and clumsiness, which occurs more frequently than language delay. Boys are much more frequently affected than girls. On meeting the young person, one is struck by the pedantic, monotonic speech and the paucity of empathy. Parents and teachers, and sometimes the child, complain about the limited ability to make friends. Parents and teachers also report intense preoccupation with circumscribed interests, which appear eccentric. Although most children with Asperger's disorder have normal intelligence, a few are mildly retarded and there may be specific learning difficulties (Klin, 1994; Ozonoff, Rogers, & Pennington, 1991).

Comorbidity in Asperger's disorder has best been described in Szatmari's (1991[vi]) review of the disorder. He suggests that there can often be an attention deficit, which may respond to stimulant treatment. Anxiety symptoms, including generalized anxiety and isolated phobias, may be present. Low self-esteem is common in adolescence and may be accompanied by depressive symptoms. Szatmari reported an increased risk of a major depressive illness developing in adolescents with Asperger's disorder, as compared with the normal adolescent population. Specific learning difficulties, particularly those affecting language comprehension and fine motor coordination, are usually present. Szatmari also reports that occasionally the child with Asperger's disorder develops severely antisocial behavior or bizarre sexual interests.

There are few outcome studies of this disorder. In a much earlier study, however, Wolff (1961) followed up 20 children with Asperger's disorder and found that the diagnosis was stable over time and that impairments in socialization and communication persisted over a number of years. Szatmari (1991[vi]), Gillberg and Steffenberg (1987), and Tantum (1988) have reported that children with Asperger's disorder are less impaired than autistic children with equivalent IQ at follow-up and spend less time in special education classes. Many of those with normal intelligence achieve well at school and have good careers. Some even marry. However, they quite often develop symptoms such as anxiety or depression in adolescence or develop features of a schizotypal personality disorder such as paranoid ideation. Schizotypal personality disorder can be very difficult to distinguish from Asperger's disorder. Szatmari (1991[vi]) helpfully suggests that obtaining a description of the developmental course of the problems is useful. He suggests that children with Asperger's disorder tend to be symptomatic when they are younger and improve to some degree during later childhood and adolescence, whereas individuals with schizotypal disorder tend to have fewer PDD symptoms earlier on. Further studies of the natural history of Asperger's disorder are required.

Treatment

Szatmari (1991[vi]) reviewed the treatment of Asperger's disorder and found that there were no controlled studies of effective treatment strategies for children with this disorder. However, Szatmari emphasized the importance of assessment, looking at the strengths of the child. In addition, education of parents and teachers about the disorder and how it differs from autism may be useful. The author suggests that improved understanding of the disorder will lead to greater acceptance of unusual behaviors. As with the study by Wolfberg and Schuler (1993[iib]) promoting social and cognitive play in children with autism, Szatmari suggests that early identification of these children and intervention aid the child's development of appropriate socialization and communication skills. Szatmari further states that clinical experience suggests that speech and language intervention are also beneficial. Social skills training may be helpful, and family therapy may be indicated where the family is overcritical toward the child. All these interventions require evaluating. There have not been sufficient studies to make any definite recommendations about treatment needs in this group of children.

Rett's Disorder

Definition

Rett's disorder is an extremely disabling condition that usually requires joint management by pediatrics and child mental health services for children with learning difficulties. Typically, a history of normal or near normal development precedes the recognition of the disorder. Autistic-like behaviors are described in the preschool years, but Rett's disorder differs from autism in certain ways. It has been described only in girls. It is characterized by stereotypic motor movements such as hand washing and wringing. Breath-holding attacks, hyperventilation, and seizures are frequent. Mental retardation is even greater than occurs in autism. Normal development and growth in the first few months is followed by developmental regression and slowing of head growth, in addition to loss of purposeful hand movements. Social and play development cease in the first 2 or 3 years, although the child remains interested in others. During middle childhood, trunk ataxia choreoathetoid movements and epileptic seizures frequently develop.

Prevalence

There has been only one study of the prevalence of Rett's disorder (Kerr & Stephenson, 1985; Trevathan & Adams, 1988). In this study the incidence of Rett's disorder in the west of Scotland was assessed by reviewing the case records and making clinical assessments of all the referrals in the area. The incidence of Rett's disorder was found to be 1 case in 30,000 live births (1 in 15,000 girls).

Treatment

Treatment of Rett's disorder has been reviewed by Perry (1991[vi]). Generally, much of the intervention with this disorder is medical, aimed at controlling seizures (Coleman, Brubaker, Hunter, & Smith, 1988[iib]; Phillipart, 1986[iib]; Trevathan & Naidu, 1988[iib]). Several authors have reported the use of behavior therapy, particularly for self-injurious behavior (Iwata, Pace, & Willis, 1986[iib]; Kerr, 1986[iib]). However, so far behavior therapy has not appeared to produce much benefit and has not been systematically evaluated. Perry (1991[vi]) remarks in his paper that music therapy has been reported to be beneficial by some authors, but it has not been systematically evaluated.

Childhood Disintegrative Disorder

Definition

In 1930 there was a report in the literature of six children who had developed normally until the age of 3–4 years and who subsequently showed developmental and behavioral regression, which recovered only to a small degree. Usually the child has learned to speak in sentences before skills are lost. Behavior then closely resembles autism, but the outcome is even worse. In only a minority of cases is an underlying neurological cause found (Volkmar, 1996b). The essential aspect of the diagnosis is apparently normal development until the age of 2 years, followed by a definite loss of previously acquired skills, with additional impairments of social functioning. This definition includes the diagnoses of dementia infantilis, disintegrative psychosis, Heller's syndrome, and symbiotic psychosis.

Prevalence

The prevalence of childhood disintegrative disorder is currently unknown. Only one study has attempted to estimate the prevalence of the disintegrative disorders in clinic-referred cases of suspected autism. In this study (Volkmar et al., 1988) 165 children were selected from referrals for assessment of possible autism. Every child completed a psychiatric and neurological examination, as well as neurological and psychological testing. Ten of the children had disintegrative disorder at follow-up (onset after a period of at least 2 years of normal development). The age of regression in these cases was between 24 and 42 months. Six (60%) of the children with disintegrative disorder had severe learning difficulties, 3 had moderate learning difficulties, and 1 had profound learning difficulties. These children exhibited a large range of behavior problems, with marked stereotypy, self-injurious behaviors, agitation, aggression, fecal smearing, and so on.

Natural History

There have been few empirical studies of the outcome of disintegrative disorders, but anecdotal evidence suggests that it is extremely poor. Volkmar et al.'s study (1988), however, did look at outcome. The 10 children were reviewed at ages 4.5–25.5 years. The study found that 3 children had some improvement and 7 had only limited improvement. Nine children were in a residential placement. Four remained mute at follow-up, 2 used single words, 1 used occasional two-word phrases, 2 spoke in sentences (although 1 of these did so only occasionally), and 1 retained idiosyncratic speech.

Treatment

It is not possible to make any specific recommendations about the treatments of the disintegrative psychoses as there are no published studies on the subject.

SUMMARY

Autism is on a spectrum of severity and is frequently highly disabling. Children with a higher IQ and more intelligible speech have a better outcome. There is often deterioration during adolescence, some of which can be attributed to onset of seizures. The prevalence of autism is 7 to 17 per 10,000 children. It is one of the least prevalent conditions seen in child mental health services, but often demands considerable resources because of the degree of disability in the more severely affected. Following a comprehensive assessment, a variety of treatment approaches should be considered and a plan tailored to the needs of the child and family. The interventions need to provide a behavior program at home and at school, incorporating parent and teacher training. Expected benefits include persisting gains in IQ, improvements in daily living skills, communication, and the ability to socialize, and a decrease of behavior problems. Studies have tended to focus on children under the age of 4 years at the time of commencing treatment, but it is unclear whether early commencement of treatment is a necessary condition for successful treatment. All the studies of behavioral interventions in autistic children have included a parent training approach. However, it is not yet clear whether this element increases effectiveness. There have been no systematic investigations into parent training groups. Despite a variety of approaches, there is no good evidence that individual social skills training significantly benefits autistic individuals

There is some evidence for physical treatments. Haloperidol may reduce aggression, hyperactivity, and preoccupations, but there is a risk of tardive dyskinesias. Psychostimulants are promising drugs for hyperactivity in children with pervasive developmental disorders. Naltrexone has also been reported in two controlled studies to improve hyperactivity and disruptive behavior, although there is no conclusive evidence that naltrexone treatment results in a reduction of self-injurious behavior. In one controlled study, clomipramine was superior to placebo in reducing autistic withdrawal and preoccupations, hyperactivity, and oppositionality and was certainly more effective than desipramine.

Asperger's disorder is characterized by the same kind of qualitative abnormalities of reciprocal social interaction that typify autism, as well as the presence of restricted, stereotyped, repetitive repertoires of interests. The essential difference from autism is the history of appropriate development of language and cognition. Most individuals with Asperger's disorder are of normal intelligence, but are often markedly clumsy. The prevalence of this disorder is higher than that of autism and is in the region of 0.9% of all boys and 0.4% of all girls. Comorbidity in Asperger's disorder is common, with increased rates of attention deficit problems and anxiety symptoms, including generalized anxiety and phobias, as compared with the general population. Low self-esteem is common in adolescence and may be accompanied by depressive symptoms. There may also be increased risk of a major depressive illness. Specific learning difficulties particularly affecting language comprehension and fine motor coordination are usually present. Many children with Asperger's disorder who have normal intelligence achieve well at school, have good careers, and some even marry. However, they quite often develop symptoms such as anxiety or depression in adolescence and early adulthood. A small number develop features of a schizotypal personality disorder such as paranoid ideation. There have not been sufficient studies to make any definite recommendations about treatment needs in children with Asperger's disorder, although most clinicians apply the same principles of treatment as they would in autism. Similarly, there is insufficient evidence to make specific recommendations for the treatment of disintegrative psychosis or Rett's disorder.

IMPLICATIONS

Children with PDD require careful and thorough assessment before interventions can be planned, because of the broad spectrum of presentations. Assessment is also vital to clarify the child's strengths and weaknesses for parents and professionals. The first line of intervention should be behavioral programs, which appear to be promising but are required to be individualized and intensive and are therefore demanding of resources. These behavioral programs should be designed for use in home and school settings, necessitating good communication between education providers, families, and health professionals. If behavioral therapies are insufficient, physical treatments may be required. The evidence is strongest for stimulant medication with comorbid attention-deficit/hyperactivity disorder (ADHD). There is no evidence to support the routine use of other medications.

There is great need for more studies of Asperger's disorder. It is relatively common, and yet very little is known about comorbidity, outcome, or effective interventions.

10

Self-Harming Disorders

This chapter discusses the severe eating disorders that occur in childhood and adolescence, and other behaviors that are known to be life threatening. Behaviors that cause accidental harm or harm through excessive repetition, such as alcohol, solvent, and drug misuse (but not cutting), are also included. The first section deals with the eating disorders, the second with suicide and deliberate self-harm, and the third with substance misuse.

EATING DISORDERS

Definition

DSM-IV defines the eating disorders, anorexia nervosa and bulimia nervosa, as follows:

Anorexia nervosa is characterized by deliberate refusal to maintain body weight above a level that is 15% *below* that expected for the individual's age and height. The diagnostic criteria also include intense fear of becoming fat even though underweight; severe restriction of food intake, often with excessive exercising; distorted perception of body image and shape; and cessation of menstruation in postmenarchal women. There are two subtypes of anorexia nervosa. In one there is regular binge eating or purging and self-induced vomiting or use of laxatives or diuretics; in the other—restricting—type, these behaviors are not present.

Many features of *bulimia nervosa* overlap those of anorexia: excessive concern with body shape and weight and use of extreme measures to control weight. Bulimia is characterized by recurrent episodes of binge eating with a feeling of lack of control over eating behavior during binges, and excessive dieting and exercise, with the use of large doses of appetite suppressants, laxatives, and/or diuretics in order to reduce weight. Despite this, weight tends to remain within the normal range. An average of at least two binges a week over a period of 3 months is required to make the diagnosis. Subtypes of bulimia nervosa are a purging type in which vomiting or purging occurs and a nonpurging type in which excessive fasting or exercise occurs without purging.

The biggest difference between anorexia and bulimia is that those with anorexia become excessively thin, whereas those with bulimia have roughly normal body weight. However, within DSM-IV, a primary diagnosis of bulimia nervosa is applied only in the absence of anorectic features. In DSM-IV, "partial syndromes" of eating disorder are recognized, which meet some but not all of the criteria for anorexia nervosa or bulimia nervosa. Examples may include women who meet the criteria for anorexia but have regular menses, or those in whom all the criteria for bulimia are met, but in whom the diagnostic behaviors occur less frequently than twice a week or over shorter periods than 3 months. DSM-IV also proposes a category for a binge eating disorder in which the compensatory behaviors characteristic of bulimia nervosa do not occur. Recognition of these variants presents a spectrum of eating disorders that may be different entities, but which may indicate merely differences in severity that may change over time in individual patients.

In general, ICD-10 pays more attention than DSM-IV to defining the core criteria. For example, ICD-10 includes—for anorexia—a Quatelet's Body Mass Index of 0.75 or less, along with the defining criteria for weight loss as greater than 15% below minimum normal weight for age and height. This can have clinical significance, as can the inclusion in ICD-10 of the widespread endocrine disorder that accompanies anorexia nervosa. ICD-10 places less emphasis on distorted perception of body image as a defining criterion of anorexia nervosa, and it also does not consider subtypes of the disorder. ICD-10 includes a possible history of an earlier episode of anorexia nervosa in the case of bulimia nervosa. Like DSM-IV, it includes a category for atypical bulimia nervosa.

Bryant-Waugh and Lask (1995) point out that in children below the age of 15, about 25% of referrals to their clinic in London present disturbances of eating that do not fit the existing diagnostic DSM-IV categories. The variants include selective eating, food-avoidance emotional disorder, and pervasive refusal syndrome. These authors recommend a flexible definition of childhood-onset eating disorders, for example "a disorder of childhood in which there is an excessive preoccupation with weight or shape, and/or food intake, and accompanied by grossly inadequate, irregular or chaotic food intake" (p. 191). Studies of children and adolescents have led to the suggestion that anorexia nervosa and bulimia nervosa may be different symptom patterns of one basic eating disorder, in which preoccupation with food and a disturbed body image are core symptoms (Van der Ham, Van Strien, & Van Engeland, 1994). But there are no reports of prepubertal bulimia nervosa. Until quite recently, very few cases with onset below the age of 14 have been noted (Schmidt, Hodes, & Treasure, 1992).

Twin studies indicate a genetic predisposition to anorexia nervosa. Heritability was found to be high, especially in restricting anorexia with adolescent onset, whereas it was almost nonexistent among patients with bulimia nervosa (Treasure & Holland, 1990). As in many other psychiatric disorders, significant events in an individual's life often precede manifestation of the disorder. In various studies, external precipitants of anorexia nervosa have been identified in 50–100% of cases, including separation and loss, family disruption, new environmental demands, direct threat to self-esteem, and in a small number of cases, physical illness (Garfinkel & Garner, 1982), but these precipitants are not specific to eating disorders.

Prevalence

Prevalence rates in young people for *anorexia nervosa* vary between 0 per 1,000 among schoolgirls in Japan (Suzuki, Morita, & Kamoshita, 1990) to 1% in English private schools (Crisp, Palmer, & Kalucy, 1976; Szmukler, 1983), and even 1.08% among Swedish adolescent girls below the age of 18 (Rastam & Gillberg, 1992). Rates depend on the way in which cases are ascertained and classified, the cultural context, whether both males and females are included in the study, and the age groups covered. In the Swedish study, the sample was small (25 subjects) and three cases were "partial" syndromes that did not meet strict diagnostic criteria. Fombonne (1995) calculated a median prevalence rate for the 15- to 20-year age group as 1.2 per 1,000. If three studies from Asia (where the rates are lower in general) are excluded, so that the figure relates essentially to young people in the Western developed world and Australia and New Zealand, the prevalence is 1.4 per 1,000. Fombonne was unable to find convincing evidence that rates have been increasing over the past 50 years.

Fairburn and Beglin (1990) caution that the methodology of detection may result in underestimation of the prevalence of eating disorders. Especially in younger children, the diagnosis may be missed (Bryant-Waugh, Knibbs, Fosson, Kaminski, & Lask, 1988). Including individuals with subthreshold diagnoses greatly increases the prevalence rates to between 5% and 15% (Herzog, Keller, Lavori, & Sacks, 1991). Using DSM-III classification criteria without the requirement of amenorrhea yielded higher figures.

Maloney et al. (Maloney, McGuire, Daniels, & Specker, 1989) found that among schoolchildren ages 7–12 years, 10.4% reported binge eating and 6% scored in the anorectic range on a child version of the Eating Attitudes Scale (ChEAT) (Garner & Garfinkel, 1979); 1.3% reported vomiting to control weight.

Both clinic and survey data show consistently higher rates for late adolescent girls. In adolescents and young adults, about 5–10% of cases occur in males (Barry & Lippman, 1990). In children, however, a number of studies have reported that between 19% and 30% of cases have been in boys (e.g., Bryant-Waugh, 1993; Fosson, Knibbs, Bryant-Waugh, & Lask, 1987; Higgs, Goodyer, & Birch, 1989). The distribution of childhood-onset anorexia nervosa between social classes seems similar to that in adults, with overrepresentation of higher social classes (Fosson et al., 1987; Gowers, Crisp, Joughin, & Bhat, 1991; Higgs et al., 1989), although this may be becoming less pronounced (Garfinkel & Garner, 1982). There are methodological problems with relating concepts of social class to those of eating disorder in different population samples. Only recently have there been reports of anorexia nervosa in adults or children from African, Asian, Caribbean, or Chinese populations. Most of these reports relate to children of migrant parents where an eating disorder may be linked to intrapersonal and intrafamilial conflicts related to the adoption of Western values (Bryant-Waugh & Lask, 1995).

Bulimia nervosa was first formally described in the late 1970s (Russell, 1979). Bulimia is less visible than anorexia; mental health professionals do not see substantial numbers of cases. The few community surveys using diagnostic interviews that have been carried out yield an average lifetime prevalence for bulimia nervosa of around 1% (Fairburn & Beglin, 1990; Fairburn, Jones, Peveler, Hope, & O'Connor, 1993a[ii]). Lifetime rates have been found to be much higher among younger than older women; these rates were 4.5% among women ages 16–24, 2.0% among those ages 25–44, and 0.4% among those ages 45–64 (Bushnell, Wells, Hornblow, Oakley-Browne, & Joyce, 1990). Lewinsohn et al. (1993) found a 1-year incidence rate of 0.75% for bulimia nervosa among a sample of 810 16-year-old schoolgirls. Earlier studies that used DSM-III criteria gave higher prevalences than those that use DSM-III-R because the revised version includes a minimum frequency of binge eating as well as measures to control weight.

Many other studies have been concerned with eating *disturbances* related to bulimia—that is, conditions assessed by a scalar approach, generally on the basis of self-completion questionnaires (Fombonne, 1995). Fairburn and Beglin (1990) have reviewed these studies. They point out that most research has been carried out with samples of convenience (generally college students at selected universities) and with self-report measures of doubtful diagnostic validity. The mean prevalence rate in studies using self-report questionnaires was 2.6% for bulimia nervosa, as opposed to 1% for diagnostic interview studies. One of the most striking results of self-report questionnaire studies is the high prevalence rates of symptomatic features of eating pathology. If a strict frequency criterion of "at least weekly" is retained, the mean prevalence rates across studies of binge eating, self-induced vomiting, and laxative misuse were, respectively, 15.7%, 2.4%, and 2.7%, whereas 29% of subjects on average said they were currently following a strict diet or fasting (Fairburn & Beglin, 1990).

Repeat self-report surveys in North America on large samples of first-year college students at two midwestern universities (Pyle, Halvorson, Neuman, & Mitchell, 1986) and a replication study in Cambridge in the United Kingdom (Cooper, Charnock, & Taylor, 1987) have given little evidence of an increase in a lifetime history of weekly binge or purging behavior (DSM-III bulimia). Studies of two large comparable samples of 14- to 18-year-olds, surveyed in 1981 and 1986, reported significant reductions in rates of dieting behaviors, in binge eating, and in excessive exercise, both currently and for prior attempts (Johnson, Tobin, & Lipkin, 1989). These authors also report changes in attitudes, with a significant decline in concern about weight among respondents (and among their friends and families) and a lower drive toward thinness. Average body weight and body dissatisfaction had remained constant across the period between 1981 and 1986. The authors speculated that attitudinal and behavioral changes reflected changes in the sociocultural context, such as the AIDS epidemic, the emergence of an antidieting literature, and increasing knowledge of the detrimental effects of eating disorders.

Comorbidity

A 3-year follow-up survey of 34 of 39 consecutively admitted adolescent inpatients (32 girls and 7 boys) fulfilling DSM-III-R criteria for anorexia nervosa found anxiety disorders (41%) and affective disorders (18%) to be the most prevalent comorbid psychiatric diagnoses, with a highly positive correlation between eating disorder and depressive psychopathology, as compared with healthy age-matched controls (Herpertz-Dahlmann & Remschmidt, 1993). Recovered anorectic young people also scored higher on depression scales than the controls. These authors conclude that disturbance of psychosexual adjustment seems to be a core symptom of anorexia nervosa (Hsu, 1990[vi]) and is likely to persist into early adulthood in spite of a good overall outcome. The findings after a 7-year follow-up of their cohort (Herpertz-Dahlmann, Wewetzer, & Remschmidt, 1995) suggested that severity of depressive symptoms at admission does not correlate with severity of depression at follow-up and that initial depressive psychopathology is not a valid prognostic indicator of outcome. However, at the time of follow-up, patients who had persisting disorder were also very likely to suffer from comorbid depression. In general, subjects with worse outcomes also had higher levels of general psychopathology (Herpertz-Dahlmann, Wewetzer, Schulz, & Remschmidt, 1996).

Steinhausen (1997) suggests that *comorbidity* may not be an appropriate term to describe the association of other psychiatric disorders with anorexia, because it is unclear to what extent these psychiatric disorders are actually coexistent or present as single disorders in individuals with a history of anorexia. Only 22.8% of women with bulimia were found to have no other lifetime history of psychiatric disorder, whereas more than half had a history of depressive disorder (Kendler et al., 1991).

Clinical Course and Outcome

Steinhausen, Rauss-Mason, and Seidel (1991) reviewed the literature in English and German from the 1950s to the 1980s (68 studies with follow-up period ranging from 1 to 33 years) on the outcome of eating disorders. Their summary of these studies' findings reported that in approximately 60% of patients, weight is restored. Normalization of menstruation occurs in approximately 55%. Eating behavior returns to normal in 44%. Twenty percent of patients have generally poor outcome, with chronic symptoms of eating disorder and poor psychosocial adaptation. Mortality was significant but has decreased in the last decade to less than 5%. These authors note wide variation between the studies, which often gave contradictory judgments on outcome and prognosis; for example, the range varies between 50% and 70% for the proportion of patients restored to normal weight, and between 30% and 70% for the establishment of normal eating behavior. For both anorexia and bulimia nervosa, severity when first coming to medical attention and longer duration of illness are the strongest predictors of a poor outcome in some follow-up studies, but these findings have not always been replicated in other investigations.

A more recent review by Steinhausen (1997) concentrates on 31 outcome studies of patients with adolescent or preadolescent onset of disorder. This review was largely restricted to anorexia because studies of samples solely with bulimia with onset during adolescence are scarce. Again, study designs and the quantity and quality of information regarding outcomes were variable. There was general agreement that good outcome means recovery from all the defining symptoms of anorexia nervosa, a fair outcome represents improvement with some residual symptoms, and a poor outcome describes long-term chronicity. Crude mortality rates were based on a total of 918 patients and ranged from 0% to 11% with a mean of 2.16% (SD = 2.88). Variations across studies were, to a large extent, dependent on the length of follow-up period. Full recovery was found among 52% overall, 29% showed some improvement, and 19% developed a chronic course of disorder. The outcome was slightly better for the core symptoms, with normalization of weight occurring in 68%, normalization of menstruation in 64%, and normalization of eating behavior in 52%. At outcome, a significant proportion suffered further psychiatric diagnoses: affective disorders (20.9%), neurotic disorders (26%), obsessive–compulsive disorders (12%), schizophrenia (6.5%), personality disorders (17.9%), and substance use disorders (18.9%).

Even more recently, Steinhausen et al. (Steinhausen, Seidel, & Metzke, 2000[vi]) have reported on a follow-up of 60 adolescent eating disordered patients (mean age 14.6 at onset of the disease) consecutively admitted between 1979 and 1988 to a child and adolescent psychiatric university department in Berlin, at a mean of 5 years and at a later mean of 11.5 years. Patients were in treatment for a mean of 33% of the initial follow-up period, but a mean of 17% of the entire 11-year follow-up period. No predictors of treatment duration were found. The mortality rate was 8.3% at the second follow-up. The distribution of abnormal Body Mass Index (BMI) reflected a trend of improvement with increasing duration of follow-up. In comparison with the 5-year follow-up, fewer patients suffered symptoms of the full clinical picture of an eating disorder at 11-year follow-up. Among the surviving patients, 80% recovered during the long-term course. There were few specific predictors of three outcome criteria: the BMI, eating disorders score, and a total outcome score. The BMI was significantly predicted by premorbid overweight at the first follow-up; at the second follow-up it was again predicted by premorbid overweight and by premorbid psychopathology and by noneating psychopathology in family members. A pathological eating disorders score was predicted by the duration of individual psychotherapy at the first follow-up and by the duration of outpatient treatment at the second follow-up. The total outcome score correlated significantly with duration of family therapy at the first follow-up and duration of inpatient treatment at the second follow-up.

Three studies of adolescents report findings at 4- (Van der Ham et al., 1994), 6- (Gillberg, Rastam, & Gillberg, 1994), and 7-year (Herpertz-Dahlmann et al., 1996) follow-up; there were no deaths in these studies. Of 25 anorectic and 24 bulimic adolescents (ages 12–21, average 16 years at intake), 47% had good, 43% intermediate, and 10% poor outcomes after 4 years. Eight percent of the anorectic patients became bulimic. At the 6-year follow-up, 51 young people with anorexia nervosa (mean age of onset 14.3 years) which included a total population of cases from one

birth cohort, were compared with a sex-, age-, and school-matched group of 51 subjects on various measures of outcome at 21 years (6.7 years after reported onset and
4.9 years after the original diagnostic study). There was no attrition. Forty-seven
percent of those with anorexia nervosa reported that they were recovered. In the
unrecovered group, all aspects of outcome were worse among those with anorexia
nervosa than in the matched comparison group. Differences between the two
groups were particularly pronounced with regard to aspects of social relationships.
Poor outcome was associated with the presence of empathy deficits, defined as
problems in understanding other people's perspectives and difficulties in interacting
reciprocally. The findings of this community-based study are similar to those of the
clinic-based (or otherwise potentially biased) samples surveyed in the paper by
Steinhausen et al. (1991). But the adolescents in the population-based cases were
found to be as abnormal as those who had applied for treatment in clinics, both at
the time of the original study and at the time of follow-up (Rastam, 1992). At 7-
year follow-up of 34 adolescents from an inpatient sample (Herpetz-Dahlmann,
1996), 1 patient had anorexia nervosa, 4 had bulimia nervosa, and 10 had eating
disorder not otherwise specified; these patients with persisting eating disorders
mostly suffered from restrictive symptoms. Both the recovered and unrecovered
young people with anorexia were similar to a control group of young people in
terms of occupational adjustment, social contacts, and dependency on family, but
differed significantly in psychosexual functioning, those with a worse outcome of
the eating disorder displaying higher levels of general psychopathology. The
authors of these studies caution that it does not seem advisable to regard normalization of eating behavior, weight, and menstrual pattern as sufficient criteria for defining successful treatment outcome. The persistence of core symptoms, in particular preoccupation with food and appearance and disturbed body image, may
increase the probability of relapse and chronicity and be associated with continuing
problems with social adaptation (Strober, Freeman, & Morrell, 1997b[v]).

North and Gowers (1999[vi]) have found that among 35 adolescents with anorexia nervosa, matched with psychiatric and community controls and followed up
at 1 and 2 years, those with anorexia with comorbid depression reported more abnormal cognitions as measured on the Eating Disorders Inventory (EDI) than the
other young people, but that those with comorbid anorexia nervosa had an equally
good outcome as compared with those with anorexia alone.

In a younger sample, with an average age of onset of anorexia nervosa of 11.7
years, followed up for a mean of 7.2 years, one child had died directly as a result of
the eating disorder, and the outcome was good in only 60% (Bryant-Waugh et al.,
1988). Among these 30 children, poor prognostic factors included early age at onset
(less than 11 years), depression during the illness, disturbed family life and one-par-
ent families, and those families in which one or both parents had been married before. It should be noted that these two studies among younger patients include all
levels of severity and a total population sample (Gillberg et al., 1994). In addition,
the young people had followed a variety of treatment approaches that are largely
not described.

Steinhausen (1997) has compared the studies of outcome in patients with age

of onset of anorexia below the age of 18 years, with 77 studies with older age of onset (Steinhausen, 2000), and found a slight trend for better global outcome and
normalization of core symptoms for the younger patients.

Because of the relatively low frequency of bulimic symptoms in younger patients, most of the knowledge about the prognostic relevance of these symptoms comes from studies on older patients, and there have been few studies so far. Three
studies of adolescent age of onset found that bulimia and purgative abuse were associated with poor outcome (Kreipe, Churchill, & Strauss, 1989; Martin, 1985;
Steiner, Mazer, & Litt, 1990). However, Steinhausen and Seidel (1993) found that
bulimia was not significantly related to outcome.

Treatment

In each section we will first discuss the treatment approaches for anorexia nervosa,
followed by those for bulimia nervosa. Methods and research outcomes differ significantly.

Physical Therapies

Weight restoration is the first major goal of any treatment for anorexia nervosa. In
most studies the need for refeeding and possibly bed rest is implicit in the treatment
of anorexia nervosa, but, of course, this depends on the stage at which treatment is
instituted in individual cases. This will apply to all children with a DSM-III diagnosis, which depends on a minimum of 25% weight loss. Unfortunately, beyond the
evidence that early intervention and hospitalization may be a positive prognostic
factor (especially among younger patients; see Bryant-Waugh et al., 1988), there is
a lack of solid empirical data to assist selection of the type and setting of treatment
intervention (Steinhausen & Glanville, 1983[v]). Certain clinical criteria, such as
severe emaciation (less than 70% of the average weight), are definite indications
for hospital treatment. Studies often do not report the exact treatments given during inpatient stays, and inpatient episodes indicate an intervention whose components, for the most part, cannot be distinguished or evaluated. However, inpatient
treatment does have certain specific advantages. These include the fostering of
what may otherwise be a fragile treatment alliance, greater awareness by the physician of complications and/or responses to intervention, and the possibility of using
a psychoeducational approach in which the patient's eating behavior is modified to
foster healthy attitudes to nutrition and to ensure the maintenance of an acceptable
weight. Outpatient treatment may be considered in cases where purging and vomiting are not part of the clinical picture, the family is very supportive, and the patient
is highly motivated and cooperative. However, high motivation for treatment is unusual; anorectic patients characteristically deny that they are ill and in need of
treatment. Denial of disorder and resistance to treatment suggests that motivational
interviewing techniques would be helpful (Vitousek, Watson, & Wilson, 1998[vi]).
No studies distinguish between the efficacy of physical treatment offered alone and
psychotherapeutic approaches offered alone; it is assumed that these should be

combined as appropriate in individual patients. In Britain, a combined approach usually depends on liaison work between a pediatrician and a child and adolescent psychiatrist. The need for inpatient care often depends on individual clinical judgment, the home background of the young person, and whether the local services can offer a specialist service outside a residential setting.

Eckert, Halmi, Marchi, Grove, and Crosby (1995[v]) found a high frequency and chronicity of bulimic symptoms among women with anorexia nervosa, plus a high rate of weight relapse (42% during the first year). These authors recommend intensive intervention to help anorectic patients restore and maintain their weight within a normal range and to decrease abnormal eating and weight control behaviors. In their 10- to 15-year follow-up of 12- to 17-year-olds, Strober et al. (1997b[v]) stressed that the good outcomes among this cohort (76% fully recovered) were likely to be due to intensive and early treatment at a university specialty service, including treatment during the follow-up. A pilot randomized study among 15 female and 1 male outpatients (ages 17–45 years), indicates that incorporation of a graded programme of exercise may increase compliance with treatment and does not reduce the short-term rate of gain in body fat or body mass index (Thien, Thomas, Markin, & Birmingham, 2000[i]).

Most patients with bulimia nervosa can be treated on an outpatient basis (Hsu, 1990[vi]; Mitchell et al., 1990[ii]), with less than 5% requiring inpatient care (Fairburn, Marcus, & Wilson, 1993b[vi]). No outcome studies so far have specifically examined the effectiveness of inpatient interventions with bulimic children and adolescents.

A pediatric day treatment program has been used as an alternative to full hospitalization for refeeding in anorectic patients. Danziger et al. (Danziger, Carcl, Varsono, Tyano, & Mimouni, 1988) treated 32 adolescents with anorexia nervosa in a day treatment program in which parents were actively involved. The adolescents initially attended the program from 8 A.M. to 10 P.M. As they approached their target weights, they were discharged and seen in outpatient sessions, three times a week until they reached target weight, and less often afterward. Initially, parents supervised the patients after meals for 1 hour to prevent vomiting, and between meals to prevent ritualistic exercising. Parents observed how staff handled the meals, and later supervised the meals themselves. Family and individual psychotherapy accompanied a structured behavior modification program. At an average of 9 months after admission, follow-up indicated that 84% had reached and retained their ideal weight, 89% had resumed menstruation, 59% had overcome body image distortions, and 88% had stopped ritualistic exercise. The involvement of parents was regarded as very helpful, although there were no formal measures of parental responses to the program.

In adults with bulimia, research has supported the effectiveness of day care programs, access to which often requires patients to have at least one failed outpatient experience (Maddocks, Kaplan, Woodside, Langdon, & Piran, 1992[v]). Such programs have been developed for children and adolescents with other disorders and may have great potential to help the more severely disturbed adolescent with bulimia nervosa.

Drug Therapies

Several types of medication have been used in the treatment of anorexia nervosa, both clinically and in controlled studies. These include the neuroleptics, appetite stimulants, and antidepressants. Research evidence of the efficacy of any of these drugs in adolescents with anorexia is very limited, and given their side effects, their clinical value may also be limited. There have been two placebo-controlled trials of antipsychotic medication in anorexia. Vandereycken and Pierloot (1982) reported that, among 18 female patients treated with pimozide or placebo in a crossover design study, there was a trend for greater daily weight gain with pimozide, but that patients' behavior was not significantly improved. Vandereycken (1984[i]) used a similar design in a placebo-controlled study of sulpiride which showed no advantage of this treatment over placebo in either the rate of weight gain or patients' behavior and attitude. Two controlled studies have looked at amitryptyline, finding no benefit as compared with placebo (Biederman et al., 1985; Halmi, Eckert, LaDu, & Cohen, 1986[v]). The appetite stimulant cyproheptadine (CYP) has been shown to have a differential effect on the anorectic–bulimic subgroup (Halmi et al., 1986[v]).

Morgan and Russell (1975) and Eckert et al. (1982[v]) have reported that although depression is common in anorexia nervosa, it is rarely severe and usually improves with weight gain. It may also respond to antidepressants. Some antidepressants that have been studied (amitriptyline, clomipramine, monoamine oxidase inhibitors (MAOIs), lithium, and fluoxetine) may have some effect on weight gain or improve dysphoria and depression (Pryor, McGilley, & Roach, 1990[vi]). Strober, Freeman, DeAntonio, Lampert, and Diamond (1997a[iv]) compared 33 patients with anorexia nervosa who received fluoxetine as part of their continuing treatment, with controls who had received identical inpatient and follow-up treatment but without fluoxetine. Analyses over 24 months following the inpatient episode failed to show that fluoxetine had a significant effect on the cumulative probability of remaining at target weight, the risk of sustained weight loss, or other clinical measures of outcome. Preliminary studies suggest that psychotherapy and fluoxetine together may be helpful in preventing relapse after weight restoration (Peterson & Mitchell, 1999[ib]). It is reported, however, that selective serotonin reuptake inhibitor (SSRI) medication has no effect on clinical symptoms of malnourished, underweight anorectic patients (Ferguson, La Via, Crossan, & Kaye, 1999[iv]).

Morgan and Russell (1975) and Hsu (1988[ib]) have reported that social anxiety, obsessive–compulsive features, and sexual fears are often present and may not respond to weight gain; Hsu (1986b[vi]) reports that patients with these disorders are usually treated with individual psychotherapy and no specific treatments appear to have been studied. Treatment compliance and personality variables may be important mediators of improved treatment outcome (Steiner et al., 1990).

There have been no randomized controlled trials in the treatment of bulimia nervosa with antidepressants in adolescents. The most recent review by Walsh (1999) of treatments in adults concludes that controlled trials of pharmacotherapy in anorexia nervosa are almost uniformly discouraging, but, on the other hand, that 15 controlled trials are quite consistent in documenting that antidepressant medication reduces the frequency of binge eating among normal-weight patients with bulimia nervosa. This review also reports that the limited data available suggest that there is a significant rate of relapse and of discontinuation of medication during the 6 months after the initial response. In two outpatient studies (Agras et al., 1992[i]; Mitchell et al., 1990[ii]), antidepressant drug therapy alone has been found to be less effective than cognitive-behavioral approaches with and without antidepressant medication.

Psychosocial Therapies

There are a variety of treatment approaches, but comparative studies that evaluate the effects of treatment are scarce. Currently, the main psychotherapeutic approaches used with adolescent anorectic patients are individual psychotherapy, behavior therapy, and family therapy. There is little doubt that young people with anorexia benefit from multifaceted treatment programs (Steinhausen, 1985[v]; Steinhausen & Seidel, 1992), but little work has been done to evaluate the effects of different components of treatment for different patients. The exceptions include most studies that report on behavioral methods.

INDIVIDUAL PSYCHOTHERAPY

Steinhausen (1995[vi]) cautions that most of the experience with individual psychotherapy comes from the treatment of adults, and that such therapy is unlikely to be of use in a young person with anorexia nervosa unless he or she has intact cognitions and sufficient motivation to undertake therapy. These are likely to be absent where the patient is emaciated, when severe depression is present, when the course of the illness is chronic, when there is severe intellectual limitation, when the family sabotages therapeutic efforts, or when the patient is a very young preadolescent. Experience derived from the treatment of adults indicates that continuing psychotherapy after discharge from hospital treatment may contribute to the prevention of relapses.

Long-term psychodynamic therapies are probably the most frequently utilized outpatient treatment for anorexia, at least in the United States (Herzog, 1995[vi]). Ego-Oriented Individual Therapy (EOIT) has been compared with Behavioral Family Systems Therapy (BFST) in a random-assignment controlled study (Robin, Bedway, Siegel, & Gilroy, 1996[vi]; Robin, Siegel, Koepke, Moye, & Tice, 1994[ii]). This study is described later in the section on family therapy.

Interpersonal Psychotherapy (IPT), a short-term, nonintrospective psychotherapy initially designed to treat depression in adults (Klerman et al., 1984[vi]) and subsequently modified to treat depression in adolescents (Mulson, Moreau, & Weissman, 1996), has recently been adapted to treat bulimia nervosa (Fairburn, 1994[vi]; Fairburn et al., 1991[ii]; Fairburn et al., 1993a[ii]). The adapted version of IPT focuses on the significant interpersonal relationship in an individual's life that appears to have caused and maintained bulimia nervosa (Robin, Gilroy, & Dennis, 1998[vi]). Little or no emphasis is placed on the patients' eating disorder symptoms or their preoccupation with weight, shape, or appearance. Treatment lasts approximately 12 weeks. A study by Fairburn et al. (1991[ii]) of 75 bulimic adults assigned to treatment conditions based on restricted randomization compared the use of IPT to cognitive-behavioral therapy (CBT) and found that both CBT and IPT were superior to behavior therapy, and both were equally effective in decreasing and eliminating bulimic symptoms at the end of the 12-month follow-up period. Inasmuch as IPT has proven to be effective with depressed adolescents (Mulson et al., 1996), it may well also prove to be helpful in adolescents with bulimia nervosa.

BEHAVIORAL THERAPIES

It has recently been recognized that for long-term improvement in patients (mainly adults) with anorexia nervosa, weight change alone is insufficient (Anderson, Morse, & Santmyer, 1985[vi]). In the last two decades, behavioral methods for the treatment of eating disorders have become increasingly popular. The main approaches are operant conditioning procedures and cognitive methods. In some instances, social skills training programs may also be used. Operant conditioning procedures may be introduced regardless of age, but cognitive methods may be more suitable for the older adolescent. There is no clear evidence from systematic research that indicates the earliest age at which cognitive therapies may be introduced. Most behavioral approaches combine operant techniques for weight gain with other treatment techniques aiming to alter irrational beliefs or body image disturbance, anxiety, poor interpersonal skills, and dysfunctional eating behavior (Garner, Olmsted, Bohr, & Garfinkel, 1982; Rosen & Leitenberg, 1982[iib]). Operant conditioning measures are more often used in the hospital setting, where it is relatively easier to control target behaviors (eating behavior and/or weight gain). The advantages of choosing one target behavior over another have been critically reviewed by Bemis (1987[vi]), as well as the choice of reinforcement schedule (Solanto, Jacobson, Heller, Golden, & Hertz, 1994). Operant conditioning has been shown to be effective in short-term weight gain, but there is no information about effects on the spectrum of pathology in young patients with anorexia nervosa (Bemis, 1987[vi]).

Lacey (1983), Lee and Rush (1986[i]), and Wolchik, Weiss, and Katzmao (1986) have shown cognitive and behavior therapy techniques to be more effective in reducing eating disorder symptoms in bulimia as compared with waiting-list controls. In anorexia, Agras, Barlow, Chapin, Abel, and Leitenberg (1974[iib]) found that information feedback, reinforcement, and the size of the meal all increased with behavior therapy. However, in a study designed to compare behavior modification and milieu therapy, Eckert, Goldberg, Halmi, Casper, and Davis (1979[i]) randomly assigned 81 patients with anorexia nervosa to behavior modification or milieu therapy for 35 days. There was no overall significant difference in weight gain between the two groups, nor was there any difference in long-term outcome.

In a controlled outcome study, Channon et al. (Channon, DeSilva, Hemsley, & Perkins, 1989[ii]) also failed to find significant differences between CBT, behavior therapy, and a no-treatment group of patients presenting with anorexia nervosa.

Williamson et al. (1989[v]) investigated the difference between inpatient and outpatient CBT using uncontrolled methods. Inpatients were more severely disturbed than outpatients. However, the study found that inpatient treatment resulted in very rapid improvement but a tendency to relapse after discharge, at 6-month follow-up. In contrast, outpatients steadily improved over the course of 6 months treatment.

Fairburn (1988[vi]) reviewed the controlled studies of psychological treatments for bulimia nervosa. Several studies have used waiting-list control groups, and all these have found no decrease in the symptomatology of patients allocated to the waiting-list group, but improvements in patients allocated to the treatment group. Generally, it appears that cognitive-behavioral treatments are beneficial in bulimia nervosa, although Fairburn questioned whether there is an obvious particular benefit of cognitive-behavioral treatments over other forms of brief psychotherapy. Kirkley, Schneider, Agras, and Bachman (1985[ii]) reported that other treatments, in particular those involving self-monitoring and education, produced similar outcomes to CBT. A recent meta-analysis of CBT studies for bulimia concludes that CBT results in significant reduction of bulimic behaviors and of cognitive distortions or attitudes associated with bulimia (Lewandowski, Gebing, Anthony, & O'Brien, 1997[ib]). This analysis was based on studies of CBT compared with other treatment approaches or waiting-list controls, or on comparisons of subjects pre- and post-treatment. Although some studies included some subjects below 18 years of age, there are probably limitations as to the extent to which the findings can be generalized to treatment approaches with children and adolescents. There have been no published studies applying CBT to children and adolescents, but, as with anorexia, it is likely that this approach may be effective with children and adolescents (typically by age 14 or 15) who have developed the level of cognitive skills and the ability to (1) think abstractly regarding attitudes and beliefs about the meaning of weight, shape, and appearance; (2) entertain alternative possible explanations to the one currently held; (3) be prepared to test alternative hypotheses through practical exercises (Turk, 1993[vi]).

A small study indicates a benefit from massage therapy in bulimic adolescents (Field et al., 1998). Twenty-four female adolescent bulimic inpatients were randomly assigned to a massage therapy group or a standard treatment (control) group. Results indicated that the massaged patients showed immediate reductions (both self-report and behavior observation) in anxiety and depression. In addition, by the last day of the therapy (approximately 5 weeks), they had lower depression scores, lower cortisol levels, higher dopamine levels, and showed improvement on several other psychological and behavioral measures. As massage therapy attenuated several major problems associated with bulimia (anxiety, depression, neuroendocrinological abnormalities, and poor self-image), it may be a useful adjunct to standard treatment.

FAMILY THERAPY

Family therapy can clearly play a part in treating a condition, such as anorexia nervosa, that has many determinants. Vandereycken (1987[vi]) suggests that family therapy should be introduced only in response to clear indications, and is almost certainly not indicated where no family dysfunction is present: in chronic patients, in those with delayed psychosocial development; in those of single-parent families, broken homes, families in which one or both parents display severe psychopathology, and families in which previous family therapeutic attempts have failed. Dare, Eisler, Russell, and Szmukler (1990[i]) have shown that, in general, family therapy is more successful than individual therapy in all but a few cases, but that one should not assume that family change is necessary to achieve individual change; techniques to achieve successful engagement and effective symptom management are most clearly associated with successful outcome and are essential. In addition, these authors caution that there may be differences between families of bulimic and anorectic patients and that, in general, the clinical approach should be sensitive to the individual reality of family dynamics and avoid assumptions (Dare, Le Grange, Eisler, & Rutherford, 1994). Todd (1985[vi]) has discussed the usefulness of combinations of family therapy with behavior modification, CBT, and individual psychotherapy. A small randomized study of 25 female adolescents requiring hospitalization has shown that although both of two groups that were offered family therapy and family group psychoeducation, respectively, achieved weight restoration following a 4-month period of treatment, the less expensive family group psychoeducation was as effective as family therapy. At 4 months, no significant change was recorded in psychological functioning of either adolescents or parents, and subsequent readmissions were reported equally among both groups (Geist, Heinmaa, Stephens, Davis, & Katzman, 2000[i]).

Gowers, Norton, Halek, and Crisp (1994[i]) reported a study of four treatment modes. Ninety subjects with DSM-III-R anorexia nervosa were randomly allocated to one inpatient and two outpatient groups, and one offering an assessment interview only. Thus, 20 patients were offered a package of outpatient individual and family psychotherapy. Compliance with treatment was acceptably high in spite of random allocation. At 2-year follow-up, 12 of the 20 were classed as well, or very nearly well, according to operational defined criteria. Statistically significant improvements over time were obtained for weight, BMI, and psychological, sexual, and socioeconomic adjustments (replicating an earlier finding of Hall & Crisp, 1983[vi]). Weight and BMI changes were significantly better than for the assessment-only group, some of whom had received extensive treatment elsewhere. At 1 year, the outpatient package seemed to be as effective as the inpatient one (Crisp et al., 1991[i]). The results of the outpatient treatment package at 3 years also suggest that the improvements in clinical status are sustained through the subsequent year. Lower weights at presentation and vomiting were associated with poorer outcome, although age and length of history were not, suggesting that patients of any age or with any length of history (up to 10 years) are likely to do well, and reflecting the currently held view that prognosis in anorexia nervosa is largely independent of age

(Hawley, 1985[iii]), perhaps because biological development is arrested by the disorder and those with anorexia are more homogeneous in terms of biological age. The authors noted, however, that a history of more than 4 years' duration may well reduce the likelihood of recovery without specialist intervention, because a poor outcome in such patients was found in the assessment-only group. They also noted that the outpatient treatment package may be replicable by nonspecialists in a general psychiatric setting, but that the contribution of the specialist service as a whole, in terms of inculcating necessary clinical skills and providing supervision of the work with anorectic patients and the specific treatment model, cannot be overestimated. The skills have been defined by Crisp et al. (1987[vi]), providing an essential grounding in the theory and application of the method of therapy with patients and their families. One of the more striking findings was that the ability to gain weight was usually evident very early in treatment, in many cases within 2 weeks of assessment, and this correlated well with subsequent outcome, both at 1- and 2-year follow-up. Thus, early failure to respond to this form of outpatient therapy may well prove to be an indication for hospital admission. The relatively good outcome for this outpatient study group raises the question of the need for admission in such cases. However, not all patients did well. Therefore, the authors stated that it is important to consider prognostic indicators for success with this treatment, and that on the basis of the relatively small sample studied, firm conclusions should probably not be drawn on the prognostic indicators found.

Only one thoroughly controlled trial has compared family therapy with individual supportive therapy in cases of anorexia and bulimia nervosa (Russell, Szmukler, Dare, & Eisler, 1987[i]). Eighty patients were included in the study, 57 with anorexia and 23 with bulimia nervosa. These patients were admitted to a specialized unit in order to restore their weight to normal. Three subgroups of patients with anorexia were studied: those with age of onset less than or equal to 18 years and duration of illness less than 3 years, age of onset less than or equal to 18 years and duration of illness more than 3 years, and age of onset of illness 19 years or older. A fourth subgroup comprised patients with bulimia nervosa. After entry into the appropriate subgroup, patients were randomly allocated to either family therapy or individual therapy. It was not possible to maintain "blindness" to the two forms of treatment, but to reduce bias, the person carrying out assessments at follow-up was not involved in the provision of treatment. The family therapy included all members of the patient's household. The individual therapy was devised as the control therapy and was made more systematic than usual clinical practice by having more frequent sessions that lasted 1 hour and were consistently supervised. This therapy was supportive, educational, and problem centered and included cognitive, interpretative, and strategic therapies. The patients allocated to the two groups were closely matched. After 1 year of psychological treatment, some of which was done on an outpatient basis following discharge from the unit, the family therapy was found to be more effective than individual therapy in patients whose illness was not chronic and had begun before the age of 19 years. In older patients, individual supportive therapy tended to be more effective than family therapy in terms of weight gain, but the improvement fell short of recovery in most patients. There

were no significant differences between the two forms of therapy in the two remaining subgroups of patients, that is, the younger chronic anorectic patients and patients with bulimia nervosa.

Positive results were also obtained with conjoint family therapy and individual
therapy in a small population of young adolescents with recent-onset anorexia
nervosa—a group that is known to have a good prognosis (Robin, Siegel, & Moye,
1995[i]). This group of 80 patients have since been followed up after 5 years and
have showed significant improvements, mainly attributable to the natural outcome
of anorexia nervosa, with improvement most evident in the early-onset and short-
history group (Eisler et al., 1997[ii]). Significant benefits attributable to the previous psychological treatments were still evident, favoring family therapy for patients
with early onset and short history of anorexia nervosa and favoring individual supportive therapy for patients with late-onset anorexia nervosa. In addition, this study
highlighted the relevance of multiple domains of family functioning (not limited to
eating-related conflict) in anorexia nervosa and in its management. Hall (1987[iii])
has also reported that family therapy is advantageous in younger patients with a recent onset of illness who live in an intact nuclear family and who have cooperative
parents.

Robin et al. (1994[ii]) compared BFST with EOIT in a random-assignment
outcome study with 37 adolescent girls meeting DSM-III-R criteria for restricting
anorexia nervosa. Each patient received 10 to 16 months of therapy and was reassessed at the end of the treatment period and at 1-, 2.5-, and 4-year follow-up. In
BFST, the family was seen conjointly, the parents were placed in control of the adolescent's eating, distorted beliefs were targeted through cognitive restructuring,
and strategic/behavioral interventions were used to change family interactions.
EOIT consisted of weekly individual sessions focusing on identifying the dynamics
underlying the self-starvation and helping the adolescent to develop the ego
strength to cope with life stresses without resorting to self-starvation. In addition,
advice was given to the parents in collateral parental sessions twice a month; parents were advised to relinquish control over eating to the therapist and patient, and
to prepare to accept a changed, more assertive adolescent. BFST produced greater
weight gain than EOIT from pre- to postassessment. Both BFST and EOIT were
found to be effective treatments for anorexia nervosa; two-thirds of the girls
reached their target weights by the end of treatment, and four-fifths of the girls in
BFST reached their target weights by 1-year follow-up. Both therapies produced
equally large improvements in eating attitudes, depressed affect, and interoceptive
awareness, maintained at 1-year follow-up, and in the limited sample of subjects
that have reached the 4-year follow-up. Family functioning was assessed through
self-report and videotaped interaction measures of general conflict and eating-
related conflict (Robin et al., 1995[i]). Neither group acknowledged any general
family conflict before or after treatment, yet both displayed high levels of negative
communication before treatment, which improved considerably after treatment.
Both groups reported and exhibited high levels of conflict over eating, which also
improved after treatment.

The absence of a no-treatment or attention-placebo control group makes it difficult to rule out the possibility that the positive changes were due to nonspecific factors in the therapeutic situation in this study (Robin et al., 1999). In addition, analyses that included several participants who were lost to follow-up revealed that although there were no differences at postassessment on BMI between participants and nonparticipants in the follow-up, nonparticipants reported more negative eating attitudes, poorer ego functioning, and more conflict over eating than participants. Furthermore, more patients treated with family therapy than with individual therapy required hospitalization, despite random assignment. Even though the amount of family and individual therapy was compared in hospitalized versus nonhospitalized patients, the intensive inpatient refeeding program may have given these adolescents an advantage. The milder starvation of the greater number of nonhospitalized patients who received EOIT may have biased the results in the opposite direction. Robin et al. (1999) concluded that parental involvement was essential to the success of their interventions with younger adolescents with anorexia nervosa, but that it is not necessary for the adolescent and the parents to be in the room together for all therapy sessions. Therapy needs to continue for a sufficient time not only to restore weight, but also to address eating attitudes, depressive affect, self-efficacy, and family relationships. Finally, they concluded that even with comprehensive multidisciplinary interventions such as those evaluated, not all adolescents with anorexia nervosa will improve: 20–30% of the adolescents did not reach their target weights, and 40–50% did not reach the 50th percentile of BMI by 1-year follow-up.

Eisler et al. compared two forms of outpatient family intervention for anorexia nervosa in a randomized treatment trial (Eisler et al., 2000). Forty adolescent patents with anorexia nervosa were randomly assigned to "conjoint family therapy" (CFT) or to "separated family therapy" (SFT), using a stratified design controlling for levels of critical comments using the Expressed Emotion index. Therapists were required to undertake both forms of treatment. The distinctiveness of the two therapies was ensured by separate supervisors conducting live supervision. Measurements were taken on admission to the study and at 3 months, 6 months, and the end of treatment. On global measure of outcome, the two forms of therapy were associated with equivalent end-of-treatment results and considerable improvement in nutritional and psychological state. For patients with high levels of maternal criticism, the SFT was superior to the CFT. Symptomatic change was also more marked with the SFT, whereas there was considerably more psychological change in the CFT group. Critical comments between parents and patients were significantly reduced and those between parents were diminished; warmth between parents increased. These authors highlight the common finding in this and the other controlled studies in adolescents that treatments that encourage parents to take charge of the adolescent's eating are effective in bringing about both symptomatic and psychological change.

Dodge, Hodes, Eisler, and Dare (1995[vi]) report an exploratory study of family therapy for bulimia nervosa in eight clinic-referred adolescents ages 14–17 years. Their approach to family therapy was based on the model developed by Eisler (1988[vi]) and Dare and Szmukler (1991[vi]), which has proven effective in the treatment of young people with anorexia nervosa. Change was measured by assessing symptomatic behaviors and global measures of family and social function prior to treatment and again 1 year later. At reassessment, bulimic behaviors were significantly reduced, although there were many continuing symptoms. The authors compare these tentative findings with the only two other studies using family therapy for bulimia nervosa that give a clear account of the outcome of treatment: the study by Russell et al. (1987[i]) showing no effect and a poor outcome in the majority of subjects, and, in contrast, a study by Schwartz et al. (1985) using a structural model of family therapy with 30 consecutive adolescent and adult bulimic referrals over a 9-month period, in which 66% of patients had achieved abstinence from bulimic symptoms or had less than one episode per month.

Summary

Eating disorders are found in about 0.1–1% of children in Western developed societies. Preoccupation with appearance, thinness, weight, and food intake is common among children of school age, but it is not possible to predict which of these children will go on to develop an eating disorder. There is little evidence to indicate that the prevalence has risen over the past 50 years. Eating disorders, a great deal more common in girls than in boys, increase in prevalence from puberty into older adolescence. They cause significant short- and long-term morbidity, with significant impairment. About 20% of young people with eating disorders remain significantly impaired over the long term and about 50% recover, and there is great variation among studies in the proportions of young people who regain and maintain normal weight, and who establish normal eating behavior and menstruation. Mortality in anorexia nervosa, with an age of onset before 18 years, is up to 11%, with a mean mortality of 2.16% across studies. There is high comorbidity between eating disorders and other psychiatric disorders, particularly depressive disorders. Heritability is high in anorexia but almost nonexistent with bulimia nervosa. Remission tends to be worse in anorexia than in bulimia. Poor outcome is associated with longer duration of illness and severity when first coming to medical attention. The probability of relapse and chronicity may also be greater in young people with eating disorder who also show pronounced deficits in empathy and thus in social relationships. Onset at a younger age may or may not indicate a better prognosis. Many patients do not receive early medical attention because the presenting symptoms and signs of anorexia nervosa in early childhood may be atypical, nor do those of normal weight with bulimia (occurring later in adolescence).

There is clinical consensus that in anorexia, independent of treatment selection, restoration of weight is the first major goal of treatment. Beyond the clinical consensus that early intervention and hospitalization (indicated for severe emaciation, for example) will have positive benefit, there is a lack of solid empirical evidence to form a rationale for the selection of the setting of treatment interventions. Medication used to treat anorexia includes neuroleptics, appetite stimulants, and antidepressants. Research evidence of the efficacy of any of these drugs in young people is very limited and, given their side effects, their clinical value may also be limited. However, antidepressants have been shown to reduce binge eating and improve weight gain, regardless of the presence of depression. Psychosocial interventions include psychotherapeutic approaches: individual psychotherapy, behavior therapy, and family therapy. Most behavioral approaches to anorexia nervosa combine operant techniques for weight gain with other treatment techniques aiming to alter irrational beliefs, disturbance of body image, anxiety, poor interpersonal skills, and dysfunctional eating behavior. Operant conditioning is more often used in the hospital setting and has been shown to be effective in short-term weight gain. No particular benefit has been found for CBT over other forms of brief psychotherapy. There is clinical consensus that multifaceted treatment programs are effective, but there has been little evaluation of the effects of different components of treatment for different patients.

At 5-year follow-up, family therapy has been shown—after admission to a specialized unit—to be more successful than individual therapy in anorectic patients with onset before the age of 19 years and whose illness is not chronic. Family change may not be necessary to achieve individual change. Individual therapy shows benefit in those with late-onset anorexia and may contribute to the prevention of relapses after discharge from hospital treatment. The evidence for the efficacy of family therapy in bulimia is equivocal. As yet there is no evidence for the efficacy of CBT for bulimia in children and adolescents.

Implications

Early recognition of young people with serious eating disorders is essential and requires education of community professionals in primary care and in schools. Research is needed to assist in identifying those young people with disturbed eating patterns who will go on to develop significant eating disorders and who might benefit from preventive interventions. Services must be available to offer rapid assessment and intensive, multifaceted, and sustained treatment programs, with inpatient care when necessary for physical rehabilitation of young people with anorexia nervosa.

Despite the clinical consensus that specialist inpatient units are needed for the treatment of eating disorders, there is no clear evidence for or against the effectiveness of specialist adolescent inpatient units over all-age eating disorder units or generic inpatient care. Given the seriousness of the disorder, such research is urgently needed.

It is important that skilled psychotherapeutic interventions are available for the treatment of young people with eating disorders: family therapy for children and young adolescents, and individual psychodynamic psychotherapy for older adolescents, with the ability to combine therapeutic interventions as indicated for individual children. Cognitive-behavioral approaches should now be tried in adolescents who present with bulimia nervosa, as adult studies suggest that they are likely to prove effective.

SUICIDE

Definition

Suicide by definition means completed suicide and refers to death that directly or indirectly results from an act that the dead person believed would result in this end. The definition of deliberate self-harm includes nonfatal or attempted suicide, but also life-threatening behaviors such as self-poisoning in which the young person does not necessarily intend to take his or her own life. Diekstra, Kienhorst, and de Wilde (1995[vi]) define *parasuicide* as

> the term originally proposed by Kreitman (1977) to cover behaviors that can vary from what are sometimes called "suicidal gestures" or "manipulative attempts" to serious but unsuccessful attempts to kill oneself. It refers to any deliberate act with non-fatal outcome that appears to cause, or actually causes, self-harm, or, without intervention from others, would have done so; this includes taking a drug in excess of its prescribed therapeutic dose. (pp. 688–689)

This definition makes no reference to intention. It also suggests that the act should be nonhabitual. A habitual user of excessive quantities of alcohol or of dangerous drugs is not considered to constitute a case of parasuicide if that person renders him- or herself unconscious, unless there is evidence of suicidal intent. Furthermore, habitual self-mutilation (cutting, piercing, head banging) is not described as parasuicide. According to Diekstra et al. (1995), there is as yet no international agreement on the precise definition of parasuicide. These authors state that most North American authors, in contrast to the majority of European researchers, continue to use the term *attempted suicide* and often require the presence of a suicidal intention for an act to be recorded as such. Self-harming behaviors are thereby regarded as symptoms or risks linked to varying types of underlying disturbance or disorder.

Incidence and Prevalence

Suicide

Suicides account for a substantial proportion of deaths among adolescents. Although in England and Wales the rate is lower than in any adult age group, suicide is one of the most important causes of death in 15- to 24-year-old males, ranking second only to motor vehicle accidents. In the United States, epidemiological data are reported in 5-year (i.e., 15–19) and 10-year (i.e., 15–24) age groups, and this shows a distinction between suicide as the second (in 15- to 19-year-olds) or as the third (15- to 24-year-olds) leading cause of death among adolescents (National Center for Health Statistics, cited in Berman & Jobes, 1995[ib]). Completed suicide is extremely rare in children under the age of 12; it becomes more common after puberty, and its incidence increases in each of the adolescent years (Moens, 1990). Parasuicide, by contrast, is a largely adolescent and early adult phenomenon and much more common in young women.

Over the period between 1980 and 1990, the suicide risk among adolescents (11–18 years) varied from about 0.04% to 0.2% among countries that report statistics to the World Health Organization (World Health Organization, 1992b). In the United States and the United Kingdom, the suicide rates in 1989, for children between 5 and 14 years of age, were 0.7 and 0.8 per 100,000, respectively, accounting for 0.3% of all deaths in this age group in the United States and 0.5% in the United Kingdom. Among 15- to 24-year-olds, the rate was 13.2 per 100,000 in the United States (13% of all deaths) and 7.6 per 100,000 in the United Kingdom (14.1% of all deaths).

The rate of suicide among male adolescents and young men increased markedly in the postwar period up to the early or mid-1980s, when an all-time high was reached in many European countries. The time trends for young females have been much less consistent. In about half the countries there was some rise, but in the other half, rates tended to fall or to remain fairly stable (Diekstra et al., 1995[vi]). Most strikingly, as the suicide rate in young men rose, the usually much higher rates in older men fell. Since the early to mid-1980s, the suicide rates in young people have leveled off or even decreased in most European countries, first in women and then in men. However, in Great Britain, rates among males ages 15–24 years were still climbing in the late 1980s (Hawton & Fagg, 1992a). For 15- to 19-year-olds the rate rose by almost 45% between 1986 and 1990 over the rates between 1976 and 1980 in young males, but the rates for teenage girls declined over the same period by 23% (Charlton et al., 1992). The continuing high rate in young men is worrisome, in light of the decreasing rates (including rates of "undetermined" deaths) in both sexes in all other age groups (McClure, 2000). For the same age group in the United States, the 1990 rate had quadrupled over the previous 40 years, and the ratio of males to females became 4.9:1. There was a 20-year gap between the United States and Britain in the increase in suicide rate among young men. In the former, the rates started to rise in the mid-1960s and in the latter, in the mid-1980s. In Britain, in 1996, rates of 0.18 and 3.90 per 100,000 were recorded for deaths due to suicide and self-inflicted injury for 10- to 14-year-old and 15- to 19-year-old males, respectively, as compared with rates of 13.25 and 15.49 per 100,000 for 20- to 24-year-old and 25- to 29-year-old males; rates for females, although much lower, showed a similar pattern. The gender gap has become more marked in recent years in all age groups: for 15- to 19-year-olds, male:female ratios were around 2:1 in the late 1970s, of the order of 3:1 in the early 1980s, and in 1990, were over 4:1.

Official statistics represent only a proportion of the total number of non-accidental self-inflicted deaths, perhaps as few as one in three in young people under the age of 20 (Madge & Harvey, 1999). A study of all officially recorded undetermined deaths found a significant deficit in the most sparsely populated districts in England and Wales and a significant excess in the most densely populated districts in young males (Saunderson, Haynes, & Langford, 1998). The number of suicides of both males and females were significantly high in densely populated districts, but the number of suicides in males was highest in the most rural areas. These authors conclude that the true extent of both completed suicide and parasuicide is almost certainly underrepresented in official statistics, and that differences in suicide methods, the likelihood of communicating suicidal intent and, perhaps, variations in access to psychiatric services may be contributory factors to observed differences between urban and rural locations in the likelihood of a death being classified as suicide.

Parasuicide

The proportion of adolescents who have engaged in acts of parasuicide is between 40 and 100 times as high as the proportion who have actually ended their own lives. Based on patient records, rates varied very widely among centers participating in a study in different countries in Europe (Diekstra, 1982; Platt et al., 1992). In most centers the rates were higher among females ages 15 and over, than among males. However, in the more recent study, the rates for males were higher than those for females. Both studies indicate that the peak ages for parasuicide fall between 15 and 44 years, but there is considerable unexplained variation between countries and sexes in the particular age with the highest rate.

All community studies report a strong preponderance of girls, and an increase of parasuicide with age throughout the adolescent period. Surveys of lifetime suicidality have generally found that teenagers in the United States report somewhat higher suicide attempt rates than their counterparts in Europe and Canada. Smith and Crawford (1986) and Harkavy-Friedman, Asnis, Boeck, and DiFiore (1987) reported lifetime attempt rates of 8.4% and 9%, respectively, for high school students based on anonymous surveys. Among 12- to 18-year-olds in Quebec, Pronovost, Cote, and Ross (1990) found a lifetime rate of 3.5%; Dutch secondary education students (ages 14–20 years) reported a 2.2% rate (Kienhorst, De Wilde, Van den Bout, Diekstra, & Wolters, 1990).

The results of community surveys suggest that patient records considerably underestimate the scale of parasuicide. Data from Oregon, the first U.S. state to require reporting of all suicide attempts requiring hospital treatment in young people under the age of 18, indicated a 0.2% hospital-treated attempt rate in 1988 (Andrus, Fleming, Heumann, & Wassell, 1991). Attempted suicide is the most common reason for acute medical admission of young people in Britain (Hawton, 1996[vi]). Hospital admissions for self-poisoning are at their highest for women in the 15- to 19-year age range and show a sharp decline with age thereafter. For men, the peak ages are in the 20s, but rates for 15- to 19-year-olds are also high. Sex ratios contrast strongly with completed suicides: although men are more likely than women to commit suicide at all ages, 70% or more of teenage hospital admissions for self-poisonings are for females (Hawton & Fagg, 1992b[v]).

Rates for parasuicide in adolescents and young adults rose steeply in the 20 years before 1975; records from centers in the United Kingdom (Hawton & Fagg, 1992a, 1992b; Hawton, O'Grady, Osborn, & Cole, 1982; Jones, 1977; Platt, Hawton, Kreitman, Fagg, & Foster, 1988) then show a steep decline, with rates in 1988 at about the same level as in 1970. Among those ages 15–19, the rates in 1988 were still clearly above the 1970 level, but considerably more so for males than for females, indicating that the female preponderance in parasuicide has reduced over the past 20 years.

Self-poisoning with barbiturates halved between 1976-77 and 1983-84, and poisonings with minor tranquilizers (the most common reason for admission) also decreased (Platt et al., 1988). More recent data from Keith Hawton's research unit at the Department of Psychiatry, Oxford University, however, show that rates of self-poisonings in older teenage girls rose steadily over the second half of the 1980s, reaching 88 per 10,000 in 1989 (Hawton & Fagg, 1992a). The Oxford data also reflect a dramatic rise in the use of paracetomol. For both sexes, paracetomol was involved in just under a quarter of self-poisonings in 1976–1977, but in almost half of those recorded in 1988–1989; by 1995, paracetomol and paracetomol compounds were used in almost two-thirds of overdoses. The Oxford team have recently reported their findings for teenage deliberate self-harm during the 11 years between 1985 and 1995 (Hawton, Fagg, Simkin, Bale, & Bond, 2000), showing an overall increase in rate of 28.1% (27.7% in males and 28.3% in females).

Many adolescent attempters experience continued disturbance after their acute attempt, and up to 50% make further attempts (Goldacre & Hawton, 1985; Mott, 1985; Otto, 1972; Shaffer, Garland, Gould, Fisher, & Trautman, 1988; Spirito, Brown, Overholser, & Fritz, 1989). Variation in further attempt rates—from 14% (Hawton et al., 1982) to 51% (Mehr, Zeltzer, & Robinson, 1981; Mehr, Zeltzer, & Robinson, 1982)—may depend to a certain extent on the length of the follow-up period. Follow-up studies indicate that 0.1–11% of attempters will eventually commit suicide. A high proportion of repeat attempts occur during the first 2 years after the initial attempt. Later suicide has been associated with greater disturbance at the time of initial contact and is many times higher in psychiatrically hospitalized patients than in outpatients (Shaffer & Piacentini, 1994). Otto (1972) reported that 70% of the attempters who ultimately completed suicide died by methods similar to those used in their initial attempts, and males are between three to seven times more likely to complete suicide. Risk factors for nonfatal repetition are similar to those for completed suicide, including male gender, poor communication, a history of previous attempts, depressive symptomatology, and hopelessness (Choquet & Menke, 1990; Pfeffer et al., 1991; Sellar, Hawton, & Goldacre, 1990).

Suicidal Ideation

Community surveys of suicidal ideation in adolescent populations (defined as high-school populations), published since 1985, were reviewed by Diekstra et al. (1995[vi]). On the assumption that retrospective questioning about suicidal ideation, "ever" or "at least once," provides some kind of estimate of the lifetime prevalence rate, this rate is estimated to fall within the range of 15–53% among adolescents and suggests that suicidal thoughts are a common phenomenon among young people. Suicidal ideation peaked in the ninth grade in a study in the Midwest (Dubow, Kausch, Blum, Reed, & Bush, 1989). Most of the studies show a clear preponderance of girls, and there is some indication of a rise in point prevalence with age, at least between 12 and 17 years of age and particularly among girls (Choquet & Menke, 1990; Diekstra, de Heus, Garnefski, de Zwart, & Van Praag, 1991). No data are available to test whether this is a function of puberty or of other changing circumstances.

Relationship between Suicide and Parasuicide Rates

The exact nature of the relationship between suicide and parasuicide remains unclear. In a number of countries, the recent decline in parasuicide rate was not accompanied by a similar decline in suicide rate. This may be because the decline was due mainly to a reduction in certain specific types of parasuicidal acts. Preliminary results from the WHO Monitoring Study (Schmidtke et al., 1996) suggest that although the proportion of the general population who have engaged in a parasuicidal act may be decreasing, the proportion of "repeaters" among those who have ever engaged in such an act may be increasing. Because the risk of fatal outcome is higher among repeaters than among first-timers, a decrease in either the prevalence or the incidence of parasuicide may not automatically lead to a decrease in the suicide rate. In addition, there is a current debate as to whether the observed decline in parasuicide rate is an artifact (Platt et al., 1988). The "true" population rate may have remained unchanged or even increased; but parasuicidal individuals or their families may have become less willing to consult medical agencies, or general practitioners may have become more likely to treat these patients themselves and less likely to refer them to hospitals or specialist centers. A few studies report that the great majority of parasuicidal acts do not lead to contact with medical agencies. A recent study in the United States (Centers for Disease Control, 1991) among students in grades 9–12 in 50 states found that 8.3% of students had engaged in a parasuicidal act and that, following this, 24% (almost the same proportion as found in an earlier Dutch study) (Diekstra, 1993) had been in contact with medical agencies.

Risk Factors and Impact of Suicidal Behavior

At the individual level, psychological autopsies suggest high rates of psychiatric disorder in adolescents who commit suicide; 90% or more showed some disorder, with affective disorders, substance misuse, and personality disorders among the most important diagnoses (Marttunen, Aro, Henriksson, & Lonnqvist, 1991). Other risk factors include disturbed family relationships, experience of suicidal behavior in the family or peer group, and access to means.

Several studies have shown that adolescents most often commit suicide during a disciplinary crisis—for example, while awaiting a punishment or other consequence of committing a crime or breaking school rules (Shaffer, 1974; Shafii, Steltz-Lenarsky, Derrick, Beckner, & Whittinghill, 1988). Other suicides occur in the context of acute depression with no obvious external precipitant. About half of all those who commit suicide had discussed or threatened suicide within 24 hours of their deaths. Previous attempts had been noted in about 50% of female and 25% of male teenage deaths (Shaffer, 1974).

Shaffer and Piacentini (1994) consider, on the basis of all the available evidence, the striking age gradient in suicide to be a function of risk factors that start to operate only in later adolescence. This applies to affective illness and alcohol abuse, two leading risk factors for suicide in adults and adolescents (Gould, Wallenstein, & Kleinman, 1990).

Formal psychiatric history is less usual in parasuicide than in completed suicides, but high levels of disturbance are reported in both the adolescents and their families. Relationship problems are common, especially among girls, and unemployment rates in the Oxford series (Hawton, Kingsbury, Steinhardt, James, & Fagg, 1999) were considerably higher than the local rates for older teenagers. Drug and alcohol problems were more frequent in males, but alcohol use at the time of the act was common in both sexes. Clinical studies suggest that antisocial and behavioral problems are also frequently present (Kerfoot, 1988).

Suicidal behavior in childhood and adolescence has been associated with adverse psychiatric and psychosocial outcomes. Otto (1972) found that suicide attempters at 10- to 15-year follow-up were much more likely than controls to be unmarried or divorced and to be listed in national registries as having criminal behavior, alcohol problems, or being in receipt of disability benefits.

Prevention of Parasuicide and Suicide

Both Diekstra et al. (1995[vi]) and Hawton (1996[vi]) discuss a variety of current approaches to the prevention of suicidal behavior in young people. They list educational programs in schools; the control and/or modification of methods used for committing suicide; efforts to reduce substance misuse; responsible media reporting of suicide; specialist services—often crisis intervention—for people seriously contemplating suicide; and aftercare programs for those who have deliberately harmed themselves. A more recent study (Thompson, Eggert, & Herting, 2000[iii]) supports the superior efficacy of indicated school-based interventions with individuals showing signs related to suicide risk as opposed to programs with high-risk groups and entire school populations.

Aftercare programs for those who have engaged in acts of parasuicide treated in hospitals have increased substantially in most countries. Most studies lack both suitable controls and adequate follow-up. A recent study, using methodologically sound design, found no effect from treatment (Allard, Marshall, & Plante, 1992[i]). One hundred fifty subjects were randomly allocated to an experimental group or to a comparison group. The intensive intervention program included an explicit treatment plan for each patient with 18 therapy appointments over 1 year, including one home visit and measures to improve attendance, and free use of outside resources such as Alcoholics Anonymous. Results showed that 22 subjects (35%) in the experimental group and 19 (30%) in the comparison group performed at least one parasuicidal act in the 2 years following randomization. Three completed suicides occurred among experimental subjects and one in the comparison group.

Crawford and Wessely (1998) report that local evidence in the United Kingdom suggests that the proportion of people who discharge themselves from the hospital before their initial assessment has been completed has more than doubled in recent years. Although those patients assessed before discharge and who receive follow-up care from specialist mental health services had the lowest repetition rate of all, no follow-up data were reported for patients managed by primary care services. Following only 33.3% participation among 129 young people admitted to Birmingham Children's Hospital after an overdose in a 15-month period, Dorer, Feehan, Vostanis, and Winkley (1999) have noted that this is a difficult population to recruit in research or to engage in treatment.

Only one trial has evaluated the outcome of treatment of a suicide attempt, in terms of repeat suicide attempts, in children and adolescents. Cotgrove, Zirinsky, Black, and Weston (1995[i]) tested an experimental approach in 105 patients ages 12.2–16.7 years (mean age 14.9 years, 85% female) admitted after deliberate self-harm. On discharge, 47 young people were randomly assigned to standard care plus an emergency (green) card acting as a passport to readmission into the local pediatric ward; 58 controls received standard care only. The percentage of repeaters after 12-month follow-up was 3 out of 47 (6.4%) in the experimental group—5 made use of their cards to gain hospital admission—and 7 out of 58 (12.1%) in the control group; the odds ratio (0.45) was not significant.

Other Outcomes

Most evaluations have been limited to the effect on probable promising outcomes, such as staying in treatment or improved family functioning. However, most evaluations of treatment following a suicide attempt suffer because of the extremely poor attendance for and compliance with treatment. Trautman, Stewart, and Morishima (1993[iv]) studied the "outpatient clinic attendance patterns" of 112 suicide attempters (ages 10–18 years) referred for follow-up services during an 18-month period. They reported an overall dropout rate of 77%, which occurred quite quickly; there was a median number of three visits before dropout. An evaluation of outpatient treatment adherence (Rotheram-Borus et al., 1996) found that the intervention program was associated with attempters being more likely to attend their initial treatment session (95.4% vs. 82.7%, $p = .018$); to attend more of the 6 treatment sessions overall (marginally significant, $p = .11$); and to complete treatment (52.3%, compared with 38.7%). In this study, 90% of eligible families were recruited and followed to compare adherence to treatment among 140 female adolescent (ages 12–18 years) suicide attempters, sequentially assigned to receive standard emergency room care and a specialized emergency room program in a busy inner-city hospital serving a predominantly disadvantaged Latino population. Although the adolescents were not randomly assigned to the two groups receiving standard or special care, no significant differences between the groups were found in age, ethnicity, or receipt of special education, nor were there any significant differences in the relevant characteristics of their mothers (e.g., marital status, primary language, age at adolescent's birth, level of education, and employment status). The specialized program included training workshops for emergency room staff, a videotape aimed at modifying families' treatment expectations, and an on-call family therapist. The CBT received by the families focused on clarifying parents' and children's beliefs and norms regarding their roles, particularly around issues of independence (Piacentini, Rotheram-Borus, & Cantwell, 1995[vi]). From the therapist's reports on this project, parental involvement appeared to be central to increasing the adolescent's adherence in the first session, but may or may not have been helpful otherwise. However, experiencing the specialized program in the emergency room directly influenced the adolescents and their mothers by reducing the adolescents' feelings of depression and suicidality, decreasing acute maternal psychiatric symptoms, increasing positive maternal attitudes toward treatment, and reshaping maternal perceptions of the ideal family as more adaptive and cohesive. Although this study demonstrated that treatment adherence could positively be increased, the authors highlight the mixed nature of the findings: In some ways those who attended appeared to have more resources than those who did not attend, but other characteristics indicated that attenders were in greater need. For example, adolescent attenders had more active suicidal behavior and lower self-esteem and rated their families as less cohesive and adaptive. Mothers who attended were more likely to be single parents and to have impulsive daughters. The mothers of adolescents who rated their families as more cohesive and adaptive were less likely to attend therapy. The authors discuss the implications for the delivery of emergency room interventions in a more recent paper (Rotheram-Borus et al., 1999[vi]).

Another study, a 6-month follow-up by structured telephone interview of 66 adolescents, 13–17 years old, was not able to locate 20% of the original sample (King, Hovey, Brand, Wilson, & Ghaziuddin, 1997[v]). Moreover, a standardized measure of treatment follow-through was not used, and there were very small numbers for some of the analyses. However, among these adolescents hospitalized on an adolescent psychiatry inpatient unit with significant suicidal thoughts, intent, or behaviors, compliance with recommended medication (66.7%) and individual therapy (50.8%) was better than compliance with parent guidance/family therapy sessions (33.3%). The most dysfunctional families and those with the least involved/affectionate father–adolescent relationships had the poorest follow-through with parent guidance/family therapy. Mothers' hostility was associated with less medication follow-up, and mothers' depressive and paranoid symptoms were linked with less adolescent individual therapy.

Harrington et al. (1998a[i]) randomly allocated patients who had engaged in acts of deliberate self-poisoning, consecutively admitted to four hospitals in Manchester. Of 162 children and adolescents under the age of 17 years, 77 were allocated to routine care and 85 to routine care plus brief family intervention. The intervention consisted of an assessment session, followed by four home-based sessions by child psychiatric social workers focusing on family communication and family problem solving. The control group received no home-based sessions. Both groups were assessed at the time of recruitment and at 2- and 6-month follow-up. The primary outcome measures were the Suicidal Ideation Questionnaire, the Hopelessness Scale, and the Family Assessment Device. An economic analysis of direct and indirect treatment costs was also undertaken. There were no significant differences in the primary outcomes between the intervention and control groups at either of the outcome assessments. Compliance with family treatment was better than that for routine care, and parents in the intervention group were significantly more satisfied with treatment at 2 months assessment ($p < .001$) than parents in the control group. A subgroup without major depression had much less suicidal ideation at both outcome assessments (analysis of covariance $p < .01$), compared with controls.

Health costs for treatment were broadly similar between subjects and controls, but at 6-month follow-up a substantial resource shift was observed in the social services sector, with the control group costing more than the intervention group as a result of increased use of foster care and residential care. These authors conclude that brief forms of intervention are likely to be effective only in subjects without major depression, who tend to have less severe forms of suicidal behavior, and that studies of more intensive forms of family intervention would be required to determine whether they are more effective in leading to better outcomes for the child (Harrington et al., 2000a). Although suicidality is associated strongly with depressive disorders, few treatment outcome studies of depressed adolescents include suicidal subjects or suicidal ideation or behavior as outcome measures. In their wide-ranging review, Miller and Glinski conclude that there is some evidence that treatment effects on suicidality are divorced from treatment effects on depression levels (Miller & Glinski, 2000[vi/ib]).

Population Approaches

Crisis intervention centers typically provide a 24-hour hotline plus referral to other mental health or social work agencies. Evaluation studies have addressed two major facets of their functioning: whether such centers attract people with an elevated risk for suicidal behavior, and whether they prevent these individuals' suicide attempts (Bridge, Potkin, Zung, & Soldo, 1977[v]; Lester, 1974). In a meta-analysis of studies addressing these two questions, Dew, Bromet, Brent, and Greenhouse (1987[ib]) drew two main conclusions. First, the centers do attract a high-risk population; center clients were much more likely to commit suicide than were members of the general population. Second, the evidence on whether the suicide rate decreases more in communities with a suicide prevention center than in those without such a center is contradictory and inconclusive; there is no indication of any marked effect, either positive or negative. Given that these centers are somewhat successful in attracting the population they are designed to help, it may be that effectiveness should be tested within specific cohorts rather than across the population as a whole. Miller, Coombs, Leeper, and Barton (1984[iii]) compared 28 center communities with 48 control communities over the period 1968–1973 and found no significant difference between them in overall change in suicide rate over time. However, the suicide rate for white females under the age of 25 showed a large and significant decrease in communities with a center as opposed to control communities. This finding, if replicated, is potentially important because young white women are the most frequent users of prevention centers and telephone emergency services.

Summary

Suicide is one of the most important causes of death in young people in the United Kingdom and the United States, especially in young males, and has, on the whole, been increasing. Although completed suicide is rare in children under the age of 12, it becomes more common after puberty and its incidence increases in each of the adolescent years. In adolescent suicides, high rates of psychiatric disorder have been found (on psychological autopsy), particularly affective disorders, substance misuse, and personality disorders. There are particularly high risks of suicide among certain groups of young people—for example, those in secure institutions and those who are homeless.

Parasuicide is largely an adolescent and early adult phenomenon and is much more common in young women. Between 40 and 100 times more adolescents engage in acts of parasuicide than those who actually end their own lives. Attempted suicide is the most common reason for acute medical admission of young people. A considerable proportion of parasuicidal adolescents repeat their attempts—usually within 2 years—and up to about 10% will eventually commit suicide. Suicidal ideation is shown to be present in about 50% of school-age children, becoming more common with increasing age. Depressive disorder is highly correlated with suicide attempts, but other factors such as associated conduct disorder (in males), adverse life events especially linked to interpersonal conflict, and access to means make it more likely that death will result. A significant proportion of young people who self-harm are not known to services, and a significant proportion discharge themselves after initial presentation.

There is some evidence that forms of brief intervention (problem solving) with the families of adolescents following a suicide attempt can alleviate adolescents' feelings of depression and suicidality and engender positive maternal attitudes toward treatment, thus enabling supportive family involvement and further compliance with specialist programs. The evidence for effective approaches to the prevention of further suicide attempts in young people is extremely limited, although there is suggestive value in issuing an emergency room card allowing continuing ready access to skilled advice and help, following initial assessment and hospital admission. Round-the-clock hotline services have not been shown to reduce the incidence of suicide attempts among the populations served.

Implications

There is clear clinical consensus that all adolescent expressions of intended suicide should be taken seriously and lead to specialist evaluation. From the evaluations of crisis intervention services, it appears to be important to be able to distinguish between young people who present with significant psychopathology, especially depression, and others whose distress is primarily in response to personal and family situations, and to offer an appropriate specialist service to each; a home visiting component may be important. Assessment of stressful life events should be one element in the evaluation of suicide risk among adolescents, particularly among those with substance abuse problems. Further research is needed on the impact of management by staff in accident and emergency departments during initial stages of treatment and on the development of greater understanding of the reasons that many choose to leave the hospital before management has been completed.

SUBSTANCE MISUSE

Definition

The substances discussed in this section are taken for their effects on mood and behavior, but have undesirable psychological consequences when taken in excess; they include alcohol, illicit and prescribed drugs, and volatile substances. Tobacco is not discussed except insofar as smoking is closely linked to the use of other drugs. It is hard to distinguish clearly between "use," often styled as "experimental" or "recreational" use, and "misuse." The World Health Organization's *Document on Nomenclature and Classification* (1981) distinguished four different aspects of alcohol and drug-related problems. *Unsanctioned use* is not approved by society, or by a group within that society. *Hazardous use* will probably lead either to dysfunctional or harmful consequences for the user. *Dysfunctional use* leads to impaired psychological or social functioning (e.g., loss of job or marital problems). *Harmful use* is known to have caused tissue damage or mental illness in a particular person. One manifestation of dysfunctional and harmful use is dependence, characterized by repeated extreme difficulty in refraining from use. It may be associated with a sense of compulsion to take the substances involved, a wish to stop in spite of continued use, tolerance to increasing amounts of the substances involved, withdrawal symptoms and the use of substances to suppress withdrawal symptoms, and rapid return to using substances even after a period of abstinence.

Both DSM-IV and ICD-10 have adopted a similar broad approach, distinguishing consumption, dependence symptoms, and adverse consequences. Within DSM-IV both substance abuse and dependency are characterized by a maladaptive pattern of substance use leading to clinically significant impairment or distress. *Dependence* is indicated by three or more of the following features occurring in the same 12-month period: (1) tolerance, marked by a need for increasing amounts of the substance, or a decreased effect from taking the same quantity of the substance; (2) withdrawal, as manifested by the characteristic withdrawal syndrome for the substance; (3) the individual's taking the substance in larger amounts or over longer periods than he or she intended; (4) a persistent desire or one or more unsuccessful attempts to cut down or control substance use; (5) a great deal of time spent in activities necessary to get the substance, taking the substance, or recovering from its effects; (6) important activities given up because of substance use; (7) continued substance use despite knowledge of personal problems caused by its use. The criteria for *abuse*—in the absence of criteria for dependence—are (1) recurrent substance use, resulting in failure to fulfill major role expectations (e.g., leading to absenteeism, or neglect of household or children); (2) recurrent use in physically hazardous situations, such as driving when impaired by substance use; (3) recurrent substance-related legal problems (e.g., arrests for disorderly conduct); (4) continued substance use despite social problems caused or exacerbated by the effects of the drug, such as fights. In children and adolescents, these classifications can rarely be clearly made. There are indications that young people *abuse* alcohol, for instance, in that alcohol and drugs are known to play a part in causing a significant proportion of traffic accidents (see below). The symptoms of *dependency*, as judged by self-report at least, appear to be less common in adolescents than in adults.

Incidence and Prevalence

Because of the difficulty in defining "cases" of alcohol and drug misuse in popula-tions, most of the data on prevalence and the incidence of new cases describe, at best, the use or consumption of substances or the consequences that can be attrib-uted to their use, and underrepresent the number of "cases" as equivalent only to users with certain kinds of problems. Silbereisen, Robins, and Rutter (1995) discuss the value of the various indicators of the use of alcohol, drugs, and volatile sub-stances by young people. Overall per capita alcohol consumption and cirrhosis of the liver have risen in most European countries since the Second World War, but it is unclear to what extent the increase applies to young people. British survey data (Duffy, 1991) covering annual assessments for 12 years since 1979, show stable rates of daily and weekly drinking for 15- to 19-year-old females. Among males of the same age, the percentages of daily drinkers and abstainers both declined slightly.

In a recent self-report study among a representative sample of 7,722 15- and 16-year-olds from 70 secondary schools in the United Kingdom, almost all pupils had drunk alcohol; 36% had smoked cigarettes in the past 30 days; 42.3% had at some time used illicit drugs, mainly cannabis; and 43% of boys and 36% of girls had tried cannabis (Miller & Plant, 1996). Cigarette smoking was more common among girls than boys, and there was a strong relationship between cigarette smoking and can-nabis use; only 6.9% of nonsmokers had ever tried cannabis, and the percentage rose with the level of smoking.

In the United States, the rate of alcohol use has tended to be stable in the past few years, although it remains high. In 1996, 26% of 8th graders reported having had a drink in the past month, compared with 40% of 10th graders and 51% of seniors. In 1995, the rate of binge drinking (five or more drinks in a row within the past 2 weeks) was 15% for 8th graders, 25% for 10th graders, and 30% for 12th graders (National Institute on Drug Abuse, 1996). These surveys omitted the 15–20% of children who are high school dropouts, who are likely to be most at risk for substance misuse, so they probably underestimate the extent of use.

Surveys consistently reveal that a significant proportion of children are drink-ing alcohol before they reach secondary school age. The proportion drinking weekly has been shown to increase evenly with age, with pronounced differences in drinking patterns between girls and boys; from 12 years onward more boys than girls are likely to be drinking (Goddard, 1996).

From a self-report study of London schoolchildren, Swadi (1988) reported that more than 10% of 11- to 16-year-olds were using alcohol as often as once a week or more. In a survey by the British Office of Population Censuses and Surveys (Goddard & Iken, 1988), 79% of 13-year-olds said that they had drunk alcohol and 29% that they usually drank once a week. By 17 years of age, 90% have consumed alcohol at least once and 62% drink in public houses (bars). At the ages of 16–17, few adolescents are categorized as heavy drinkers, but, overall, a substantial minor-ity of young people do drink heavily. Three recent surveys in the United Kingdom have noted that 2–7% of males were drinking more than 50 units a week and 1–4% of females were drinking more than 31 units a week (Foster, Wilmot, & Dobbs, 1990; Goddard & Iken, 1988; Plant, Peck, & Samuel, 1985). By the ages of 18–24,

20% of men and 5% of women drank at levels that are widely accepted to be detrimental. Overall, there appears to be no strong association between adolescent and adult drinking, although in the 1958 British birth cohort, the 16-year-olds who drank most and most frequently were most likely to drink most heavily at 23 years (Ghodsian & Power, 1987).

On the basis of longitudinal research data in the United States, Kandel and Faust (1975) proposed that heavy alcohol use is sometimes a first step in a substance-abusing career. The more heavily involved an adolescent is in alcohol, the greater are the chances of drug use. Swadi (1988) found that among those who drink more than once a week, 34% have used drugs repeatedly, compared to 22% among those who only drink once a week, and 2% among those who never drank. However, Robson (1996) comments on a recent trend in the U.K. youth scene to use illicit drugs and alcohol recreationally and alternately, depending on circumstances, and argues that the escalation theory, which suggests that use of a drug such as cannabis may inexorably lead to, or in some way cause, a progression to "hard drugs," does not bear critical examination. Most people who try cannabis never move to any other drug. However, a large majority of heroin addicts have histories of earlier experimentation with cannabis, and most have used alcohol and tobacco before that. This cannot be construed as a causative sequence, but the use of cannabis can bring a large number of otherwise law-abiding young people into contact with the criminal underworld.

Recent reports from the University of Exeter school-based surveys indicate that almost a third of 15-year-olds have experimented with illegal drugs (Schools Health Education Unit, 1994). The results from different studies on drug use are relatively consistent (e.g., Zoccolillo, Vitaro, & Tremblay, 1999, in Quebec, Canada), although there is some variation depending on the methods used, and in many instances the studies have not been validated against other measures of drug use. In Roker's study (1995) of 2,000 young people in southeast England, 35% of 15- and 16-year-olds report having used cannabis, whereas only 5.5% report having used ecstasy. Cannabis had been used by 3–5% of children ages 11–16 years in two large-scale surveys in the United Kingdom (Health Education Authority, 1992). In older teenagers, the rate rises to 17% according to the British Crime Survey (Mott, 1985). This was still lower than the high (but declining) rates in the United States. The American High School Survey reports that in 1980, 60% of seniors had tried cannabis but by 1991 this had fallen to 37% who had ever used, with 14% having used cannabis in the previous month (National Institute on Drug Abuse, 1996).

Estimates of the misuse of volatile substances range from 3 to 11% in children at secondary school (Chadwick, Anderson, Bland, & Ramsey, 1989; Edeh, 1989; Swadi, 1988). School-based surveys of the use of a range of drugs (e.g., Wright & Pearl, 1995) show that use of heroin and cocaine is probably below 1%, but there are some localities of higher-prevalence drug use where heroin and cocaine may each be used by some 2% of secondary school children. The United Kingdom has seen a recent dramatic increase of interest in hallucinogens in young people, fed by the music culture of rave parties (Farrell, 1989; Pearson, Ditton, Newcombe, & Gilman, 1991).

Miller and Plant note a large rise in all types of drug experimentation since 1989 (Miller & Plant, 1996). Knowledge of drug use and offers of drugs to 14- and 15-year-olds have increased (Wright & Pearl, 1995). Farrell and Taylor (1994[vi]) summarize the overall picture in the United Kingdom as appearing

> to be one of high initiation to tobacco and alcohol with high levels of regular consumption and experimentation with solvents, cannabis and more recently, hallucinogens, but low rates of heroin and cocaine use. The pattern emerging from the US studies is that of a falling prevalence of new initiates to illicit drug use but also local pockets of high-density problem drug use associated with a complex range of social problems. (p. 530)

Comorbidity

Kessler et al. (1996) note that most studies finding co-occurrence of substance use disorder (SUD) and other psychiatric disorders and/or behavior problems are cross-sectional, but that even when one disorder demonstrably precedes another, causality cannot be implied and clinical prediction cannot be made.

Epidemiological studies reveal a high prevalence of comorbidity of substance misuse with psychiatric disorders (Bukstein, Brent, & Kaminer, 1989). In clinic populations, the more severe the problems with substance use, the greater the likelihood of coexistent psychiatric disorder. Anxiety disorders, affective disorders, and antisocial personality are most common. However, a follow-up of preschool children in the San Francisco Bay Area to the age of 18 found a U-shaped relationship between psychological health and frequent users of substances, experimenters, and abstainers, with experimenters being the most healthy (Shedler & Block, 1990). The authors suggest that these findings indicate that problem drug use is a symptom, not a cause, of personal and social maladjustment and that in experimenters, drug use appears to reflect age-appropriate and developmentally understandable experimentation. Colder and Chassin (1999) also found that in 15- to 17-year-olds, problem use was associated with fundamental family disruptions and poor psychosocial functioning, and moderate use reflected unconventionality and socialization specific to alcohol, challenging the assumption that adolescent alcohol use and problem use represent a continuum.

Many risk factors for adolescent drug abuse also predict other adolescent problem behaviors (Hawkins et al., 1988, Jenson, Catalano, & Lishner, in Hawkins et al., 1992). There is evidence that adolescent drug abuse correlates with delinquency, teenage pregnancy, and school misbehavior and dropout (Elliott, Huizinga, & Menard, 1988; Jessor & Jessor, 1977; Zabin et al., 1986). Alcohol and drug use have been associated with major depression in college students (Deykin, Levy, & Wells, 1987). A few studies have noted that in comorbidity with anxiety disorders, nearly 40% of high school seniors appear to use drugs to "relax and relieve tension." Hovens et al. (1994) found that among adolescent substance abusers with co-occurring psychiatric disorder, overanxious disorder predominated in the young women and conduct disorder in the young men. Lavik, Clausen, and Pedersen (1991) have noted a strong relationship between eating disorders and alcohol misuse. A report on the psychiatric diagnosis of adolescents who have recently been detoxified and then referred to psychiatric inpatient services, showed that 42% had a conduct disorder, 35% had major depression, and 21% had a combination of attention deficit, hyperactivity, and impulsive disorder. Educational delay and personality difficulties were common, although the most frequent diagnostic cluster in the sample was attention deficit disorder (ADD) with hyperactivity and conduct disorder (CD) (DeMilio, 1989).

Population studies are congruent with clinic studies in finding an association between CD and adolescent SUD. In New Zealand, the Dunedin Multidisciplinary Health and Development Study gathered mental health data on young people at ages 11, 13, 15, 18, and 21 (Newman et al., 1996). The prevalence of DSM-III-R SUDs at age 21 was 9.8% for alcohol dependence and 9.6% for marijuana dependence, with rates nearly three times higher in young men than in young women. Among those with SUDs, 43.2% had a history of CD at younger ages; 38.1% had a previous history of depressive disorder, 29% of anxiety disorder, 11% of ADD, and 21.9% had no history of previous disorder.

Among a group of 349 adolescent psychiatrically referred outpatients, 11% met full criteria for an SUD by parental report (Wilens, Biederman, Abrantes, & Spencer, 1997). Controlling for age, adolescents with SUDs had higher risk for mood and disruptive behavioral disorders as compared with psychiatric controls, with the onset of psychopathology preceding the onset of the SUD by at least 1 year in the majority of cases. Those with SUD had lower overall functioning, more school dysfunction, and more psychiatric hospitalizations than those with psychiatric disorders only.

A case–control study of adolescent inpatients who had been sexually abused indicated that they may well be at higher risk for substance abuse, and that this may relate to particular coping styles and strategies that are developed by these young people (Singer, Petchers, & Hussey, 1989).

Clinical Presentation

There is little information about service use to indicate the problems that present in young drug users. Since 1990, the proportion of drug addicts who are known to the authorities aged under 25 has increased by 20% (H.M. Government Statistical Service, 1994). There has also been a substantial increase in young people under 25 who have been found guilty of drug-related offenses.

Young people rarely present simply as users of substances, although substantial problems may arise from experimental use, such as the deaths that can result from first-time solvent inhalation. The most important effect of alcohol on young adults' physical health is in the area of accidental and nonaccidental injury. About a third of accident fatalities in 16- to 19-year-olds are found to be associated with alcohol (U.S. Department of Transportation, 1993). This finding is likely to underestimate deaths associated with alcohol in this age group, because teenagers have more accidents at low blood-alcohol levels than adults (British Paediatric Association and the Royal College of Physicians, 1995[vi]). In the United Kingdom there has been an improvement in alcohol-related mortality between 1982 and 1992, which may partly be due to a decline in drunk driving (Department of Transport, 1993). Alcohol and drugs can affect all areas of functioning and may be a precipitant to both suicide and deliberate self-harm (Kerfoot & Huxley, 1995). One-third of adolescents who commit suicide are intoxicated at the time of death, and a further number are under the influence of drugs (Brent, 1987). Studies in a number of countries have found that the percentage change in alcohol consumption has the single highest correlation with changes in suicide rates (Diekstra, 1989). Alcohol misuse may be the determining factor in the recent rise in male suicides (Williams & Morgan, 1994). In addition, many young people who deliberately harm themselves also misuse alcohol and drugs. The rates reported range from 13% to 42%, depending on the sample and the definition of misuse (Hawton et al., 1982; Spirito et al., 1989).

Substance misuse may go unrecognized, as an aggravating or precipitating factor, when young people seek help with social and psychiatric problems. Because children and young people who are drinking excessively or misusing drugs may not be accessible through conventional services, they may be prepared to discuss their drug use in the context of other issues where they perceive themselves to be in greater need of help. For example, they may seek help at voluntary or local authority agencies set up to advise young people with housing problems and agencies providing advice on family planning. Local authority and voluntary agency youth workers attached to clubs and recreational centers for young people may be another point of contact for those with problems of drinking and drug use.

There is evidence that young people with comorbid psychiatric symptomatology who are in substance abuse treatment programs may well not be receiving mental health treatment. This has been shown clearly, at least in groups who are marginalized in other respects, such as Native Americans (Novins, Beals, Shore, & Manson, 1996). Studies of adolescents (Kaminer, Tarter, Bukstein, & Kabene, 1992[iv]) suggest that comorbidity does influence treatment outcome.

Early onset of legal or illegal recreational drug use, as well as significant escalation in the teenage years, are bad prognostic signs. Regular or heavy consumption of these drugs during adolescence has a strong association with later alcohol and drug abuse; mental and physical problems; difficult family, social, and sexual relationships; and disruption of education and employment. A 20-year longitudinal population-representative study has shown that childhood aggression was related to both young adult drug use and delinquency, and that there was stability of drug use and delinquency between early adolescence and young adulthood (Brook, Whiteman, Finch, & Cohen, 1996). Drug use during early adolescence impacted on delinquency not only in early adolescence, but also in late adolescence and young adulthood.

The correlations between tobacco, alcohol, and cannabis use were studied in a birth cohort of New Zealand children at age 16 (Lynskey, Fergusson, & Horwood, 1998). About 54% of the correlations could be explained by a factor representing the individual's vulnerability to substance use—that is, the extent of association with delinquent or substance-using peers, novelty seeking, and parental illicit drug use. Similar findings have emerged from a sample of 1,687 adolescents living in mixed urban/rural communities in Colombia, South America (Brook et al., 1998). There were some notable gender differences among the findings of this study, as elsewhere (e.g., Farrell & White, 1998; Lifrak, McKay, Rostain, Alterman, & O'Brien, 1997), with a stronger relationship between peer pressure and use among girls than boys. The relation between adolescent alcohol use and peer alcohol use is not simple (Curran, Stice, & Chassin, 1997). Over a 3-year period in a community-based sample of 363 Hispanic and Caucasian adolescents, peer alcohol use predicted later increases in alcohol use in the index adolescents, and alcohol use in the index adolescents predicted later increases in peer alcohol use. These authors point out that if earlier peer group affiliation is predictive of later adolescent substance use (peer socialization), then the peer group is an important focus for interventions, but that if adolescents begin to use illicit substances and then affiliate with substance-using peers, peer group intervention may be misplaced.

Treatment

Physical Therapies

The use in adolescents of pharmacological agents to counteract or decrease the subjective reinforcing effects of a substance, or as aversion agents (e.g., disulfiram), has received minimal attention in the literature. Substitution therapy includes the use of opioid agonists (e.g., methadone) for heroin addiction and naltrexone for alcohol dependence. In the absence of evidence demonstrating the safety and efficacy of pharmacotherapy to decrease the subjective effects of a substance, the use of these agents in adolescents should be reserved for only the most severely dependent who have been resistant to other treatment. Different treatment approaches apply to specific drugs. The management of opiate withdrawal by methadone treatment in adults has been extensively evaluated. Farrell and Taylor (1994[vi]) conclude that methadone has been demonstrated to be moderately effective as a maintenance treatment over the longer term in those who are dependent on opiates, but it is of limited use in those with a short history—in most young people, in other words.

The high prevalence of comorbid psychiatric disorders means that many adolescents may require pharmacotherapeutic agents directed toward these disorders. Potential targets for pharmacological treatment are depression, ADHD, severe aggressive behavior, and anxiety disorders. Unfortunately, there are few data demonstrating the efficacy of pharmacological agents prescribed for adolescents with SUD and comorbid psychiatric disorders, although several studies in adult populations suggest the efficacy of a variety of agents. Geller et al. (Geller, Cooper, Watts, Cosby, & Fox, 1992[i]) found lithium to be moderately efficacious in treating adolescents with comorbid major mood disorders and recently published results from a double-blind, placebo-controlled, random allocation trial of lithium for adolescents with bipolar disorder and secondary substance dependency (Geller et al., 1998[i]). However, the sample in this study was small and unrepresentative, and there was no follow-up of the modest improvements.

Psychosocial Therapies

Patient-centered approaches to treatment in young people have received little research attention. Moreover, many approaches used in adults, such as cue exposure for the prevention of relapse in alcohol, heroin and cocaine dependence, and harm minimization (e.g., minimizing the risk of transmission of HIV infection from contaminated injecting equipment among injecting drug users), have not been applied.

Although the effectiveness of interpersonal and psychodynamic therapies for adolescents is suggested by case reports and clinical experience, controlled studies of these methods in adolescent populations are lacking. Adolescent peer group therapy (Fisher & Bentley, 1996[ii]), cognitive-behavioral approaches such as rehearsal and social control contracting (Azrin et al., 1994[ii]), problem-solving and coping skills training (Hawkins, Jenson, Catalano, & Wells, 1991[ii]), and relapse prevention techniques (Catalano, Hawkins, Wells, Miller, & Brewer, 1990[vi]; Myers, Brown, & Mott, 1993[v]) show promise, at least for the few months after discharge from treatment (Weinberg, Rahdert, Colliver, & Glantz, 1998[ib]). Many treatment programs for adolescents use behavioral therapies, such as operant conditioning (i.e., rewarding and punishing for appropriate and inappropriate behavior, respectively), as part of an inpatient or residential behavior management program.

Approaches to treatment have mainly been based on social learning theory and cognitive-behavioral therapy. A significant proportion of adolescents with SUDs report cognitive distortions and negative internalized self-statements. Although cognitive therapy has yet to be systematically studied, cognitive approaches show effects with adolescents treated for depression (Stanton & Shadish, 1997[ib]). Interventions aimed at cognitive aspects of coping have also been shown to be useful in preventing relapse in adolescents following treatment for substance abuse (Myers et al., 1993[v]). This study recruited 80 teenagers consecutively admitted to two inpatient adolescent drug and alcohol treatment programs in San Diego, California. Both programs were based on the Alcoholics Anonymous 12-step treatment approach and had similar lengths of stay of about 4–6 weeks; none of the subjects left treatment prematurely. Analyses were conducted on 57 adolescents after exclusion of individuals who evidenced low commitment to change, who were institutionalized following treatment, or for whom outcome data (at 6 months) were unreliable. In contrast with earlier findings, which suggested the importance of social support and problem-focused coping in managing the immediate demands of a relapse-risk situation (Myers & Brown, 1990), the current results suggest that cognitive strategies such as wishful thinking may play a greater role in relapse-risk situations than has previously been appreciated. On the basis of findings in their earlier study, Myers and Brown (Myers et al., 1993[v]) offer an interpretation positing that a teenager's cognitive approach might influence his or her active coping efforts by reducing his or her situational appraisal of stress; that is, that wishful thinking may act to diminish vigilance by averting the focus from the demands of the actual situation, thus decreasing the likelihood of using an active coping response.

Family-oriented therapies have received most attention in clinical research on treatment for adolescents with SUDs. In a meta-analysis and literature review, Stanton and Shadish (1997[ib]) support the superiority of family therapy (but not family psychoeducation or support groups) for adolescent SUDs over other modalities and note that family treatment can enhance the effectiveness of other approaches.

One of several theory-based models of family therapy shown to be efficacious in improving parent–adolescent relationships, and in turn reducing adolescent drug use, is structural–strategic family therapy (SSFT) (Joanning, Quinn, & Mullen, 1992[ii]; Lewis, Piercy, Sprenkle, & Trepper, 1990[ii]; Szapocznik et al., 1988[i]). SSFT refers to treatments that involve all family members (whether present or not at therapeutic sessions), because drug and alcohol abuse are understood as being related to dysfunctional family structures (e.g., over- or underinvolvement) and interactional patterns (e.g., conflict avoidance) and has as a primary focus the therapeutic alliance between therapist and family members.

Skills training for the parents of drug-abusing adolescents is frequently associated with family therapy. This approach aims to reduce the adolescent's drug use by eliciting changes in the parents' or caretaker's family management practices (Schmidt et al., 1996[v]). These authors showed moderate to excellent improvement in parenting in two-thirds of 29 parents of drug-abusing adolescents, following a course of 16 sessions of multidimensional family therapy. Chi-square goodness-of-fit analyses revealed a statistically significant association between improvement in parenting and reduction in adolescent drug use and behavior problems. Joanning et al. (1992[ii]) conducted a pretest–posttest comparison of the effectiveness of three models of adolescent drug abuse treatment: Family Systems Therapy (FST), Adolescent Group Therapy (AGT), and Family Drug Education (FDE). Families, consisting of at least one parent and one drug-abusing adolescent, were randomly assigned to FST (40), AGT (52), and FDE (42). Analyses were carried out when at least 23 families in each treatment condition had completed the intervention and been posttested immediately following treatment and 6 months later. Among families assigned to AGT, 29 adolescents dropped out of treatment, tending to do so early. Because only the adolescent was treated, families, especially parents, were not invested in or did not fully understand the treatment, were unwilling to bring their children to treatment, challenged the method of treatment, or refused to complete posttest assessments. A lower incidence of these problems was found with the other two treatment conditions. The findings suggest that FST may be helpful in limiting behavior related to adolescent drug use, and that AGT and FDE may not. The incidence of drug use and problem behaviors among adolescents receiving FST appeared to have dropped at posttest, and this reduction was significantly greater than among those receiving AGT and FDE. The three treatment conditions had virtually no impact on family functioning as assessed via traditional self-report measures. However, adolescents in all treatment conditions reported improved communication between themselves and their parents. However, these findings can only be indicative, because of several methodological weaknesses: There was no no-treatment control group; ratings of adolescent behavior were obtained from parents' and therapists' perceptions and were not a direct measure of drug use; different therapists conducted each of the three treatment conditions, possibly with differing degrees of competence; and the adolescent sample contained a mix of occasional and regular drug users whose outcomes were not analyzed separately.

The willingness of the adolescent and his or her family to cooperate with treatment will influence the approach to treatment. A randomized controlled trial of a strategy for engaging adolescent drug users and their families in therapy used a strategic, structural systems engagement intervention to overcome resistance, based on an identified pattern of interactions that interfere with entry into treatment (Szapocznik et al., 1988[i]). Among 108 Hispanic families, 93% of those receiving the intervention engaged with treatment, compared with 42% of controls, and 77% completed treatment, compared with 25% of controls. The ratings were carried out blind.

The British Paediatric Association (BPA) and Royal College of Physicians' (RCP) report, *Alcohol and the Young* (1995[vi]), stated that "at the present time, as far as we can ascertain, there are virtually *no* appropriate secondary care services for young people with alcohol and drug problems in the UK" (p. 50). A few residential treatment facilities exist, but the actual benefit of a containing environment in achieving beneficial outcomes has not been shown (Rosenthal, 1989[vi]). The BPA/RCP committee set out recommendations for services with regard to organization, assessment of young people, treatment approaches, and realistic outcomes, not confined to "cure."

The American Academy of Child and Adolescent Psychiatry (AACAP) has published *Practice Parameters for the Assessment and Treatment of Children and Adolescents with Substance Abuse Disorders* (1997b). This also stresses the importance of assessment for the presence of disorders and of the young person's problems, as well as the commonly found difficulties in carrying out detailed and comprehensive assessment with young people who tend to deny or minimize their problems.

A summary of the AACAP Practice Parameters (AACAP Work Group on Quality Issues, 1998[vi]) states that the primary goal for the treatment of adolescents with SUDs is achieving and maintaining abstinence from substance use. But although abstinence is the explicit long-term goal, it is important to recognize both the chronicity of SUDs in some adolescents and its self-limited nature in others; thus, there may be acceptable interim goals. However, "controlled" use of a substance of abuse should never be an explicit goal in the treatment of adolescents.

Community treatment includes programs such as school-based counseling and self-help groups, as well as prosocial organizations and recreational opportunities (e.g., sports, wilderness experiences) that offer supervised activities in a drug-free environment. These activities may augment outpatient treatment or follow long-term treatment in other settings to facilitate the adolescent's drug-free lifestyle.

Self-help groups are important adjuncts to the treatment of SUDs in adolescents. Referral to self-help groups is appropriate at all levels of care.

Comprehensive community-based treatments, such as multisystemic therapy (MST), may be an effective model for violent, chronic juvenile offenders and other youths with complex substance-related problems. Using social–ecological models of behavior, MST targets individual, family, peer, school, and community factors associated with substance use and other deviant behaviors. Studies of MST have shown reductions in substance use and other deviant behaviors (see Henggeler et al., 1998[vi], and Chapter 5 on conduct disorder).

Summary

A significant proportion of primary school children drink regularly. About 30% of 15-year-olds drink alcohol at least weekly, with between 2% and 7% of adolescent males reporting heavy drinking (and half this rate among adolescent girls). The rates increase with age, and there are pronounced differences in drinking patterns between girls and boys; from 12 years onward more boys than girls drink heavily. Almost a third of 15-year-olds have also experimented with illegal drugs. The use of heroin and cocaine is low, probably below 1%, but it is possibly used by some 2% of secondary school children in some localities in Britain. There seems to have been a large rise in all types of drug experimentation in the past decade.

Most illicit drug use among teenagers is experimental and short-term. A majority of adolescents will not sustain measurable long-term harm from transient and short-term use. Use of cigarettes and alcohol, and to a lesser extent cannabis, tends to be more protracted. Alcohol and drugs can affect all areas of functioning, and their use may be associated with accidental injury and death, as well as suicide and deliberate self-harm. Regular or heavy consumption during adolescence has a strong association with later alcohol and drug abuse; mental and physical problems; difficult family, social, and sexual relationships; and disruption of education and employment.

Family and peers are key influences on the likelihood of adolescent substance use and abuse. Nonstandard family structures, early childhood exposure to alcohol, and peers involved in substance use are associated with increased likelihood. Positive relations with parents act as protective factors for subsequent substance use. Young people rarely present simply as users of substances. There is very high comorbidity between problems with substance misuse and psychiatric disorders, the most common being depression, anxiety, and conduct disorders.

The primary goal of most treatment programs has been to achieve and maintain abstinence from substance use. Among the important characteristics of successful treatment programs are sufficient duration, intensiveness, and comprehensiveness; the presence of aftercare or follow-up treatment; sensitivity to the cultural, racial, and socioeconomic realities of adolescents and their families; family involvement; collaboration with social service agencies; promotion of prosocial activities and a drug-free lifestyle; and involvement in self-help groups.

Psychosocial treatments based on social learning theory and cognitive approaches appear to be more effective than no treatment or treatment as usual. Family therapy has been shown to be superior to other treatment modalities. Comprehensive community-based treatments such as MST, which combines these interventions, have been shown to be particularly efficacious in reducing substance abuse. The use of pharmacological agents in adolescents to counteract or decrease the subjective reinforcing effects of a substance or as aversion agents has received minimal attention in the literature.

The high prevalence of comorbid psychiatric disorders means that treatment may also be given for depression, ADHD, severe aggressive behavior, and anxiety disorders. Studies of adults suggest the efficacy of various agents, although there is little evidence relating to adolescents with SUD and comorbid psychiatric disorders.

Implications

The high prevalence of substance use problems in adolescence indicates a need for special services. This is further justified by the powerful associations of substance use with mental health problems and other health risks. Treatment centers should aim to offer comprehensive services of appropriate intensity for the disorder, have adequate provision for follow-up, and be integrated with the family, the community, and other service providers, in order to promote lifestyle change. Services should incorporate provision for family-based treatments, as well as strong community outreach, and be able to offer cognitive and social learning theory-based approaches. The development of skills in providing MST across services appears to us desirable. In light of the high comorbidity, substance use services should be integrated with other forms of psychiatric service provision.

11

Children with Physical Symptoms

This chapter covers a range of problems at the complex interface between psyche and soma. In recent years, interest in this area has led to the development of new subspecializations in health psychology and liaison psychiatry. Within these specializations are a number of distinct areas of clinical activity. This chapter reviews research on treatment interventions in three broad areas: children with physical symptoms with no identifiable cause; the management of pain and discomfort associated with physical illness; and the management of physical disorder using psychological techniques, including the prevention of adverse psychosocial sequelae of chronic physical disease.

The subject of children with physical symptoms for which there is no identifiable physical cause is a complex area that is distinguished by the almost complete lack of well-conducted research into either etiology or treatment, despite the regularity and frequency of attendance of such children in pediatric clinics. Much care must be taken in the psychological management of such children, as some will prove to have undetected organic disease. It is not always easy to decide in which group to place certain types of somatic complaint. In this chapter, headache, which as Garralda (1992) has pointed out, has better-established physiological concomitants and fewer psychological associations, has been included with other chronic illnesses and not with unexplained physical symptoms. Chronic fatigue syndromes have been included in the "unexplained" category. To some extent these are arbitrary decisions, which may prove incorrect as knowledge of the etiology of all of the conditions discussed in this chapter advances.

Irrespective of physical diagnosis, children with physical symptoms may experience pain and discomfort related either to their underlying conditions or to the investigative and treatment procedures employed in the management of their situations. As a result, there is a body of research concerning preparation of children for potentially painful procedures, as well as research into improving children's strategies for dealing with painful procedures. The second following section of this chapter addresses this work, which has tended to focus on pain management (e.g., coping with injections) irrespective of diagnostic group.

Children whose physical symptoms have clear and well-recognized organic causes, as in chronic illnesses such as asthma, diabetes, migraine, and cancer, are at significantly greater risk of developing psychiatric disorder. Psychosocial factors may be involved in precipitating the onset of such diseases or worsening their course by exacerbating existing symptoms or interfering with compliance with treatment regimes. Research in this area has tended to focus on ways in which the child, and less frequently, the family, can manage the illness better. Research has usually been carried out on children within specific diagnostic categories and, despite the recognized risk of psychiatric disorder, has focused on physical, but not psychological outcomes.

Only children with unexplained physical symptoms will meet criteria for recognized psychiatric disorders (somatization disorder, undifferentiated somatoform disorder, conversion disorder, pain disorder, and hypochondriasis). Children undergoing painful procedures or with chronic illness may have diagnosable psychiatric disorders, but the research presented here concerns either the psychological management of their physical symptoms or efforts to prevent the development of psychiatric disorder. Chronic physical illness is a general risk factor for psychiatric disorder, but does not predict particular types of disorder. The management of such disorders is likely to be easier if the treating clinician has a good working knowledge of the child's chronic illness and its management and works closely with the child's pediatrician. However, broadly speaking, psychiatric treatment is the same as for any child presenting with similar problems. The reader is therefore referred to the other relevant chapters in this volume.

PHYSICAL SYMPTOMS WITH NO IDENTIFIABLE PHYSICAL CAUSE

Children may exhibit a wide range of apparently inexplicable physical symptoms, from seemingly innocuous and rather vague aches and pains, to more severe paralyses and other neurological disturbances. The field has been well reviewed recently (Benjamin & Eminson, 1992; Campo & Fritsch, 1994; Fritz, Fritsch, & Hagino, 1997; Garralda, 1992; Garralda, 1996; Lask & Fosson, 1989), with all reviewers commenting on the lack of empirical research.

Definitions

Neither of the two major disease classification systems have specific diagnostic criteria for children and adolescents. Presumably due to a lack of child-based empirical research, adult definitions are applied to children. ICD-10 (World Health Organization, 1993) and DSM-IV (American Psychiatric Association, 1994) have very similar diagnostic groupings for unexplained physical symptomatology. Somatization disorder requires a range of physical symptoms (eight in DSM-IV, six in ICD-10) that cannot be explained by a known medical condition and are not feigned. These symptoms must cause distress and, in ICD-10, help seeking. ICD-10 also requires that the symptoms be present for at least 2 years and has a separate category—somatoform autonomic dysfunction—for symptoms primarily related to the autonomic nervous system. Undifferentiated somatoform disorder in both classifications refers to similar presentations but with fewer physical complaints. Pain disorder (DSM-IV) and somatoform pain disorder (ICD-10) describe the presentation of persistent pain in the absence of an adequate physiological explanation (although a painful physical condition may be present) where psychological factors are thought to be involved in the onset or maintenance of the pain. Hypochondriasis refers to a persistent, nondelusional belief that a physical illness is present. This belief causes significant distress and is not affected by medical reassurance that there is no such illness. DSM-IV includes a separate category of body dysmorphic disorder describing imagined defects in physical appearance. This is included within the ICD-10 category of hypochondriacal disorder. Finally, both classifications describe conversion disorders in which motor or sensory function is impaired, suggesting a neurological diagnosis, but in which there is no evidence of a physical diagnosis. DSM-IV requires that psychological factors be associated with the symptoms. ICD-10, which includes dissociative (conversion) disorders in a separate category from somatoform disorders along with other dissociative conditions, requires a convincing relationship in time between the onset of physical symptoms and psychological stressors.

Chronic fatigue syndromes are included in this section, although it is recognized that the etiology of these conditions is uncertain and controversial. Fatigue continuing after an apparent viral illness has long been recognized. Recently there has been an increase in interest in this area and an apparent increase in cases presenting to health services. Carter, Edwards, Kronenberger, Michalczyk, and Marshall (1995) recently described a series of children with chronic fatigue syndromes who scored highly on somatization and depression ratings. They concluded that psychological evaluation is warranted in chronic fatigue syndromes. There are consensus criteria for diagnosis from the U.S. Centers for Disease Control (Fukuda et al., 1994) and from Oxford (Sharpe et al., 1991). A Joint Working Group of the British Royal Colleges of Physicians, Psychiatrists and General Practitioners (1996) has recently comprehensively reviewed the available literature. In diagnostic terms, children with chronic fatigue would probably be diagnosed as having undifferentiated somatoform disorder, although within ICD-10 the criteria for neurasthenia would also seem to describe children with chronic fatigue.

Prevalence

Estimates of prevalence are difficult to interpret because of differing definitions of somatization, the different measures used, and the lack of information about children's concomitant physical status. The lack of appropriate child-centered diagnostic criteria is another factor. Offord et al. (1987), in a large-scale epidemiological survey of 3,294 children (Ontario Child Health Study, OCHS), found negligible rates of somatization in children under the age of 11 years.

More evidence is available for older children and adolescents. In 12- to 16-year-olds in the OCHS, 11% of girls and 5% of boys were identified as meeting

DSM-III-R criteria for somatization disorder (Offord et al., 1987). In a Finnish sample of more than 2,000 14- to 15-year-olds, Aro, Paronen, and Aro (1987) found 13% of girls and 6% of boys reporting frequent psychosomatic symptoms at all three separate assessments over an 18-month period. Garber, Walker, and Zeman (1991) sampled 540 children and adolescents and found that somatic symptom reporting increased with age and that girls reported substantially more symptoms than boys. The commonest symptoms were headache, low energy, sore muscles, nausea, stomach and back pains, blurred vision, and weakness. In the 2 weeks prior to completing a questionnaire, 15% reported four or more symptoms and 1%, 13 or more. Reporting of somatic symptoms was positively correlated with reports of anxiety and depression and negatively correlated with perceived self-competence. At the time of the study, 13 or more symptoms were required to fulfill the criteria for DSM-III-R diagnosis. This figure has been reduced to 8 symptoms in DSM-IV.

Eminson, Benjamin, Shortall, and Woods (1996) investigated 805 11- to 16-year-olds for lifetime prevalence of physical symptoms. Overall, 95% indicated that their health had been good for most of their lives. Symptom reporting increased with age, with girls having a median of 6 symptoms and boys, 5 symptoms; 10% of girls and 7% of boys had a lifetime prevalence of 13 or more symptoms. The most common symptoms were a lump in the throat (52%), dizziness (42%), heart pounding (40%), various aches and pains (joints, head, abdomen, chest: 30%), nausea (30%), blurred vision (26%), and a bad taste in the mouth (26%). There was an association between highly reported symptoms and attitudes to illness associated with mental distress, preoccupation with health, and fears about illness.

The aforementioned studies concern children in the community. In general practice there is evidence that psychological factors contribute to about one-fifth (17%) of children's attendances (Garralda & Bailey, 1987) and to nearly half (47%) of consultations in pediatric clinics (Garralda & Bailey, 1990).

Accurate estimations of prevalence of particular conditions are rare. Recurrent abdominal pain in 6-year-olds has been reported at around 25% in one epidemiological study (Faull & Nicol, 1986). Conversion disorders are reportedly very rare under the age of 5 years and unusual before 11 years of age (Goodyer, 1981[vi]).

Clinical Presentation

Children with unexplained physical symptoms may present with a variety of problems, ranging from seemingly straightforward recurrent abdominal pains and vague headaches to serious disturbances of neurological function—for example, disturbances of gait and motor function, sensory impairments, and pseudoseizures. Affected children, their families, and sometimes their pediatricians, see problems in terms of biological causes and explanations and are often reluctant to consider psychological/psychiatric explanations and referrals. As a result, children may have had symptoms for months or even years at the time of initial referral to mental health services. Families have often sought multiple investigations and assessments in an attempt to find a medical explanation for the problem. These investigations in themselves may have been harmful to the child. Some of these children are extremely disabled at the time of referral to mental health services and may have been absent from normal peer activities and education for weeks, months, or even years.

Garralda (1992) summarized a range of possible etiological factors associated with somatizing disorders generally. However, these factors are derived from anecdotal accounts and presentations of case series and are therefore of dubious validity. Garralda concludes that physical illnesses often precede or co-exist with such disorders. Associated psychiatric disorders are present in one-third to one-half of the children. Emotional disorders are more common than conduct problems. The children are often described as conscientious/obsessional or as sensitive, insecure, and anxious and may have difficulties with peer and social relationships. The children's families are often described as preoccupied with health issues. There is evidence that under stress, mothers consult medical practitioners more frequently about their children. Children with conversion disorders are often reported to have had a "model" available to them with similar symptoms (Grattan-Smith, Fairley, & Procopis, 1988[vi]). In a small minority there is evidence of major family dysfunction, with sexual abuse in particular being cited as a possible etiological factor.

Campo and Fritsch (1994) comment on the likelihood that somatization peaks in late childhood or early adolescence and that although recurrent abdominal pain is common in younger children, headache and limb pain become more frequent with increasing age. Sex ratios are about equal, with the exception of pseudoneurological symptoms, in which girls outnumber boys. They conclude that there is limited evidence for a substantial genetic contribution to the problem, despite the apparent clustering in families. Parents of children with somatization disorders may have more psychiatric symptoms and more physical symptoms than controls. The children themselves are more likely to have psychiatric disorders, particularly anxiety and panic disorders. Adverse life events, traumatic events such as abuse, and experience of physical illness seem to be associated with somatization. Campo and Fritsch also raise the possibility of the physician's role in maintaining somatization through needless overinvestigation. Case series of conversion disorder (e.g., Goodyer, 1981[vi]) also refer to the adverse effects of overinvestigation by pediatricians in maintaining or exacerbating symptoms, although reports of organic disease being mistaken for psychiatric disorder go some way toward explaining why clinicians may wish to continue to investigate (Rivinus, Jamison, & Graham, 1975).

Little is known of longer-term outcomes or of the natural history of children with somatizing disorders. Accurate prognosis is difficult, given the many differing criteria used for diagnosis in the studies cited. Some figures are available for the more severe conversion disorders. In Goodyer's (1981[vi]) series, 10 out of 13 (66%) were symptom free at 12 months and only 1 of the remaining 3 still had conversion symptoms. He notes that the children took about the same amount of time to recover, irrespective of length of illness before treatment commenced. Leslie (1988[vi]) states that 17 out of 20 (85%) children were symptom free within 3 months of treatment, but gives only a very sketchy outline of treatment. In Grattan-Smith's series (1988[vi]), 32 out of 52 (62%) had either completely recovered or improved noticeably at discharge. Goodyer and Mitchell (1989) followed up 93 children with somatic disorders. Children with pseudoseizures had the poorest outcome, with 40% unchanged since discharge. In contrast, 85% of all other presenting children were judged to have improved since discharge from psychiatric treatment.

Benjamin and Eminson (1992), in summarizing prognosis, note that the roots of much adult illness behavior seem to lie in childhood and family experiences, but that the best that can be said about the future of children with somatizing symptoms is that "many children do not suffer from them during the follow-up periods but others do and are also vulnerable to develop new symptoms." In adult populations, unexplained symptoms are "severe, persistent, and disabling, with considerable personal, social and healthcare costs" (Mayou & Sharpe, 1997, p. 561). Evidence is in shorter supply for children, but the reviews available also suggest that children with somatizing disorders are frequent utilizers of health care services.

Treatment

There are very few controlled trials of any form of treatment for somatization disorders in children. Those that do exist are for recurrent abdominal pain and are described in the following paragraphs. Some controlled studies have been carried out for fatigue syndromes, but these have been on largely adult populations. There are no methodologically adequate trials of treatment for conversion disorders, but numerous anecdotal accounts.

Recurrent Abdominal Pain

PHYSICAL THERAPIES

Feldman et al. (1985[i]) evaluated a physical treatment, namely, the use of dietary fiber, for recurrent abdominal pain (RAP). Fifty-two children, ages 5–15, were recruited from private physicians; they did not therefore constitute a representative sample. They had to have had at least one episode of pain per week for 2 months and no evidence of weight loss or organic disease to meet entry criteria. After baseline measurements, subjects were randomly allocated to receive fiber (10 g/day) or placebo cookies for 6 weeks. The design was double-blind and included checks on treatment compliance. Clinically significant improvement was set at a reduction in attacks of 50%. Significantly more of the treatment group met this criterion than the control group.

COGNITIVE-BEHAVIORAL THERAPIES

Sanders et al. (1989[i]; Sanders, Shepherd, Cleghorn, & Woolford, 1994[i]) have carried out a series of experiments to evaluate cognitive-behavioral treatments for RAP. In the first study (Sanders et al., 1989[i]), 16 children ages 6–12 years were randomly allocated to either a cognitive-behavioral intervention or a waiting-list control group. The intervention consisted of eight sessions for children and their mothers. Explanations of children's pain behaviors were presented and discussed with mothers. Parents were advised to ignore nonverbal pain behaviors and distract children into other activities that could then be praised. Children were taught progressive muscular relaxation and a cognitive coping strategy that included self-monitoring of pain, and given advice on making positive self-coping statements, self-distraction, and the use of relaxation. Both groups improved, but at 3-month follow-up, significantly more children in the intervention group were pain free. Children in the treated group responded more quickly than controls, and effects were more likely to generalize to the school setting.

In a further study (Sanders et al., 1994[i]) the authors comment on caregiving practices that may maintain or reinforce pain behavior in children. They cite sympathy and attention, expression of concern, and nurturance contingent on pain; external help seeking, expressions of anger or criticism; avoidance of nonpreferred activities; and parental modeling. This second study randomly allocated children to either a cognitive-behavioral family intervention or standard pediatric care. The intervention comprised six 50-minute sessions for children and parents and included an explanation of RAP and a rationale for treatment, contingency management training for parents, and self-management training for children. This study was methodologically stronger than the 1989 study. The sample was larger (44 children, ages 7–14 years) and included a longer follow-up period (12 months) because of the episodic nature of RAP. In addition, the control group received an intervention, albeit only 4–6 sessions of standard pediatric care providing general reassurance and care. Baseline measures were also taken of parental expectations, and this factor was controlled for in the subsequent analysis of results. Both interventions reduced pain (intensity and frequency), but children in the intervention group were significantly more likely to be pain free immediately posttreatment and at 6 months on self-report, and at 12 months on parental report. The intervention group also reported lower rates of relapse and less interference by pain in daily living at 12 months. These differences were not due to pretreatment differences in parental expectations. There was no evidence of symptom substitution; other symptoms decreased as the pain decreased. Active self-coping in the child and parenting likely to promote adaptive coping were predictors of pain behavior posttreatment as predicted.

BEHAVIORAL THERAPIES

No other significant studies of treatment of RAP have been found. However, a brief, uncontrolled evaluation of a behavioral treatment for toddler diarrhea (Furnell & Dutton, 1986[vi]) may be relevant, given the evidence that some children with RAP may have had longstanding physical complaints. Twenty-nine consecutively referred toddlers (mean age 22 months) were offered a behavioral intervention (mean length 2 months/six sessions) aimed at decreasing behavior difficulties generally, and therefore the child's overall levels of arousal. Sessions focused on discussion of parental anxiety, potential domestic and personal stress and attitudes toward parenting, in addition to providing practical advice about behavioral management. Overall, 20 of the 21 parents accepting treatment reported resolution of the diarrhea within 2 months, with concomitant decrease in other behavioral symptoms. Improvement was maintained at 6-month follow-up.

Conversion Disorders

No controlled studies of the treatment of conversion disorder in children exist, but there are numerous case series and studies in the literature. The sudden onset and variability of symptoms and presentation to physical health services, followed by variable patterns of investigation before referral to mental health services, have made the organization of randomized controlled trials of treatment particularly difficult. Early interest in psychodynamic models and treatments has given way to explanations that are rooted in social learning theory and that make use of concepts such as the sick role and abnormal illness behavior.

In the absence of controlled trials, all that can be reported is the advice of experts distilled from reports of case series. The management plans described have seeming face validity but are themselves based on a number of unproven assumptions—for example, that families should always be involved in treatment. There are a number of common features in the management programs described in recent case series (Dubowitz & Hersov, 1976[vi]; Goodyer, 1981[vi]; Grattan-Smith et al., 1988[vi]; Leslie, 1988[vi]; Thomson & Sills, 1988[vi]). These suggest that assessment and management should be carried out jointly by pediatricians and mental health professionals working closely together. Parents, and sometimes the whole family, should be closely involved; treatment should not focus just on the child. Liaison with schools is also seen as vital. Physical investigation must be thorough and prompt, and seen to be so by the family, but should cease once organic disease has been excluded. Reassurance concerning the absence of serious organic disorder should be followed by an explanation for the symptoms that acknowledges their reality but provides an alternative rationale to that of pure organic disorder—such explanations are commonly based on descriptions of "anxiety" or "tension." The treatment focus is thus on rehabilitation and improving function irrespective of the cause of dysfunction. An active program of physical rehabilitation with graded activity and reintroduction of normal behaviors, for example, school attendance, needs to be started as soon as practically possible. Many authors advocate physiotherapy as part of this program and as a means of providing an "escape with honor" for the child. Improvements are positively reinforced and illness behavior ignored as much as possible.

Chronic Fatigue Syndromes

Controlled evaluations of treatment for adults with chronic fatigue syndromes are starting to appear. There seems to be some evidence for the usefulness of graded aerobic exercise (Fulcher & White, 1997[i]) and cognitive-behavioral therapy (CBT) (Sharpe et al., 1996[i]). No controlled studies have been found evaluating treatment for children and young people. Therefore, as with conversion disorders, the advice of experts is presented here. Vereker (1992[vi]) describes a series of 10 consecutive cases of children, ages 10–16 years when referred to a child psychiatry clinic. Following exclusion of other organic disease, parents and children were reassured, their concerns and the seriousness of the situation acknowledged, and alternative explanations of symptomatology and rationales for treatment offered. An active rehabilitation program was started, with graded increases in activity in all areas of the child's life. Vereker comments on the importance of school attendance, even if not for the full school day, and the need for the child to avoid social isolation if at all possible. In 4 cases in which symptoms caused physical restriction and/or the child had been housebound for some time, admission to a pediatric ward was arranged to enable rehabilitation to proceed. In 4 cases in which parents were convinced that their child's illness was purely physical and that active rehabilitation would be harmful, they refused treatment. In all of the remaining cases, the rehabilitation regime brought about substantial improvements. Marcovitch (1997[vi]) also suggests that active rehabilitation will work in children. He emphasizes the crucial role that school can play and the need to draw up individualized rehabilitation plans. The broad principles of treatment as suggested by Vereker (1992[vi]) and Marcovitch (1997[vi]) are not dissimilar to the suggested treatment approaches for the management of conversion disorders.

Summary and Implications

The changing definitions of somatizing disorders and the lack of developmentally appropriate diagnostic criteria hamper the interpretation of the few research findings that exist. Somatizing disorders are commonly encountered in clinical practice and are often very disabling, with treatment involving high costs, but accurate data concerning prevalence, etiology, treatment, and prognosis are lacking. Physical treatment with dietary fiber may be effective in recurrent abdominal pain, but this finding needs replication. CBTs promoting active self-coping have been shown to be effective in the management of recurrent abdominal pain, but these findings also need replication.

No randomized controlled trials have investigated treatment of conversion disorders or chronic fatigue syndromes in children. Expert advice regarding the management of these conditions recommends techniques similar to the cognitive-behavioral approaches to recurrent abdominal pain, but these have not been systematically evaluated.

Developmentally appropriate diagnostic criteria for somatizing disorders are needed to facilitate further research. Further research into the treatment of these disorders is urgently needed to guide clinical practice.

PREPARATION FOR PAINFUL PROCEDURES

The development of children's understanding of pain, the measurement of pain, and the influence of the family have been reviewed by McGrath (1995[vi]). Memory for pain as evidenced by anticipatory fear is present from 6 months of age, and by 18 months children can recognize pain in others and utilize basic coping strategies such as seeking cuddles. Nevertheless, children under 5 years find it difficult to understand needle procedures, and younger children typically have more pain from needle procedures than older children. There are obvious difficulties in measuring pain, but reliable self-report measures exist and can be supplemented by observational methods and physiological methods. Yet there are problems with interpreting the findings: Is behavioral distress such as screaming a sign of pain or an indication of "active coping"? Self-report is difficult under the age of 5 years. The family may significantly influence children's experience of pain, with some types of pain tending to aggregate in families. Mechanisms are unclear, but there is support for the role of modeling (Osborne, Hatcher, & Richtsmeier, 1989) and reinforcement (Dunn-Geier, McGrath, Rourke, Latter, & D'Astous, 1986).

Treatment

Lansdown and Sokel (1993[vi]) review the literature on pain management and provide useful and practical advice for clinicians who have to help children prepare for, and cope with, painful procedures. Younger children tend to use passive rather than active means of relieving pain and rely on others, usually parents. Older children will use more active methods such as rubbing the affected part, but left to their own devices; children rarely develop self-initiated coping strategies (Gaffney & Dunne, 1986; Gaffney & Dunne, 1987). Lansdown and Sokel emphasize the importance of preparation, with information giving (both sensory and procedural); rehearsal, using play and drawing as well as role play; and modeling. Simple interventions include permission to make a noise and distraction. More complex interventions encourage the child to participate, increasing the child's sense of mastery and control, and utilize cognitive-behavioral techniques such as relaxation and the use of imagery and self-instruction.

Children need to undergo similar painful procedures for different diagnostic conditions. This section is organized into subsections concerning the procedures rather than clinical diagnoses. There has been considerable research into this area; only recent and well-conducted studies that have implications for practice are presented here.

Venipuncture and Injections

BEHAVIORAL THERAPIES

Even simple procedures such as venipuncture can produce high levels of distress in children (Humphrey, Boon, Linden Van den Heuvell, & Van de Wiel, 1992). Distraction is an effective treatment for pain and distress associated with venipuncture, particularly in younger children. Vessey, Carlson, and McGill (1994[i]) randomly allocated 100 children (mean age 7 years, 4 months) due for routine venipuncture, to either the standard procedure (comfort using touch and soft voices by nursing staff) or a simple distraction technique using a kaleidoscope. Younger children reported more pain and were observed in more distress, but irrespective of age, children in the distraction group reported significantly less pain and were observed to show less behavioral distress. Even in newborn infants, there are techniques to reduce behavioral distress. Campos (1994[i]) randomly allocated 60 newborns (mean age 51.5 hours) to one of three groups following a routine heelstick procedure: rocking at 30 cycles per minute, sitting on the experimenter's lap with a pacifier, and routine care (i.e., being placed in a crib and covered with a blanket). Observers blind to the hypotheses of the trial viewed videotapes of the children to check the reliability of ratings. Both rocking and the use of the pacifier reduced physiological measures of distress (heart rate) and crying, but the pacifier produced a sleeping baby (its removal provoked further arousal) whereas the rocking produced a calm, but alert, baby.

Rainwater, Sweet, Elliott, and Bowers (1988[vi]) used systematic desensitization for treating needle phobias in 26 children (ages 7–20 years) with diabetes. Although this was not a randomized trial or even a suitable single-case design, the authors did use a standardized treatment protocol and achieved a very high success rate. Only 1 child failed to complete treatment (due to transport problems), and in the remaining 25 children, 35 of the 38 reported fear responses were successfully treated, with improvements maintained at 1-year follow-up. This seemingly cost-effective intervention required an average of 2–4 sessions, depending on the skill of the clinician (student therapists required more sessions).

COGNITIVE-BEHAVIORAL THERAPIES

In older children, cognitive-behavioral packages have been used to reduce anticipatory fear during self-administered insulin injections. Moore, Geffken, and Royal (1995[iib]) describe an intervention in two girls, ages 11 and 13 years. The package consisted of breathing exercises before and during injections, watching a short video of a peer self-injecting without obvious pain or anxiety prior to injections, pacing (counting slowly out loud as a distraction during injections), and positive reinforcement for using these methods. An ABAB, single-case design was used. The package substantially reduced the time needed for injections and the behaviors indicative of distress, with a return to longer times and more distress when the package was not used.

Bauchner, Vinci, and Ariane (1994) interviewed 91 school-age children (mean age 10.2 years) and 111 adolescents (mean age 14.4 years). Of the school-age children, 83% wanted parents present during a painful procedure, but so did 47% of the adolescents. Bauchner et al. (1994) describe a series of three studies in an emergency department. In the first, 78% of 250 parents wanted to be present if their child needed blood drawn. In the second, only 60% of 50 parents of infants (mean age 12 months) actually stayed during venipuncture or cannulation. Less than half of the parents who stayed had been asked to stay, and 38% of those who did not stay had been asked to leave by the child's doctor. Finally, Bauchner et al. randomized 300 parents of children under 3 years to three conditions: present and taught a specific intervention, present but given no specific instructions, and not present during a procedure. The purpose of this study was to evaluate how easily parents could be taught a simple intervention consisting of comfort using touch, and distracting talk. Parents in the intervention group learned the intervention easily, found it helpful, and reported high levels of satisfaction with care. Levels of children's distress were not reported.

Parents may not always be helpful for children undergoing painful procedures. Parental agitation, reassurance, and apologies to the child may precede child distress during painful procedures (Blount et al., 1989; Bush & Cockrell, 1987). To examine the differential effects of parental behavior on children, Gonzalez, Routh, and Armstrong (1993[i]) recruited 42 parent–child dyads in which the child (age 3–7 years) was due for a routine intramuscular injection, and randomly assigned them to three conditions: parental reassurance, parental distraction (nonprocedural talk), and control (no specific advice). Mothers in the first two groups were given oral instructions, watched a videotape, and had an opportunity to practice their distracting or reassuring strategies with a research assistant. Mothers in these groups were prompted to continue with their strategy while the child was having the injection. Subsequent rating of the mothers' behaviors by blind raters confirmed that they used predominantly reassuring or distracting strategies. Mothers in the control group used both strategies but to a much lesser degree. Child self-reports of distress were similar across all three groups, but ratings by observers blind to group assignment indicated significant reduction in behavioral correlates of distress in the distraction group as compared with the reassurance and control groups.

Manne, Bakeman, Jacobsen, Gorfinkle, and Redd (1994[i]) also examined the involvement of parents during painful procedures and looked at other factors influencing the success or otherwise of distraction techniques. They recruited 36 children (mean age 5 years, 3 months) with cancer and due for routine venipuncture. The children and parents were then randomly allocated to two groups, both of which were to use a simple distraction technique. In one group, parents were instructed to coach the child in the technique (paced breathing using a party blower) and to praise child cooperation. In the other, nurses were instructed to assist the parent in coaching the child. Training for parents consisted of a 10-minute session, with parent and child, prior to venipuncture and involved oral instruction, modeling, and role play. Nurses had a 1-hour training session including a theoretical overview, oral instructions, video demonstrations, and role play. Parents carried out the instructions given and were more likely to get the child to use the distraction technique than were nurses. Use of the technique was associated with less crying during the procedure. Specific prompts about use of the blower were more effective than general encouragement. Older age and less initial distress also predicted more blower use and less subsequent distress. The role of the nurses was difficult to evaluate, as they did not follow instructions. Nurses in both groups did some coaching but were as likely to coach the child directly as to coach the parent in helping the child.

Bone Marrow Aspiration and Lumbar Punctures

COGNITIVE-BEHAVIORAL THERAPIES

Ellis and Spanos (1994[vi]) review cognitive-behavioral interventions for children's distress during bone marrow aspirations (BMA) and lumbar punctures (LP). They quote the Consensus Conference on Management of Childhood Cancer Pain, which said that childhood pain is not managed effectively and recommended that in children over 5 years, individualized packages should utilize both behavioral and pharmacological interventions either alone or in combination (Zeltzer et al., 1990[vi]). Jay et al. (1985[iia]) describe the development and evaluation of a cognitive-behavioral intervention for BMA or LP. The intervention involved breathing exercises and positive imagery techniques, watching filmed models, behavioral rehearsal, and positive reinforcement. Parents were present during the procedure and encouraged to coach the child in using the techniques. Five cases are presented, using a multiple baseline and a single-case design, and conclusions are drawn about the possible efficacy of the intervention. A repeated measures, counterbalanced design (i.e., where all children received all three interventions but in different orders) was then used to evaluate the intervention further in comparison with a pharmacological intervention (Valium) and a minimum treatment–attention control condition. The study included 73 children (ages 3–13 years), 56 of whom completed all three intervention conditions (Jay et al., 1987[i]). Children in the intervention group had significantly lower pain ratings, behavioral distress, and pulse and blood pressure measures, than either of the other two groups. However, as Ellis and Spanos (1994[vi]) point out, these results were for overall ratings of the entire procedure. When broken down into component phases, there were not always significant between-group differences for each phase of the procedure. This highlights a problem with interpreting such research—namely, the possibility that different interventions may be more effective for different phases of painful procedures, for example, anticipatory distress and the actual encounter. Further evidence of this problem is found in another study (Jay, Elliott, Fitzgibbons, Woody, & Siegel, 1995[i]), which compares this intervention with general anaesthesia. Eighteen children (mean age 6 years) were randomly allocated to either the cognitive-behavioral intervention (CBT) described earlier or to a general anesthetic (GA). Observational and self-report measures were used and indicated that although there was more observed behavioral distress in the first minute of the procedure for the CBT group, there were more 24-hour postprocedure behavioral adjustment problems reported by parents in the GA group. There were no differences in the self-reported pain, fear, or pulse rates between the two groups, or differences in anticipation of the next BMA. Parent preferences and stress levels were similar in each group, and it was not possible to predict which children would prefer which intervention. The CBT intervention did, however, take up considerably less time and may therefore be more cost-effective.

Kazak et al. (1996[i]) note that many studies evaluate CBT as an alternative to pharmacological interventions and report on a randomized controlled study comparing drugs only with a combination of drugs and CBT techniques. The study involved 92 children, with newly diagnosed leukemia and due to undergo BMA or LP, and samples were stratified by age (mean age 5 years). The psychological component of the intervention was developed collaboratively with parents, who were trained to assume a primary role in coaching children in the use of age-appropriate distraction, guided imagery, and relaxation techniques.

Mothers and nurses reported lower ratings of child distress in the combined intervention group as compared with the drug-only group, but no significant differences were found on other measures—for example, parent distress and quality of life. Staff could not be blind to the interventions offered, but attempts were made to inform staff about the project in a way that gave equal weight to the possible advantages of each method. Younger children, as expected, showed less anticipatory distress but more distress during the procedure, irrespective of intervention offered.

HYPNOTIC INTERVENTIONS

Hypnotic techniques offer an alternative to cognitive-behavioral methods for distress during painful procedures. Ellis and Spanos (1994[vi]) and Genius (1995[vi]) have reviewed these. Ellis and Spanos highlight some of the theoretical controversies surrounding hypnosis, most important of which concerns the failure to identify physiological or behavioral markers that accurately reflect a hypnotic state. There are no standardized procedures in clinical hypnosis, which further hampers effective evaluation. Many of the techniques described—for example, the use of guided imagery—seem very similar to aspects of the cognitive-behavioral packages described earlier. Nevertheless, techniques described as hypnotic have been shown to be effective in pain reduction. Zeltzer and LeBaron (1982[i]) randomly allocated 33 children (mean age 10 years), due to undergo BMA and/or LP, to one of two conditions: deep breathing, distraction, and practice (nonhypnosis) and therapist-assisted guided imagery (hypnosis). Both interventions reduced pain during BMA and LP, but the "hypnosis" produced significantly greater effects. Wall and Womack (1989[i]) also randomly allocated 20 children (age range 5–18 years), due to undergo BMA or LP, to two conditions: hypnosis with a standard induction procedure followed by relaxation, and visual imagery with a self-chosen distraction procedure. Both interventions were effective in reducing pain, but there were no significant between-group differences.

Burns

There are fewer studies investigating other forms of painful procedure than there are studies of the procedures already discussed. Kavanagh (1983[ii]) describes a small study in which cognitive-behavioral techniques were used to alleviate distress during the changing of dressings for burn patients. Consecutive admissions to a burn unit received a standard intervention (nursing control and use of distraction) for a period of time, after which new admissions received an experimental approach emphasizing predictability and mastery, and which involved the child more. Numbers were small (nine in total), but the children receiving the experimental approach did show significantly less maladaptive behavior in the first 2 weeks of hospitalization and less depression at discharge. There were many methodological problems, but most tended to reduce the power to detect group differences, suggesting that this approach merits further evaluation.

Chemotherapy

Hypnosis has been used to reduce the distress, and nausea and vomiting, associated with chemotherapy for cancer patients. This is a serious problem, and in some pediatric samples is associated with 30–60% noncompliance with oral chemotherapy. Zeltzer, Dolgin, LeBaron, and LeBaron (1991[i]) randomly allocated 54 children (ages 5–17 years) to one of three conditions: hypnosis, support (cognitive distraction and relaxation), and an attention control. Hypnosis consisted of therapist-assisted guided positive imagery. The hypnosis group showed a significantly greater reduction in somatic symptoms associated with chemotherapy than either of the other two groups. The distraction/support group stayed about the same, whereas the attention control group got worse over time. None of the interventions had any significant impact on the functional variables measured, such as school attendance or behavior. Jacknow, Tschann, Link, and Boyce (1994[i]) also investigated hypnosis for chemotherapy-related nausea and vomiting, using a randomized controlled, single-blind design. Twenty children (mean age 12 years) were allocated to either a hypnosis intervention (using medication only when required as a supplement) or a medication-based regime to combat side effects. Although the two groups did not differ in nausea and vomiting at subsequent chemotherapy, the group treated with hypnosis did use less medication and have significantly less anticipatory nausea and vomiting.

Summary and Implications

Even common and simple procedures such as venipuncture can produce significant distress in children. Research in this area is made difficult by the problems of measuring pain and the responses to it, particularly in younger children. Most studies investigate only symptomatic relief, but it is encouraging to see the emergence of studies using randomized, controlled designs to investigate the underlying mechanisms of action of different interventions.

Simple behavioral interventions, such as rocking in newborns and distraction in younger children, are effective in reducing distress. In older children, cognitive-behavioral strategies that promote more active coping and give the child a sense of mastery and predictability have been repeatedly shown to be very effective in reducing procedural distress. Cognitive-behavioral interventions may also be effective as an adjunct to pharmacological treatments.

Parental presence may help reduce procedural distress if parents can be coached to promote distraction and/or active coping, but may increase distress if parents are agitated or uncertain. Interventions should therefore usually involve parents, not just children. Yet there is evidence that parents are often not invited to be present during painful procedures, let alone involved in their management.

Hypnotic interventions are difficult to define and have much in common with cognitive-behavioral interventions that incorporate relaxation training. Most studies have not been well designed, but there is some evidence that these approaches can be effective in reducing procedural pain and the somatic symptoms associated with chemotherapy.

Different interventions may be more effective for different phases of painful procedures. For example, GA may eliminate all observed distress during a procedure, but is less effective than CBT at reducing postprocedural distress. Different coping strategies may be more useful for some children than others. Interventions should involve parents who can support the child's use of coping strategies, but if the parents are too distressed by this, then it is helpful to designate a member of staff to take this role. It is likely that interventions need to be fitted to particular types or stages of procedure as well as to particular individuals, and that multimodal interventions are often appropriate. Further research is urgently needed to inform this process.

CHILDREN WITH CHRONIC ILLNESS

Prevalence

Chronic illness and disability are common in children and adolescents. One of the best recent epidemiological studies is the OCHS (Boyle et al., 1987). Cadman et al. (1987) report on the questionnaire responses concerning 3,294 children ages 4–16 years, from a representative, stratified sample of 1,869 Ontario families. Overall, 1.9% had a chronic limitation of function (limited in activity, mobility, self-care, or social role for more than 6 months) without having a chronic illness or medical condition; 14% of children had a chronic illness without limitation of function, and 3.7% had both a chronic illness and limitation of function. In all, 19.6% of children had either limited function, chronic illness, or both—a finding that fits with other studies of the prevalence of chronic illness in child populations. These chronic health problems were slightly more common in boys, in older children, and in the two lowest quintiles of family income. Children with chronic health problems were also much higher users of mental health and social services.

Psychosocial Impact of Chronic Illness

Children with chronic health problems are more likely to have psychiatric disorder. Rutter et al. (1970b) found that the risk of psychiatric disorder doubled if chronic illness was present, and increased by a factor of 5 if the chronic illness involved the central nervous system. In the OCHS, 14.1% of healthy children had psychiatric disorder, as compared with 23.4% of those with chronic illness (odds ratio 2.1) and 32.6% of those with chronic illness and limitation of function (odds ratio 3.4) (Cadman et al., 1986). Lavigne and Faier-Routman (1992) concluded from a meta-analysis of 87 studies that children with physical disorders show increased risk for overall adjustment problems and may show more internalizing problems. They also concluded that children with physical disorders had significantly lower self-concepts.

Chronic illness in childhood can impact significantly on family members. Sabbeth and Leventhal (1984) reviewed the literature on marital adjustment in parents of chronically ill children. Rates of divorce were no higher than in control groups, but marital distress was higher, suggesting that parents may stay together despite the increased disharmony linked with childhood illness. However, most of this evidence comes from cross-sectional studies. One study that followed up, prospectively, mothers of newly diagnosed children with diabetes found that they had only a short period of self-resolving depression after diagnosis and then seemed to be reasonably well adjusted. Maternal emotional distress was associated not with medical aspects of the disease, but with how bothersome and difficult they found its management, and was predicted by maternal distress immediately after diagnosis (Kovacs et al., 1990). There is some evidence for increased risks of behavioral and emotional disturbance in the siblings of chronically ill children (Garrison & McQuiston, 1989).

Pless and Nolan (1991) favor a noncategorical approach, suggesting that similarities of experience for children with chronic illness outweigh the differences due to particular diagnoses. While acknowledging that diseases affecting the neurological or sensory systems may lead to greater levels of problems, they identify a range of risk factors for psychosocial dysfunction that cross diagnostic boundaries, including severity, visibility, predictability, age of onset and duration, and pattern of medical care. Patterson and Blum (1996) have also reviewed the literature and enumerated risk and protective factors for adverse psychosocial outcomes. They identified disease factors (invisibility, remitting–relenting course, and uncertainty all predict greater risk), child factors (male gender, temperament, and low intelligence predict greater risk), family factors (clear boundaries and cohesiveness protect from risk), and community factors (family involvement with informal support networks predicts lower risk) as the key variables.

Little is known about the longer-term psychosocial sequelae of chronic illness. Pless, Cripps, Davies, and Wadsworth (1989) report on the findings from follow-up of a representative birth cohort at 15, 26, and 36 years. At 26, young adults with experience of chronic illness had been treated medically for emotional disorders significantly more than had healthy members of a comparison group. At 36, all cohort members were interviewed with the use of the Present State Examination, a standardized diagnostic interview. Women who had experienced chronic illness in childhood were significantly more likely to have higher scores. This study also revealed that children with chronic illness from lower social groups had reduced life chances (educational achievement, employment opportunities) as compared with similarly ill children from higher social groups. Pless, Power, and Peckham (1993) followed up another national birth cohort until the age of 23, when all subjects were interviewed; methods and outcome measures were more sophisticated than in the earlier study. Men with experience of chronic physical illness had significantly higher relative risks for abnormal scores on the Malaise Inventory, specialist psychological care, poor educational qualifications, periods of unemployment, and poor socialization. These studies provide some support for the notion that adverse psychosocial effects of chronic illness may continue past childhood and into adulthood.

Treatment

An increasing number of intervention studies are being reported concerning children with chronic illness and their families. Helping children and their families to cope with chronic illness is a complex task that requires the clinician to understand something of the child's and family's beliefs, attitudes and knowledge about the illness, and its treatment and outcome. Kibby, Tyc, and Mulhern (1998[ib]) have conducted the only meta-analysis of psychological interventions for children and adolescents with chronic medical conditions. Forty-two studies published between 1990 and 1995 met their inclusion criteria, predominantly behavioral and cognitive-behavioral interventions targeted at either disease management, or less commonly, at reducing the emotional distress associated with disease. They included some studies without control groups and report a mean effect size (ES) for interventions of 1.12 and evidence that in those studies that included follow-up (only 22%), benefits were maintained over time. Treatment often requires major behavioral changes. It is therefore not surprising that the majority of reported studies in this field use cognitive and behavioral techniques, emphasizing the need to change patterns of thinking and behaving. Such interventions are often time-limited and relatively easy to describe and standardize, as compared with individual psychodynamic and systemic therapies, providing another reason that there may be fewer of these latter studies in the literature. We describe some of the more methodologically sound studies that attempt to explore these issues. Where a large number of studies have been published in a specific area, presentation has been biased toward those with particular clinical implications.

Asthma

Asthma is now one of the major common chronic diseases in industrialized countries and is the most common chronic disease of childhood. A recent self-report survey of 12- to 14-year-olds in Great Britain found a prevalence of 21%, including those ever having had a diagnosis of asthma (Kaur et al., 1998). Asthma accounts for up to 2,000 deaths a year in England and Wales. Morbidity has risen over the last two decades. The existing effective treatments involve the regular use of inhalers and the avoidance of precipitants such as allergens. Compliance with management strategies is not always complete.

COGNITIVE-BEHAVIORAL THERAPIES

Lehrer, Sargunaraj, and Hochron (1992[vi]) have reviewed and categorized psychological treatment approaches in asthma into three broad groups: multicomponent psychoeducational programs (discussed later), interventions aimed specifically at stress reduction (usually relaxation and biofeedback), and family therapy approaches. Psychoeducational programs usually go beyond the mere imparting of knowledge. Evans and Mellins (1991[vi]) reviewed educational programs and described the typical components of such packages. They usually provide extensive learning opportunities for child and family (typically four to eight 1-hour sessions), share similar curricula, and develop active partnerships with clinic staff. The curricula in such programs commonly include information about the etiology and treatment of asthma, early recognition of attacks and prompt initiation of treatment, the importance of remaining calm, recognition of the need for emergency care, identification and recognition of potential triggers and reduction of exposure to them, normalization of home and school activities, dealing with peer problems, and communicating effectively with family and professionals. Active teaching of problem-solving strategies is often included, as are components aimed at relaxation and stress reduction.

Lewis, Rachelefsky, Lewis, de la Sota, and Kaplan (1984[i]) report an early evaluation of one such program: Asthma Care Training (ACT) for Kids. Sixty-five children with severe asthma, ages 7–12 years, were randomly assigned to either an intervention group or a control treatment consisting of three 1½-hour educational sessions (delivered to groups of 10–12 families). The intervention consisted of five 1-hour sessions, delivered to children and parents in separate groups (coming together for the last 15 minutes of each session), and was aimed at increasing active decision making by the family in relation to asthma care. Sessions covered knowledge of asthma, environmental control of triggers, medication, decision making, and "balanced living." Raters interviewed the family on the telephone at 3, 6, and 12 months and spoke to parents and children separately, but were not blind to group status. One year after the intervention there was no difference in knowledge between the two groups, but parental reports of child dependence and trouble with asthma in the preceding 3 months were significantly reduced in the intervention group. In addition, children in the intervention group had made fewer emergency room visits and been hospitalized less because of asthma than those in the control group. Qualitative data from the study suggested that intervention group families reported better communication within the family. The authors suggested that the program was not only clinically effective but also cost-effective, with the savings from reduced hospitalization and emergency visits far outweighing the costs of delivering the intervention. However, there are significant flaws in the study, particularly regarding the means of collecting data at follow-up.

Other studies evaluating psychoeducational interventions are similar. Lehrer et al. (1992[vi]) in their review conclude that psychoeducational approaches produce increased medication compliance, greater perceived self-competence in managing symptoms, and decreased use of medical services, despite the fact that most studies have been carried out on small, unrepresentative populations, resulted in high dropout rates, and do not seem to devote enough time to training children in the more effective behavioral change techniques.

Other ways of delivering educational programs are being explored. Taggart et al. (1991[vi]) describe a self-management program delivered to 40 6- to 12-year-old children while they were in the hospital following admission for asthma. The program is brief and has three components. First, written and play materials for children and parents cover the nature of asthma, recognition of and avoidance of potential triggers, the need to acknowledge feelings associated with asthma, and information about treatments. Second, a 10-minute videotape presents three strategies for self-management: recognition and avoidance of triggers, recognition of early signs, and early treatment. Another videotape uses puppets to present some of the feelings associated with asthma and some of the restrictions imposed by the illness. This is used to facilitate group discussion. Finally, the written and video material is discussed in a 15–30-minute session with the nurse. A randomized, controlled evaluation was not deemed possible in the acute setting. Instead, children were used as their own controls, and comparisons were made of data collected before and after the intervention. Data were collected at admission and by telephone 3 months later by interviewers who were not blind to group status. The program significantly increased children's knowledge, expected responses to early warning signs of asthma (the children were better able to identify early warning signs and take appropriate steps) and internal locus of control (they felt they had more personal control over their illness).

Computerized educational programs are also being developed. Given the power and availability of modern computers, these should be capable of delivering standardized packages with the necessary degree of interaction required for some of the behavior change techniques, but these packages have not yet been systematically evaluated. Rubin et al. (1986[i]) report an evaluation of a basic educational package, delivered by computer to children with asthma. Sixty-five children, ages 7–12 years, were randomly allocated to the educational package or to playing computer games for an equivalent length of time. Unsurprisingly, the group that received the educational package showed significantly more knowledge than the control group. This study at least demonstrated the acceptability of such methods in children and paved the way for further work.

Colland (1993[i]) carried out a large randomized, controlled trial of a multifaceted self-management program for children with asthma. The intervention comprised 10 weekly group sessions (6–8 per group) lasting 1 hour each. It aimed to increase knowledge, acceptance of illness and treatment, self-efficacy, and the use of appropriate self-management techniques. This study is especially important because of a number of methodological strengths not present in other evaluations of CBT in asthma. Numbers were relatively large: 112 children, ages 8–13, who met the agreed-upon eligibility criteria, and who were recruited from six clinics around the country in an attempt to gain a more representative sample from which to generalize. The study focused on children in a particular age range; the program materials were designed to be appropriate for children at this developmental level. Moreover, the study looked only at children who were having difficulties with asthma management as defined by scores on a standardized test of asthma coping. Subjects were allocated to three groups: intervention, information control, and no treatment. Measures were taken after treatment and at 6- and 12-month follow-up. Children in the intervention group improved significantly on both psychological and medical out-come variables at posttreatment and 6 months after treatment, as compared with either of the two control groups. Children who had received the intervention also had more knowledge of asthma and less state anxiety posttreatment, but only knowledge remained significantly improved 6 months later. Only minimal informa-tion is given about results at 12-month follow-up, but it is suggested that improve-ments were maintained. There were no dropouts from the program, suggesting high user acceptability.

Evans et al. (1999[i]) randomly allocated 1,033 children from inner cities, ages 5–11 years, with moderate to severe asthma, to standard care with or without an educational intervention. The intervention comprised two group sessions for asthma education and one individual session for the children's caretakers within 2 months of baseline measures. The sessions covered asthma triggers and environ-mental control, as well as problem-solving and communication strategies, and were delivered by asthma counselors (master's-level social workers), who then visited caretakers at least every 2 months, with telephone contact in the alternate months, for a period of 1 year. The exact number and length of the contacts and the content of individual sessions were tailored to the families' needs, based on scores on the Asthma Risk Assessment Tool. Families were contacted every 2 months and asked to recall the number of symptom days (wheeze, loss of sleep, or reduction in play caused by asthma) in the preceding 2 weeks. Subjects had significantly fewer symp-tom days than controls and were hospitalized less. These improvements were main-tained during the 1-year follow-up period. This study incorporates the cognitive behavioral as well as educational elements of psychoeducational programs into the routine clinical care of a large number of children in deprived inner-city areas. The intervention was of low intensity and yet appears to be effective; it therefore has considerable implications for routine service delivery.

Lehrer et al.'s (1992[vi]) second group of interventions concerned relaxation and stress management. They reported that a number of studies of progressive mus-cular relaxation had shown statistically significant increased pulmonary function, although not always achieving clinical significance. Vasquez and Buceta (1993a, 1993b, 1993c [ii]) describe an attempt to evaluate the effectiveness of the relax-ation component of self-management programs. Twenty-seven children (ages 8–13) with light to moderate asthma were allocated to three groups, matched with re-spect to age, sex, and severity of asthma. The first group took part in an asthma self-management program (six 1-hour sessions comprising education, identification of triggers, and encouragement to comply), the second received this program plus re-laxation training, and the third was a no-treatment control. Baseline measures and ratings at 6 and 12 months were by self-report. The self-management program in-creased the frequency of asthma care behavior, but no significant changes were ob-served in clinical or pulmonary function variables. However, when the comparison was restricted to subjects displaying a low level of self-care practices, the self-man-agement program proved to be effective in reducing attack duration, negative con-sequences of asthma for the child, and the level of therapeutic response to attacks.

Adding the relaxation technique to the self-management program did not im-prove the treatment's efficacy. However, state anxiety and spirometric data for both treatment groups, obtained before and after each session with the therapist, showed that relaxation reduced state anxiety while not modifying basal spirometric values. Further analysis of the data indicated that attack duration decreased significantly in those patients whose attacks were precipitated by emotional triggers and who received the self-management plus relaxation intervention, and their peak expiratory flow rate improved as compared with that of patients in all other groups. This small study had no credible attention control, and it is unclear whether subjects were randomly allocated. Nevertheless, it illustrates the need to look beyond simple group differences and investigate to ascertain which children are likely to respond to which components of particular interventions.

Relaxation may influence asthma in a number of ways. There is some evidence that the use of electromyographic biofeedback to reduce facial muscle tension is associated with improved pulmonary function in the short term. Kotses et al. (1991[i]) randomly allocated 33 children with asthma, ages 7–16, to two regimes, one designed to reduce facial muscle tension and the other to keep it stable. Baseline measures were taken, followed by 8 weeks of training (weekly sessions lasting 20 minutes), during which children were encouraged to practice exercises at home. Those children who had training to reduce facial tension did indeed achieve this objective. At 5-months follow-up they also showed significantly improved pulmonary function, decreased anxiety, and increased positive attitudes toward asthma.

Although the Colland (1993[i]) study included psychological outcome measures, only one methodologically sound study has sought specifically to investigate the impact of psychoeducational and stress reduction packages on children's psychological status as opposed to their physical condition. In this important study, Perrin, MacLean, Gortmaker, and Asher (1992[i]) randomly allocated 81 children with asthma ages 6–14, to two groups. The subjects were nonrepresentative recruits from community pediatric practice. They were mostly white and middle class. The intervention group received a combined education and stress management program (four 2-hour sessions comprising education about asthma for the parents and child, and stress management training for the child alone). The stress management component consisted of sessions on relaxation, contingency coping, and problem solving. The second group included waiting-list controls and received no treatment. Only 56 of the 81 subjects completed the study, but these 56 were not significantly different on baseline measures from the dropouts. The intervention brought about a significant decrease in total behavior and internalizing scores on the Child Behavior Checklist (CBCL) and an increase in the child's involvement in chores around the house and in daily activities. There was no association between the children's scores on knowledge of asthma and their psychological status. The increased risk of psychological problems in children with asthma may be linked to difficulties in coping with their experience of negative life events (MacLean, Perrin, Gortmaker, & Pierre, 1992). After the intervention, there was no longer an association between the experience of negative life events and CBCL scores in the intervention group. Such an association still existed in the control group, suggesting that the intervention may have reduced psychological dysfunction by enabling the child to cope better with adverse life events.

FAMILY AND SYSTEMIC THERAPIES

There has been interest in family and systemic treatments for children with chronic illness for many years since Liebman, Minuchin, and Baker's (1974[vi]) description of the use of structural family therapy in treating intractable asthma. This influential paper describes earlier work on asthma concerning the separation of the child from the parents, and characterizes families who respond poorly to their child's asthma as intrusive, overinvolved, overprotective, and conflict avoiding. Seven cases of effective family therapy are described. Few controlled trials have explored these suggestions further. Lask and Matthew (1979[i]) randomly allocated 33 families (with 37 children, ages 4–14) to six sessions of family therapy over 4 months, or to a no-treatment control condition. The children had relatively severe asthma, but it is unclear how they were recruited. Few details of the therapeutic intervention are given. At 1-year follow-up, children in the experimental group had significantly improved scores on some, but not all, measures of respiratory function (thoracic gas volume and daily wheeze scores). No rating was made of either individual child or family psychological function. Gustafsson et al. (Gustafsson, Kjellman, & Cederblad, 1986[i]) also randomly allocated children with the most severe cases of asthma, attending a large pediatric outpatient department, to either family therapy sessions or to a no-treatment control condition. Numbers were small (of the 20 most severe cases, only 17 children were randomly allocated to one of the two conditions), and there is only a brief description of the intervention, which lasted up to 8 months but with the number of sessions ranging from 2 to 21. Nevertheless, the experimental group improved significantly in general pediatric assessment, peak expiratory flow, medication usage, and daily functioning.

Diabetes

Diabetes mellitus affects 1–3% of the population. About 25% of sufferers have the insulin-dependent type (IDDM). IDDM is one of the most common endocrine disorders of childhood, with 1 in 800 children affected. Successful management involves once or twice daily injections of insulin, regular testing of blood and urine, and strict dietary control. Sufferers have to live with the knowledge that the disease carries with it the risk of serious long-term complications such as myocardial infarction, gangrene, renal failure, and blindness, and that life expectancy is reduced. There is evidence that maintenance of very good blood glucose control can significantly reduce the risks of long-term complications of the illness.

COGNITIVE-BEHAVIORAL THERAPIES

Boardway, Delamater, Tomakowsky, and Gutai (1993[i]) evaluated the effects of stress management training for adolescents (12–17 years) with a history of poor control of their diabetes. Subjects were randomly assigned to either a stress management intervention or to a no-treatment control group. The intervention consisted of 13 group sessions over 6 months, covering the identification of stressful situations associated with diabetes and the management of these situations using a prob-lem-solving approach. Role play, modeling, and discussion were used in the group to promote effective problem solving. Numbers were small, with only one interven-tion group (9 subjects) and one control group (10 subjects); these represented only about half of the adolescents identified who fitted the original inclusion criteria. Diabetes-specific stress was reduced significantly in the intervention group and was maintained at 3-month follow-up, but metabolic control, regimen adherence, self-efficacy, and general coping styles were unchanged. Like many studies in this field, the focus of this study was too narrow: there is evidence of change in the targeted outcome measures, but not enough clinically relevant outcomes were targeted.

The same research team have also reported on an intervention designed to pro-mote self-management of diabetes (Delamater et al., 1990[i]). Most diabetic chil-dren will receive some self-management training soon after diagnosis. An impor-tant component of this is the use of self-monitoring of blood glucose (SMBG) to inform decisions about diet, exercise, and insulin requirements. In this study all children ages 3–16 with newly diagnosed IDDM were randomly allocated to one of three conditions: routine care, routine care plus supportive counseling, and routine care plus self-management training. Supportive counseling sessions focused on ad-justment to the diagnosis, on family coping, and on providing emotional support. Self-management training sessions focused specifically on SMBG and taking appro-priate action in the light of results. Sessions included education, problem solving, role play, and homework evaluation. Both types of intervention comprised seven sessions in the first 4 months postdiagnosis and then booster sessions at 6 and 12 months. The interventions are of interest because they are family focused and tar-geted at children immediately after diagnosis, a time when one might expect inter-vention to be most effective. The children in the self-management group had sig-nificantly lower HbA_1 scores (a measure of glycosylated hemoglobin that is said to reflect overall blood glucose levels and therefore overall diabetic control) at 1 and 2 years postdiagnosis than those in the group receiving routine care. The scores of the children whose families received supportive counseling were intermediate between the other two groups. Although not significantly different from those of the self-management training group, the HbA_1 scores of the counseling group had dropped enough to suggest a clinically significant difference. This study also had a narrow focus, with no attempt made to investigate any psychosocial outcomes.

Some investigators have explored the effect of cognitive-behavioral interven-tions targeted at parents or families, concerning young people's diabetic control. Guthrie, Sargent, Speelman, and Parks (1990[ii]) recruited parents who had scores of more than 300 on the Holmes and Rahe Life Stress Scale (Holmes & Rahe, 1967) and who had children with diabetes present for more than 2 years. Parents were alternately allocated to relaxation therapy (10 weekly sessions of muscular re-laxation using temperature biofeedback) or to a no-treatment control. Dropout from the study was high; it was difficult to persuade parents in the intervention group to continue with all the sessions, and control parents soon realized that they were in the no-treatment group and defaulted. As a result, only nine subjects and three controls completed all monitored sessions (there were 10 in each group at the start of the study). Nevertheless, the HbA_{1c} of the children of parents who received relaxation training reduced significantly over 3 months, with no significant change in the control group. However, although children in both groups had raised HbA_{1c} levels, those of the experimental group were higher, and even after intervention were higher, than those of the control group pre-intervention.

Satin, la-Greca, Zigo, and Skyler (1989[i]) evaluated the effects of a family-oriented group intervention. The study randomly allocated 32 adolescents with diabetes (mean age 14.6 years) and their families to one of three conditions: a multifamily group, a multifamily group with parent simulation exercise, and a no-treatment waiting-list control. Participating families were volunteers, primarily from middle-income levels. The multifamily group intervention consisted of six weekly sessions (90 minutes each) covering the emotional impact of diabetes and diabetes-related problems. Families were encouraged to communicate with each other and to develop new problem-solving strategies to deal with these problems. Discussion and role play were used in the groups. In addition, in some families, parents were asked to simulate diabetes for 1 week, with their adolescent diabetic children taking responsibility for their "care." HbA_{1c} for young people in the multifamily plus simulation intervention group had decreased significantly at the end of treatment, but not at 6-month follow-up, as compared with that of other intervention group and the control group. HbA_{1c} levels before treatment in all groups were equal and more than double the levels normally expected. Analysis of later groups only (earlier groups were larger; later groups were restricted to just three or four families) showed that HbA_{1c} improvements were maintained at 6-month follow-up and that the adolescents with diabetes perceived a "teenager with diabetes" significantly more positively. This latter finding may reflect more positive self-concepts and self-esteem in the adolescents with diabetes as a result of the intervention.

Some studies have tried to use cognitive-behavioral methods to improve social skills and peer relationships. The underlying rationale is that children with chronic illness face high peer pressures, which conflict with the demands of illness management. Training is usually in groups and utilizes role playing of specific situations. Kaplan, Chadwick, and Schimmel (1985[i]), in a pilot study, randomly allocated 21 volunteers (ages 13–18) at a summer camp for young people with diabetes to a "social learning program" or to a discussion group control condition. The social learning program consisted of facilitated group discussion concerning adverse peer influences on management of diabetes. A problem-solving approach was taught to address these situations, and the solutions generated were rehearsed in role plays and discussed. The intervention took place on a daily basis during the 3-week camp. At 4-months follow-up the experimental group had lower HbA_1 scores. This decrease was not associated with knowledge scores relating to diabetes but was significantly associated with self-reported diabetes self-care.

Follansbee, La Greca, and Citrin (1983[i]) also randomly assigned adolescents with diabetes (48 young people, ages 12–16) to either coping skills training or a discussion group control condition. Both groups' compliance with medication and control increased significantly, but only in the experimental group was this associated with significant increases in assertion and decreases in aggression.

FAMILY AND SYSTEMIC THERAPIES

There are fewer well-designed studies of family and systemic therapies in diabetes. Wysocki et al. (2000[i]) randomly allocated 119 adolescents (ages 12–17) with IDDM and reporting parent–adolescent conflict on standardized questionnaires at levels that could impede family management, to one of three treatments: standard treatment, educational support, or Behavioral Family Systems Therapy (BFST). The sample had poor diabetic control as measured by glycated hemoglobin. This was a well-designed study with careful monitoring of treatment integrity. However, despite the relatively large sample size, the three groups differed significantly after randomization on a number of demographic variables and in terms of levels of family conflict. Immediately posttreatment, there were no significant changes in glycated hemoglobin or diabetes-specific psychological adjustment, but suggestions of improvements in parent–adolescent relationships and diabetes-related conflict in those who had received BFST. This study is unusual because it attempts to show that change in presumed underlying mechanisms (parent–adolescent conflict) can influence disease-related functioning and diabetic control; it is unfortunate that group differences following randomization make interpretation of the findings difficult. In a similar study, a less intensive intervention that focused on improving parental involvement in diabetes management while reducing conflict demonstrated reductions in diabetes-related conflict and a trend toward improved diabetic control (Anderson, Brackett, Ho, & Laffel, 1999). In this study 85 children (mean age 12.6 years) with IDDM were randomly allocated to standard care, an attention control group, or a "teamwork intervention." The third condition comprised four 20–30-minute sessions integrated into routine ambulatory appointments and focused on the importance of parent–teenager shared responsibility for diabetes tasks while avoiding conflict. These sessions were supported by written materials. The attention control group received "traditional diabetes education." During the 12-month study period, parent involvement in diabetes fell away in the two control groups but was maintained in the intervention group, yet with significantly less diabetes-related conflict reported. In the 12 months after the study period adolescents in the intervention group had a 2.4 times greater chance of improving their diabetic control than those in the comparison group, a difference that was just short of statistical significance.

INDIVIDUAL PSYCHODYNAMIC THERAPIES

Despite numerous case reports, there have been almost no methodologically sound evaluations of individual psychodynamic treatments in the management of chronic illness. The exception is the study by Moran, Fonagy, Kurtz, Bolton, and Brook (1991[ii]), which examined the impact of intensive psychoanalytic psychotherapy on children with diabetes that was very hard to control, necessitating admission to a pediatric hospital. The children were consecutively admitted to two hospitals meeting pre-agreed criteria for hard-to-control diabetes (22 children over 3 years, ages 7–19). All the children admitted to one hospital (11) received psychoanalytic psychotherapy three to five times weekly for the duration of their stay (mean length of stay 15 weeks, range 5–28 weeks). Children at the other hospital received routine medical care. A mental health worker regularly saw parents of the children receiving psychotherapy. At 1-year follow-up the children in the experimental group showed significant reductions in HbA_1 scores and in insulin requirements.

Headache

Classic migraine headaches are recurrent and usually unilateral. They are preceded by sensory, motor, and mood disturbances and are often accompanied by nausea or vomiting. Approximately 4–7% of school-age children suffer from migraine, with frequency increasing with age and a substantial proportion continuing to suffer into adult life (Hermann, Kim, & Blanchard, 1995[vi]). Tension headaches are bilateral and described as causing feelings of tightness or constriction. They are not associated with nausea and vomiting and may be exacerbated by stress. Approximately 80% of all headaches are tension headaches (Williamson, Baker, & Cubic, 1993[vi]).

The literature on intervention studies in children has been reviewed recently. Hermann et al. (1995[vi]) report a meta-analysis of 17 studies (only 9 of which used a control group design) concerning what they describe as pediatric migraine. Williamson et al. (1993[vi]) review 20 studies, some of which they report as concerning tension headache but which Hermann et al. describe as concerning migraine. Overall, most studies investigating psychological interventions gave a positive outcome, with support for thermal biofeedback and progressive muscular relaxation, either alone or in combination, as superior to other psychological treatments (cognitive therapy alone, or autogenic training). However, the review reports a dearth of good-quality studies comparing psychological interventions with credible no-treatment controls. There is evidence of substantial placebo effects with spontaneous remission rates of 30–40% of children in some studies. Waiting-list controls are commonly used, but the expectation of participants that they will not improve until they receive the intervention must influence overall outcome, calling this design into question. Many studies examine volunteer recruits from school or community settings, which makes it difficult to assess the findings' applicability to referred populations.

A well-designed study by McGrath et al. (1988[i]) randomly allocated 99 children ages 9–17 (referred to a migraine clinic), to a relaxation intervention or a nonspecific, attention control intervention. Both treatments were manualized, and checks were made on the integrity of treatment delivery and on the credibility of the treatments to the subjects. Headache intensity decreased in both groups, but immediately after treatment and at 3- and 12-month follow-up the groups did not differ significantly. However, in a further study (McGrath et al., 1992[i]), 87 referred children ages 11–18 were randomly allocated to a relaxation and coping program delivered either by manual and audiotape or by a therapist, or to a placebo-control group. In this study, both treatment interventions were superior to placebo on overall measures of headache and tests of clinical significance (reduction in headache by 50% or more). Improvements were maintained at 12-month follow-up. The addition of a coping skills element to the intervention is a notable difference between this and the earlier study.

Because of the cost of delivering relaxation and skin temperature biofeedback training to young people with migraine, some studies have evaluated ways of delivering the intervention in different settings or in a self-help format. Larsson and Melin (1988[i]) randomly allocated adolescents (16–18 years) to relaxation training, an attention control group, or a self-monitoring, no-treatment control group. Subjects were volunteers, not a referred clinic population. All students in the relaxation group had initial sessions in groups at school, and then some had therapist-assisted individual sessions and others had a self-help program comprising a manual and audiotapes. Both forms of relaxation were superior to controls in reducing headache. The partial self-help regime was as effective as the therapist-assisted program. Other studies, albeit with volunteer subjects and waiting-list controls who received no treatment, have shown the equivalence of therapist-assisted programs to fully self-administered programs (Larsson, Daleflod, Hakansson, & Melin, 1987[i]) and have also demonstrated the equivalence of programs delivered in school settings to those in clinic settings (Osterhaus et al., 1993[ii]).

A possible mechanism for the effectiveness of treatments involving a relaxation component is described by Van der Helm-Hylkema, Orlebeke, Enting, Thijssen, and Van Ree (1990), who examined various biological markers in a group of 20 subjects receiving relaxation and skin temperature biofeedback for common migraine, as compared with matched waiting-list controls. Headache intensity and duration in both groups had decreased at 9-month follow-up, but in the experimental group, decreases in headache indices were associated with increases in levels of beta-endorphin, a substance known to be decreased in adults with classic migraine.

Juvenile Rheumatoid Arthritis

Less work has been directed specifically at children with the painful condition of arthritis. Lavigne et al. (1992[vi]) evaluated a six-session package that taught relaxation using electromyogram and temperature biofeedback to the child and instructed mothers in behavioral techniques to promote compliance with physical treatment and school attendance. Eight children (ages 10–17 years) were involved in a multiple-baseline, across-subjects design. Both children and parents reported the program's efficacy in reducing painful symptoms.

Cancer

Varni, Katz, Colegrove, and Dolgin (1993[i]) investigated the impact of social skills training on the psychosocial adjustment and perceived social support of children with newly diagnosed cancer. Sixty-four children (ages 5–13), undergoing a school reintegration program, were randomly allocated to either a social skills training group (three 60-minute individual sessions on problem solving, assertiveness, and handling teasing, plus two follow-up sessions) or a no-treatment control condition.

At 9-month follow-up, the children in the intervention group reported higher perceived classmate and teacher social support and their parents reported a decrease in internalizing and externalizing behavior problems and an increase in school competence. These gains were greater than those at 6 months, suggesting an enduring effect of the intervention.

Interventions That Target More Than One Diagnostic Group

The majority of interventions so far described have targeted the child with chronic illness and have addressed specific individual diagnoses. Most have sought to alter physical outcomes or specific illness-related behaviors, such as compliance. Many of these approaches have the indirect effect of providing psychosocial support of a general kind for parents themselves, but relatively few make this an explicit aim, and fewer still state specifically how they do so. A small group of studies seek to intervene in the families of children with chronic illness generally. These studies may aim to alter illness-related parameters, but more often seek to change or prevent adverse psychosocial outcomes. This section reviews studies relating specifically to children with chronic illness.

Most of the few studies completed have methodological problems. For example, Michielutte, Patterson, and Herndon (1981[ii]) evaluated a home visiting program in which a pediatric nurse tried to give general psychosocial support to families of children with cancer, postdischarge, to improve parental coping, interpersonal relationships, and family function. Seventy families were involved, but without random allocation to home visiting or control groups. The intervention's nature and frequency are unclear, and the nurse had no counseling training. Most parents rated the service useful, but only 1 of 7 measures of parental emotional reactions (anger) and 2 of 13 measures of family functioning differentiated the intervention group by the end of the research. Fife (1978[i]) compared a behavioral approach with a nondirective approach to tackle the specific problem of parental overprotectiveness in leukemia. Subjects were randomly allocated, but numbers were small (16 in total), and neither approach was found to be superior. Marteau, Gillespie, and Swift (1987[vi]) evaluated the effects of a weekend meeting for parents of children with diabetes and found a high level of satisfaction with the occasion and increased parental confidence in looking after their children, maintained 3 months later. The study, like many others of this kind, did not include control groups with which to compare those involved in the particular intervention.

Those studies with adequate methodology are suggestive of benefit, but not conclusively. Pless and Satterwhite (1972[i]) looked at nonprofessional family counselors. In their study, 97 families with children with a diverse range of chronic illnesses were randomly allocated to receive either home visiting or no treatment. Potential counselors responded to advertisements and were mainly mothers of children with a chronic illness. After a brief training period (five 6-hour sessions), they visited families at a frequency determined by negotiation with the families. It is unclear how much time was spent with families, but their activities included listening to parents talk about the stresses of raising their children and advising them appropriately, facilitating family relations, educating them about the illness, coordinating service agencies, and acting as advocates. After 1 year, significantly more of the children in the intervention group were rated as improved in psychological status as compared with those in the control group. Positive outcome was more likely if the families were of "low risk" and if more than five visits were carried out in the year of the study. The counselors were also very favorably received by parents, usually mothers, and dropout rates were low.

Stein and Jessop (1984[i]) compared a home care program including monitoring and provision of health care, advocacy, education, and support, with standard care. In the program, 219 children, with a diverse range of chronic illnesses meeting pre-agreed criteria, were recruited from local pediatric clinics and randomly allocated to experimental and no-treatment control groups. The sample was not representative; the subjects were largely of lower socioeconomic status and from ethnic minority groups. The minimum intervention consisted of one home assessment visit and six contacts in 6 months, but nursing staff negotiated with parents to determine the exact frequency of visits. Assessment was not blind, and although the aim of the service was to provide a whole-family approach, encompassing both the biomedical and the psychosocial, it was not made clear how this was done, what training the pediatric and nursing staff were given, nor what the determinants were of the changes observed. Six months into treatment, there were significant effects on the child's psychological adjustment and on the mother's satisfaction with care in the home care experimental condition. Twelve months after treatment commenced, mothers in the experimental group were still more satisfied with care, but only children whose families had received the intervention for the full year maintained statistically significant improvements in psychological adjustment. There were also trends for improvement in the mother's psychiatric status. Stein and Jessop (1991[i]) report on this program's long-term effects . Five years later, they interviewed 68% of the original sample (mean age 12 years) and found that the children in the experimental group had significantly better psychological adjustment than the controls, and that adjustment 5 years later was better than at the end of treatment.

Nolan, Zvagulis, and Pless (1987[i]) report on a well-designed, randomized, controlled trial of social work support, in which 345 children were randomly allocated to a social work intervention or to a no-treatment control condition. Families received social work support for 6 months and were evaluated 4 months after treatment ended. There was no evidence of preventive or therapeutic effects of the intervention on children's behavior problems, social functioning, or self-esteem, or on maternal psychological functioning or the impact of the illness on the family. However, it is unclear whether the social workers had actually been trained appropriately in counseling. Relatively few of the families found the intervention benefited either themselves (57%) or their children (42%), but this may be due to the intervention's low intensity; the average number of personal contacts with the families in the 6-month period was only three (range 2–13).

Ireys, Silver, Stein, Bencivenga, and Koeber (1991[i]) report preliminary findings concerning an evaluation of parent support. The study randomly allocated 95 mothers of children with chronic health problems, ages 5–9 years, to experimental and no-treatment control groups. The intervention was implemented by mothers from the community with experience in rearing children with health problems, who provided biweekly phone contact and regular face-to-face contact for 1 year. These contacts provided information, emotional support, and affirmation of the mothers' skills. Analysis of results 6 months into the intervention showed significant increases in self-esteem and self-efficacy in the experimental group. A later randomized controlled intervention with 193 mothers of children (ages 7–11 years) with chronic illness also significantly decreased maternal anxiety as measured by the Psychiatric Symptom Index. Depression scores were not reduced by the intervention (Ireys et al., 2001[i]). Ireys, Sills, Kolodner, and Walsh (1996[i]) describe a similar project for mothers of children with juvenile rheumatoid arthritis. Forty-five mothers were randomly assigned to receive support from experienced mentors (mothers with experience of caring for children with arthritis) or to a no-treatment control group. Mentors had a 30-hour training program and regular ongoing supervision. The intervention, which lasted 15 months, was intended to provide informational, affirmational, and emotional support by means of telephone, face-to-face, and occasional group contacts. At the end of treatment, the groups did not differ significantly on the outcome measures of social support and mental health status, although the trends favored the experimental group.

Coupey, Bauman, Lauby, Koeber, and Stein (1991[i]) reported preliminary findings of an intervention aimed at adolescents with a range of different chronic illnesses. In this intervention, 140 adolescents (ages 14–17, 70% with chronic illness) were randomly allocated to either a 2-month social skills training and 4-month job placement, or to a no-treatment control. The treatment group showed significant increases in self-esteem and decreased psychiatric symptoms at the end of the intervention.

In one of the few studies in this field exploring service-level outcomes, Gustafsson and Svedin (1988[ii]) have looked at the cost-effectiveness of mental health liaison to pediatric services. They compared 42 children (ages 1–16 years), consecutively referred to the liaison service with "psychosomatic or somatic disorders," with age- and diagnosis-matched controls. The liaison service comprised weekly consultation to the pediatric nursing group, family therapy for the family, and individual therapy for selected children. Only minimal information is given concerning the nature and length of treatment. Days in the hospital per year before and after treatment were calculated for the treated group and compared with days in the hospital per year for the matched controls over similar time periods. Total costs of delivering care, both pediatric and psychiatric, were also calculated. The authors conclude that the liaison service significantly reduces the number of days in the hospital and overall costs of treatment. There are serious problems with the method (lack of definition of subjects and intervention, retrospective nature of data collection, adequacy of controls), and therefore with the conclusions, but this study at least attempts to consider service-level outcomes, not just symptomatic relief.

Only one large study of suitably rigorous methodology has looked at family-based interventions aimed at reducing psychosocial symptoms in children with a broad range of chronic illnesses. In this study, Pless et al. (1994[i]) recruited 1,069 children ages 4–16 years from nine specialty clinics. After investigators traced problems, screened for eligibility criteria regarding degree of chronicity and functional impairment, and obtained informed consent, 332 children were stratified by clinic and randomly allocated to either an intervention group or a no-treatment control group that received standard clinic care. The 1-year intervention was provided by nurses and designed to be incorporated easily into the existing workload of nurses in the speciality clinics. The nurses were required to make a minimum of 12 contacts with each family during the course of the study. In fact, the average number of contacts was 15, with a mean duration of 21 minutes; 76% of contacts were by telephone. Analysis of nursing logs indicated that their activities, which were based on the McGill model of nursing (Gottlieb & Rowat, 1987), included relationship building, gathering information about families' needs, providing support, increasing knowledge or enabling families to view situations differently, improving family problem solving, and helping families to acquire appropriate resources and/or contact appropriate services. Where indicated, nurses liaised, on behalf of the family, with clinics and with schools. No information is given about the training the nurses received prior to the intervention or about supervision during the intervention. Despite the relatively low level of input, children in the experimental group showed significant improvements in psychosocial adjustment (less dependent, anxious, and depressed) and in self-worth.

Summary and Implications

The majority of interventions relating to chronic illness are psychological interventions directed at improving physical outcomes. Far fewer attempt to prevent or reduce the adverse psychosocial sequelae of chronic illness. Most studies are directed at the children themselves, but some target parents. Very few address the problems of siblings or look at families as a whole, as opposed to the children or parents as individuals within the family.

The existing research is difficult to interpret—sample sizes are usually small, and within-sample variation is often high. Subjects are often volunteers, and not enough studies include at-risk children. Common difficulties include wide age ranges and differences in the timing of the intervention in relation to the time of diagnosis. Thus, even when the sample consists of children of broadly similar age, some of these children have had their chronic illness for many years and others for only a few months. It seems likely that such variance will impact significantly on the outcome of therapeutic interventions. Attempts at randomized controlled trials have suffered from a lack of credible no-treatment control groups.

Education alone for children with chronic illness increases knowledge about that illness, but is insufficient to bring about changes in illness management. Multicomponent cognitive-behavioral interventions, including various combinations of education, trigger recognition, relaxation, problem-solving skills, and stress reduction, have been shown to be effective in improving physical status in a number of different diagnostic groups, although it is unclear whether relaxation is an essential component of these packages. In at least one study, a similar multi-component cognitive-behavioral intervention has been shown to be effective in reducing psychological disorder. The mechanism for this may be via an increase in the young person's ability to cope with negative life events. There is some evidence that systemic family therapies are effective in improving physical status in asthma. Cognitive-behavioral interventions targeted at families rather than individuals have also been shown to be effective in improving physical status in diabetes. These programs seem to work regardless of the evidence of psychological difficulties in the child, including difficulties directly related to the illness. Interventions focused on improving family functioning reduce diabetes-related family conflict, but have not yet been shown to reliably improve diabetic control. There is a tentative suggestion that psychoanalytic psychotherapy may be effective in the management of hard-to-control diabetes, but this finding has not been replicated and is of unknown relevance to other illness groups.

There is increasing evidence that broad-based interventions aimed at providing education and support, delivered in the community by nurses with minimal training in psychological intervention, may prevent later adverse physical and psychological outcomes.

Further research needs to focus on exploring which components of multicomponent packages are effective and which children are most suited to which interventions. Most of the work to date has focused on "pathology" and investigated interventions to improve the functioning of poorly coping children and families. As most studies are directed at the children themselves, and very few address the problems of siblings or parents or look at families as a whole, more research is needed to develop effective interventions that involve the whole family. Not enough work has explored the attributes of well-functioning children and families.

12

Specific Developmental Disorders

Specific developmental disorders (SDDs) are difficulties with particular areas of cognitive functioning, which constitute by far the most common reason for provision of special educational help (American Academy of Child and Adolescent Psychiatry, 1998b[vi]), although in many cases the original reason for consultation may have been a behavioral problem or school refusal. SDDs are very often associated with Axis I disorders, and there is a continuing complex relationship between Axis I and Axis II problems over time; thus, specific developmental difficulties can lead to secondary emotional and behavioral problems in later childhood or adolescence. There has long been controversy over whether learning disabilities should be defined by discrepancy between IQ and achievement, or between age and achievement, in the specific areas at issue. A consensus appears to have emerged in favour of the age–achievement discrepancy, which effectively means that children whose achievement levels are very scattered but at an average-to-superior level throughout will not be regarded as needing intervention, whereas a child with consistently poor achievement as compared with peers will be regarded as having several disabilities requiring services (e.g., Toppelberg & Shapiro, 2000).

Just as in Axis I disorders, it is essential to explore issues of comorbidity and contributing contextual factors. In the case of learning disabilities, such factors will clearly include educational considerations such as quality of education provided, number of changes of school, frequent absences from school, neglect at home, and so on. Assessment also needs to take account of the child's cultural and linguistic background and experiences, as well as the possible effects of Axis I disorders (for instance, attention deficits or anxiety), in interpreting intelligence and attainment scores.

DEFINITIONS

SDDs involve delays or abnormalities affecting capacities that would normally have appeared by the age that the child has reached.

In DSM-IV and in ICD-10, these disorders cover communication (expressive and/or receptive language, or articulation), motor skills, and learning (reading, mathematics, written expression, or other academic skills). In the case of learning disorders, achievement within the area of disorder should be substantially below that expected, given the child's age, IQ, educational opportunities, and relevant sensory capacities. (IQ testing should be carried out individually, by an appropriately trained clinician, and in such a way that the developmental capacities in question are not directly required. Testing of the capacities being evaluated must similarly be carried out individually and interpreted by a person with appropriate diagnostic experience.) "Substantially below" is usually interpreted as two or more standard deviations (SDs) below the expected level, although one SD may be accepted as more appropriate, for instance, where there is doubt as to the validity of the IQ testing (e.g., the impairment has had a significant impact on performance in a test of general intelligence). The impairment must also significantly interfere with either academic achievement or activities of daily living.

Receptive, expressive, and mixed receptive/expressive language disorders are diagnosed according to very similar criteria to those of the learning disorders. The articulation disorders, phonological disorder and stuttering, are defined by abnormal forms of speech, rather than by delay in development, as well as by the criterion that the impairment must be handicapping to normal activities and not sufficiently explained by low IQ, sensory impairment, or environmental factors. Similarly, developmental coordination disorder is defined as difficulties with activities requiring motor coordination, in comparison with the level expected, given the child's age, IQ, and medical condition. The impairment must also significantly interfere with either academic achievement or activities of daily living.

In this decade, research has suggested that it may not be useful to distinguish between children with a specific developmental delay (i.e. discrepancy between overall IQ and performance in a given area) and those with similar poor performance in, say, reading, which is not significantly behind their overall cognitive level (e.g., Beitchman & Young, 1997[ib]; Shaywitz, Fletcher, Holahan, & Shaywitz, 1992a; Shaywitz, Escobar, Shaywitz, Fletcher, & Makuch, 1992b). It seems that the mechanisms involved and the needs of both groups may be similar (e.g., Bishop, 1994[ib]), and requiring a substantial IQ–achievement discrepancy risks preventing children who achieve poorly across a wide range of skills from benefiting from the services available to those with more limited impairment, who may include children of high IQ with only average achievement in one area. Beitchman and Young (1997[ib]), in a recent and authoritative review, recommend that if a child is not functioning below the expected level for age or grade, he or she is not likely to require special help and should not be regarded as learning disordered, even though there may be a substantial IQ–achievement discrepancy in one, or more than one, area.

Similarly, the Practice Parameters issued by the American Academy of Child and Adolescent Psychiatry (AACAP, 1998[vi]) recommend that children be included where there is a significant discrepancy between age and achievement, rather than between IQ and achievement. They point out that the trend in research is toward domain-specific assessment and remedial help, which allows early detection and assistance for any child performing below age-appropriate levels within any given domain, regardless of whether the child also has difficulties in other domains. The IQ–achievement criterion required a child to have fallen significantly behind his or her expected level in educational attainment before the cutoff was passed and special help was made available.

PREVALENCE

As with other disorders, the prevalence of SDDs varies with the sampling criteria, the tests used, and the definitions applied (e.g., Kavale & Forness, 1995; Myers & Hammill, 1992). The AACAP Practice Parameters (1998b[vi]) report that 10–20% of children and adolescents show at least one SDD. In the United States, 4–5% of the school-age population is receiving special educational help for learning disabilities. The majority of these children show reading disorder, and 90% show a written-language-based disorder of either reading or expressive writing or both (Denckla, 1991). A similar pattern was shown in an epidemiological study of 9- and 10-year-olds (Lewis, Hitch, & Walker, 1994). A very useful overview by Kavale and Forness (1995) estimates the prevalence of reading disorder at around 4%, with a range in different samples from 2–10%. Developmental disorder of written expression seems to occur with similar frequency, with boys three times more likely to meet criteria. Mathematics disorder is reported to be shown by 1–6% of children, and in this case girls may be more often affected. Figures for the prevalence of developmental language disorder range from 1% to 13% (Cantwell & Baker, 1991; Tomblin et al., 1997), but some have cautioned that the higher figure would overestimate those requiring intervention (Bishop, 1994[ib]). For speech and language delays alone, the median prevalence figure is 5.9% (Law, Boyle, Harris, Harkness, & Nye, 1998).

Both expressive and receptive language disorders, and reading disorders, have consistently been reported to be more common in boys, although recent studies have found no difference between the rates of reading disorder in boys and girls of grade (primary) school age (Flynn & Rahbar, 1994; Shaywitz, Shaywitz, Fletcher, & Escobar, 1990). The review by Beitchman and Young (1997[ib]) suggests that the sex difference usually reported in clinical samples may be the result of referral bias, with teachers referring disruptive boys for evaluation but not referring the girls with similar reading problems but without disruptive behavior. This suggestion has been supported by epidemiological studies (Prior, Smart, Sanson, & Oberklaid, 1999).

CLINICAL PRESENTATION

SDDs range from mild impairment—which may be easy to miss but may lead to serious difficulties over time, and which require sophisticated, domain-specific diagnostic testing to reveal the problem—to abnormalities that would be very obvious to anyone meeting the child or observing him or her attempting to use particular academic skills. The child may show particular deficits that would be abnormal at any age, or may simply have the performance typical of a younger child.

The child may well not have been referred because of learning or language difficulties at all, but for behavioral problems (perhaps particularly in regard to school attendance or compliance), which are associated—in a third of cases, or in some studies many more—with one or more SDDs (Cohen et al., 2000; Kauffman, 1997). It is important to be aware that some behavioral problems may be more part of a developmental disability than a secondary, psychiatric disorder. For example, children with language-based memory deficit (LMD), which is characterized by poor sequencing and verbal memory, may appear to show attention deficit disorder (ADD) because they do not remember what they are supposed to be doing. These children may well seem bright and capable because of their good associative language ability, so that their failure to follow through on tasks and instructions seems like laziness or inattention (Richman & Eliason, 1992, p. 543). Alternatively, the child may become school phobic, or defiant or aggressive, perhaps partly in response to the anxiety or frustration caused by the developmental difficulty. The SDD itself may not have been recognized (Cohen, Davine, Horodesky, Lipsett, & Isaacson, 1993a). A more recent study by Cohen and her colleagues (Cohen et al., 1998b) replicated and extended the previous report. They assessed 380 children ages 7–14, consecutively referred to child psychiatric services, 38% of whom had a previously identified language impairment. They found that of the 235 children referred for psychiatric treatment who had not been regarded as showing an SDD, 41% also met stringent criteria for one or more of these disorders.

These striking findings about the level of unsuspected SDD among children referred for psychiatric evaluation raise the question of the impact of diagnosis. There seems to be evidence that at the kindergarten stage, children with an identified disorder showed lower self-esteem than those whose disorder had not previously been diagnosed (Vaughn, Hogan, Kouzekani, & Shapiro, 1990). However, among children of school age, this pattern was found to be reversed (Ribner, 1978). Thus, it may be that having an unrecognized learning disorder has a negative effect on self-esteem over time. Cohen et al.'s 1993a study showed that 4- to 12-year-old children with undiagnosed learning disorders were more likely to show externalizing symptoms (attention deficit, aggression, and delinquency) than were their diagnosed counterparts. However, their later study (Cohen, Barwick, Horodezky, Vallance, & Im, 1998a; Cohen et al., 1998b) did not replicate that result; what it did show was a high level of psychopathology in both groups, and, interestingly, a deficit in social cognition (especially emotion decoding and social problem solving) associated with language disorder, whether recognized or not. In contrast, a meta-analytic study of developmental coordination disorder (marked clumsiness) (Wilson & McKenzie, 1998) demonstrated that this problem was associated with pervasive deficits in information processing, particularly problems in visuospatial processing.

It is worth keeping in mind that although a child who sustains a brain injury or disease, with consequent cognitive impairments, tends to be extensively investigated and monitored, a child with perhaps a similar degree of developmental cognitive impairment may either be undiagnosed or misdiagnosed as emotionally or behaviorally disordered (Richman & Eliason, 1992).

There is clear evidence that at least some SDDs have a strong genetic component, with the risk for first-degree relatives being 5–10 times higher than for the general population (see Bishop, 2001). Although environmental influences (talking and reading to children) are known to help normal language acquisition, there is no evidence that language or learning disorders are generally the result of a lack of environmental stimulation or support (Bishop, North, & Donlan, 1995; Tomblin & Buckwalter, 1994). Many studies have shown local brain abnormalities, both structural and functional, in patients with SDDs; this evidence is comprehensively summarized and discussed by Filipek (1999).

Comorbidity

SDDs tend to be found together, particularly reading and writing disorders, and reading and language disorders. Early language disorder is associated with higher rates of later learning disorders, even if the language disorder improves (Torgesen, Wagner, & Rashotte, 1994; Wallach & Butler, 1994). There is also substantial comorbidity with Axis I disorders; estimates agree in suggesting that about 50% of both epidemiological samples and groups of children referred for SDDs also show Axis I disorders (Cantwell & Baker, 1991; Rutter et al., 1970b; Toppelberg & Shapiro, 2000). Attention-deficit/hyperactivity disorder (ADHD) is especially frequent (Beitchman, Nair, Clegg, Ferguson, & Patel, 1986; Chadwick, Taylor, Taylor, Heptinstall, & Danckaerts, 1999; Hinshaw, 1992a), and it appears that it is attention problems rather than conduct disorders that are associated with reading disorders (Frick et al., 1991; Taylor et al., 1991). There is recently emerging evidence (Prior et al., 1999) that, developmentally, behavioral problems most often precede learning difficulties, and that there are specific associations between learning difficulties and behavior problems; mathematical problems may be associated with internalizing disorders, particularly among girls. Interestingly, in the study by Prior et al., literacy problems were also associated with many internalizing, as well as the well-recognized externalizing, symptoms.

Natural History

The long-term outcome of learning and language disorders offers a mixed picture, and one complicated by the fact that many studies have included children who had received treatment. An excellent systematic review of speech and language delays in children up to 7 years (Law et al., 1998) gave a median persistence figure for untreated children, followed up for several years, as 38% and 66% persistence, depending on whether children had speech or other language problems, or both. Children of 2–3 years whose expressive language is poorly developed, but whose comprehension is normal, generally acquire normal expression over the following year (Law et al., 1998; Thal, 1991). Further work has suggested that this good prognosis applies where children are moderately impaired; on the other hand, where a 2-year-old has a spoken vocabulary of 8 words or fewer, improvement is far less likely. Most longer-term follow-up studies, investigating impairment into the school years, have shown good recovery from early delay in expressive language (Bishop & Edmundson, 1987; Whitehurst, Fischel, & Lonigan, 1991); however, another study by Rescorla and Schwartz (1990) gave dissenting conclusions. Bishop (1994[ib]) offers a useful summary of this picture for the clinician: Children of 2 years whose vocabularies include fewer than 50 words should be monitored; those whose vocabularies include fewer than 8 words at 2 years, whose comprehension is also poor, or who remain well below normal limits at age 2½, should be offered intervention. Bishop and Edmundson (1987) have given further guidance for children approaching school age: Four-year-olds who can retell the gist of a simple story are likely to have a good outcome, whereas those who confuse the sequence have a poorer prognosis.

There have been at least two long-term follow-up studies of children with severe speech and language disorders, who were educated at a special school offering intensive remedial help (Griffiths, 1969; Haynes & Naidoo, 1991). In both studies, about half of the children had language abilities within the normal range when assessed in adolescence or adulthood, but there were sometimes related educational and psychiatric difficulties that had persisted. Other follow-up studies have confirmed that severe speech and language disorders in childhood do tend to have significant adverse long-term effects (Clegg, Hollis, & Rutter, 1999; Johnson et al., 1999; Stothard, Snowling, Bishop, Chipchase, & Kaplan, 1998). A recent pair of papers by Howlin et al. (Howlin, Mawhood, & Rutter, 2000; Mawhood, Howlin, & Rutter, 2000) reports on a careful follow-up into young adulthood of 47 people who had suffered from either autism or developmental receptive language disorder at 7–8 years of age. The two groups had been matched on both nonverbal IQ and expressive language. In adulthood, it was found that although the autism group still had more severe and pervasive problems, the language impairment group had developed similar though less severe social deficits; 75% had moderate or severe social problems. Their cognitive and linguistic difficulties had become more similar to those of the individuals with autism.

An important long-term follow-up of a very large community sample of 5-year-olds with speech and language disorders has recently been reported by Beitchman et al. (2001). At the first stage (Beitchman et al., 1986), 1,655 children were recruited for screening, of whom 142 passed through a rigorous selection procedure. These children were matched with the same number of children from the same sample, whose speech and language were normal. The majority of this combined sample (244/284) agreed to follow-up at age 19, with the follow-up including psychiatric assessment. The children with language-impairment were more likely to refuse follow-up. The study found that children who had language impairment had significantly raised rates of later anxiety disorders (mainly social phobia) and antisocial personality disorders. However, those children who had only a speech impairment at 5 years did not differ from the controls. Nearly all of these psychiatric disorders started after the screening for language problems at age 5.

Well-designed follow-up studies have shown that reading disabilities tend to persist into adolescence and adulthood (see Chadwick et al., 1999; Maughan, 1995). It appears that although reading comprehension and word recognition usually improve (very much influenced by how much continued exposure there is to reading materials), phonological coding continues to be a problem into adulthood (Bruck, 1992; Pennington, Van-Orden, Smith, Green, & Haith, 1990). It particularly affects spelling and the reading of unfamiliar words (Scarborough, 1984). Reading also remains slower than average (Denckla, 1993). Overall, higher IQ and milder childhood severity of disorder are the best predictors of young adult reading ability (Maughan, 1995). Later educational and occupational achievement are further heavily influenced by social class and parental support (O'Connor & Spreen, 1988). Children with SDDs drop out of school, in the United States, at a rate 50% higher than average (U.S. Department of Education, 1995).

The behavioral and emotional difficulties strongly associated with childhood reading disorder are less evident by young adulthood; raised rates of psychosocial problems are reported in some samples (e.g., Spreen, 1987), but not others (e.g., Bruck, 1985). However, there is evidence that early language or learning disorder predicts later development of an Axis I condition (Bruck, 1985; McGee, Feehan, Williams, & Anderson, 1992). For example, Cantwell and Baker (1991) demonstrated that children with an SDD who did not show any Axis I disorder were more likely than their peers to develop an Axis I disorder over the following 4–5 years. Similarly, Beitchman et al. (1986) found that language disorders predicted later anxiety symptoms in girls. (An important recent study by Chadwick et al. (1999) showed that the well-known association between early reading retardation and later hyperactivity was unlikely to be due to hyperactivity arising *de novo* as a response to educational failure.) It seems that most of this morbidity occurs in adolescence and does not persist into adult maladjustment or delinquency (see Maughan, Pickles, Hagell, Rutter, & Yule, 1996).

There is much less evidence on the medium- or long-term outcome of other SDDs, although nonverbal learning disabilities (NVLD; Denckla, 1991), characterized mainly by visuospatial impairment and difficulty in acquiring mathematical skills, seem to have a fairly poor prognosis. What evidence there is (reviewed by Beitchman & Young, 1997[ib]) shows persistence and even worsening of the disorder over time, together with a raised incidence of social and emotional problems, especially internalizing disorders (Denckla, 1991; Semrud-Clikeman & Hynd, 1990).

TREATMENT

The main interventions used for SDDs are provided by the school psychological service and remedial education services, in the case of academic skills disorders, and by speech therapists for other speech and language disorders, rather than by mental health professionals. These approaches are not described or evaluated in full detail here, but the clinician should be aware that where evaluations have been carried out, there are doubts as to whether traditional speech therapy and remedial educational approaches produce durable and generalizable benefits (Bishop, 1994[ib]; Lyon & Cutting, 1998[vi]; Maughan & Yule, 1994[vi]).

In contrast to this skeptical view, an authoritative systematic review of the outcome of speech therapy for early speech and language delays (Law et al., 1998) concluded that 9/10 randomized controlled trials (RCTs) found statistically significant improvements with intervention; parent-administered intervention was as effective as that provided by the clinician; 10/12 quasi-experimental design studies and a number of investigations using experimental single-case designs also showed a significant impact of treatment. Although the studies tended to have very small sample sizes and there were some common methodological problems (e.g., the use of raw scores instead of standardized scores, thus confounding maturational and treatment effects), the studies taken together yielded median effect sizes (ESs) in the region of 1.0, strongest for enhancement of expressive language and weakest for receptive (comprehension) problems. Thus, the average treated child might move from the 5th to the 25th percentile on a standard language test.

To complicate the picture further, we have a recent, more negative report (Glogowska, Roulstone, Enderby, & Peters, 2000[i]) of an RCT involving 159 preschool children attending 16 community speech and language clinics in Bristol, United Kingdom. The children were allocated to either one-to-one speech and language therapy as normally provided in the clinic, or to "watchful waiting." The children were reassessed after 12 months by research therapists blind to initial results, and with an attempt to make them blind to treatment condition. The therapy group showed significantly greater improvement on only one of the five outcome measures, although there was a significantly greater chance that the treated children would no longer meet criteria for receiving treatment (62% still met these criteria, whereas 77% of the untreated children did). The authors concluded that treatment as usually provided was largely ineffective, and that clinicians should reconsider the appropriateness of current practice in terms of timing, nature, or intensity. Given that most children, even in the treated group, continued to meet criteria for inclusion after 12 months, it was clear that these preschool language problems had not resolved spontaneously, and the question therefore arises whether a different treatment strategy could have helped them more.

The only traditional mental health treatment that seems to have been evaluated for an SDD is psychoanalytic psychotherapy. Heinicke (1965) reported a study of a sample of children ages 7–10 with developmental reading disorders with comorbid emotional symptoms. These children received psychodynamic therapy, either one or four sessions per week, for 2 years. Greater improvement was found in the group receiving more frequent therapy. Heinicke and Ramsey-Klee (1986[iii]) extended this study, using the results of the first to try to maximize the impacts of different treatment frequencies. They introduced a third group, matched to the first two, who received therapy once a week for the first year and four times a week for the second. Outcome was measured in terms of the referral problem (reading level) and general academic performance, together with a standardized psychodynamic diagnostic profile. At termination of therapy, the groups did not differ significantly, but at 1-year follow-up, the groups that had received treatment either four times a week throughout, or once a week followed by four times a week, showed continued improvements on all measures, beyond those of the once-a-week group. It therefore seemed that more intensive treatment, for at least part of the therapy period, had a more lasting beneficial effect.

There were some methodological difficulties with this study, reflecting the methods prevalent in all outcome research 35 years ago. Diagnostic characteristics of the sample were poorly described, the projective tests and the interview for elic-iting diagnostic details were of unknown reliability, and the therapy was not fully specified but just stated to be analytically oriented. Nevertheless, this study was a rare attempt to do three things: (1) to evaluate the effectiveness of intensive and nonintensive psychodynamic therapy for emotional and learning disturbances (which have been repeatedly shown to be intertwined); (2) to isolate the impact of treatment frequency, which is of interest in a variety of therapies, and particu-larly—for practical and theoretical reasons—in psychodynamic treatment; and (3) to measure change in both objective, service-relevant ways, and ways that reflected the theoretical perspective. In all these respects, the study broke new ground.

Much more recently, various psychological approaches have evolved, based on cognitive, cognitive-behavioral, task-analytic, neuropsychological, and construc-tivist models, although these approaches in fact overlap, with differences largely in emphasis (Hallahan, Kauffman, & Lloyd, 1996[vi]). These approaches are reviewed by Lyon and Cutting, who see them as more promising than traditional, mainly ed-ucationally based methods. Neither model has been adequately evaluated, however. Lyon and Cutting note that "a review of the literature related to both LDs (learning disabilities) as a general category and to domain-specific LDs (e.g., dyslexia) indi-cates that until recently no single teaching method, treatment intervention, or combination of methods has been found to yield clinically significant, long-term gains" (Lyon & Cutting, 1998[vi], p. 479). The authors detail the existing litera-ture's methodological limitations, which should offer constructive guidance for future studies.

One carefully designed experimental study (Nelson, Camarata, Welsh, Butkov-sky, & Camarata, 1996) will serve as a good example of work that could throw much more light on the treatment of specific developmental disorders. This is a case series of seven children with language disorder, ages 4.7–6.7 years, matched with seven younger (2.2–4.2 years) children whose language development was nor-mal, and comparable to that of the children with language disorder. For each child, six linguistic abilities were identified, three of which were absent and three partially developed. These target capacities were paired. The speech therapist then worked in one of three ways with each pair: no treatment, imitative treatment, or conversa-tional recasting. Thus, each child was equally exposed to each approach, but only some of the child's speech difficulties were addressed. It was found that conversa-tional recasting was a more effective strategy for both the disordered and the nor-mal group, although imitative learning has previously been regarded as the proce-dure of choice.

Even if not asked to provide direct treatment for SDDs, clinicians may play a number of useful roles: contributing to assessment; treating associated disorders such as emotional or behavioral problems, including school refusal and poor peer relationships; and educating and advising children, parents, and teachers about the children's difficulties. The assessment of children with SDDs needs to include comprehensive neuropsychological testing, not simply to ascertain whether a child does have an SDD, but to examine the child's specific strengths and weaknesses, both within the area of difficulty and in other areas. Without this specificity, parents, teachers, and other professionals involved with the child may make counterproductive assumptions about his or her limitations. In other words,

> it is usually essential to know at least as much about what a child with LD (Learning Disability) *can* do as it is to know what he or she *cannot* do, if the clinician's goal is to design an appropriate treatment/intervention plan. Most treatment plans for children with LD usually combine a direct attack on the deficits and the exploitation of the child's assets and strengths that are probably going to be useful in compensatory intervention strategies. (Rourke & Del Dotto, 1992[vi], p. 524).

No systematic studies of direct clinical treatments for SDDs themselves, other than the work of Heinicke on psychoanalytic psychotherapy, were discovered in this review, so the treatment guidelines that follow are based on expert opinion (American Academy of Child and Adolescent Psychiatry, 1998b[vi]; Beitchman & Young, 1997[ib]).

No medication has been demonstrated to be beneficial for SDDs, and generally medication is not used in these cases. However, pharmacotherapy may have an important role, for instance, in managing comorbid ADHD (Gittelman, 1983[vi]), and there is a suggestion that piracetam might improve comprehension in children with reading disability(Wilsher, 1991). Beitchman and Young (1997[ib]), however, recommend that any attempts at pharmacotherapy for SDDs should be regarded as experimental.

Psychotherapeutic or other psychological therapies (such as social skills training) may be helpful in managing associated problems, such as demoralization, poor social skills, or social avoidance. It may be important, particularly in severe cases, for the material and activities used in therapy to be adapted to the SDD, with less reliance on verbal activity than might be usual. Support groups for children with SDDs may be helpful (Falik, 1995[vi]).

Bishop (1994[ib]) gives some useful and sensitive guidance about the counseling of parents to facilitate the understanding and management of children with speech and language disorders. She discusses at what age speech therapy should begin for a child and suggests that from the point of view of maximal language gains, the earlier speech therapy starts the better. However, from the perspective of limited resources and of reducing anxiety and self-consciousness in the child, this may be better left until it is clear that the problem is not improving at an acceptable rate. As with all intervention, the essential issue is whether the child will be better off, on balance, with or without specialist involvement. Bishop helpfully outlines advice that should be given to parents, even if the child is not directly treated:

(1) The problem is not a result of an inadequate environment, (2) the child should not be coerced, for instance, by withholding a reward until a sentence is said correctly, (3) in the case of language disorders, all communication by the child, verbal or nonverbal, should be accepted and encouraged.

SUMMARY

At present, there is a discrepancy between DSM criteria for SDDs and the consensus in the research and clinical literature about the appropriate definition of these disorders. DSM definitions require a substantial gap between actual achievement and predicted level based on IQ and age, not explained by contextual factors. Expert opinion favours criteria based on a gap between age and achievement, rather than between mental age and achievement. If adopted, this change would cause some shift of professional attention from brighter children with circumscribed disabilities to children with a lower overall level and perhaps multiple areas of cognitive difficulty.

SDDs very commonly present together with other developmental disorders and with Axis I disorders. They seem to be more strongly related to genetic and/ or neurological abnormalities than to environmental factors. SDDs differ from each other, but, broadly speaking, moderate levels of disability have been found to be associated both with continuing developmental disorder and with the development of Axis I disorders, both emotional and disruptive. There is a high rate of undiagnosed SDD, especially among children referred to clinics for behavioral problems.

Interventions for these disorders have largely been carried out by speech therapists, remedial teachers, or educational psychologists, rather than by mental health professionals. Studies of the effectiveness of these interventions have given somewhat mixed results, broadly positive across many small studies and suggesting that parents could be taught to deliver therapy just as effectively—for certain delays—as professional therapists. However, a recent large-scale study of speech therapy gave negative results. Expert opinion has tended to be that speech and language therapies do not make a long-term or generalized impact, but this clearly needs further investigation and clarification of the discrepant findings. Newer strategies, based on research on underlying psychological deficits and tailored to individual cognitive strengths and weaknesses, do seem promising but have not been properly evaluated as yet.

Clinicians have important roles in monitoring children referred for Axis I disorders for co-existing Axis II problems, in contributing to thorough assessments of a wide range of capacities, and in advising parents and others on the complex relationships between emotional, behavioral, and cognitive problems.

Medication and forms of psychotherapy may have useful roles in managing associated emotional or behavioral symptoms, but there is little convincing evidence yet that they directly improve the SDD. There is evidence from one early study that psychodynamic therapy, particularly if delivered intensively after the first stage, can have a beneficial impact on reading retardation coupled with emotional disturbance.

IMPLICATIONS

Children referred for psychiatric evaluation should be screened for indications of SDDs. Children should be considered to show developmental disabilities warranting assessment if they are falling substantially behind an age-appropriate level of cognitive performance in academic skills, language development, or motor coordination. Parents, teachers, and children need information about the precise deficits and strengths in children's abilities, and about ways of helping children to address and compensate for their limitations. It is probably wise to wait before offering treatment to 2- to 3-year-old children, who often spontaneously improve considerably. There is evidence that for expressive language problems, parents can make effective therapists, and speech and language therapists should probably be trained to provide more indirect treatment.

To the extent that they are involved in managing children with SDDs, clinicians need to collaborate with those devising programs based on developmental and cognitive psychology, to integrate these programs with other interventions required for Axis I conditions, and to evaluate the effectiveness of programs for treatment of SDDs.

More research will be needed, both to elucidate the nature of these disorders and to evaluate treatment strategies. It would be worthwhile to explore the contribution of psychodynamic psychotherapy further, whether alone or in combination with educational measures.

13

Conclusions and Implications

The previous chapters presented an appraisal of outcome research relevant to the treatment of childhood mental disorder. This chapter attempts to integrate some of the most consistent findings in order to facilitate their application in clinical settings. This is not an easy task. In the first chapter we reviewed in some detail the complexities surrounding the generalizability of outcome data. In particular, we drew attention to the difficulties encountered by researchers when attempting to balance the need for experimental control sufficient for drawing logical inferences and the need to represent ordinary clinical work in research to a level that makes findings relevant to service delivery settings. Here we will focus on three issues. First, we consider the practical problems involved in interpreting the research evidence presented in this volume. Second, we briefly highlight the main findings from the review, describing the treatments for each diagnostic category that appear to be supported by the current evidence base. We also highlight some limitations of the current literature, with suggestions for specific areas where the evidence base is extremely thin and further research is urgently needed. Finally, we consider some generic implications that were suggested by the review of literature.

INTERPRETING RESEARCH EVIDENCE

The Perspectives of Funders, Clinicians, and Researchers

From the *clinician's* standpoint, research of almost any sort, but particularly outcome research, has profound intrinsic limitations. Clinicians frequently refer to the complexity of the problems they face in the service delivery setting, where choice of treatment is a decision-making process guided by patient characteristics (age, diagnosis, chronicity, IQ), family and social circumstances (resources available to the family, parental conflicts, educational background of the parents, psychiatric and health problems in the parents), and treatment protocols available to the service (length of waiting list, skill mix of the team, clinical resources available). Decisions need to be made concerning the appropriateness of treatment, likely outcomes without treatment, the kind of treatment likely to be accepted, the professional who can provide the treatment, the appropriate treatment setting, the temporal course of the treatment and modifications to the treatment in light of treatment response, and the impact of the treatment on the child and on other members of the family (Mash, 1998; Schroeder & Gordon, 1991). Each case is different and extremely complex, the answers to the child's and the family's problems not at all obvious. Attempts to "prescribe" treatment on the basis of diagnosis are irrelevant because they are simplistic. The assignation of diagnostic labels may seem an irrelevant burden imposed by extraneous pressure.

In contrast, *funders* may be expected to be concerned with the identification of treatments that are cost-effective in relation to specific disorders. In principle, knowing the case mix of a specific service and having research evidence that pertains to treatment modalities in relation to different conditions, funders should be able to dictate the kinds of services that should be offered and the ideal skill mix within a specific agency. In reality, funders rarely have outcomes as a central focus. Their concern is cost minimization, and therefore the cheapest way of bringing about legitimate termination of an illness episode is best. Although inferences may be drawn from research on this issue, no definitive conclusions can be reached, because outcome research is rarely concerned with long-term cost savings and does not have legitimate requests for further services as a key outcome criterion. Nevertheless, funders and service planners may look at outcome research with a view to influencing service delivery. At this level, however, what they look for is evidence clearly indicating which treatments to reimburse and what skill mix they should recruit. In doing this, they cannot afford to pay heed to the many qualifications and limitations that researchers tend to impose on their findings. This kind of cookbook approach to planning, of course, can set funders against groups of providers and may undermine the goal of strengthening the research base of everyday clinical practice.

The perspective of the *researcher* is different again. Most likely, the researcher's priorities are generated equally by the research funding bodies and by genuine intellectual curiosity. The purse strings of research funders are mostly controlled by fellow researchers who are familiar with the pitfalls of outcome investigation, and require adherence to the agreed-upon canons that are aimed at minimizing ambiguity and maximizing the potential for causal inference linking improvement and intervention. This will be easier to achieve with some treatments and clinical populations than others. Research questions asked will follow the funding bias for unequivocal conclusions, creating areas of vacuum in the literature from both the funders' and the clinicians' perspective. We have been aware throughout this review that questions easiest to answer were answered most often, and in these domains, answers achieved considerable sophistication. In domains where populations were less accessible or treatments more complex to implement, the answers are still outstanding and the research literature remains thin. The researcher's priorities are not less pragmatic or intellectually more pure than the considerations governing the decision making of funders or clinicians. Each is simply concerned with a different aspect of the change process.

Whereas the clinician's priority is the achievement of change itself, the researcher is concerned with unequivocally establishing what has led to change, and the funder is concerned with the cost of change and the likely recurrence of this expenditure in the foreseeable future, as well as how costs expended on one group impact on services that may be offered to others. This disjunction of priorities has, in the past, generated general dissatisfaction among many clinicians, who felt that their concerns were hardly considered; many researchers, who felt that their findings were frequently ignored or scarcely attended to; and funders of clinical services, who were confused between claims and counterclaims of researchers and practitioners.

A Tentative Framework for Integrating Research Findings into Practice

In interpreting the evidence summarized in this review, we have found the framework provided by Alan Kazdin (Kazdin, 1997a; Kazdin & Kendall, 1998) the most helpful for conceptualizing the competing needs of clinicians, funders, and researchers. At the heart of this integration is the implicit guidance that a consistently applied theoretical framework provides. Kazdin's model proposes seven steps in the development of effective treatment: (1) the conceptualization of the dysfunction in terms of key aspects, processes, and mechanisms relating to the development and course of the disorder, (2) empirical testing that validates these hypothesized processes, (3) development of a theoretical or conceptual framework that links a treatment method to the processes and mechanisms hypothesized to underpin the disorder, (4) the operationalization of the treatment method whereby procedures to be applied are codified to make measurement possible and provide evidence that treatment has taken place, (5) carrying out outcome studies that test the effectiveness of the treatment across the full range of the hierarchy of evidence, as well as process outcome studies that explore key treatment components, necessary treatment length, and efficacy relative to other treatments, (6) carrying out experimental studies to determine whether the processes and mechanisms hypothesized are indeed the ones that are involved in the mediation of treatment effects, and (7) establishing the boundary conditions by identifying characteristics of the child, the parents, the family system, the social environment, and other attributes with which the treatment procedure interacts.

We recognize that this is a statement of an ideal rather than a state of affairs that is readily expectable in relation to any disorder or any particular mode of therapy. Nevertheless, Kazdin's "developmental" framework for treatment development is not only pan-theoretical but also incorporates the diverse concerns of clinicians, funders, and researchers. The clinician's concerns are recognized in the need for the clear formulation and establishment of boundaries within which any treatment should be applied. The legitimate concern of funders may be particularly associated with tests of treatment outcome, and researchers may be most invested in empirical tests of psychopathological and treatment models. With the adoption of such an integrated model of treatment development, the priorities of all stakeholders can be met without the need for three different types of inquiry to address the priorities of each. What is needed now is for stakeholders to join forces in establishing specific treatment approaches within a matrix of treatment methods and treatment evaluations across these seven criteria.

SUMMARY OF THE EVIDENCE BASE FOR INTERVENTIONS IN CHILD AND ADOLESCENT MENTAL HEALTH SERVICES

The spread of randomized controlled trials (RCTs) across the different diagnostic groupings in child and adolescent mental health is patchy. There are relatively large numbers of well-conducted RCTs evaluating psychopharmacological treatments and cognitive-behavioral treatments for particular childhood problems, presumably due to the relative ease of conducting well-designed studies in these areas. However, even in these two areas of intervention, we identified large gaps in the evidence base. In this summary, evidence is grouped by type of intervention. If no reference is made to certain diagnostic groups within a particular section, it should be assumed that no evidence exists to evaluate that type of intervention for that diagnosis.

Psychopharmacological Treatments

Anxiety

Although expert opinion has recommended cognitive-behavioral therapy (CBT) as a first-line treatment for obsessive–compulsive disorder (OCD) on the basis of open trials, so far RCT evidence is available to support only the usefulness of medication; selective serotonin reuptake inhibitors (SSRIs) appear to be significantly more effective than either placebo or other types of antidepressant or anxiolytic medication. Approximately half the patients with OCD in trials of SSRIs show clinically significant improvement.

However, although they are fairly commonly prescribed, there has been little research on the efficacy of benzodiazepines, SSRIs, or beta-blockers for anxiety symptoms in children or adolescents other than for OCD.

Depression

The number and quality of RCTs evaluating the efficacy of medication in depression are poor but improving. Studies currently suggest that tricyclic antidepressants are of little value, whereas SSRIs show promise. SSRIs also seem to be safer.

Conduct Problems and Delinquency

Although medication cannot be justified as the first line of treatment for severe conduct problems, a considerable amount of research has explored the potential value of psychopharmacological treatments. The evidence is strongest for psychostimulant medication for oppositional disorder, in conjunction with psychosocial treatments such as parent training. Psychostimulants have been shown to reduce antisocial behaviors in children and adolescents with diagnoses of comorbid attention-deficit/hyperactivity and conduct disorder (ADHD–ADD/CD), independent of the effect of these medications on attention deficit and hyperactivity symptoms. Combinations of psychosocial and stimulant treatments have also been tried, and there are some indications that the two in combination may have broader and longer-lasting effects than either one alone.

Experimental approaches have looked at lithium, clonidine, anticonvulsants, and neuroleptics in the treatment of conduct disorder (CD). Lithium is likely to be less desirable than methylphenidate in the treatment of milder forms of antisocial behavior, but may be appropriate for the pharmacological treatment of explosive, severely aggressive manifestations of CD. However, in view of the complexities of the treatment protocol, substantial side effects, and limited advantage over placebo, this treatment should be restricted to very cooperative families where other treatments for explosive aggressive behavior have failed. Small-scale open trials have shown clonidine to improve destructive and aggressive behavior, but evidence at the moment is suggestive rather than compelling. Anticonvulsants have been tried and found useful in the treatment of impulsive behavior in open trials, but better-controlled investigations have reported more equivocal findings, including substantial side effects.

Traditional neuroleptics appear to be effective in reducing aggressiveness, but their efficacy is associated with sedation and interference with learning, as well as more severe side effects. Atypical antipsychotics show promise in the reduction of aggressiveness and may be less likely to be associated with unwanted effects, although this picture is rapidly changing.

In conclusion, there is insufficient evidence to justify the use of psychopharmacological treatments as the first line of treatment in conduct problems. However, medication may be appropriate in the management of comorbid psychiatric disorders associated with aggression, particularly ADHD.

Attention-Deficit/Hyperactivity Disorders

Large numbers of well-conducted trials have provided evidence not only about the efficacy of medication in ADHD, but also about the appropriate prescribing regime. If diagnostic criteria are met and the behavior problems are pervasive in at least two different types of setting, a trial of medication should be the first line of intervention in these problems.

There is compelling evidence that stimulant medication should be the first-choice treatment. Stimulants (methylphenidate, dexamphetamine) have been demonstrated to be effective with inattention, hyperactivity, and impulsivity in the classroom, irrespective of age and with any comorbid condition. Early studies suggested that stimulants were less effective for children with comorbid depression and/or anxiety, but findings from recent studies lead us to conclude that, at least for anxiety, this is not the case. The evidence is somewhat less compelling for the impact of stimulants on academic performance, and there is no evidence that prosocial behaviors increase with their use. There is no evidence as to who will respond well to stimulants and no evidence of serious, irreversible side effects. As it is not possible to predict which dose will be effective, dosage should be increased within safe limits until an effect is achieved. There is no evidence of abuse of their medication in adolescence by individuals with ADHD.

There is no evidence that the trial of other drugs during this phase is particularly helpful. However, if there is no or only partial resolution of symptoms, other medication should be considered. There is less compelling but still good evidence for the effectiveness of clonidine, tricyclics, monoamine oxidase inhibitors (MAOIs), and carbamazepine, although it should be noted that these drugs all have more serious side effects than the stimulants. If stimulants are ineffective, they can be discontinued and replaced with tricyclic antidepressants, clonidine, or SSRIs. Some experts recommend adding clonidine to stimulants, but there is as yet no good evidence for or against this. If stimulants aggravate emotional problems (for example, anxiety), then tricyclics should always be considered. However, there is no evidence for the superior effectiveness of antipsychotics or tricyclic antidepressants in combination with stimulants.

Effective monitoring of the size of the dose of medication is needed to minimize adverse side effects of drug treatment, and there should be annual trials of drug holidays to see whether the medication is still required.

Tourette's Disorder

In the absence of comorbid problems, evidence supports haloperidol or clonidine as the treatments of choice, with little to choose between them, in the treatment of Tourette's disorder. There are significant side effects from haloperidol, including neurological symptoms such as rigidity and tremor. Clonidine may lead to ECG changes as well as inducing drowsiness. A potential second-line treatment is pimozide, which is less sedating than haloperidol but has a greater risk of ECG abnormalities. As children with Tourette's disorder are usually referred because of the distress and embarrassment caused by the tics, deciding whether to use medication requires careful thought, because of the risk of side effects and the fact that tics do not worsen if left untreated. It is important that these considerations be relayed to children and parents so that fully informed consent to treatment is given.

In the presence of comorbid attention deficit disorder (ADD), methylphenidate, clonidine, and tricyclic antidepressants have all been shown to be effective, albeit in only a very limited number of trials. Currently, clonidine is probably the first choice of drug, although methylphenidate is the least likely drug to lead to troublesome side effects. Early evidence that methylphenidate routinely exacerbated tics has not been confirmed. Drug treatments for tics, as for all disorders, require regular monitoring, particularly as the treatment of the comorbid disorder may have an impact on the severity of the tics and most of the recommended drugs have a significant risk of side effects.

Schizophrenia

There are very few well-conducted trials of pharmacological treatments for children with schizophrenia. Traditional neuroleptic medication has been demonstrated to reduce acute positive symptoms, but there are relatively few trials with children. Side effects of neuroleptic medication can be serious and must be regularly monitored. As yet, there is little empirical evidence of the superiority of atypical over traditional neuroleptic medication for children with schizophrenia, and, again, there are concerns about the side effects of these drugs. In the absence of empirical data, best practice guidelines are frequently based on extrapolation from adult studies and/or the consensus of child clinicians. Best practice advice suggests the use of neuroleptic medication with close monitoring of side effects, which should continue well beyond the acute phase.

Bipolar Disorders

Some evidence supports the use of lithium in the acute phase of bipolar disorder, but there are no controlled studies of its long-term prophylactic use. No good studies support the use of neuroleptics, although best practice reviews suggest their use. Anticonvulsants are used in adult patients to prevent recurrence and may be effective in the maintenance treatment of children and adolescents. There is no evidence to support the use of benzodiazepines in children with bipolar disorder.

Pervasive Developmental Disorders

There is limited evidence to support the use of medication in pervasive developmental disorders (PDD). If behavioral therapies are insufficient, physical treatments are sometimes used. A diagnostic approach that identifies treatable comorbid conditions should guide practice. The evidence is strongest for stimulant medication with comorbid ADHD. There is no evidence to support the routine use of other medications. Haloperidol has been used to reduce aggression, hyperactivity, and preoccupations, but its use raises similar concerns to those described for the use of neuroleptics in CD.

In more experimental studies, naltrexone has been reported in two controlled studies to improve hyperactivity and disruptive behavior, although there is no conclusive evidence that it results in a reduction of self-injurious behavior. In one controlled study, clomipramine was superior to placebo in reducing autistic withdrawal and preoccupations, hyperactivity and oppositionality, and was more effective than desipramine.

Eating Disorders

Medication used in the treatment of anorexia includes neuroleptics, appetite stimulants, and antidepressants. Research evidence of the efficacy of any of these drugs in young people is very limited and, given their side effects, their clinical value may also be limited. Antidepressants have been shown to improve binge eating (also in bulimia nervosa) and weight gain, regardless of the presence of depression. There is no evidence that any one antidepressant is more effective than any other, and limited data suggest a significant rate of discontinuation of medication and of relapse.

Substance Misuse

The use of pharmacological agents to counteract or decrease the subjective rein-forcing effects of a substance or to act as aversion agents, in treating adolescents with substance misuse, has received minimal attention in the literature. Methadone has been demonstrated to be moderately effective as a maintenance treatment over the longer term in those who are dependent on opiates, but is of limited use in those with a short history (i.e., most young people).

Specific Developmental Disorders

Medication may have a useful role in managing associated emotional or behavioral symptoms, but there is no convincing evidence that psychopharmacological treat-ments directly improve specific developmental disorder (SDD).

Other Physical Treatments

Electroconvulsive Therapy

There is no systematic evidence for or against the use of electroconvulsive therapy (ECT) in children and young people with schizophrenia or with bipolar disorder.

Diet

Although there is no good evidence for the blanket exclusion of additives and colorings in a child's diet, there is evidence that the exclusion of certain foods from the diet is effective in the treatment of ADHD in a selective group of children with complex problems. No particular foods are implicated, and each child has to be carefully assessed for evidence of an adverse reaction to a particular food item. If parents have not noticed a specific adverse reaction to a particular food, then the evidence does not usually warrant the effort involved in imposing a selective exclu-sion diet. Adherence to the dietary regime requires exceptionally strong parental commitment for effective implementation.

There is evidence from one study that a high-fibre diet leads to a reduction in episodes of recurrent abdominal pain over a 6-week period, but this finding needs to be replicated.

Cognitive-Behavioral Treatments (Including Problem-Solving Skills Training and Social Skills Training)

Anxiety

Specific CBT packages have been shown to be effective in the treatment of gener-alized anxiety disorders and simple phobias, and the improvements appear to be well maintained. Exposure has usually been assumed to be a central aspect of the efficacy of such treatments. However, recent studies have cast doubt on this; therapeutic support without exposure was found to be equally effective in two well-designed studies of the treatment of school phobia. Where exposure treatment is used, it may well be more effective and humane to use a gradual, rather than a "flooding," approach. There is evidence that CBT can be successfully provided in groups and that including family members is beneficial where there are family problems.

CBT-based treatments are used commonly in the treatment of OCD in clinical settings, but although promising, their efficacy has not as yet been convincingly demonstrated. It seems likely that a combination of CBT and medication is needed to reduce entrenched OCD, and maintenance is a serious issue. Current trials are addressing this issue.

Depression

The evidence base supports CBT as a treatment for depression, whether provided individually or in a group. However, family problems can reduce the efficacy of CBT and may also need to be addressed. Providing longer courses of CBT (or booster sessions) in cases of nonresponse to a standard length of treatment seems to promote recovery. In studies to date, CBT has been shown to be more effective than tricyclic medication. However, it seems possible that CBT is less effective in more severe cases, where medication may be required instead or in addition. In a good example of the value of RCTs in exploring underlying mechanisms of disorder, CBT has not been shown to be more effective in cases where there are greater cognitive distortions. Thus the benefits of CBT are apparently not explained by a reduction in negative cognitions.

Social skills training has not yet been shown to be an effective treatment for depressive disorders, although it may be helpful in reducing residual social skills deficits when mood has lifted, perhaps reducing the strong likelihood of relapse. The same may be true for other approaches, such as family and individual therapies that address risk factors for further episodes, whether rooted in personality or family functioning.

Conduct Problems and Delinquency

Problem-solving skills training is the most rigorously investigated singular approach to the cognitive-behavioral treatment of conduct problems. Its effectiveness in combination with parent training has been demonstrated by two independent studies and seems to be the treatment of choice for conduct problems in school-aged children ages 8–12. Recent reports support the effectiveness of the treatment in the ordinary clinic context, as well as in less representative university clinic settings.

Mild conduct problems are ameliorated with the help of training in social skills and anger management coping skills, but there is no evidence for the use of these approaches on their own with more chronic and severe cases.

A number of treatment packages that combine a range of individual skills-oriented techniques (including anger management) appear promising and have been tried with delinquent youth. However, evidence for efficacy on outcomes of social concern, such as arrest or conviction rates, is limited, the most effective combination of specific techniques has not yet been identified, and results on long-term outcomes are equivocal. Interventions based on the traditional principles of punishment and deterrence have not been adequately tested, but effectiveness studies indicate that there is at least a possibility of adverse outcomes from these interventions.

Cognitive-behavioral treatments of adolescents with conduct problems administered in groups could worsen the young persons' problems.

Attention-Deficit/Hyperactivity Disorder

If there is an unsatisfactory or insufficient response to physical treatment for ADHD, then psychosocial treatments should be added. The most compelling evidence is for parent training (see the following discussion) or behavioral therapy. Behavior therapy programs have been shown to improve on-task behavior and reduce disruptive behavior, but with little evidence of generalization across settings. On their own they are less effective than stimulant medication, but can prevent a need for higher doses of medication. There is no good evidence that CBT is effective on its own, and its effective component may be the behavioral one. There is no evidence that social skills intervention leads to an improvement in poor relationships in children with ADHD.

Pervasive Developmental Disorders

Evidence suggests that the first line of intervention in PDD should be behavioral. However, programs need to be individualized and intensive and are therefore demanding of resources. They also need to take place in home and school settings, necessitating good communication between educators, families, and health professionals and a component of parent and teacher training. Demonstrated benefits include persisting gains in IQ; improvements in daily living skills, communication, and the ability to socialize; and a decrease in behavior problems.

Studies have tended to focus on children under the age of 4 years at the time of commencing treatment, but it is unclear whether early commencement of treatment is a necessary condition for successful treatment.

Despite a variety of approaches, there is no good evidence that individual social skills training significantly benefits individuals with autism.

Eating Disorders

Operant conditioning techniques have been used in hospital settings for anorexia nervosa and have been shown to be effective in short-term weight gain. They are often used in combination with other cognitive techniques aimed at altering irrational beliefs, disturbance of body image, anxiety, poor interpersonal skills, and dysfunctional eating behavior. However, although in adults CBT has been shown to be effective for bulimia, there is, as yet, no evidence for its over other forms of brief psychotherapy in children and adolescents.

Suicide

There is some evidence that brief cognitive–behavioral interventions focusing on problem solving with the families of adolescents following a suicide attempt can decrease adolescents' feelings of depression and suicidality and increase positive maternal attitudes toward treatment, thus enabling supportive family involvement and further compliance with specialist programs.

Education programs targeted at high-risk adolescents that promote personal control, problem solving, and coping skills are promising in reducing suicide risk behaviors, depression, hopelessness, stress, and anger. However, the evidence for effective cognitive-behavioral interventions in preventing suicide is not compelling.

Substance Misuse

Psychosocial treatments based on social learning theory and cognitive approaches appear to be more effective for adolescents with substance misuse than no treatment or treatment as usual, but these have yet to be systematically studied.

Physical Symptoms

In a unique study of unexplained physical symptoms, a package of cognitive-behavioral techniques, including progressive muscular relaxation, self-monitoring, distraction, and positive self-statements by children, and distraction and contingency management of pain and non-pain behaviors by parents, has been shown to be effective in the management of recurrent abdominal pain.

A range of cognitive-behavioral interventions, for different developmental levels, have been shown to be effective in different aspects of the management of acute and chronic pain. For example, general anaesthesia is less effective than CBT at reducing postprocedural distress. Rocking of newborns and distraction in younger children are effective in reducing distress. In older children, cognitive-behavioral strategies that promote more active coping and give the child a sense of mastery and predictability reduce procedural distress. It is difficult to know whether hypnosis is functionally different from CBT incorporating relaxation training, but there is some suggestive evidence that hypnosis can be effective in reducing procedural pain and the somatic symptoms associated with chemotherapy. Cognitive-behavioral interventions may also be effective as an adjunct to pharmacological treatments.

In children with chronic illness, education alone increases knowledge about that illness but is insufficient to bring about changes in illness management. Cognitive-behavioral techniques have been shown to be effective in improving physical outcomes in asthma, diabetes, headaches, and other chronic illnesses, but with slightly different specific interventions for each illness group. Cognitive-behavioral interventions targeted at families rather than individuals have also been shown to be effective in diabetes.

These programs seem to work regardless of the evidence of psychological difficulties in the child, including difficulties directly related to the illness. It is not clear whether the effect is directly on the physical symptoms or via a psychological impact, and further work is needed to determine which components of the complex packages evaluated are the most effective. It is unclear, for example, whether relaxation is an essential component of these interventions.

Parent Skills Training

Conduct Problems and Delinquency

There is accumulating evidence that parent training programs generally may be applied in a wide range of conduct problems and effectively delivered in various settings. Good manuals and videotape support are also available. For younger children with conduct problems, parent training approaches should be the intervention of choice. On average, about two-thirds of children under 10 whose parents participate in parent training improve. However, many outcome domains have been neglected in these studies, including peer relations, social competence, academic functioning, and participation in activities. Observed abnormalities in families' interaction patterns, associated with conduct problems, provide an important empirical foundation for parent training. Evidence that changing these patterns has the power to alter the child's behavior is very strong.

Larger effects (fewer dropouts, greater gains and better maintenance) tend to be found for parent training when the children are younger. More difficult and older children above the age of 8 require adjunctive treatment to parent training, to handle problems in the family or, with older children, to address the cognitive (particularly problem-solving) deficits in the child.

Evidence for the long-term maintenance of treatment gains is limited. Interventions that have evidence of long-term gain are also those requiring the highest therapeutic input and greatest client commitment. Evidence for generalization beyond the home to other settings (to school, with teachers or peers) is just beginning to be demonstrated.

Although parent training appears to be a powerful intervention, it makes substantial demands on the families. These demands include reviewing educational material, systematically observing the child, implementing reinforcement procedures, maintaining telephone contact with the therapist, and attending clinic sessions. These requirements may be overwhelming for some families, who may either fail to begin or prematurely discontinue treatment. Factors shown to be associated with failure to benefit substantially from the programs include parental socioeconomic disadvantage, psychiatric difficulties in parents (drug and alcohol problems, depression, personality difficulties), marital/relationship difficulties, low levels of social support, comorbidity in the child (unmedicated hyperactivity, language disorders, mental retardation), and severity of conduct problems. Adjunctive treatments such as social problem-solving skills training for single parents, partner support training for families with marital discord, and community-based treatment for high-risk and immigrant families generally facilitate parent training.

Parent training is also culturally highly sensitive. Methods of child control are strongly culture-bound. Although ethnicity has not been shown to influence outcome in all studies, parent training may not have generalized beyond the United States, partly because of the cultural specificity of many of its implicit assumptions. However, a replication study in the United Kingdom strongly supports the generalizability of the approach.

Specific programs found to be effective include Helping the Non-compliant Child (Forehand & McMahon, 1981), Videotape Modeling Group Discussion (Webster-Stratton, 1996a), the Oregon Social Learning Center Program (Patterson, 1976), and Parent–Child Interaction Therapy (Eyberg et al., 1995). These programs differ in terms of the amount of therapeutic input required, but data on which may be more or less suitable to what type of clinical population is at the moment lacking.

The effectiveness of parent training has been assessed in adolescents with delinquency. Although trials show statistically significant gains associated with these programs, such gains are of low clinical significance and the evidence does not justify the general implementation of parent training programs for adolescents with CD.

Attention-Deficit/Hyperactivity Disorder

If there is unsatisfactory/insufficient response to physical treatment in children with ADHD, then psychosocial treatments should be added. The most compelling evidence is for parent training, which is effective in improving compliance with instructions. Not all families are able to persist with the approach, however.

Pervasive Developmental Disorders

All the studies of behavioral interventions in children with autism have included a parent training approach. However, there have been no systematic investigations into parent training groups, and it is not yet clear whether this element of the intervention increases the effectiveness of behavioral interventions.

Physical Symptoms

Parental presence may be helpful in reducing procedural distress in children with physical symptoms if parents can be coached to promote distraction and/or active coping. If parents are agitated or uncertain, the child's distress may increase, and it may be more helpful to elicit support for the child from a member of staff. There is evidence that parents are often not invited to be present during painful procedures, let alone involved in their management.

Psychodynamic Therapies

Psychodynamic therapies have only recently begun to be evaluated using well-designed studies, despite being widely used in clinical settings. The development of manualized forms of psychodynamic therapies, and more appropriate outcome measures, would be useful steps toward more widespread, systematic evaluation.

Anxiety

There is some evidence that psychodynamic psychotherapy can be effective in the treatment of children with anxiety disorders, but research is needed on which children specifically benefit from psychodynamic psychotherapies. For instance, it could be that children who are hard to help with the use of other treatments are able to respond to these techniques, but as yet the required research has not been done to clarify this.

Depression

Individual child psychotherapy has not yet been shown to be an effective treatment for depression, but Interpersonal Psychotherapy, adapted for adolescents (IPT-A), is a promising treatment for adolescent depression.

Conduct Disorders and Delinquency

Psychodynamic treatments have not been demonstrated to be effective for children with conduct problems relative to untreated or alternative treatment control groups. Rates of clinically significant improvement appear to be lower in psychodynamic therapy than in other treatments, whereas treatment length and number of sessions are greater.

Attention-Deficit/Hyperactivity Disorder

There is no evidence either for or against the effectiveness of psychodynamic therapy in children with ADHD.

Physical Symptoms

There is a tentative suggestion that psychoanalytic psychotherapy may be effective in the management of hard-to-control diabetes, but this finding has not been replicated and is of unknown relevance to other illness groups.

Specific Developmental Disorders

There is some evidence, from an early study, that psychodynamic therapy, particularly if delivered intensively, can have a beneficial impact on reading retardation that is coupled with emotional disturbance.

Family/Systemic Therapies

As with psychodynamic therapies, family and systemic therapies have generally not been evaluated with the use of well-designed studies, despite their widespread use in clinical settings. The development of manualized forms of treatment is a useful first step toward more systematic evaluation. Family therapy, or parent work in parallel with individual treatment for the child, has been included as a condition in four RCTs. Neither approach has been convincingly shown to be more effective than general support or routine care, but family therapy in particular needs to be manualized for effective evaluation to be conducted.

Functional family therapy (FFT) has been shown to be effective in reducing recidivism in adolescents who have multiply offended. It is a very promising treatment and considerably less demanding of staff time than multisystemic therapy (MST). Its evaluation in an effectiveness/clinic setting seems opportune.

At 5-year follow-up, family therapy has been shown—after admission to a specialized unit—to be more successful than individual therapy in young people with anorexia nervosa. This was true for patients with onset before the age of 19 years and whose illness was not chronic. Family change may not be necessary, however, to achieve individual change. The evidence for the efficacy of family therapy in bulimia is equivocal. Family therapy has been shown to be superior to other treatment modalities in reducing substance misuse.

There is some evidence that systemic family therapies are effective in improving physical status in children with asthma. The same studies suggest that family therapy may be a cost-effective form of treatment, as compared with usual physical treatment regimes.

No studies have so far examined the effectiveness of family therapy for childhood anxiety disorders. There is no evidence either for or against the effectiveness of systemic therapy in ADHD.

Multimodal Interventions

There is increasing interest in developing and evaluating packages of care that comprise a range of physical and psychological treatment interventions.

A package known as multisystemic therapy (MST) is the most effective treatment for delinquent adolescents in reducing recidivism and improving individual and family pathology. This approach includes individualized assessment to determine the particular factors involved in a youth's delinquent behavior, followed by a combination of family therapy and behavioral techniques targeted at the young person, the family, the school, and the community. It has also been shown to be particularly efficacious in reducing substance abuse. It is substantially more effective than individual treatment, even for quite troubled and disorganized families. MST shares a particular strength with other systemic family approaches in reducing attrition rates in this highly volatile group.

Multimodal treatments have not yet consistently demonstrated superiority over other interventions in children with ADHD and CD but there are a number of trials in progress.

Interventions in School Settings

Conduct Problems and Delinquency

There is clear evidence that classroom contingency management methods are effective in controlling the behavior of children with conduct problems in that setting, but they have not yet been shown to generalize beyond the classroom situation or beyond the termination of the programs. Parent-administered reinforcements may enhance classroom contingency management in universal or selective prevention programs. However, the modification of teachers' behavior is unlikely by itself to cause clinically significant outcomes in individuals with severe conduct problems.

The enhancement of social competence in schoolwide programs appears to have only modest and temporary effects on CD. Whole-school implementation of antiviolence (antibullying) programs show promise in reducing the level of aggression within schools, but their effect on the prevalence of aggressive behavior of clinical severity is not known.

School-based approaches to the management of delinquency have considerable potential, but studies to date have failed to demonstrate powerful positive effects.

Attention-Deficit/Hyperactivity Disorder

There is evidence that further educational input is required to help children with ADHD, with delayed attainments, to catch up, but there is no evidence for the efficacy of particular educational approaches.

Hospitalization/Alternative Care Settings

Conduct Problems and Delinquency

A number of alternative settings for treatment have been evaluated in relation to attempts to reduce delinquency. Group homes operated according to behavioral principles are less costly and perhaps more effective at reducing criminal behavior than ordinary group homes, but the superior effects dissipate once young people leave the programs. The integration of a training program for carefully selected foster parents, with problem-solving skills and anger management skills training for delinquent adolescents, has been shown by several studies to be a powerful therapeutic tool, reducing behavior problems as well as recidivism.

Day hospitalization represents a promising approach to severe conduct disorder and delinquency, as it preserves links with community and family while removing the adolescent from the context within which the problem behaviors originated. However, available evidence only partially fulfills the promise of this approach, with most studies reporting either equivocal findings or basing conclusions on rather heterogeneous samples.

It should be noted that none of these approaches are as effective as MST and are all likely to be more costly.

Schizophrenia, Bipolar Disorder, and Eating Disorders

In the absence of empirical data, best practice guidelines usually suggest admission as part of the assessment process for schizophrenia and severe bipolar disorders. However, there is no evidence either for or against the effectiveness of treatment in residential settings.

There is also a clinical consensus that hospitalization is indicated for severe weight loss in anorexia nervosa, preferably in specialist inpatient units. There is, however, a lack of empirical evidence to form a rationale for the selection of the best setting for treatment interventions, and there is no evidence for or against the effectiveness of specialist adolescent inpatient units over all-age eating disorder units or generic inpatient care.

Implications for Service Delivery

Assessment

Outcome research is usually organized around diagnostic groups; however, if diagnostic systems are used, most children's predicaments are found to involve more than one diagnosis. Irrespective of the major presenting problem, comorbid disorders are frequent, and therefore services must be organized to allow for comprehensive assessment of the child, the family, and the child's environmental context in every case. In many cases multiple treatments will be needed. If services are not organized around multidisciplinary teams, there should be clear procedures for accessing expertise from a range of relevant professionals.

Clinicians have important roles in monitoring children referred for Axis I disorders for co-existing Axis II problems, contributing to thorough assessments of a wide range of capacities, and advising parents and others on the complex relationships between emotional, behavioral, and cognitive problems. Services should therefore ensure that all children referred for mental health evaluation should be screened for indications of specific developmental disorders.

Psychopharmacological Treatments

There is clear evidence for the effectiveness of medication for the treatment of OCD, ADHD, and tics. High levels of comorbidity also mean that the likelihood of these problems being present in children with other main presenting problems is high. Services must therefore include child and adolescent psychiatrists with expertise in the use of psychopharmacological treatments. This is already the case in some areas, but by no means in all.

Psychological Treatments

Although there is clear evidence to support cognitive-behavioral interventions as the treatment of choice for generalized anxiety and phobias, depression, CD in older children, and for some physical symptoms, there is no such thing as generic behavior therapy or CBT to be used in treating these disorders. Instead, there are particular packages that have been at least partly validated for children with specific problems and at particular developmental stages. Services will therefore need trained therapists with the capacity to flexibly apply cognitive-behavioral strategies to particular situations.

Although less evidence supports family systemic and psychodynamic treatments, this is often due to a paucity of well-conducted research in these areas. There is evidence that family systemic therapy is the treatment of choice in anorexia nervosa, and it may have a role in the treatment of depression, some physical symptoms, and CD. Family systemic therapy skills are also an essential component of MST. There is little evidence either for or against the effectiveness of psychodynamic therapies, but there are some suggestions that they may be useful, particularly in situations where other treatments have failed. There is also emerging evidence that brief forms of psychosocial treatments, such as interpersonal therapy, may be effective in treating depression. Services need to ensure that children and families have access to these forms of therapy as well as cognitive-behavioral treatments, pending further evidence regarding their effectiveness.

Multiagency Working

Services should recognize that many of the factors associated with poor outcome (socioeconomic disadvantage, parental psychiatric disorder, etc.) also make it difficult for families and adolescents themselves to engage and remain in treatment. More intensive, multicomponent, community-based interventions involving more than one agency may be needed for such families. This approach requires local agencies (health, social welfare, juvenile justice, education, and the voluntary sector) to work together in delivering integrated programs of care.

Early Recognition and Long-Term Care

There is evidence that for many children and adolescents with mental health problems, early recognition and treatment can improve prognosis and reduce subsequent morbidity. Mental health professionals need to be involved in training professionals in other services who come into regular contact with children so as to facilitate the early identification of psychiatric disorder. It may be worthwhile to screen for some undiagnosed disorders, such as anxiety, given their prevalence and the evidence of secondary problems in peer relationships and academic performance.

The long-term and relapsing nature of many conditions requires services to be organized to remain involved with some children and families over long periods of time while retaining the capacity to respond to acute crises.

Conduct Disorder

All services for children under the age of 8 should have some kind of parent training program. The evidence is strongest for the Webster-Stratton videotape modeling group discussion, which is also the most cost-effective. Community-based treatments are cheaper and, as found in some studies, more effective than clinic-based treatments, and therefore the integration of parent training programs with local activities should be explored.

Older children with CD will need access to cognitive-behavioral interventions that focus on enhancing problem-solving skills.

There is also evidence that behavioral interventions, although not generalizing beyond the classroom setting, can be very effective in reducing externalizing behaviors in the classroom. Educational services therefore need staff who can implement such programs.

Delinquency

MST is the most effective treatment for delinquent adolescents in reducing recidivism and improving individual and family pathology. It is a multilevel, relatively intensive, community-based, highly structured and well-integrated program focusing on goals proximal to offending behavior—for example, family monitoring and supervision of the adolescent. MST is substantially more effective than individual treatment even for quite troubled and disorganized families, and it also reduces attrition rates. There is evidence that psychosocial treatment strategies can be effectively integrated with juvenile justice provision. There is no evidence to support the sentencing programs that involve incarceration.

Nevertheless, these are difficult problems to treat, and there is a need for a specialist set of services, well integrated with the local juvenile justice, social welfare, and educational systems, if effective interventions are to be delivered.

Attention-Deficit/Hyperactivity Disorder

The outcome of attention deficit problems is poor if untreated, but effective treatments exist. Services must be organized so that adequately trained staff can assess, treat, and monitor treatment over long periods, continuing throughout the school years. Given the large numbers of children involved and the need for specialist skills, monitoring by specialist clinics may be helpful. Thought should be given to early case identification services and early intervention to reduce education underachievement.

Residential and Day Care Facilities

There is no empirical evidence either for or against the use of residential and day treatment facilities. However, there is clinical consensus that the severity and complexity of some disorders (schizophrenia, bipolar disorder, severe eating disorders, severe depression with high suicide risk, and others) may require access to inpatient and day patient treatment units. For many of these severe and complex conditions, services must also allow for the assessment and exclusion of organic conditions.

Physical Symptoms

There is strong evidence that a variety of psychological treatments can have a positive impact on physical symptoms, whether of unknown (and presumed psychological) origin or associated with the presence of diagnosed chronic physical illness or disability. However, pediatric services have often not acted on research evidence that could significantly improve the quality of life of children in their care. For example, despite the evidence that parental presence may be helpful in reducing procedural distress if parents can be coached to promote distraction and/or active coping, there is evidence that parents are often not even invited to be present during painful procedures, let alone involved in their management. In developing multiagency responses in the community for mental health problems, clinical settings must not neglect working jointly with pediatric services for children with physical symptoms.

Implications for Training

Some of the interventions for which there is the strongest evidence are complex and require specialist training—for example, MST for delinquency, CBT for anxiety disorders and depression, parent training for CD, problem-solving interventions for older children with CD, family and systemic therapy interventions, interpersonal therapy in depression, and many more.

In many parts of the world such training is not widely available at present, making it unlikely that the clinicians are providing the treatments validated by research. Training in the provision of effective psychosocial therapies needs to be far more readily available through affordable and locally based training. The existence of more properly trained therapists delivering treatments validated by research would also facilitate further well-conducted research.

Implications for Further Research

Areas Where There Is No or Very Limited Evidence

There are a number of areas within child and adolescent mental health where there is a startling and worrying lack of evidence to guide practice. The areas where there is least evidence are not always those where problems are less common or less severe. Further research into these areas is urgently needed to guide clinical practice.

Very few outcome studies examine the role of medication in the treatment of children and adolescents with schizophrenia and bipolar disorder. Particular attention should be paid to the role of newer antipsychotic medications and anticonvulsants for bipolar disorders. There are no systematic evaluations of psychosocial treatments in schizophrenia and bipolar disorder. Given that most children and adolescents live within families, it is particularly important to study the possible usefulness of family-based interventions. Similarly, there is insufficient evidence to provide any empirically based guidelines for the treatment of children and adolescents with schizoaffective disorder. Most clinicians extrapolate from evidence concerning the treatment of adult psychosis in managing young people with these problems.

Asperger's disorder is relatively common, and yet very little is known about comorbidity, outcome, or effective intervention. It is not possible, from the evidence base, to make any definite recommendations about treatment in children with Asperger's disorder. Most clinicians apply the same principles of treatment as they would in autism. Similarly, there is insufficient evidence to make specific recommendations regarding the treatment of disintegrative psychosis or Rett's disorder.

No randomized, controlled trials have investigated the treatment of conversion disorders or chronic fatigue syndromes in children. Expert advice regarding the management of these conditions recommends techniques similar to the cognitive-behavioral approaches to recurrent abdominal pain, with the addition of graded reintroduction of normal activities, but these have not been systematically evaluated.

Strategies for intervention in SDDs have mainly been offered by speech and language therapists or educational psychologists, rather than mental health practitioners. There is conflicting evidence as to their effectiveness, but there are some findings that parents can be helped by training to be effective therapists for their children. Newer strategies, based on research on underlying psychological deficits and tailored to individual cognitive strengths and weaknesses, seem promising but have not yet been properly evaluated.

There is little or no empirical evidence to guide decisions about location of treatment and when specialist residential or day care facilities might be needed. Given the cost of these facilities, research is needed to provide clearer guidance for service development.

Areas Where Further Research Is Needed

There is clearly a need to conduct further research into the origins and treatment of a wide range of child and adolescent mental health problems. This review has identified a number of areas where existing research has suggested specific topics for further work that may have a significant impact on the organization and delivery of treatment services.

GENERIC ISSUES

The very high placebo response observed in some child and adolescent patients makes demonstration of efficacy of all treatments problematic. In addition, the large difference in outcome between clinically referred depressed adolescents and those recruited through advertisement, a difference not attributable to greater severity, indicates that findings on efficacy in nonreferred samples cannot confidently be extrapolated to clinical groups. As there is also a high rate of remission among children in inactive control conditions, it may be wise to offer brief supportive therapy as the first-line treatment, followed by psychological treatment or medication only if the child fails to improve.

Outcome measures should cover more domains than that of symptomatology; a treatment may be more effective in the long run if it has a beneficial impact across other domains of functioning, even if the effect on symptoms is no greater.

Psychodynamic and family therapies should be manualized as a step toward systematic evaluation of these widely used approaches.

Most of the work to date has focused on "pathology" and investigated interventions to improve the functioning of poorly coping children and families. Not enough work has explored the attributes of well-functioning children and families.

Further research needs to focus on exploring which components of multicomponent packages are effective and which children are most suited to which interventions.

ANXIETY

As a substantial proportion (about half) of children with OCD fail to show clinically significant, sustained improvement even with the best-supported medication, there is a need to continue to work on effective psychosocial treatments for this condition. In particular, controlled studies of CBT are needed.

It would be valuable to explore the replicated finding that therapeutic support is as effective as CBT in the treatment of school phobia. This contradicts the generally accepted view that exposure is a central element in the cognitive-behavioral treatment of anxiety disorders, and it therefore requires further evaluation.

DEPRESSION

Inasmuch as research has shown a variety of treatment packages to be effective in treating depression in children, further research is needed to identify the elements that are most helpful in particular clinical situations, and to compare active treatments to each other rather than to inactive conditions such as a waiting-list control.

As the benefits of CBT are apparently not attributable to a reduction in negative cognitions, the mechanism of effectiveness needs to be explored.

CONDUCT PROBLEMS AND DELINQUENCY

Current priorities for research in the area of conduct problems and delinquency include a need for more precise indications for titrating and combining treatment modalities, effective extensions of programs to community settings, and the development of effective dissemination strategies, as inadequate implementations appear to have poorer outcomes. There is a suggestion that interventions may be more effective for children at younger ages, but this has not been substantiated in longitudinal studies. A high research priority is the development and evaluation of a cost-effective treatment approach to handle conduct problems of adolescence (particularly those with early childhood onset). Evidence-based treatments for this group are not widely available outside specialist centers.

ATTENTION-DEFICIT/HYPERACTIVITY DISORDER

Given the significant proportion of children with ADHD who are nonresponders to methylphenidate, further studies exploring combination treatments should be undertaken. Although we know that methylphenidate and other medications are effective, it is less clear as to how long treatment should continue.

More research is needed into effective educational interventions addressing the educational underachievement of many children with this disorder.

TOURETTE'S DISORDER

Further randomized controlled studies of medication for children with Tourette's disorder are urgently required, especially of the drugs with lower risks of side effects such as the SSRIs, selective MAOIs and atypical neuroleptics.

EATING DISORDERS

Given the high prevalence of young people with disturbed eating patterns in the community, research is needed to assist in identifying and intervening with those young people who will go on to develop significant eating disorders.

SUICIDE

Further research is needed into the impact of management by staff in accident and emergency departments during the initial stages of treatment of young people who have attempted suicide, the development of a greater understanding of why many choose to leave hospital before management has been completed, and—more generally—how to avert further suicide attempts over the longer term.

TRENDS IN THE DEVELOPMENT OF THERAPEUTIC APPROACHES IN CHILD AND FAMILY DISORDERS

In the course of this review, we noted a number of important trends in therapeutic approaches dictated by the emerging evidence. These trends are discussed in the following paragraphs.

Emphasis on the biological determinants of mental disorder and on the interaction of biological and psychosocial factors has increased. There is greater sensitivity to developmental considerations in the design and implementation of both physical and psychosocial treatment strategies, and a heightened interest in combining intervention strategies, both in terms of coupling physical and psychosocial treatments and in linking different treatment modalities (behavioral, cognitive, systemic, etc.). Awareness of increasingly specific sets of childhood and family problems has led to a proliferation of treatment operationalizations (manuals).

Increasing awareness of having to consider the system within which the child functions (the family, the school, the neighborhood, etc.) has led to a heightened interest in developing packages of interventions targeted at different people in the dysfunctional system, using different treatment approaches, and involving multiple agencies as service providers. It has also produced increasing concern about the child's social interactions and social functioning, rather than simply symptom-focused goals. There is an increased tendency across different treatment orientations to offer treatment in the context of the entire family, rather than focusing on the individual child. Mental health interventions have been extended from traditional inpatient and outpatient settings to more community-focused environs.

Increasingly, attention has been paid to social and demographic needs as well as the constraints imposed by health care delivery systems and the demands of everyday practice. Sensitivity to the role of ethnic, cultural, and biological factors as moderators of treatment effects has increased. There has been a growing awareness of the accountability of clinicians for the choice of treatments, including the evidence base for the treatment and its costs, leading to an emphasis on pharmacological and brief psychosocial treatments. More emphasis has been placed on treatment as a collaborative decision-making process between clients and clinicians.

It is beyond the scope of this summary to explore these emerging trends in detail. However, we regard a number of the issues raised as pivotal in evaluating the literature on effectiveness.

The Implicit Systemic Developmental Model and Its Implications

It seems to us that there is an emergent pan-theoretical model in child and adolescent mental health intervention, which draws its inspiration from a combination of biological, systems, cognitive-behavioral, and psychodynamic perspectives. Although these sources are not inevitably acknowledged and are very rarely acknowledged simultaneously, they permeate the application of the developmental psychopathology framework to treatment interventions (e.g., Alexander et al., 1996[vi]; Cicchetti & Cohen, 1995; Henggeler et al., 1998[vi]; Howard & Kendall, 1996a; Mash, 1998; Sameroff, 1995, 1998). We believe that this approach is a response to the burgeoning research literature on the naturalistic and experimental treatment outcome of childhood mental disorder. This new approach appears to us to be, at least for the moment, mostly implicit, to be inferred from attitudes rather than explicitly declared. It is most evident in the "how" of interventions, rather than the "what." It tends to guide the objectives of intervention strategies rather than the procedures of interventions themselves. It affects the scope and manner of service delivery rather than the content of the service. It reflects the active and immediate concerns of clinicians with clients, rather than their formal training and traditional attitudes. In the following section we review emergent themes from this review in the light of this model.

First, the child is rarely viewed as an individual. Rather, problem behaviors, either of the child or at the family level, are formulated in terms of interrelated and interreacting response systems and subsystems that regulate the child's behavior and which simultaneously exert a regulating influence on others within the same system. This tendency is as evident in modern psychoanalytic perspectives (e.g., Hauser, Powers, Noan, & Jacobson, 1984; Renik, 1993) as in cognitive-behavioral ones (Howard & Kendall, 1996a). The need to take an ecological approach is increasingly recognized, even when the focus is on a single aspect, such as the child's conduct problems, communication problems, or learning difficulties. A quarter of a century's research in developmental psychopathology confirms the view that specific problem behaviors are likely to be the consequence of heterogenous causal determinants, including the transactional interaction of biological predisposition with lived experience. It follows that the impact of an intervention cannot be assessed in terms of any single target variable, but a wide range of outcomes need to be considered, including the impact of changes in one relationship (subsystem) on other relationships within the same system (Emde & Robinson, 2000). Family systems are dynamic rather than stable entities. The child's dysfunction and family system interact in ways that are often difficult to predict. Finally, family systems are developmental entities. Their history creates predispositions in relation to, and expectations about, the future. The past does not determine the present, but rather interacts with it. The future can be altered only through addressing the interaction and not merely by addressing either the past or the present (Garbarino, 1995).

There are still many important differences between the contents of different approaches to the treatment of childhood problems. Historically, the differences between psychosocial treatment approaches have been so great that in the 1970s a special U.S. congressional inquiry was set up to determine whether psychosocial treatments had any claim to efficacy at all (Office of Technology Assessment, 1980). However, the high level of agreement on the guiding principles of treatment interventions for children is a clear sign of the emergent systemic perspective embracing all these orientations, including the now powerful biological approach.

What are the manifestations of this implicit systemic model on treatment approaches taken as a whole? Here we discuss some of the key points.

The Developmental Framework and the Merging of Preventive and Treatment Approaches

Conceptualizations of childhood disturbance and treatment have increasingly attempted to formulate, elaborate, anticipate, and modify the natural history of childhood disorders. Historically, child psychiatry has always had a considerable interest in the epidemiology of disorders (e.g., Rutter, 1997; Sameroff, 1998), and it is hardly surprising that as interest in treatment interventions has developed, it has built on this tradition. Even more important, perhaps, has been the emerging interest in developmental psychopathology as the organizing discipline in understanding child mental disorder (Cicchetti & Cohen, 1995; Toth & Cicchetti, 1999). Developmental psychopathology views development as involving progressive reorganizations in response to changing environmental demands and conceptualizes psycho-pathology as a breakdown of the child's and family's coping responses when adaptation is demanded of them.

Developmental psychopathology has forced outcome investigators to compare the posttreatment development of treated children with that of those developing normally. As a result, several treatment approaches that generated strong pre–post differences in measured behavior were found to be wanting. For example, in one study of integrated CBT for adolescents with ADHD, improvement following treatment was found in the majority of treated individuals to fall short of substantial improvements when it was assessed against the functioning of normal children (Barkley et al., 1992). In studies of problem-solving training for children with disordered conduct, the majority of successfully treated children were still found to function outside the norms for a nonclinical population 1 year after treatment termination (Kazdin et al., 1987b[i]). These considerations echo child psychoanalyst Anna Freud's statement that the aim of her intervention is to return the child to "the path of normal development" (Freud, 1965). Clearly, interventions are increasingly judged against this developmental objective.

Developmental considerations deeply permeate the outcome literature. Developmental stage (in general, rather inadequately assessed in terms of the child's chronological age) has been found to interact with the type of treatment. For example, a meta-analysis of CBT interventions found significantly larger effect sizes (ESs) for adolescents (ages 11–13) than for younger children (7–11 years) (Durlak et al., 1991). Similarly, medication effects depend on the child's biological capacity to metabolize specific pharmacological agents, and developmental pharmacokinetic and pharmacodynamic considerations are of great current concern (Vitiello & Jensen, 1997). Researchers are increasingly attempting to adjust their intervention to the child's developmental stage (biological, social, cognitive, and contextual). Maximizing the effectiveness of both biological and psychosocial interventions will depend on the full integration of developmental findings with the treatment literature.

THE WIDENING OF TREATMENT OBJECTIVES AND THE EMERGENT INTEGRATION OF THERAPIES

Psychosocial interventions in particular, but perhaps also medical interventions, are changing their foci in line with the implicit systemic model. The change is perhaps clearest in the evolution of behavioral treatments. These have moved from an approach firmly rooted in positivistic learning theory that denied the importance of all processes beyond those entailed in classical and operant conditioning, to an orientation that, at least implicitly (and sometimes explicitly; e.g., Howard & Kendall, 1996a; Meichenbaum, 1997), recognizes the importance of the child's and parents' feelings and thoughts (emotions and cognitions) as determinants of behavior. This shift has quickly led to a broadening of CBT interventions to include disorders that are principally affective in nature (e.g., depression). More important, in our view, among clinicians within this orientation there is increased concern with the emotional environment of the child. This environment includes communication patterns in the family (Gottman, Katz, & Hooven, 1997), which have thus far been the predominant concern of family therapists. A further example is the recognition of the importance of metacognitive controls in childhood disorders (Fonagy & Target, 1996; Howard & Kendall, 1996a).

The clearest implication of the implicit systemic model is that treatment objectives cannot be restricted to the child's symptomatic distress. Early behavioral interventions were widely known for addressing problems in an extremely narrow way (e.g., specific anxieties) and measuring progress with highly reactive instruments (e.g., anxiety in terms of avoidance of a phobic stimulus). This approach does not fit with the emerging implicit systemic model. Our review illustrates how treatment approaches rooted in a cognitive-behavioral tradition increasingly aim to influence the child's functioning within his or her family or peer group through the development of capacities, skills, and competencies that may maintain improvements in social relationships (Hoagwood et al., 1996). Comparisons of the effectiveness of pharmacological preparations will also require more sensitive measures of outcome than the degree of symptomatic change can provide, otherwise specific drug effects will be difficult to establish.

To achieve this goal, interventions aimed at specific problems with the child often need to be supplemented by additional procedures aimed at improving family functioning. For example, parent training for children with CD is more effective in the long term if a partner support component is added (Dadds et al., 1987[i]). Similarly, adding a family component to a treatment that focuses on problem solving, emotion management, communication, and interaction skills significantly enhances the effectiveness of treatment of children with anxiety problems (Barrett et al., 1996[i]). The notion that childhood problems are best seen in terms of the interrelation of response systems implies that treatment goals must focus on the development of psychological capacities within the child and within the family system that reduce dysfunction and improve adaptation in the long term. In Alan Kazdin's formulation (1997a), the outcomes must include child and family functioning, as well as outcomes of social importance.

More generally, the shifts in treatment objectives have brought about something of an integration between psychosocial treatment approaches. This integration has not produced the evolution of overarching theories, as some had hoped (e.g., Goldfried, 1995). Nor has there been an integration of techniques, as others had anticipated (e.g., Wachtel, 1977, 1987). Rather, there is increasing agreement across orientations concerning the clinical priorities in approaching families with problems. Convergence in techniques may be expected to be a consequence of integration at the level of the formulation of the clinical problem. We anticipate that it may become increasingly difficult to distinguish psychosocial approaches in future reviews. Perhaps the increasing specialization of treatment packages is a reaction to a reduction in the heterogeneity of treatment orientations.

A clear implication of the emergent systemic model is that treatments need not occur within the traditional setting of clinics and consulting rooms. If it is recognized that the child's disorder is a function of numerous interrelated response systems, then it clearly follows that the range of treatment settings as well as treatment agents has, in the past, been unnecessarily restricted. Outcome studies increasingly demonstrate that the most effective places for treatment delivery may not be either inpatient or outpatient settings. The community (Cunningham et al., 1995[i]), foster homes (Chamberlain, 1998[vi]), the school (Kolvin et al., 1981; Olweus, 1996[v]), summer camps (Pelham & Hoza, 1996b), and homes (Patterson & Forgatch, 1987[vi]) may be ideal contexts for intervention because of the unequivocal presence of the systemic pathogens in these environments. By the same token, the administrator of the intervention need not be the therapist. Administrators may be peers (mentoring approaches), teachers (Hops & Walker, 1988), parents (Forehand & Long, 1988[ii]), or foster parents (Chamberlain, 1998[vi]).

The Moderation of the Radical Goals of Treatment

A more subtle implication of the recognition of powerful biological and developmental determinants has been the moderation of some of the radical goals of psychosocial treatments. The early phase in the development of any novel treatment approach is characterized by a certain therapeutic optimism verging on grandiosity. This was certainly true for both psychoanalysis and behavior therapy in their respective heydays. In contrast, modern cognitive-behavioral therapists tend increasingly to focus on helping clients accept rather than control their thoughts and feelings (Jacobson & Christensen, 1996). This trend is perhaps clearest in the cognitive-behavioral approach to the treatment of schizophrenia (Kuipers et al., 1998), which has not so far been extended to childhood psychosis. Nevertheless, we note that recent cognitive-behavioral approaches to children with ADHD include helping parents accept their reactions to their child's condition, while also providing them with alternative coping strategies (Barkley, 1997). A number of disorders are at least partially irreversible as a consequence of the interaction between biological predisposition and the sensitivity of brain development to environmental influence during the early years; the implicit systemic approach suggests that psychosocial interventions (like medical ones) for childhood mental disorder may be forced to abandon the implicit notion of cure in favour of the treatment goal of more balanced functioning of subsystems within a systemic model. The relatively disappointing results of many trials that report long-term follow-ups speak eloquently to this issue.

The Decline of Generic Therapies and the Emergence of Specialist Treatments

Perhaps linked to the implicit assumption that developmental and situational demands may be quite specific at particular ages with particular groups in particular settings, the popularity of generic therapies has declined. In addition, there has been increased specialization. Neither physical nor psychosocial treatment can be regarded as generically effective. Specific programs based on particular principles are shown to be valid and useful with particular subgroups within a diagnostic category. Statements such as "cognitive-behavioral therapy is effective" are inherently suspect without accompanying specification of the particular permutation of techniques that were subjected to evaluation. This shift has major implications for training, as it can no longer be regarded to be adequate to offer training in the general principles of a particular brand-name approach, such as systemic family therapy, without also offering training in particular techniques brought together to deliver a specific program of intervention.

Here, of course, there may be major paradoxes. An individual with generic training in clinical psychology with a cognitive-behavioral orientation may not be in the best position to deliver a specific cognitive-behavioral program. In fact, the evidence suggests the contrary. Therapists in MST tend to be master's-level clinicians with no training in approaches other than MST (Borduin, 1999[vi]). Two eminent cognitive-behavioral therapists at a recent meeting of the American Academy of Child and Adolescent Psychiatry both informally expressed a preference for recruiting therapists with generic psychodynamic training for their trials in preference to individuals whose generic training was cognitive-behavioral. Despite the anecdotal nature of such evidence, there is no doubt that the increasing specialization of therapeutic programs presents a major challenge for the continued training of child mental health professionals. Effective interventions appear to require comprehensive knowledge of the specific parameters of particular treatment interventions and particular clusters of problems.

Multicomponent Interventions and Multidisciplinary Work

The recognition that problems are unlikely to have a single cause has foregrounded treatment intervention with multiple components. The so-called combined therapies include the integration of pharmacological and psychosocial treatments (Arnold, Abikoff, & Wells, 1997; Piacentini & Graae, 1997) as well as the combination of intervention strategies rooted in separate frames of reference, particularly systemic and cognitive-behavioral (Henggeler et al., 1999). Kazdin (1996a[vi]) has eloquently outlined the dangers of such combined and multimodal treatments.

In the course of this review, we were frequently confronted with the multidisciplinary character of many formulations and interventions. This was clear across most of the disorders scrutinized. The interconnected influences of physical, behavioral, educational, and social factors are clear in the treatment of ADHD (e.g., Multimodal Treatment Study of Children with ADHD Cooperative Group, 1999), anxiety disorders (e.g., Piacentini & Graae, 1997), childhood depression (e.g., Kazdin & Marciano, 1998), disorders of conduct (e.g., Kazdin, in press), and in the case of children with chronic physical illnesses (e.g., Johnson & Rodrigue, 1997).

The multidisciplinary perspective is notable both at the level of formulation and at the level of treatment delivery. A wide range of professionals are, and arguably need to be, involved in the delivery of mental health services to children and adolescents. Moderators of treatment outcome frequently include learning disabilities, implying the need for the involvement of educators. Both diagnostic considerations and effective use of drug treatments call for the involvement of child psychiatrists and pediatricians. A wide range of child mental health specialists have been shown to be helpful in delivering well-designed cognitive-behavioral programs (nurses, psychologists, social workers), although psychologists and child psychiatrists appear to play a key role in both designing and evaluating these interventions (e.g., Kazdin, 1998). Many treatment programs, notably MST (e.g., Borduin, 1999[vi]), demonstrate the importance of attending to the social needs of families with children or adolescents with mental disorder, clearly identifying a need for social work involvement. A reinforcement of the emphasis on interdisciplinary work is one of the key implications of this review.

THE CHRONIC CARE MODEL

It follows from the general systemic formulation of childhood disorders that brief treatments can have only limited effects. The dynamic systems in which children and adolescents with mental disorders live will tend to return to states of equilibrium, which frequently rekindle the dysfunctional behaviors of the children. This problem has been increasingly recognized by those designing innovative intervention programs. Kazdin (1997a), for example, proposed that disorders such as ADHD and early-onset CD may require continuing care in much the same way that juvenile-onset diabetes mellitus requires continuous administration of insulin. The need for interventions of greater intensity is more readily recognized in the case of disorders with great manifest severity such as childhood autism. The psychosocial intervention models that can titrate long-term interventions in an economic way have not yet been developed and represent a challenge for the future. Unfortunately, the emphasis on short-term interventions that followed the radical and optimistic agenda of early behavioral intervention has, to some degree, immunized funders against considering long-term treatments, particularly long-term and relatively intensive treatments. Equally pertinent and similarly underdeveloped is the "dental care" model suggested by Kazdin, whereby children and their families with chronic disorders are seen for regular checkups every 6 months. Treatment is offered on an as-needed basis as emerging developmental issues highlight new aspects of the child's and the family's problems.

Sensitivity to Contextual Effects and Individual Differences

The implicit systemic developmental model has focused the attention of researchers on individual differences in the manifestation of childhood disorders and the need to take these into consideration as moderators of the effectiveness of treatments. For example, the systemic perspective helped highlight the key role of parental psychopathology (maternal depression, parental substance misuse, marital conflict, abnormal parental attributional styles and parenting attitudes, etc.) in determining treatment outcome (e.g., Brent et al., 1999[i]; Dadds et al., 1987[i]; Frick et al., 1992). As all interventions with children rely extensively on the involvement of family members (from seeking professional help for the child, through administering medication, to acting as agents of change in parent training programs), it is clear that the presence of mental disorder in family members can strongly impact the likelihood of achieving successful treatment results. The successful treatment of the parent's disorder may be an essential precondition of the child's benefiting from treatment. In one study of parent training for children with ADHD, children with mothers who had ADHD were found to benefit more if the mother's ADHD was medicated as part of the treatment (Evans, Vallano, & Pelham, 1994).

Similarly, the systemic approach brings gender and cultural issues to the fore. For example, there have been a number of suggestions that the parenting values of specific ethnic groups should be considered in designing parent training programs (Forehand & Kotchick, 1996; Iwamasa, 1996). Evidently, parenting values will be quite different according to socioeconomic status, religious beliefs, and ethnic group. Similarly, recognition that the treatment of pathology exists within a system has drawn attention to cultural issues concerning gender. For example, gender differences are marked in the development of disruptive behavior. Anxiety is closely connected to disruptive behavior problems in girls but not in boys (Zahn-Waxler, Cole, Welsh, & Fox, 1995), and girls show a higher incidence of comorbid disorders (Zahn-Waxler, 1993). Further, although boys tend not to be upset by aggressive social exchanges, girls report high levels of distress (Crick, 1995). Whereas boys express anger directly, girls tend to do so indirectly, via verbal insults, gossip, tattling, ostracism, or threatening to withdraw friendship (Crick, Bigbee, & Howes, 1996). Findings such as these imply that treatment interventions for conduct problems may need to be modified according to both race and gender.

User Empowerment

In conducting this review, we have become aware of an increasing concern, on the part of clinicians and researchers, with the views of the families and the children who participate in evaluations. In our view it follows from the increased sensitivity to systemic and contextual factors in both the causation and remediation of childhood abnormality that the model of service delivery should move away from one focused on the "mental health expert" to one oriented toward achieving a collaborative relationship between the child, the family, and the clinician. The models reviewed in considering treatments for conduct problems (e.g., Henggeler et al., 1994; Webster-Stratton & Herbert, 1994) provide good examples of this collaborative decision-making perspective on the treatment of childhood disorders. It seems to us that within the implicit systemic framework, treatment strategies are applied as part of a flexible and collaborative enterprise jointly undertaken by the clinician and the family that enables the treatment to evolve, given certain generic strategies inherent to the approach, with at least partial participation of the client in decision making and full sensitivity to the varying needs of the family at different treatment phases.

This more flexible approach presents a new problem for evaluation. Although, on one hand, we recognize that treatments are unlikely to be effective without this kind of flexibility, we are also cognizant of the risk of compromising the standardization of treatment administration, which is essential in outcome research. We see flexibility and standardization as in opposition only at particular phases of treatment development. As a treatment approach matures, decision processes can become increasingly explicit; the decision tree (algorithm) approach frequently adopted in pharmacological trials is an example. Nevertheless, the need for flexibility brings with it a need for more detailed explication of decision-making processes than has perhaps been the case in the past. If user empowerment is an essential precondition to effective treatment, the development of explicitly stated algorithms for psychosocial treatments should be a priority.

SUMMARY

Based on our review, we have arrived at a number of assumptions and attributes that we believe increasingly characterize treatment research in the field of child and adolescent mental health.

1. The commitment to a coherent and consistent theoretical framework to guide practice that links models of pathology and treatment at least at the conceptual level
2. The recognition of the multiple causation of childhood disorder (although different orientations may privilege different levels of such an analysis
3. The recognition of the importance of bidirectional (reciprocal) influences
4. The recognition of the importance of neurobiological processes and that both drugs and psychosocial treatments can achieve changes by changing the brain
5. The recognition that a unique emphasis on either past (distal) or present (proximal) factors is inadequate
6. The recognition that adequate assessment must include information concerning development and knowledge of the population of children showing similar problems (incidence, prevalence, biological factors, system parameters)
7. Reliance on a multimethod approach in assessment and treatment
8. Commitment to the comprehensive evaluation of outcomes
9. A dialectic between an ideographic emphasis and a population-based approach
10. The involvement of the family in the treatment
11. The recognition of the importance of both emotions and cognitions in both causation and treatment

12. The recognition of the need to develop operational rules (manuals) for the implementation of treatments
13. The use of techniques specific to client groups and to developmental stages (e.g., preschool, adolescence)
14. The recognition of the key role played by social interactional processes between therapist and clients as part of treatment
15. A wish to explore the biological, psychological, and interpersonal processes that generate change
16. A concern with the generalization of outcomes both across settings and across time
17. The recognition of the need for measures of change across a number of domains
18. A concern with the experience of users of services
19. A concern with the wider social context of the families, including cultural factors

Appendix 1

Glossary of Psychopharmacological and Other Physical Treatments

This glossary provides a brief explanation and description of common psychopharmacological and other physical treatments for those not familiar with their use. It is not intended to be used as a guide for prescribing. Examples of common drugs from each major grouping are given, but this is not intended to be a complete list. Anyone wishing to prescribe medication for a child mental health disorder is strongly urged to consult his or her local prescribing guidance, which will contain far more detailed information about indications, contraindications, side effects, and appropriate dosages. It should be noted that because of the relative lack of experience of using these drugs in young people, a number of them are not officially licensed for use with children, despite being widely used.

ANTIPSYCHOTICS

Antipsychotic drugs are also known as major tranquilizers or neuroleptics. Traditional neuroleptics are all dopamine agonists and have similar therapeutic effects. Choice of which agent to use is often determined by the particular side effect profile of the different drugs and the tolerance of individual patients to particular drugs. Commonly used drugs are *chlorpromazine, thioridazine,* and *trifluoperazine* (phenothiazines), *haloperidol* and *droperidol* (butyrophenones), *sulpiride* (a benzamide), and *pimozide* (a diphenylbutyl-piperidine). Most antipsychotics can be administered orally or by intramuscular injection. Long-acting depot injections of major tranquilizers are rarely used in children and young people.

These drugs are used for the treatment of schizophrenia and other schizophreniform psychoses, mania, movement disorders such as tics, and, more experimentally, in the treatment of aggressive, overactive, and antisocial behaviors. *Pimozide* and *haloperidol* are the most commonly used antipsychotics in the treatment of Tourette's disorder.

Acute dystonic reactions (oculogyric crises, muscle spasms, etc.) and dyskinesias may occur on commencing treatment, or when dosages are increased, and seem particularly common in children and younger adults. Movement-related side effects—tremor, rigidity, and slowing of movements (extrapyramidal or "parkinsonian" features)—may occur with regular treatment and, in turn, can be treated with anticholinergic drugs such as procyclidine or orphenadrine. Other side effects include skin rashes, gastric disturbances, photosensitivity, cholestatic jaundice, postural hypotension, leucopenia and, more rarely, agranulocytosis, and obesity. Periodic blood counts and tests of renal and liver function are necessary if children are prescribed these drugs.

Pimozide carries an important additional risk of ECG changes, which appear to occur in approximately 20% of children taking the treatment. It should be withdrawn if there is T wave inversion or the development of U waves, and the ECG should be checked before any increase in dose, as well as prior to initiating treatment, and at regular intervals every few months.

Neuroleptic malignant syndrome (hyperthermia, muscle rigidity, autonomic instability, and altered consciousness) is rare but may occur with all antipsychotic medications. Tardive dyskinesia (rhythmical involuntary movements of the tongue, face, or mouth) is associated with longer-term treatment, but may occur in young people.

ATYPICAL ANTIPSYCHOTICS

Clozapine is a newer, "atypical" antipsychotic with markedly reduced extrapyramidal side effects. It has antiserotinergic properties and weak dopamine blocking activity at all but the D_4 receptor. However, it does have other potentially serious side effects, including neutropenias and agranulocytosis, seizures, and cardiac problems. It should not be prescribed without regular and careful blood monitoring. Because its potential value is compromised by its side effects, a new generation of atypical antipsychotics has been developed, characterized by their ability to be antagonists at 5-HT_{2A} receptors as well as at the more traditional D_2 receptor. These include such drugs as *risperidone*, *olanzapine*, and *amisulpride*.

PSYCHOSTIMULANTS

Methylphenidate and *dexamphetamine* are centrally acting stimulant drugs used for the treatment of attention deficit and hyperactivity disorders and conduct disorders (CD). They interact with catecholaminergic neurones and affect many areas of the central nervous system (CNS). It is unclear how they exert their effect at the receptor level, although there have been several hypotheses in the literature with some authors suggesting that noradrenaline is the primary mediator and others that the primary mediator is dopamine. *Methylphenidate* and *dexamphetamine* are both fast-acting drugs. They are rapidly absorbed after oral ingestion (in tablet form) and have an onset of action within the first hour. The duration of effect is no more than 4 hours.

Side effects are common and dose related, but rarely serious, and include dysphoria with episodes of unexplained weeping, irritability, abdominal pain and headache, difficulty in sleeping, and appetite suppression. Careful management of the dosage regime can reduce problems with appetite suppression and insomnia, as the drugs have a very short half-life and are eliminated quickly from the body. Thus, if the last dose is at least 4 hours before meals and before bedtime, these side effects can be largely eliminated.

Early reports suggested that stimulants should be avoided in children with comorbid seizures because they were thought to lower the seizure threshold. Recent practice suggests that if the seizure disorder is adequately treated, stimulants are safe to use. Similarly, early suggestions that stimulant medication exacerbated tics may have been ill founded.

Regular use over time with high dosages leads to significant growth retardation, but catch-up growth occurs on cessation of treatment so that final height is rarely significantly affected. There may be increases in heart rate and/or blood pressure. Probably the most severe side effect is the precipitation of a psychosis, but this is very rare in children and young people.

Height, weight, pulse, and blood pressure should be monitored regularly.

ANTIDEPRESSANTS

Tricyclic Antidepressants

The most common drugs in the tricyclic antidepressant group are *imipramine, lofepramine,* and *nortriptyline,* which are less sedating, and *amitriptylline, dothiepin,* and *clomipramine,* which are more sedating. They are used in the treatment of depression, obsessive–compulsive disorders (OCDs), attention deficit and hyperactivity disorders and tics. *Clomipramine* is particularly indicated in OCDs. These drugs have a variety of pharmacological actions, including alpha-adrenergic, antihistaminic, and anticholinergic activity. Their main mode of action is thought to be related to their ability to inhibit the reuptake of noradrenaline and serotonin (5HT). They are taken orally, and although side effects may be immediate, therapeutic effects may not be apparent for some 2 to 3 weeks.

Tricyclic antidepressants have frequent and potentially serious side effects, which include dry mouth, sweating, constipation, blurred vision, weight gain, hypertension, and cardiac arrhythmias. They are particularly dangerous in overdose. Blood pressure, pulse, and ECG monitoring should be carried out routinely if tricyclics are prescribed. There is a small risk of mania developing in patients successfully treated for depression, necessitating close monitoring of the mental state.

Selective Serotonin Reuptake Inhibitors

Because of the side effects of tricyclic antidepressants, a newer generation of selective serotonin (5-hydroxytryptamine, 5HT) reuptake inhibitors (SSRIs) have been developed, including *fluoxetine, paroxetine,* and *sertraline.* Side effects still occur (gastric disturbances, rashes, drowsiness, sweating, and tremor) but cardiotoxic problems are much less common. As with tricyclics, the possibility of mania developing as depression lifts needs to guarded against.

Monoamine Oxidase Inhibitors

Monoamine-oxidase inhibitors (MAOIs), as their name suggests, inhibit monoamine oxidase, thus causing an increase in levels of amine transmitters. *Phenelzine* and *isocarboxide* are the commonest irreversible MAOIs. *Moclobemide* is said to act by reversible inhibition of monoamine oxidase A and is therefore known as a reversible MAOI.

These drugs are used in the treatment of depression and anxiety and taken orally. Side effects include postural hypotension, dizziness, drowsiness, insomnia, fatigue, agitation and tremor, and anticholinergic effects such as dry mouth, constipation and other gastric disturbance, and blurred vision. More rarely, there may be liver problems and leucopenias.

As metabolism of some amines is inhibited by sympathomimetic drugs, and the pressor effect of tyramine in food is potentiated, interactions with foods and other drugs, including other antidepressants, can be very dangerous, and great caution must be exercised. Reversible MAOIs such as *moclobemide* cause less potentiation of tyramine, but caution is still needed.

LITHIUM

Lithium is an alkali metal with effects on (1) ion channels, (2) serotonin, dopamine and norepinephrine transmitter systems, and (3) second messenger. It is usually administered orally.

Lithium is used in the acute management of mania and in the long-term prophylactic treatment of bipolar disorders. It is also used, although much less commonly, in the treatment of severe aggressive conduct disorder, in which it is reported to reduce "explosiveness."

Children seem to tolerate lithium well, and few side effects are reported in the studies mentioned earlier. Commonly reported side effects are nausea, vomiting, diarrhea, tremor, polyuria, weight gain, headache, and fatigue. Thyroid and renal changes are common with polyuria and polydipsia. Rarer side effects can include arrhythmias, leucocytosis, muscle weakness, and exacerbation of skin conditions. Lithium has been reported to alter EEG patterns.

Serum lithium levels need to be monitored weekly on commencement of therapy, but once stabilized, lithium levels, as well as renal and thyroid function, should be monitored every 3–6 months.

ANTICONVULSANTS

The anticonvulsants *sodium valproate* and *carbamazepine* are used in the treatment of bipolar disorders (BPDs), especially in combination with lithium in treatment-resistant patients and in the treatment of aggressive outbursts.

Sodium valproate is administered orally. Its mode of action is unclear but is thought to involve potentiation of the inhibitory action of gamma amino-butyric acid (GABA).

Side effects of carbamazepine are significant and include lethargy, thrombocytopenia, liver dysfunction, ataxia, and tremor. Liver function should be monitored routinely when *sodium valproate* is prescribed.

Carbamazepine's mode of action is unclear. It too is administered orally. Side effects include dizziness, ataxia, drowsiness, headache, diplopia, skin rashes, leucopenia, liver dysfunction, and gastric disturbances. Patients prescribed *carbamazepine* should have regular blood monitoring.

BENZODIAZEPINES

The benzodiazepines are also known as minor tranquilizers. Benzodiazepines such as *diazepam*, *lorazepam*, *alprazolam*, and *clonazepam* have been used in the treatment of night terrors and parasomnias because of their action in reducing the amount of time spent in stage 4 sleep, and in support of behavioral anxiety management programs. Benzodiazepines have been tried in the management of aggressive behavior, but there is a risk that their disinhibiting effects may make such behavior worse.

There is little evidence to support the use of benzodiazepines with child mental health problems, and when used they are usually held to be effective only in the very short term.

BETA-BLOCKERS

Beta-blockers such as *propranolol* and *oxprenolol* block beta-adrenoreceptors and have been used in the treatment of the somatic symptoms of anxiety, and more experimentally in the treatment of aggression. Tablets are taken orally, and potential side effects include mood changes, dizziness, sleep disturbance, hypoglycemia, skin rashes, and gastric upsets. Caution must be exercised in administering these drugs to those with cardiac problems and those taking medication for cardiac problems, because of the influence on cardiovascular function.

More important, *propranolol* can cause bronchospasm and is therefore contraindicated if there is a history of asthma.

CLONIDINE AND GUANFACINE

Clonidine is an alpha-2 agonist most commonly used in the treatment of hypertension.

It has been used in the treatment of attention deficit and hyperactivity disorders, in the treatment of tics in children with Tourette's disorder, and, more experimentally, in the treatment of resistant CDs.

Side effects are not severe, the most frequent being drowsiness. Irritability has also been reported, especially in the early weeks of treatment. ECG changes such as prolongation of the P-R interval may occur and require an ECG prior to initiating treatment as well as during treatment. Blood pressure monitoring is required at the higher dosages.

A related drug to *clonidine* is *guanfacine*, which has a longer half-life than *clonidine* and is less sedating. It is also more selective in its binding with the alpha-receptors and does not bind with the alpha-1 receptors. It has been used in the treatment of attention deficit and hyperactivity disorders.

PIRACETAM

Nootropil (*piracetam*) has been used experimentally in the treatment of specific reading disorders. It is taken orally, and side effects are rare, but include somnolence and insomnia, weight gain, hyperkinesia, depression, rashes, and gastric upset.

ELECTROCONVULSIVE THERAPY

Electroconvulsive therapy (ECT) is only rarely used in children and adolescents, and there are no adequate controlled trials. Its use is controversial and tends to be considered in the presence of severe and disabling symptomatology when all other treatment approaches have failed. Under appropriate anesthesia, brief pulses of electricity are delivered for a fixed, brief period of time in order to induce a convulsion. The current is delivered via electrodes placed on the client's head either bilaterally or unilaterally to the nondominant hemisphere. Physical complications are rare, but include cardiac arrhythmias, hypertension, chest infections and emboli, dislocations due to insufficient muscle relaxation, and prolonged seizures. Psychological testing indicates a significant but short and rapidly decreasing retrograde amnesia and some anterograde amnesia for about 24 hours after each treatment. There is no clear evidence of long-lasting memory problems. The most troublesome side effect is headache, which may last for some hours after treatment.

Appendix 2

Search Terms

Search term	Related clinical term
abuse	physical emotional $\left.\right\}$ abuse sexual
academic	academic skills disorder academic problems/difficulties
acculturation	acculturation problem
addiction	drug and alcohol addiction
adjustment	adjustment disorder
affective	affective disorder
agoraphobic	agoraphobic disorder
anorexia	anorexia nervosa
antisocial	antisocial personality disorder antisocial behavior
overanxious	overanxious disorder
Asperger's	Asperger's disorder
autism	autism
bereavement	bereavement problems
bipolar	bipolar disorder
borderline	borderline personality disorder
bulimia	bulimia nervosa
bullying	conduct disorder, ODD
childhood disintegrative disorder	childhood disintegrative disorder

Search term	Related clinical term
communication	communication problems/difficulties/disorder
conduct	conduct disorder/problems
conversion	conversion disorder
cyclothym*	cyclothymic disorder
delirium	delirium disorder
delusion*	delusional disorder, delusions
delinqu*	delinquency
depression	depression
development*	development, developmental
disruptive	disruptive behavior
dissociat*	dissociation, dissociative
dysthym*	dysthymia, dysthymic disorder
eating	eating disorders
encopresis	encopresis disorder
enuresis	enuresis disorder
epilepsy	seizure disorder
feeding	feeding problems
failure to thrive	failure to thrive
gender	gender identity disorder
hyperactivity	hyperactivity, ADHD
hypochondria*	hypochondria
hypomania	hypomania, hypomania disorder
hysteria	hysteria
identity	identity problems
impulse control	impulsivity
intermittent explosive disorder	intermittent explosive disorder
kleptomania stealing	kleptomania
language	language delay/language disorders
learning	learning difficulties/disabilities
mania	mania, manic episodes, manic depression

Search term	Related clinical term
mental retardation	mental retardation
mixed episode	mixed episode
mood	mood disorders
motor	motor skills disorder, motor problems
Munchhausen by proxy syndrome (MBPS)	Munchhausen by proxy syndrome (MBPS)
neurolepsy	neurolepsy problems
neglect	problems of neglect
nightmare*	nightmares, nightmare disorders
obsessive–compulsive	obsessive–compulsive disorder (OCD)
offend*	young offenders
pain	pain disorder, difficulties with pain
panic	panic disorder, panic attack
paranoi*	problems related to paranoia
patholog*, psychopathology	pathological, pathology
personality	personality problems, disorders
pervasive developmental delay	pervasive developmental delay (PDD)
phobia*	phobic disorders
phonological	phonological disorders
psychotic	psychosis, psychotic disorders
posttraumatic	posttraumatic stress disorders
reading	reading disorders, reading difficulties
relational relationship	relationship disorders
Rett's	Rett's disorder
schizo*	schizophrenia, schizotypal/schizoaffective, schizoid/schizophrenic disorder
school refusal	school refusal
sexual disorder*	sexual problems, sexually inappropriate behavior, sexual behavior, sexual difficulties
self-harm	self-harm
separation anxiety	anxiety disorders

Search term	Related clinical term
sleep*	sleepwalking disorder, sleep disorders
insomnia	
dyssomnia	
parasomnia	
somat*	somatic problems
psychosomat*	somatoform disorder
somatoform	
specific	specific developmental disorders
stereotypic	stereotypic movement disorder
stuttering	speech disorders
suicide	suicide and self-harm
substance abuse	drug/alcohol abuse/dependence
substance dependence	
tic	tics, Tourette's
trichotillomania	trichotillomania
Tourette's	Tourette's disorder
pyromania	firesetting
fire*	
truan*	truancy

Note. Using the asterisks (that are next to some terms) in the search engine means it will search for all words beginning with that term.

References

AACAP Official Action. (1997). Practice parameters for the assessment and treatment of children, adolescents, and adults with attention deficit/hyperactivity disorder. *Journal of the American Academy of Child and Adolescent Psychiatry, 36*(Suppl.), 85S–121S.

AACAP Work Group on Quality Issues. (1998). Summary of the practice parameters for the assessment and treatment of children and adolescents with substance abuse disorders. *Journal of the American Academy of Child and Adolescent Psychiatry, 37*, 122–126.

Aber, J. A., Brown, J. L., & Henrich, C. C. (1999). *Teaching conflict resolution: An effective school based approach to violence prevention.* New York: National Center for Children in Poverty.

Abidin, R. R. (1997). Parenting Stress Index: A measure of the parent–child system. In C. P. Zalaquett & R. J. Wood (Eds.), *Evaluating stress: A book of resources* (pp. 277–291). Lanham, MD: Scarecrow Press.

Abikoff, H. (1991). Cognitive training in ADHD children: Less to it than meets the eye. *Journal of Learning Disabilities, 24*, 205–209.

Abikoff, H., Ganeles, D., Reiter, G., Blum, C., Foley, C., & Klein, G. R. (1988). Cognitive training in academically deficient ADDH boys receiving stimulant medication. *Journal of Abnormal Child Psychology, 16*, 411–432.

Abikoff, H., & Gittelman, R. (1985). The normalizing effects of methylphenidate on the classroom behaviour of ADDH children. *Journal of Abnormal Child Psychology, 13*, 33–44.

Abikoff, H., Klein, R., Klass, E., & Ganeles, D. (1987, October). *Methylphenidate in the treatment of conduct disordered children.* Paper presented at the symposium "Diagnosis and treatment issues in children with disruptive behavior disorders", conducted at the annual meeting of the American Academy of Child and Adolescent Psychiatry, Washington, DC.

Abikoff, H., & Hechtman, L. (1996). Multimodal therapy and stimulants in the treatment of children with attention deficit hyperactivity disorder. In E. D. Hibbs & P. S. Jensen (Eds.), *Psychosocial treatments for child and adolescent disorders: Empirically based strategies for clinical practice* (pp. 341–369). Washington, DC: American Psychological Association.

Abikoff, H., & Klein, R. G. (1992). Attention-deficit hyperactivity and conduct disorder: Comorbidity and implications for treatment. *Journal of Consulting and Clinical Psychology, 60*, 881–892.

Ablon, J. S., & Jones, E. E. (1998). How expert clinicians' prototypes of an ideal treatment correlate with outcome in psychodynamic and cognitive-behavioral therapy. *Psychotherapy Research, 8*, 71–83.

Abramowitz, A. J. (1994). Classroom interventions for disruptive behavior disorders. *Child and Adolescent Psychiatric Clinics of North America, 3*, 343–360.

Abramowitz, A. J., & O'Leary, S. G. (1991). Behavioral interventions for the classroom: Implications for students with ADHD. *School Psychology Review, 20*, 220–234.

Achenbach, T. M. (1988). Integrating assessment and taxonomy. In M. Rutter & A. H. Tuma (Eds.), *Assessment and diagnosis in child psychopathology* (pp. 300–343). New York: Guilford Press.

Achenbach, T. M. (1991a). *Manual for the Child Behavior Checklist/4–8 and 1991 Profile.* Burlington: University of Vermont, Department of Psychiatry.

Achenbach, T. M. (1991b). *Manual for the Teacher Report Form and Profile.* Burlington: University of Vermont, Department of Psychiatry.

Achenbach, T. M. (1991c). *Manual for the Youth Self-Report and 1991 Profile.* Burlington: University of Vermont, Department of Psychiatry.

Achenbach, T. M. (1995). Diagnosis, assessment, and comorbidity in psychosocial treatment research. *Journal of Abnormal Child Psychology, 23,* 45–64.

Achenbach, T. M., & Edelbrock, C. S. (1981). Behavioral problems and competencies reported by parents of children aged four through sixteen. *Monographs of the Society for Research in Child Development, 46,* 1–82.

Achenbach, T. M., & Edelbrock, C. S. (1983a). *Manual for the Child Behavior Checklist and Revised Child Behavior Profile.* Burlington: University of Vermont, Department of Psychiatry.

Achenbach, T. M., & Edelbrock, C. S. (1983b). *Manual for the Child Behavior Checklist and Revised Child Behavior Profile.* Burlington: Department of Psychiatry, University of Vermont.

Achenbach, T. M., & Edelbrock, C. S. (1986). *Manual for the Teacher's Report Form and Teacher Version of the Child Behavior Profile.* Burlington: University of Vermont, Department of Psychiatry.

Achenbach, T. M., & Edelbrock, C. S. (1987). *Manual for the Youth Self-Report and Profile.* Burlington: University of Vermont, Department of Psychiatry.

Achenbach, T. M., & Howell, C. T. (1993). Are American children's problems getting worse?: A 13-year comparison. *Journal of the American Academy of Child and Adolescent Psychiatry, 32,* 1145–1154.

Achenbach, T. M., Howell, C. T., McConaughy, S. H., & Stanger, C. (1995a). Six-year predictors of problems in a national sample of children and youth: II. Signs of disturbance. *Journal of the American Academy of Child and Adolescent Psychiatry, 34,* 488–498.

Achenbach, T. M., Howell, C. T., McConaughy, S. H., & Stanger, C. (1995b). Six-year predictors of problems in a national sample: I. Cross-informant syndromes. *Journal of the American Academy of Child and Adolescent Psychiatry, 34,* 336–347.

Achenbach, T. M., Howell, C. T., McConaughy, S. H., & Stanger, C. (1995c). Six-year predictors of problems in a national sample: III. Transitions to young adult syndromes. *Journal of the American Academy of Child and Adolescent Psychiatry, 34,* 658–669.

Achenbach, T. M., McConaughy, S. H., & Howell, C. T. (1987). Child/adolescent behavioral and emotional problems: Implications of crossinformant correlations for situational specificity. *Psychological Bulletin, 101,* 213–232.

Adams, M., Kutcher, S., Antoniw, E., & Bird, D. (1996). Diagnostic utility of endocrine and neuroimaging screening tests in first onset adolescent psychosis. *Journal of the American Academy of Child Adolescent Psychiatry, 35,* 67–73.

Addis, M., Wade, W., & Hatgis, W. (1999). Barriers to dissemination of evidence based practices: Addressing practitioners' concerns about manual based psychotherapies. *Clinical Psychology: Science and Practice, 6,* 430–411.

Adler, R., Nunn, R., Northam, E., Lebnan, V., & Ross, R. (1994). Secondary prevention of childhood firesetting. *Journal of the American Academy of Child and Adolescent Psychiatry, 33,* 1194–1204.

Agras, W. S., Barlow, D. H., Chapin, H. N., Abel, G. G., & Leitenberg, H. (1974). Behavior modification of anorexia nervosa. *Archives of General Psychiatry, 30,* 279–286.

Agras, W. S., Rossiter, E., Arnow, B., Telch, C. F., Raeburn, S. D., Schneider, J., Bruce, B., Perl, M., & Koran, L. (1992). Pharmacologic and cognitive-behavioral treatment for bulimia nervosa: A controlled comparison. *American Journal of Psychiatry, 149,* 82–87.

Al Ansari, A., Gouthro, S., Ahmad, K., & Steele, C. (1996). Hospital-based behavior modification program for adolescents: Evaluation and predictors of outcome. *Adolescence, 31,* 469–476.

Albano, A. M., Marten, P. A., Holt, C. S., Heimberg, R. G., & Barlow, D. H. (1995). Cognitive-behavioral group treatment for social phobia in adolescents: A preliminary study. *Journal of Nervous and Mental Disease, 183,* 649–656.

Alderman, J., Wolkow, R., Chung, M., & Johnston, H. F. (1998). Sertraline treatment of children and adolescents with obsessive–compulsive disorder or depression: Pharmacokinetics, tolerability and efficacy. *Journal of the American Academy of Child and Adolescent Psychiatry, 37,* 386–394.

Alessi, N., Naylor, M. W., Ghaziuddin, M., & Zubieta, J. K. (1994). Update on lithium carbonate therapy in children and adolescents. *Journal of the American Academy of Child and Adolescent Psychiatry, 33,* 291–304.

Alexander, J. F., Barton, C., Schiavo, R. S., & Parsons, B. V. (1976). Systems-behavioral intervention with families of delinquents: Therapist characteristics, family behavior, and outcome. *Journal of Consulting and Clinical Psychology, 44,* 656–664.

Alexander, J. F., & Parsons, B. V. (1973). Short-term behavioral intervention with delinquent families: Impact on family process and recidivism. *Journal of Abnormal Psychology, 81,* 219–225.

Alexander, J. F., & Parsons, B. V. (1982). *Functional family therapy.* Monterey, CA: Brooks/Cole.

Alexander, J. F., Waldron, H. B., Newberry, A. M., & Liddle, N. (1988). Family approaches to treating delinquents. In E. W. Nunnally, C. S. Chilman, & F. M. Cox (Eds.), *Mental illness, delinquency, addictions and neglect* (pp. 128–146). Newbury Park, CA: Sage.

Alexander, J. G., Jameson, P. B., Newell, R. M., & Gunderson, D. (1996). Changing cognitive schemas: A necessary antecedent to changing behaviors in dysfunctional families? In K. S. Dobson & K. D. Craig (Eds.), *Advances in cognitive-behavioral therapy* (pp. 174–192). Thousand Oaks, CA: Sage.

Allard, R., Marshall, M., & Plante, M. C. (1992). Intensive follow-up does not decrease the risk of repeat suicide attempts. *Suicide and Life-threatening Behavior, 22,* 303–314.

Allen, A. J., Leonard, H., & Swedo, S. E. (1995). Current knowledge of medications for the treatment of childhood anxiety disorders. *Journal of the American Academy of Child and Adolescent Psychiatry, 34,* 976–986.

Allen, J. P., & Land, D. (1999). Attachment in adolescence. In J. Cassidy & P. R. Shaver (Eds.), *Handbook of attachment: Theory, research, and clinical applications* (pp. 319–335). New York: Guilford Press.

Alto, J. L., & Frankenberger, W. (1995). Effects of methylphenidate on academic achievement from first to second grade. *International Journal of Disability, Development and Education, 42,* 259–273.

Aman, M. G. (1982). Stimulant drug effects in developmental disorders and hyperactivity: Toward a resolution of disparate findings. *Journal of Autism and Developmental Disorders, 12,* 385–398.

Aman, M. G., Findling, R. L., & Derivan, A. (1999, October). *Risperidone versus placebo for severe conduct disorder in children with mental retardation.* Paper presented at the American College of Clinical Pharmacy Annual Meeting, Kansas City, MO.

Aman, M. G., Kern, R. A., McGhee, D. E., & Arnold, L. E. (1993a). Fenfluramine and methylphenidate in children with mental retardation and attention deficit hyperactivity disorder: Laboratory effects. *Journal of Autism and Developmental Disorders, 23,* 491–506.

Aman, M. G., Kern, R. A., McGhee, D. E., & Arnold, L. E. (1993b). Fenfluramine and methylphenidate in children with mental retardation and ADHD: Clinical and side effects. *Journal of the American Academy of Child and Adolescent Psychiatry, 32,* 851–859.

Aman, M. G., Marks, R. E., Turbott, S. H., Wilsher, C. P., & Merry, S. N. (1991). Methylphenidate and thioridazine in the treatment of intellectually subaverage children: Effects on cognitive–motor performance. *Journal of the American Academy of Child and Adolescent Psychiatry, 30,* 246–256.

Ambrosini, P. J. (2000). A review of pharmacotherapy of major depression in children and adolescents. *Psychiatric Services, 51,* 627–633.

Ambrosini, P. J., Bianchi, M. D., Rabinovitch, H., & Elia, J. (1993). Antidepressant treatments in children and adolescents: I. Affective disorders. *Journal of the American Academy of Child and Adolescent Psychiatry, 32,* 1–6.

Ambrosini, P. J., Wagner, K. D., Biederman, J., Glick, I., Tan, C., Elia, J., Hebeler, J. R., Rabinovitch, H., Lock, J., & Geller, D. (1999). Multicenter open-label sertraline study in adolescent outpatients with major depression. *Journal of the American Academy of Child and Adolescent Psychiatry, 38,* 566–572.

American Academy of Child and Adolescent Psychiatry. (1997a). Practice parameters for the assessment and treatment of children and adolescents with anxiety disorders. *Journal of the American Academy of Child and Adolescent Psychiatry, 36*(Suppl.), 69S–84S.

American Academy of Child and Adolescent Psychiatry. (1997b). Practice parameters for the assessment and treatment of children and adolescents with substance use disorders. *Journal of the American Academy of Child and Adolescent Psychiatry, 36*(10, Suppl.), 140–156.

American Academy of Child and Adolescent Psychiatry. (1998a). Practice parameters for the assessment and treatment of children and adolescents with depressive disorders. *Journal of the American Academy of Child and Adolescent Psychiatry, 37*(10, Suppl.), 63S–83S.

American Academy of Child and Adolescent Psychiatry. (1998b). Practice parameters for the assessment and treatment of children and adolescents with language and learning disorders. *Journal of the American Academy of Child and Adolescent Psychiatry, 37*(Suppl.), 46S–62S.

American Academy of Child and Adolescent Psychiatry. (1998c). Practice parameters for the assessment and treatment of children and adolescents with obsessive–compulsive disorder. *Journal of the American Academy of Child and Adolescent Psychiatry, 37*(10, Suppl.), 27S–45S.

American Academy of Child and Adolescent Psychiatry. (1999). Practice parameters for the assessment of children, adolescents and adults with autism and other pervasive developmental disorders. *Journal of the American Academy of Child and Adolescent Psychiatry, 38*(Suppl.), 32S–54S.

American Academy of Pediatrics Committee on Drugs. (1996). Unapproved uses of approved drugs: The physician, the package insert, and the Food and Drug Administration: Subject review. *Pediatrics, 98*, 143–145.

American Psychiatric Association. (1952). *Diagnostic and statistical manual of mental disorders.* Washington, DC: Author.

American Psychiatric Association. (1987). *Diagnostic and statistical manual of mental disorders* (3rd ed., rev.). Washington, DC: Author.

American Psychiatric Association. (1994). *Diagnostic and statistical manual of mental disorders* (4th ed.). Washington, DC: Author.

Anastopoulos, A. D., DuPaul, G. J., & Barkley, G. J. (1991). Stimulant medication and parent training therapies for attention deficit-hyperactivity disorder. *Journal of Learning Disabilities, 24*, 210–218.

Anastopoulos, A. D., Shelton, T. L., DuPaul, G. J., & Guevremont, D. C. (1993). Parent training for attention-deficit hyperactivity disorder: Its impact on parent functioning. *Journal of Abnormal Child Psychology, 21*, 581–596.

Anderson, A. E., Morse, C. L., & Santmyer, K. S. (1985). Inpatient treatment for anorexia nervosa. In D. M. Garner & P. E. Garfinkel (Eds.), *Handbook of psychotherapy for anorexia nervosa and bulimia* (pp. 311–333). New York: Guilford Press.

Anderson, B. J., Brackett, J., Ho, J., & Laffel, L. M. B. (1999). An office-based intervention to maintain parent–adolescent teamwork in diabetes management: Impact on parent involvement, family conflict, and subsequent glycemic control. *Diabetes Care, 22*, 713–721.

Anderson, J. C., Williams, S., McGee, R., & Silva, P. A. (1987). DSM-III disorders in preadolescent children: Prevalence in a large sample from the general population. *Archives of General Psychiatry, 44*, 69–76.

Anderson, L. T., Campbell, M., Grega, D. M., Perry, R., Small, A. M., & Green, W. H. (1984). Haloperidol in the treatment of infantile autism: Effects on learning and behavioral symptoms. *American Journal of Psychiatry, 141*, 1195–1202.

Anderson, S. R., Avery, D. L., DiPeitro, E. K., Edwards, G. L., & Christian, W. P. (1987). Intensive home based early intervention with autistic children. *Education and Treatment of Children, 10*, 352–366.

Andreasen, N. (1982). *The scales for the assessment of positive and negative symptoms.* Iowa City: University of Iowa.

Andrews, D., Zinger, I., Hoge, R., Bonta, J., Gendreau, P., & Cullen, F. (1990). Does correctional treatment work? A clinically relevant and psychologically informed meta-analysis. *Criminology, 28*, 369–404.

Andrews, D. A., & Bonton, J. (1994). *The psychology of criminal conduct.* Cincinnati, OH: Anderson.

Andrus, J. K., Fleming, D. W., Heumann, M. A., & Wassell, J. T. (1991). Surveillance of at-tempted suicide among adolescents in Oregon, 1988. *American Journal of Public Health, 81,* 1067–1069.

Angold, A., & Costello, E. J. (1995). A test–retest reliability study of child-reported symptoms and diagnoses using the Child and Adolescent Psychiatric Assessment (CAPA-C). *Psychological Medicine, 25,* 755–762.

Angold, A., & Costello, E. J. (1996). Toward establishing an empirical basis for the diagnosis of oppositional defiant disorder. *Journal of the American Academy of Child and Adolescent Psychiatry, 35,* 1205–1212.

Angold, A., Costello, E. J., Farmer, E. M., Burns, B. J., & Erkanli, A. (1999). Impaired, but undiag-nosed. *Journal of the American Academy of Child and Adolescent Psychiatry, 38,* 129–137.

Angold, A., Erklanis, A., Costello, E. J., & Rutter, M. (1996). Precision, reliability and accuracy in the dating of symptom onsets in child and adolescent psychopathology. *Journal of Child Psy-chology and Psychiatry, 37,* 657–664.

Angold, A., Weissman, M., John, K., Merikangas, K., Prusoff, B., Wickramaratne, I., Gammon, G., & Warner, V. (1987). Parent and child reports of depressive symptoms in children at low and high risk of depression. *Journal of Child Psychology and Psychiatry, 28,* 901–909.

Anonymous. (1992). Cross design synthesis: A new strategy for studying medical outcomes. *Lancet, 340,* 944–946.

Aos, S., Phipps, P., Barnoski, R., & Lieb, R. (1999). *The comparative costs and benefits of programs to re-duce crime: A review of national research findings with implications for Washington state.* Olympia, WA: Washington State Institute for Public Policy.

Apter, A., Bernhout, E., & Tyano, S. (1984). Severe obsessive–compulsive disorder in adolescence: A report of eight cases. *Journal of Adolescence, 7,* 349–358.

Apter, A., Pauls, D. L., & Bleich, A. (1993a). An epidemiological study of Gilles de la Tourette's syn-drome in Israel. *Archives of General Psychiatry, 50,* 734–738.

Apter, A., Ratzoni, G., King, R. A., Weizman, A., Iancu, I., Binder, M., & Riddle, M. A. (1993b). Fluvoxamine open-label treatment of adolescent inpatients with obsessive–compulsive disor-der or depression. *Journal of the American Academy of Child and Adolescent Psychiatry, 33,* 342–348.

Arbuthnot, J., & Gordon, D. A. (1986). Behavioral and cognitive effects of a moral reasoning devel-opment intervention for high-risk behavior-disordered adolescents. *Journal of Consulting and Clinical Psychology, 54,* 208–216.

Armbruster, P., & Kazdin, A. E. (1994). Attrition in child psychotherapy. In T. H. Ollendick & R. J. Prinz (Eds.), *Advances in clinical child psychology* (Vol. 16, pp. 81–108). New York: Plenum Press.

Armenteros, J. L., Whitaker, A. H., Welikson, M., Stedge, D. J., & Gorman, J. (1997). Risperidone in adolescents with schizophrenia: An open pilot study. *Journal of the American Academy of Child and Adolescent Psychiatry, 36,* 694–700.

Arnold, J. E., Levine, A. G., & Patterson, G. R. (1975). Changes in sibling behavior following family intervention. *Journal of Consulting and Clinical Psychology, 43,* 683–688.

Arnold, J. E., O'Leary, S. G., Wolff, L. S., & Acker, M. M. (1993). The Parenting Scale: A measure of dysfunctional parenting in discipline situations. *Psychological Assessment, 5,* 137–144.

Arnold, L. E., Abikoff, H. B., & Wells, K. C. (1997). National Institute of Mental Health Collabora-tive Multimodal Treatment Study of Children with ADHD (the MTA): Design challenges and choices. *Archives of General Psychiatry, 54,* 865–868.

Arnold, L. E., Stoff, D. M., Cook, E., Cohen, D. J., Kruesi, M., Wright, C., Hattab, J., Graham, P., Zametkin, A., Castellanos, F. X., McMahon, W., & Leckman, J. F. (1995). Ethical issues in bi-ological psychiatric research with children and adolescents. *Journal of the American Academy of Child and Adolescent Psychiatry, 34,* 929–939.

Aro, H., Paronen, O., & Aro, S. (1987). Psychosomatic symptoms among 14–16-year-old Finnish adolescents. *Social Psychiatry, 22,* 171–176.

Asarnow, J. R. (1994). Childhood-onset schizophrenia. *Journal of Child Psychology and Psychiatry, 35,* 1345–1371.

Asarnow, J. R., Jaycox, L. H., & Tompson, M. C. (2001). Depression in youth: Psychosocial interventions. *Journal of Clinical Child Psychology, 30*, 33–47.

Asarnow, J. R., Tompson, M., Hamilton, E. B., Goldstein, M. J., & Gurthrie, D. (1994). Family expressed emotion, childhood onset depression, and childhood schizophrenia spectrum disorders: Is expressed emotion a non-specific correlate of child psychopathology or a specific risk factor for depression? *Journal of Abnormal Child Psychology, 22*, 129–146.

Asher, S. R., & Dodge, K. A. (1986). Identifying children who are rejected by their peers. *Developmental Psychology, 22*, 444–449.

Asperger, H. (1944). Autistischen Psychopathen in Kindesalter. *Archiv fur Psychiatrie und Nervenkrankheiten, 177*, 76–136.

Associated Marine Institutes. (1999). *1999 Recidivism Study*. Tampa, FL: Author.

Audit Commission. (1996). *Misspent youth*. London: Her Majesty's Stationery Office.

August, G. J., Ostrander, R., & Bloomquist, M. J. (1992). Attention deficit hyperactivity disorder: An epidemiological screening method. *American Journal of Orthopsychiatry, 62*, 387–396.

Ayllon, T., Garber, S., & Pisor, K. (1975). The elimination of discipline problems through a combined school–home motivational system. *Behavior Therapy, 6*, 616–626.

Azrin, N. H., McMahon, P. T., Donohue, V. A., Besalel, V. A., Lapinski, K. J., Kogan, E. S., Acierno, R. E., & Galloway, E. (1994). Behaviour therapy for drug abuse: A controlled treatment outcome study. *Behaviour Research and Therapy, 32*, 857–866.

Azrin, N. H., & Peterson, A. L. (1988). Habit reversal for the treatment of Tourette syndrome. *Behaviour Research and Therapy, 11*, 347–355.

Azrin, N. H., & Peterson, A. L. (1990). Treatment of Tourette syndrome by habit reversal: A waiting-list control group comparison. *Behavior Therapy, 21*, 305–318.

Baer, A., & Nietzel, M. T. (1991). Cognitive and behavioral treatment of impulsivity in children: A meta-analytic review of the outcome literature. *Journal of Clinical Child Psychology, 20*, 400–412.

Baer, D. M. (1993). Quasi-random assignment can be as convincing as random assignment. *American Journal on Mental Retardation, 97*, 373–375.

Bailey, A. J., Bolton, P., Butler, L., Le Couteur, A., Murphy, M., Webb, T., & Rutter, M. (1993). Prevalence of the fragile X anomaly amongst autistic twins and singletons. *Journal of Child Psychology and Psychiatry, 34*, 673–688.

Bailey, A. J., Le Couteur, A., Gottesman, I., Bolton, P., Simonoff, E., Yuzda, E., & Rutter, M. (1995). Autism as a strongly genetic disorder: Evidence from a British twin study. *Psychological Medicine, 25*, 63–77.

Ballenger, J. C., Reus, V. I., & Post, R. M. (1982). The "atypical" clinical picture of adolescent mania. *American Journal of Psychiatry, 139*, 602–606.

Balthazor, M. J., Wagner, R. K., & Pelham, W. E. (1991). The specificity of the effects of stimulant medication on classroom-learning-related measures of cognitive processing for attention deficit disorder children. *Journal of Abnormal Child Psychology, 19*, 35–52.

Bandura, A. (1977). *Social learning theory*. Englewood Cliffs, NJ: Prentice-Hall.

Bank, L., Marlowe, J. H., Reid, J. B., Patterson, G. R., & Weinrott, M. R. (1991). A comparative evaluation of parent-training interventions for families of chronic delinquents. *Journal of Abnormal Child Psychology, 19*, 15–33.

Barabasz, A. F. (1973). Group desensitization of test anxiety in elementary school. *Journal of Psychology, 83*, 295–301.

Barkley, R. A. (1981). *Hyperactive children: A handbook for diagnosis and treatment*. New York: Guilford Press.

Barkley, R. A. (1987). *Defiant children: A clinician's manual for parent training*. New York: Guilford Press.

Barkley, R. A. (1988). The effects of methylphenidate on the interactions of pre-school children with their mothers. *Journal of the American Academy of Child and Adolescent Psychiatry, 27*, 336–341.

Barkley, R. A. (1990). *Attention-deficit/hyperactivity disorder: A handbook for diagnosis and treatment*. New York: Guilford Press.

Barkley, R. A. (1997). *ADHD and the nature of self-control.* New York: Guilford Press.

Barkley, R. A., DuPaul, G. J., & McMurray, M. B. (1990a). Comprehensive evaluation of attention deficit disorder with and without hyperactivity as defined by research criteria. *Journal of Consulting and Clinical Psychology, 58,* 775–789.

Barkley, R. A., Fischer, M., Edelbrock, C., & Smallish, L. (1991). The adolescent outcome of hyperactive children diagnosed by research criteria: III. Mother–child interactions, family conflicts and maternal psychopathology. *Journal of Child Psychology and Psychiatry and Allied Disciplines, 32,* 233–255.

Barkley, R. A., Guevremont, D. C., Anastopoulos, A. D., & Fletcher, K. E. (1992). A comparison of three family therapy programs for treating family conflicts in adolescents with ADHD. *Journal of Consulting and Clinical Psychology, 60,* 450–462.

Barkley, R. A., Karlsson, J., Strzelecki, E., & Murphy, J. V. (1984). Effects of age and Ritalin dosage on mother–child interactions of hyperactive children. *Journal of Consulting and Clinical Psychology, 52,* 750–758.

Barkley, R. A., McMurray, M. B., Edelbrock, C. C., & Robbins, K. (1989). The response of aggressive and nonaggressive ADHD children to two doses of methylphenidate. *Journal of the American Academy of Child and Adolescent Psychiatry, 28,* 873–881.

Barkley, R. A., McMurray, M. B., Edelbrock, C. S., & Robbins, K. (1990b). Side effects of methylphenidate in children with attention-deficit hyperactivity disorder: A systemic, placebo-controlled evaluation. *Pediatrics, 86,* 184–192.

Barkley, R. A., Shelton, T. L., Crosswait, C. C., Moorehouse, M., Fletcher, K., Barrett, S., Jenkins, L., & Metevia, L. (2000). Multi-method psycho-educational intervention for preschool children with disruptive behavior: Preliminary results at post-treatment. *Journal of Child Psychology and Psychiatry, 41,* 319–332.

Barnes, J. (1998). Mental health promotion: A developmental perspective. *Psychology, Health and Medicine, 3,* 55–69.

Baron-Cohen, S., Allen, J., & Gillberg, C. (1992). Can autism be detected at 18 months? The needle, the haystack, and the CHAT. *British Journal of Psychiatry, 161,* 839–843.

Baron-Cohen, S., Leslie, A. M., & Frith, U. (1986). Mechanical, behavioural and intentional understanding of picture stories in autistic children. *British Journal of Developmental Psychology, 4,* 113–125.

Baron-Cohen, S., Tager-Flusberg, H., & Cohen, D. J. (1993). *Understanding other minds: Perspectives from autism.* Oxford: Oxford University Press.

Barrett, M. L., Berney, T. P., Bhate, S., Famuyiwa, O. O., Fundudis, T., Kolvin, I., & Tyrer, S. (1991). Diagnosing childhood depression: Who should be interviewed—parent or child? *British Journal of Psychiatry, 159*(Suppl. 11), 22–28.

Barrett, P. M., Dadds, M. R., & Rapee, R. M. (1996). Family treatment for childhood anxiety: A controlled trial. *Journal of Consulting and Clinical Psychology, 64,* 333–342.

Barrickman, L., Noyes, R., Kuperman, S., Schumacher, E., & Verda, M. (1991). Treatment of ADHD with fluoxetine: A preliminary report. *Journal of the American Academy of Child and Adolescent Psychiatry, 30,* 762–767.

Barrickman, L. L., Perry, P. J., Allen, A. J., Kuperman, S., Arndt, S. V., Herrmann, K. J., & Schumacher, E. (1995). Bupropion versus methylphenidate in the treatment of attention-deficit/hyperactivity disorder. *Journal of the American Academy of Child and Adolescent Psychiatry, 34,* 649–657.

Barrios, B. A., & O'Dell, S. L. (1989). Fears and anxieties. In E. J. Mash & R. A. Barkley (Eds.), *Treatment of childhood disorders* (pp. 167–221). New York: Guilford Press.

Barry, A., & Lippman, B. (1990). Anorexia nervosa in males. *Postgraduate Medicine, 87,* 161–165.

Bartak, L., & Rutter, M. (1976). Differences between mentally retarded and normal intelligence autistic children. *Journal of Autism and Childhood Schizophrenia, 6,* 109–120.

Barth, R. P. (1991). An experimental evaluation of in-home child abuse prevention services. *Child Abuse and Neglect, 15,* 363–375.

Barton, C., Alexander, J. F., Waldron, H., Turner, C. W., & Warburton, J. (1985). Generalizing treatment effects of Functional Family Therapy: Three replications. *American Journal of Family Therapy, 13,* 16–26.

Basile, V. C., Motta, R. W., & Allison, D. B. (1995). Antecedent exercise as a treatment for disruptive behaviour: Testing hypothesized mechanisms of action. *Behavioral Interventions, 10,* 119–140.

Bauchner, H., Vinci, R., & Ariane, M. (1994). Teaching parents how to comfort their children during common medical procedures. *Archives of Disease in Childhood, 70,* 548–550.

Baum, C. G., & Forehand, R. (1981). Long-term follow-up assessment of parent training by use of multiple outcome measure. *Behavior Therapy, 12,* 643–652.

Baum, C. G., Reyna McGlone, C. L., & Ollendick, T. H. (1986, November). *The efficacy of behavioral parent training: Behavioral parent training plus clinical self-control training, and a modified STEP program with children referred for noncompliance.* Paper presented at the meeting of the Association for Advancement of Behavior Therapy, Chicago.

Bauman, M. (1991). Microscopic neuro-anatomic abnormalities in autism. *Pediatrics, 31,* 791–796.

Baumgaertel, A., Wolraich, M. L., & Dietrich, M. (1995). Comparison of diagnostic criteria for attention deficit disorders in a German elementary school. *Journal of the American Academy of Child and Adolescent Psychiatry, 34,* 629–638.

Beardslee, W. R., Wright, E. J., Salt, P., Drezner, K., Gladstone, T. R., Versage, E. M., & Rothberg, P. C. (1997). Examination of children's responses to two preventive intervention strategies over time. *Journal of the American Academy of Child and Adolescent Psychiatry, 36,* 196–204.

Beck, A. T., Ward, C. H., Mendelson, M., Mock, J., & Erbaugh, J. (1961). An inventory for measuring depression. *Archives of General Psychiatry, 4,* 561–571.

Beecham, J. K. (1995). Collecting and estimating costs. In M. R. J. Knapp (Ed.), *The economic evaluation of mental health care* (pp. 61–82). Aldershot, UK: Arena.

Beecham, J. K., & Knapp, M. R. J. (1992). Costing psychiatric options. In G. Thornicroft, C. Brewin, & J. Wing (Eds.), *Measuring mental health needs* (pp. 163–183). Oxford: Oxford University Press.

Beidel, D. C., & Turner, S. M. (1997). At risk for anxiety: I. Psychopathology in the offspring of anxious parents. *Journal of the American Academy of Child and Adolescent Psychiatry, 36,* 918–924.

Beidel, D. C., Turner, S. M., & Morris, T. L. (1999). Psychopathology of childhood social phobia. *Journal of the American Academy of Child and Adolescent Psychiatry, 38,* 643–650.

Beidel, D. C., Turner, S. M., & Morris, T. L. (2000). Behavioral treatment of childhood social phobia. *Journal of Consulting and Clinical Psychology, 68,* 1072–1080.

Beitchman, J. H., Nair, R., Clegg, M., Ferguson, B., & Patel, P. G. (1986). Prevalence of psychiatric disorders in children with speech and language disorders. *Journal of the American Academy of Child Psychiatry, 25,* 528–535.

Beitchman, J. H., Wilson, B., Johnson, C. J., Atkinson, L., Young, A., Adlaf, E., Escobar, M., & Douglas, L. (2001). Fourteen-year follow-up of speech/language-impaired and control children: Psychiatric outcome. *Journal of the American Academy of Child and Adolescent Psychiatry, 40,* 75–82.

Beitchman, J. H., & Young, A. R. (1997). Learning disorders with a special emphasis on reading disorders: A review of the past 10 years. *Journal of the American Academy of Child and Adolescent Psychiatry, 36,* 1020–1032.

Bell-Dolan, D. J., Last, C. G., & Strauss, C. C. (1990). Symptoms of anxiety disorders in normal children. *Journal of the American Academy of Child Psychiatry, 29,* 759–765.

Bemis, K. M. (1987). The present status of operant conditioning for the treatment of anorexia nervosa. *Behavior Modification, 11,* 432–463.

Benjamin, S., & Eminson, D. M. (1992). Abnormal illness behaviour: Childhood experiences and long-term consequences. *International Review of Psychiatry, 4,* 55–70.

Bennett, D. S., & Gibbons, T. A. (2000). Efficacy of child cognitive-behavioral interventions for antisocial behavior: A meta-analysis. *Child and Family Behavior Therapy, 22,* 1–15.

Bergeron, L., Valla, J. P., & Breton, J. J. (1992). Pilot study for the Quebec Child Mental Health survey: Part I. Measurement of prevalence estimates among 6 to 14 year olds. *Canadian Journal of Psychiatry, 37,* 374–380.

Berman, A. L., & Jobes, D. A. (1995). Suicide prevention in adolescents (age 12–18): A population perspective. *Suicide and Life-Threatening Behavior, 25,* 143–154.

Bernal, G., Bonilla, J., & Bellido, C. (1995). Ecological validity and cultural sensitivity for outcome research: Issues for the cultural adaptation and development of psychosocial treatments with Hispanics. *Journal of Abnormal Child Psychology, 23,* 67–82.

Bernal, M. E., Klinnert, M. D., & Schultz, L. A. (1980). Outcome evaluation of behavioral parent training and client-centered parent counseling for children with conduct problems. *Journal of Applied Behavior Analysis, 13,* 677–691.

Berney, T., Kolvin, I., Bhate, S. R., Garside, R. F., Jeans, J., Kay, B., & Scarth, L. (1981). School phobia: A therapeutic trial with clomipramine and short-term outcome. *British Journal of Psychiatry, 138,* 110–118.

Bernier, J. C., & Siegel, D. H. (1994). Attention deficit hyperactivity disorder: A family and ecological systems perspective. *Families in Society, 75,* 142–151.

Bernstein, G. A., & Borchardt, C. M. (1991). Anxiety disorders of childhood and adolescence: A critical review. *Journal of the American Academy of Child and Adolescent Psychiatry, 30,* 519–532.

Bernstein, G. A., Borchardt, C. M., Perwien, A. R., Crosby, R. D., Kushner, M. G., Thuras, P. D., & Last, C. G. (2000). Imipramine plus cognitive-behavioral therapy in the treatment of school refusal. *Journal of the American Academy of Child and Adolescent Psychiatry, 39,* 276–283.

Bernstein, G. A., Garfinkel, B. D., & Borchardt, C. M. (1990). Comparative studies of pharmacotherapy for school refusal. *Journal of the American Academy of Child and Adolescent Psychiatry, 29,* 773–781.

Bernstein, G. A., Hektner, J. M., Borchardt, C. M., & McMillan, M. H. (2001). Treatment of school refusal: One-year follow-up. *Journal of the American Academy of Child and Adolescent Psychiatry, 40,* 206–213.

Bertagnoli, M. W., & Borchardt, C. M. (1990). A review of ECT for children and adolescents. *Journal of the American Academy of Child and Adolescent Psychiatry, 29,* 302–307.

Bettelheim, B. (1967). *The empty fortress.* New York: Free Press.

Bhadrinath, B. R. (1998). Olanzapine in Tourette syndrome (letter). *British Journal of Psychiatry, 172,* 366.

Bickman, L. (1996). A continuum of care: More is not always better. *American Psychologist, 51,* 689–701.

Bickman, L., Guthrie, P. R., Foster, E. M., Lambert, E. W., Summerfelt, W. T., Breda, C. S., & Heflinger, C. A. (1996). *Evaluating managed mental health services: The Fort Bragg experiment.* New York: Plenum Press.

Biederman, J. (1987). Clonazepam in the treatment of prepubertal children with panic-like symptoms. *Journal of Clinical Psychiatry, 48*(Suppl.), 38–42.

Biederman, J. (1991). Sudden death in children treated with a tricyclic anti-depressant: Commentary. *Journal of the American Academy of Child and Adolescent Psychiatry, 30,* 495–497.

Biederman, J., Baldessarini, R., Wright, V., Keenan, K., & Faraone, S. (1993a). A double-blind placebo-controlled study of desipramine in the treatment of attention deficit disorder: III. Lack of impact of comorbidity and family history factors on clinical response. *Journal of the American Academy of Child and Adolescent Psychiatry, 32,* 199–204.

Biederman, J., Baldessarini, R. J., Wright, V., Knee, D., & Harmatz, J. S. (1989). A double-blind placebo-controlled study of desipramine in the treatment of ADD: I. Efficacy. *Journal of the American Academy of Child and Adolescent Psychiatry, 28,* 777–784.

Biederman, J., Faraone, S., & Lelon, E. (1995). Psychiatric comorbidity among referred juveniles with major depression: Fact or artifact? *Journal of the American Academy of Child and Adolescent Psychiatry, 34,* 579–590.

Biederman, J., Faraone, S., Milberger, S., Curtis, S., Chen, L., Marrs, A., Ouellette, C., Moore, P., & Spencer, T. (1996). Predictors of persistence and remission of ADHD into adolescence: Results from a four-year prospective follow-up study. *Journal of the American Academy of Child and Adolescent Psychiatry, 35,* 343–351.

Biederman, J., Faraone, S. V., Doyle, A., Lehman, B. K., Kraus, I., Perrin, J., & Tsuang, M. T. (1993b). Convergence of the Child Behavior Checklist with structured interview-based psychiatric diagnoses of ADHD children with and without comorbidity. *Journal of Child Psychology and Psychiatry, 34,* 1242–1251.

Biederman, J., Faraone, S. V., Keenan, K., Benjamin, J., Krifcher, B., Moore, C., Sprich-Buckminster, S., Ugaglia, K., Jellinek, M. S., & Steingard, R. (1992). Further evidence for family-genetic risk factors in attention deficit hyperactivity disorder. Patterns of comorbidity in probands and relatives psychiatrically and pediatrically referred samples. *Archives of General Psychiatry, 49,* 728–738.

Biederman, J., Gastfriend, D. R., & Jellinek, M. S. (1986). Desipramine in the treatment of children with attention deficit disorder. *Journal of Clinical Psychopharmacology, 6,* 359–363.

Biederman, J., Herzog, D. B., Rivinus, T. M., Harper, G. P., Ferber, R. A., Rosenbaum, J. F., Harmatz, J. S., Tondorf, R., Orsulak, P. J., & Schildkraut, J. J. (1985). Amitriptyline in the treatment of anorexia nervosa: A double-blind, placebo-controlled study. *Journal of Clinical Psychopharmacology, 5,* 10–16.

Biederman, J., Newcorn, J., & Sprich, S. (1991). Comorbidity of attention deficit hyperactivity disorder with conduct, depressive, anxiety and other disorders. *American Journal of Psychiatry, 148,* 564–577.

Biederman, J., Wilens, T., Mick, E., Spencer, T., & Faraone, S. V. (1999). Pharmacotherapy of attention deficit hyperactivity disorder reduces risk for substance use disorder. *Pediatrics, 102,* 1–5.

Bierman, K. L. (1989). Improving the peer relationships of rejected children. In G. G. Lahey & A. E. Kazdin (Eds.), *Advances in clinical child psychology* (Vol. 12, pp. 53–84). New York: Plenum Press.

Bierman, K. L., Miller, C. M., & Stabb, S. D. (1987). Improving the social behavior and peer acceptance of rejected boys: Effects of social skills training with instructions and prohibitions. *Journal of Consulting and Clinical Psychology, 55,* 194–200.

Bierman, K. L., & Welsh, J. A. (1997). Social relationship deficits. In E. J. Mash & L. G. Terdal (Eds.), *Assessment of childhood disorders* (3rd ed., pp. 328–365). New York: Guilford Press.

Bird, H. R. (1996). Epidemiology of childhood disorders in a cross-cultural context. *Journal of Child Psychology and Psychiatry, 37,* 35–49.

Bird, H. R., Canino, G., Rubio-Stipec, M., Gould, M. S., Ribera, J., Sesman, M., Woodbury, M., Huertas-Goldman, S., Pagan, A., Sanchez-Lacy, A., & Moscoso, M. (1988). Estimates of the prevalence of childhood maladjustment in a community survey of Puerto Rico: The use of combined measures. *Archives of General Psychiatry, 45,* 1120–1126.

Bird, H. R., Yager, T., Staghezza, B., Gould, M. S., Canino, G., & Rubio-Stipec, M. (1990). Impairment in the epidemiological measurement of childhood psychopathology in the community. *Journal of the American Academy of Child and Adolescent Psychiatry, 29,* 796–803.

Birmaher, B., Baker, R., & Kapur, S. (1992). Clozapine for the treatment of adolescents with schizophrenia. *Journal of the American Academy of Child and Adolescent Psychiatry, 31,* 160–164.

Birmaher, B., Brent, D. A., Kolko, D., Baugher, M., Bridge, J., Holder, D., Iyengar, S., & Ulloa, R. E. (2000). Clinical outcome after short-term psychotherapy for adolescents with major depressive disorder. *Archives of General Psychiatry, 57,* 29–36.

Birmaher, B., Quintana, H., & Greenhill, L. L. (1988). Methylphenidate treatment of hyperactive autistic children. *Journal of the American Academy of Child and Adolescent Psychiatry, 27,* 248–251.

Birmaher, B., Ryan, N. D., Williamson, D., Brent, D. A., Kaufman, J., Dahl, R. E., Perel, J., & Nelson, B. (1996a). Childhood and adolescent depression: A review of the past 10 years. Part I. *Journal of the American Academy of Child and Adolescent Psychiatry, 35,* 1427–1439.

Birmaher, B., Ryan, N. D., Williamson, D. E., Brent, D. A., & Kaufman, J. (1996b). Childhood and adolescent depression: A review of the past 10 years. Part II. *Journal of the American Academy of Child and Adolescent Psychiatry, 35,* 1575–1583.

Birmaher, B., Waterman, G. S., Ryan, N., Cully, M., Balach, L., Ingram, J., & Brodsky, M. (1994). Fluoxetine for childhood anxiety disorders. *Journal of the American Academy of Child and Adolescent Psychiatry, 33,* 993–999.

Birmaher, B., Waterman, G. S., Ryan, N. D., Perel, J., McNabb, J., Balach, L., Beaudry, M. B., Nasr,

F. N., Karambelkar, J., Elterich, G., Quintana, H., Williamson, D. E., & Rao, U. (1998). Randomized, controlled trial of amitryptyline versus placebo for adolescents with "treatment resistant" major depression. *Journal of the American Academy of Child and Adolescent Psychiatry, 37,* 527–535.

Birnbrauer, J. S., & Leach, D. J. (1993). The Murdoch early intervention program after two years. *Behavior Change, 10,* 63–74.

Bishop, D. M., Frazier, C. E., Lanza-Kaduce, L., & Winner, L. (1996). The transfer of juveniles to criminal court: Does it make a difference? *Crime and Delinquency, 42,* 171–191.

Bishop, D. V. (1994). Is specific language impairment a valid diagnostic category? Genetic and psycholinguistic evidence. *Philosophical Transactions of the Royal Society of London. Series B: Biological Sciences, 346,* 105–11.

Bishop, D. V. (2001). Genetic influences on language impairment and literacy problems in children: Same or different? *Journal of Child Psychology and Psychiatry, 42,* 189–198.

Bishop, D. V., & Edmundson, A. (1987). Language impaired 4 year olds: Distinguishing transient from persistent impairment. *Journal of Speech and Hearing Disorders, 52,* 156–173.

Bishop, D. V., North, T., & Donlan, C. (1995). Genetic basis of specific language impairment: Evidence from a twin study. *Developmental Medicine and Child Neurology, 37,* 56–71.

Bjerregaard, B., & Smith, C. (1993). Gender differences in gang participation, delinquency, and substance use. *Journal of Quantitative Criminology, 9,* 329–355.

Black, B., & Uhde, T. W. (1994). Treatment of elective mutism with fluoxetine: A double-blind, placebo-controlled study. *Journal of the American Academy of Child and Adolescent Psychiatry, 33,* 1000–1006.

Black, N. (1996). Why we need observational studies to evaluate the effectiveness of health care. *British Medical Journal, 312,* 1215–1218.

Blagg, N. R., & Yule, W. (1984). The behavioural treatment of school refusal: A comparative study. *Behaviour Research and Therapy, 22,* 119–127.

Blanchard, E. B. (1970). Relative contributions of modeling, informational influences, and physical contact in extinction of phobic behavior. *Journal of Abnormal Psychology, 76,* 55–61.

Blechman, E. A., Dumas, J. E., & Prinz, R. J. (1994). Prosocial coping by youth exposed to violence. *Journal of Child and Adolescent Group Therapy, 4,* 205–227.

Blechman, E. A., Prinz, R. J., & Dumas, J. E. (1995). Coping, competence, and aggression prevention: Part 1. Developmental model. *Applied and Preventive Psychology, 4,* 211–232.

Block, J. (1978). Effects of a rational emotive mental health program on poorly achieving, disruptive high school students. *Journal of Counseling Psychology, 25,* 61–65.

Block, J., Block, J. H., & Gjerde, P. F. (1988). Parental functioning and the home environment in families of divorce: Prospective and concurrent analyses. *Journal of the American Academy of Child and Adolescent Psychiatry, 27,* 207–213.

Block, J. H., Block, J., & Gjerde, P. F. (1986). The personality of children prior to divorce. *Child Development, 57,* 827–840.

Bloom, A. S., Russell, L. J., Weisskopf, B., & Blackerby, J. L. (1988). Methylphenidate induced delusional disorder in a child with attention deficit disorder with hyperactivity. *Journal of the American Academy of Child and Adolescent Psychiatry, 27,* 88–89.

Blount, R. L., Corbin, S. M., Sturges, J. W., Wolfe, V. V., Prater, J. M., & James, L. D. (1989). The relationship between adults' behavior and child coping and distress during BMA/LP procedures: A sequential analysis. *Behavior Therapy, 20,* 585–601.

Blum, N. J., Mauk, J. E., McComas, J. J., & Mace, F. C. (1996). Separate and combined effects of methylphenidate and a behavioral intervention on disruptive behavior in children with mental retardation. *Journal of Applied Behavior Analysis, 29,* 305–319.

Boardway, R. H., Delamater, A. M., Tomakowsky, J., & Gutai, J. P. (1993). Stress management training for adolescents with diabetes. *Journal of Pediatric Psychology, 18,* 29–45.

Bolton, D., Collins, S., & Steinberg, D. (1983). The treatment of obsessive–compulsive disorder in adolescence: A report of fifteen cases. *British Journal of Psychiatry, 142,* 456–464.

Bolton, P., & Rutter, M. (1990). Genetic influences in autism. *International Review of Psychiatry, 2,* 67–80.

Bone, M., & Meltzer, H. (1989). The prevalence of disability among children. *OPCS Surveys of Disability in Great Britain. Report 3.* London: Her Majesty's Stationery Office.

Borduin, C. M. (1999). Multisystemic treatment of criminality and violence in adolescents. *Journal of the American Academy for Child and Adolescent Psychiatry, 38,* 242–249.

Borduin, C. M., Henggler, S. W., Blaske, D. M., & Stein, R. (1990). Multisystemic treatment of adolescent sexual offenders. *International Journal of Offender Therapy and Comparative Criminology, 34,* 105–113.

Borduin, C. M., Mann, B. J., Cone, L. T., Henggeler, S. W., Fucci, B. R., Blaske, D. M., & Williams, R. A. (1995). Multisystemic treatment of serious juvenile offenders: Long-term prevention of criminality and violence. *Journal of Consulting and Clinical Psychology, 63,* 569–578.

Borison, R. L., Arg, L., & Hamilton, W. J. (1983). Treatment approaches in Gilles de la Tourette syndrome. *Brain Research Bulletin, 11,* 205–208.

Bornstein, R. A., Stefl, M. E., & Hammond, L. (1990). A survey of Tourette syndrome patients and their families: The 1987 Ohio Tourette Survey. *Journal of Neuropsychiatry and Clinical Neuroscience, 2,* 275–281.

Botteron, K. N., & Geller, B. (1995). Pharmacologic treatment of childhood and adolescent mania. *Child and Adolescent Psychiatric Clinics of North America, 4,* 283–304.

Boulton, M. J., & Flemington, I. (1996). The effects of a short video intervention on secondary school pupils' involvement in definitions of and attitudes toward bullying. *School Psychology International, 17,* 331–345.

Bowen, R. C., Offord, D. R., & Boyle, M. H. (1990). The prevalence of overanxious disorder and separation anxiety disorder: Results from the Ontario Child Health Study. *Journal of the American Academy of Child and Adolescent Psychiatry, 29,* 753–758.

Bowring, M. A., & Kovacs, M. (1992). Difficulties in diagnosing manic disorders among children and adolescents. *Journal of Child and Adolescent Psychiatry, 31,* 611–614.

Boyle, M. H., & Offord, D. R. (1991). Psychiatric disorder and substance use in adolescence. *Canadian Journal of Psychiatry, 36,* 699–705.

Boyle, M. H., Offord, D. R., Hofmann, H. G., Catlin, G. P., Byles, J. A., Cadman, D. T., Crawford, J. W., Links, P. S., Rae-Grant, N. I., & Szatmari, P. (1987). Ontario Child Health Study. *Archives of General Psychiatry, 44,* 826–831.

Boyle, M. H., Offord, D. R., Racine, Y. A., Szatmari, P., Sanford, M., & Fleming, J. E. (1997). Adequacy of interviews vs. checklists for classifying childhood psychiatric disorder based on parent reports. *Archives of General Psychiatry, 54,* 793–799.

Bozarth, J. D., & Roberts, R. R. (1972). Signifying significant significance. *American Psychologist, 27,* 774–775.

Bradley, S., Brody, J., Landy, S., Tallett, S., Watson, W., Shea, B., & Stephens, D. (1999). *Brief psychoeducational parenting program: An evaluation.* Paper presented at the 46th Annual Meeting of the American Academy of Child and Adolescent Psychiatry, Chicago.

Brandenburg, N. A., Friedman, R. M., & Silver, S. E. (1990). The epidemiology of childhood psychiatric disorders: Prevalence findings from recent studies. *Journal of the American Academy of Child and Adolescent Psychiatry, 29,* 76–83.

Brecher, M. (1999). *Use of risperidone for conduct disorder in children with mental retardation.* Paper presented at the 46th Annual Meeting of the American Academy of Child and Adolescent Psychiatry, Chicago.

Breen, M. J., & Altepeter, T. S. (1990). *Disruptive behavior disorders in children: Treatment-focused assessment.* New York: Guilford Press.

Breiner, J. L., & Forehand, R. (1981). An assessment of the effects of parent training on clinic-referred children's school behavior. *Behavioral Assessment, 3,* 31–42.

Brent, D. (1987). Correlates of medical lethality of suicide attempts in children and adolescents. *Journal of the American Academy of Child and Adolescent Psychiatry, 26,* 87–91.

Brent, D. A., Holder, D., Kolko, D., Birmaher, B., Baugher, M., Roth, C., Iyengar, S., & Johnson, B. A. (1997). A clinical psychotherapy trial for adolescent depression comparing cognitive, family, and supportive therapy. *Archives of General Psychiatry, 54,* 877–885.

Brent, D. A., Kolko, D., Birmaher, B., Baugher, M., & Bridge, J. (1999). A clinical trial for adolescent depression: Predictors of additional treatment in the acute and follow-up phases of the trial. *Journal of the American Academy of Child and Adolescent Psychiatry, 38,* 263–270.

Brent, D. A., Kolko, D., Birmaher, B., Baugher, M., Bridge, J., Roth, C., & Holder, D. (1998). Predictors of treatment efficacy in a clinical trial of three psychosocial treatments for adolescent depression. *Journal of the American Academy of Child and Adolescent Psychiatry, 37,* 906–914.

Brent, D. A., Roth, C. M., Holder, D. P., Kolko, D. J., Birmaher, B., Johnson, B. A., & Schweers, J. A. (1996). Psychosocial interventions for treating adolescent suicidal depression: A comparison of three psychosocial interventions. In E. D. Hibbs & P. S. Jensen (Eds.), *Psychosocial treatments for child and adolescent disorders: Empirically based strategies for clinical practice* (pp. 187–206). Washington, DC: American Psychological Association.

Brestan, E. V., & Eyberg, S. M. (1998). Effective psychosocial treatments of conduct-disordered children and adolescents: 29 years, 82 studies, and 5,272 kids. *Journal of Clinical Child Psychology, 27,* 180–189.

Brestan, E. V., Eyberg, S. M., Boggs, S. R., & Algina, J. (1997). Parent–child interaction therapy: Parents' perceptions of untreated siblings. *Child and Family Behavior Therapy, 19,* 13–28.

Bridge, T. P., Potkin, S. G., Zung, W. W., & Soldo, B. J. (1977). Suicide prevention centers: Ecological study of effectiveness. *Journal of Nervous and Mental Disease, 164,* 18–24.

British Paediatric Association and the Royal College of Physicians. (1995). *Alcohol and the young.* London: Royal College of Physicians.

Bronfenbrenner, U. (1979). *The ecology of human development: Experiments by nature and design.* Cambridge, MA: Harvard University Press.

Brook, J. S., Brook, D. W., De La Rosa, M., Duque, L. F., Rodriguez, E., Montoya, I. D., & Whiteman, M. (1998). Pathways to marijuana use among adolescents: Cultural/ecological, family, peer, and personality influences. *Journal of the American Academy of Child and Adolescent Psychiatry, 37,* 759–766.

Brook, J. S., Whiteman, M., Finch, S. J., & Cohen, P. (1996). Yound adult drug use and delinquency: Childhood antecedents and adolescent mediators. *Journal of the American Academy of Child and Adolescent Psychiatry, 35,* 1584–1592.

Brooks, R. B., & Snow, D. L. (1972). Two case illustrations of the use of behavior modification techniques in the school setting. *Behavior Therapy, 3,* 100–103.

Brown, R. T., Madan-Swain, A., & Baldwin, K. A. (1991). Gender differences in a clinic-referred sample of attention-deficit-disordered children. *Child Psychiatry and Human Development, 22,* 111–128.

Brown, R. T., Wynne, M. E., & Medenis, R. (1985). Methylphenidate and cognitive therapy: A comparison of treatment approaches with hyperactive boys. *Journal of Abnormal Child Psychology, 13,* 69–87.

Brown, R. T., Wynne, M. E., & Slimmer, L. W. (1984). Attention deficit disorder and the effect of methylphenidate on attention, behavioral, and cardiovascular functioning. *Journal of Clinical Psychiatry, 45,* 473–476.

Bruck, M. (1985). The adult functioning of children with specific learning disabilities: A follow-up study. *Advances in Applied Developmental Psychology, 1,* 91–129.

Bruck, M. (1992). Persistence of dyslexics' phonological deficits. *Developmental Psychology, 28,* 874–886.

Bruun, R. D. (1984). Gille de la Tourette's syndrome. An overview of clinical experience. *Journal of the American Academy of Child and Adolescent Psychiatry, 23,* 126–133.

Bruun, R. D. (1988). The natural history of Tourette's syndrome. In D. J. Cohen (Ed.), *Tourette's syndrome and tic disorders* (pp. 21–40). New York: Wiley.

Bryant-Waugh, R. (1993). Anorexia nervosa in young boys. *Neuropsychiatre de l'Enfance et de l'Adolescence, 41,* 287–290.

Bryant-Waugh, R., Knibbs, J., Fosson, A., Kaminski, Z., & Lask, B. (1988). Long-term follow-up of patients with early onset anorexia nervosa. *Archives of Disease in Childhood, 63,* 5–9.

Bryant-Waugh, R., & Lask, B. (1995). Annotation: Eating disorders in children. *Journal of Child Psychology and Psychiatry, 36,* 191–202.

Bryson, S. (1997). Epidemiology of autism: Overview and issues outstanding. In D. J. Cohen & F. R.

Volkmar (Eds.), *Handbook of autism and pervasive developmental disorders* (pp. 41–46). New York: Wiley.

Buitelaar, J. K. (2000). Open-label treatment with risperidone of 26 psychiatrically hospitalized children and adolescents with mixed diagnoses and aggressive behavior. *Journal of Child and Adolescent Psychopharmacology, 10,* 19–26.

Bukstein, O. G., Brent, D. A., & Kaminer, Y. (1989). Comorbidity of substance abuse and other psychiatric disorders in adolescents. *American Journal of Psychiatry, 146,* 1131–1141.

Bukstein, O. G., & Kolko, D. J. (1998). Effects of methylphenidate on aggressive urban children with attention deficit hyperactivity disorder. *Journal of Clinical Child Psychology, 27,* 340–351.

Burns, B. J., Costello, E. J., Angold, A., Tweed, D., Stangl, D., Farmer, E. M. Z., & Erkanli, A. (1995). Children's mental health service use across service sectors. *Health Affairs, 14,* 147–159.

Bush, J. P., & Cockrell, C. S. (1987). Maternal factors predicting behaviors in the pediatric clinic. *Journal of Pediatric Psychology, 12,* 505–518.

Bushnell, J. A., Wells, J. E., Hornblow, A. R., Oakley-Browne, M. A., & Joyce, P. (1990). Prevalence of three bulimia syndromes in the general population. *Psychological Medicine, 20,* 671–680.

Buydens-Branchey, L., Branchey, M. H., & Noumair, D. (1989). Age of alcoholism onset. I. Relationship to psychopathology. *Archives of General Psychiatry, 46,* 225–230.

Cadman, D., Boyle, M. H., Offord, D. R., Szatmari, P., Rae-Grant, N. I., Crawford, J., & Byles, J. (1986). Chronic illness and functional limitation in Ontario children: Findings of the Ontario Child Health Study. *Canadian Medical Association Journal, 135,* 761–767.

Cadman, D., Boyle, M. H., Szatmari, P., & Offord, D. R. (1987). Chronic illness, disability, and mental and social well-being: Findings of the Ontario Child Health Study. *Pediatrics, 79,* 805–813.

Cadoret, R. J., Troughton, E., Merchant, L. M., & Whitters, A. (1990). Early life psychosocial events and adult affective symptoms. In L. Robins & M. Rutter (Eds.), *Straight and devious pathways from childhood to adulthood* (pp. 300–313). Cambridge: Cambridge University Press.

Caine, E. D., Polinsky, R. J., Kartzinel, R., & Ebert, M. H. (1979). The trial use of clozapine for abnormal involuntary movement disorders. *American Journal of Psychiatry, 136,* 317–320.

Campbell, M., Adams, P. B., Small, A. M., Curren, E. L., Overall, J. E., Lowell, T., Anderson, P. D., Lynch, N., & Perry, R. (1988). Efficacy and safety of fenfluramine in autistic children. *Journal of the American Academy of Child and Adolescent Psychiatry, 27,* 434–439.

Campbell, M., Adams, P. B., Small, A. M., Kafantaris, V., Silva, R. R., Shell, J., Perry, R., & Overall, J. E. (1995). Lithium in hospitalized aggressive children with conduct disorder: A double-blind and placebo-controlled study. *Journal of the American Academy of Child and Adolescent Psychiatry, 34,* 445–453.

Campbell, M., Anderson, L. T., Meier, M., Cohen, I. L., Small, A. M., Samit, C., & Sacher, E. J. (1978). A comparison of haloperidol and behavior therapy and their interaction in autistic children. *Journal of the American Academy of Child and Adolescent Psychiatry, 17,* 640–655.

Campbell, M., Anderson, L. T., Small, A. M., Adams, P., Gonzalez, N. M., & Ernst, M. (1993). Naltrexone in autistic children: Behavioral symptoms and attentional learning. *Journal of the American Academy of Child and Adolescent Psychiatry, 32,* 1283–1291.

Campbell, M., Anderson, L. T., Small, A., Locascio, J., Lynch, N., & Choroco, M. (1990). Naltrexone in autistic children: A double-blind and placebo-controlled study. *Psychopharmacology Bulletin, 26,* 130–135.

Campbell, M., & Cueva, J. E. (1995a). Psychopharmacology in child and adolescent psychiatry: A review of the past seven years. Part I. *Journal of the American Academy of Child and Adolescent Psychiatry, 34,* 1124–1132.

Campbell, M., & Cueva, J. E. (1995b). Psychopharmacology in child and adolescent psychiatry: A review of the past seven years. Part II. *Journal of the American Academy of Child and Adolescent Psychiatry, 34,* 1262–1272.

Campbell, M., Friedman, E., Green, W. H., Collins, P. J., Small, A. M., & Breuer, H. (1975). Blood serotonin in schizophrenic children: A preliminary study. *International Pharmacopsychiatry, 10,* 213–221.

Campbell, M., & Gonzalez, N. M. (1996). Overview of neuroleptic use in child psychiatric disorders.

In G. Haugland & M. Richardson (Ed.), *Use of neuroleptics in children* (pp. 1–22). *Clinical practice, No. 37*. Washington, DC: American Psychiatric Press.

Campbell, M., Gonzalez, N. M., & Silva, R. (1992). The pharmacologic treatment of conduct disorders and rage outbursts. *Psychiatric Clinics of North America, 15*, 69–85.

Campbell, M., Schopler, E., Cueva, J. E., & Hallin, A. (1996). Treatment of autistic disorder. *Journal of the American Academy of Child and Adolescent Psychiatry, 35*, 134–143.

Campbell, M., Small, A. M., Green, W. H., Jennings, S. J., Perry, R., Bennett, W. G., & Anderson, L. (1984). Behavioral efficacy of haloperidol and lithium carbonate. *Archives of General Psychiatry, 41*, 650–656.

Campbell, S. B. (1995). Behavior problems in preschool children: A review of recent research. *Journal of Child Psychology and Psychiatry and Allied Disciplines, 36*, 113–149.

Campbell, S. B., & Ewing, L. J. (1990). Follow-up of hard to manage preschoolers: Adjustment at age 9 and predictors of continuing symptoms. *Journal of Child Psychology and Psychiatry, 31*, 871–889.

Campbell, S. B., Ewing, L. J., Breaux, A. M., & Szumowski, E. K. (1986). Parent referred problem three-year-olds: Follow-up at school entry. *Journal of Child Psychology and Psychiatry and Allied Disciplines, 27*, 475–488.

Campis, L. K., Lyman, R. D., & Prentice-Dunn, S. (1986). The Parental Locus of Control Scale: Development and validation. *Journal of Clinical Child Psychology, 15*, 260–267.

Campo, J. V., & Fritsch, S. L. (1994). Somatization in children and adolescents. *Journal of the American Academy of Child and Adolescent Psychiatry, 33*, 1223–1235.

Campos, R. G. (1994). Rocking and pacifiers: Two comforting interventions for heelstick pain. *Research in Nursing and Health, 17*, 321–331.

Cantwell, D. P. (1996a). Attention deficit disorder: A review of the past 10 years. *Journal of the American Academy of Child and Adolescent Psychiatry, 35*, 978–987.

Cantwell, D. P. (1996b). Classification of child and adolescent psychopathology. *Journal of Child Psychology and Psychiatry, 37*, 3–12.

Cantwell, D. P., & Baker, L. (1987). Prevalence and type of psychiatric disorder and developmental disorders in three speech and language groups. *Journal of Communication Disorders, 20*, 151–160.

Cantwell, D. P., & Baker, L. (1989). Stability and natural history of DSM-III childhood diagnoses. *Journal of the American Academy of Child Adolescent Psychiatry, 28*, 691–700.

Cantwell, D. P., & Baker, L. (1991). Association between attention deficit-hyperactivity disorder and learning disorders. *Journal of Learning Disabilities, 24*, 88–95.

Cantwell, D. P., & Baker, L. (1992). Attention deficit disorder with and without hyperactivity: A review and comparison of matched groups. *Journal of the American Academy of Child and Adolescent Psychiatry, 31*, 432–438.

Cantwell, D. P., Baker, L., & Rutter, M. (1978). A comparative study of infantile autism and specific developmental receptive language disorder: IV. Analysis of syntax and language function. *Journal of Child Psychology and Psychiatry and Allied Disciplines, 19*, 351–362.

Cantwell, D. P., & Rutter, M. (1994). Classification: Conceptual issues and substantive findings. In M. Rutter, E. Taylor, & L. Hersov (Eds.), *Child and Adolescent Psychiatry: Modern Approaches* (3rd ed., pp. 3–21). Oxford, UK: Blackwell Scientific.

Caplan, R. (1994). Thought disorder in childhood. *Journal of the American Academy of Child and Adolescent Psychiatry, 33*, 605–615.

Carlson, C. L., Pelham, W. E., Milich, R., & Dixon, J. (1992a). Single and combined effects of methylphenidate and behavior therapy on the classroom performance of children with attention-deficit hyperactivity disorder. *Journal of Abnormal Child Psychology, 20*, 213–232.

Carlson, C. L., Pelham, W. E., Milich, R., & Dixon, J. (1992b). Single and combined effects of methylphenidate and behavior therapy on the classroom performance of children with attention deficit hyperactivity disorder. *Journal of Abnormal Child Psychology, 20*, 213–232.

Carlson, C. L., Pelham, W. E., Swanson, J. M., & Wagner, J. L. (1991). A divided attention analysis of the effects of methylphenidate on the arithmetic performance of children with attention deficit hyperactivity disorder. *Journal of Child Psychology and Psychiatry and Allied Disciplines*, *32*, 463–471.

Carlson, G. A. (1990). Child and adolescent mania: Diagnostic considerations. *Journal of Child Psychology and Psychiatry*, *31*, 331–341.

Carlson, G. A., Davenport, Y. B., & Jamieson, K. (1977). A comparison of outcome in adolescent- and late-onset bipolar manic depressive illness. *American Journal of Psychiatry*, *134*, 919–922.

Carlson, G. A., & Strober, M. (1978). Manic–depressive illness in early adolescence. A study of clinical and diagnostic characteristics in six cases. *Journal of the American Academy of Child and Adolescent Psychiatry*, *17*, 138–153.

Carlson, J. S., Kratochwill, T. R., & Johnston, H. F. (1999). Sertraline treatment of five children diagnosed with selective mutism: A single-case research trial. *Journal of Child and Adolescent Psychopharmacology*, *9*, 293–306.

Carlsson, E., & Sroufe, L. A. (1995). Contribution of attachment theory to developmental psychopathology. In D. Cicchetti & D. J. Cohen (Eds.), *Developmental psychopathology. Vol. 1: Theory and methods* (pp. 581–617). New York: Wiley.

Caron, C., & Rutter, M. (1991). Comorbidity in child psychopathology: Concepts, issues and research strategies. *Journal of Child Psychology and Psychiatry*, *32*, 1063–1080.

Carpenter, R. L., & Apter, S. J. (1988). Research integration of cognitive–emotional interventions for behaviorally disordered children and youth. In M. C. Wang, M. C. Reynolds, & H. J. Walberg (Eds.), *Handbook of special education research and practice* (Vol. 2). Oxford: Pergamon Press.

Carpenter, W. R., & Kirkpatrick, J. (1988). The heterogeneity of the long-term course of schizophrenia. *Schizophrenia Bulletin*, *14*, 645–652.

Carter, A. S., & Pauls, D. L. (1991). Preliminary results of a prospective family study of Tourette's syndrome. *Psychiatric Genetics*, *2*, 26–27.

Carter, B. D., Edwards, J. F., Kronenberger, W. G., Michalczyk, L., & Marshall, G. S. (1995). Case control study of chronic fatigue in pediatric patients. *Pediatrics*, *95*, 179–186.

Carter, C. M., Urbanowicz, M., Hemsley, R., Mantilla, L., Strobel, S., Graham, P. J., & Taylor, E. (1993). Effects of a few food diet in attention deficit disorder. *Archives of Diseases in Childhood*, *69*, 564–568.

Casat, C. D., Pleasants, D. Z., & Van Wyck Fleet, J. (1987). A double-blind trial of buprorion in children with attention deficit disorder. *Psychopharmacology Bulletin*, *23*, 120–122.

Casey, R. J., & Berman, J. S. (1985). The outcome of psychotherapy with children. *Psychological Bulletin*, *98*, 388–400.

Castellanos, F. X., Giedo, J. N., Elia, J., Marsh, W. L., Ritchie, G. F., Hamburger, S. D., & Rapaport, J. L. (1997). Controlled stimulant treatment of ADHD and comorbid Tourette's syndrome: Effects of stimulant and dose. *Journal of the American Academy of Child and Adolescent Psychiatry*, *36*, 589–596.

Castonguay, L., Goldfried, M., Wiser, S., Raue, P., & Hayes, A. M. (1996). Predicting the effect of cognitive therapy for depression: A study of unique and common factors. *Journal of Consulting and Clinical Psychology*, *64*, 497–504.

Catalano, R. F., Berglund, M. L., Ryan, J. A. M., Lonczac, H. S., & Hawkins, J. D. (1999). *Positive youth development in the United States: Research findings on evaluations of the Positive Youth Development Programs* (Report to the U.S. Department of Health and Human Services, Office of the Assistant Secretary for Planning and Evaluation and National Institute for Child Health and Human Development). Seattle: Social Development Research Group.

Catalano, R. F., Hawkins, J. D., Wells, E. A., Miller, J. L., & Brewer, D. D. (1990). Evaluation of the effectiveness of adolescent drug abuse treatment, assessment of risks for relapse, and promising approaches for relapse prevention. *International Journal of Addiction*, *25*, 1085–1140.

Cawthron, P., James, A., Dell, J., & Seagroatt, V. (1994). Adolescent onset psychosis. A clinical and outcome study. *Journal of Child Psychology and Psychiatry*, *35*, 1321–1332.

Ceci, S. J., & Bruck, M. (1993). Suggestibility of the child witness: A historical review and synthesis. *Psychological Bulletin*, *113*, 403–439.

Ceci, S. J., Huffman, M. L. C., Smith, E., & Loftus, E. F. (1996). Repeatedly thinking about a non-event: Source misattributions among preschoolers. In K. Pezdek & W. P. Banks (Eds.), *The Recovered Memory/False Memory Debate* (pp. 225–244). San Diego, CA: Academic Press.

Cederblad, M., & Rahim, S. I. A. (1986). Effects of rapid urbanization on child behaviour and health in a part of Khartoum, Sudan: I. Socio-economic changes 1965–1980. *Social Science and Medicine, 22*, 713–721.

Celiberti, D. A., & Harris, S. L. (1993). Behavioral intervention for siblings of children with autism: A focus on skills to enhance play. *Behavior Therapy, 24*, 573–599.

Centers for Disease Control. (1991). From the Centers for Disease Control: Attempted suicide among high school students—United States, 1990. *Journal of the American Medical Association, 266*, 1911–1912.

Chadwick, O., Anderson, R., Bland, M., & Ramsey, J. (1989). Neuropsychological consequences of volatile substance abuse: A population based study of secondary school pupils. *British Medical Journal, 298*, 1679–1683.

Chadwick, O., Taylor, E., Taylor, A., Heptinstall, E., & Danckaerts, M. (1999). Hyperactivity and reading disability: A longitudinal study of the nature of the association. *Journal of Child Psychology and Psychiatry, 40*, 1039–1050.

Chamberlain, P. (1990). *Teaching and supporting families: A model for reunification of children with their families.* Grant No. 90CW0994. Washington, DC: Administration for Children, Youth and Families, Child Welfare Services, Human Development Services, U.S. Department of Health and Human Services.

Chamberlain, P. (1994). *Family connections.* Eugene, OR: Castalia.

Chamberlain, P. (1996). Intensified foster care: Multi-level treatment for adolescents with conduct disorders in out-of-home care. In E. D. Hibbs & P. S. Jensen (Eds.), *Psychosocial treatments for child and adolescent disorders: Empirically based strategies for clinical practice* (pp. 475–490). Washington, DC: American Psychological Association.

Chamberlain, P. (1998). Treatment foster care. *Office of Juvenile Justice and Delinquency Prevention: Juvenile Justice Bulletin, December*, 1–11.

Chamberlain, P., & Moore, K. J. (1998a). A clinical model for parenting juvenile offenders: A comparison of group care versus family care. *Clinical Child Psychology and Psychiatry, 3*, 375–386.

Chamberlain, P., & Moore, K. J. (1998b). Models of community treatment for serious juvenile offenders. In J. Crane (Ed.), *Social programs that really work.* New York: Russell Sage Foundation.

Chamberlain, P., Moreland, S., & Reid, K. (1992). Enhanced services and stipends for foster parents: Effects on retention rates and outcomes for children. *Child Welfare, 71*, 387–401.

Chamberlain, P., & Reid, J. B. (1991). Using a specialized foster care treatment model for children and adolescents leaving the state mental hospital. *Journal of Community Psychology, 19*, 266–276.

Chamberlain, P., & Reid, J. B. (1994). Differences in risk factors and adjustment for male and female delinquents in treatment foster care. *Journal of Child and Family Studies, 3*, 23–39.

Chamberlain, P., & Reid, J. B. (1998). Comparison of two community alternatives to incarceration for chronic juvenile offenders. *Journal of Consulting and Clinical Psychology, 66*, 624–633.

Chamberlain, P., & Rozicky, J. G. (1995). The effectiveness of family therapy in the treatment of adolescents with conduct disorders and delinquency. *Journal of Marital and Family Therapy, 21*, 441–459.

Chambers, W. J., Puig-Antich, J., Hirsch, M., Paez, P., Ambrosini, P. J., Tabrizi, M. A., & Davies, M. (1985). The assessment of affective disorders in children and adolescents by semi-structured interview: Test–retest reliability of the Schedule for Affective Disorders and Schizophrenia for school-age children, present episode version. *Archives of General Psychiatry, 42*, 696–702.

Chambless, D. L., & Hollon, S. (1998). Defining empirically supported therapies. *Journal of Consulting and Clinical Psychology, 66*, 7–18.

Chambless, D. L., Sanderson, W. C., Shoham, V., Johnson, S. B., Pope, K. S., Crits-Christoph, P., Baker, M., Johnson, B., Woods, S. R., Sue, S., Beutler, L., Williams, D. A., & McCurry, S. (1996). An update on clinically validated therapies. *Clinical Psychologist, 49*, 5–18.

Champion, L. A., Goodall, G. M., & Rutter, M. (1995). Behavioural problems in childhood and stressors in early adult life: A 20 year follow-up of London school children. *Psychological Medicine, 25,* 231–246.

Chandler, M., & Moran, T. (1990). Psychopathy and moral development: A comparative study of delinquent and nondelinquent youth. *Development and Psychopathology, 2,* 227–246.

Channon, S., DeSilva, P., Hemsley, D., & Perkins, R. A. (1989). A controlled trial of cognitive-behavioural and behavioural treatment of anorexia nervosa. *Behaviour Research and Therapy, 27,* 529–535.

Chappell, P. B., Riddle, M. A., Scahill, L., Lynch, K. A., Schultz, R., Arnstein, A., Leckman, J. F., & Cohen, D. J. (1995). Guanfacine treatment of comorbid attention-deficit hyperactivity disorder and Tourette's syndrome: Preliminary clinical experience. *Journal of the American Academy of Child and Adolescent Psychiatry, 34,* 1140–1146.

Charlton, J., Kelly, S., Dunnell, K., Evans, B., Jenkins, R., & Wallis, R. (1992). *Trends in suicide deaths in England and Wales. Population Trends, 69.* London: Her Majesty's Stationery Office.

Chess, S. (1971). Autism in children with congenital rubella. *Journal of Autism and Childhood Schizophrenia, 1,* 33–47.

Chesson, R., Harding, L., Hart, C., & O'Loughlin, V. (1997). Do parents and children have common perceptions of admission, treatment and outcome in a child psychiatry unit? *Clinical Child Psychology and Psychiatry, 2,* 251–270.

Chiesa, M., & Fonagy, P. (1999). From the efficacy to the effectiveness model in psychotherapy research: The APP multi–centre project. *Psychoanalytic Psychotherapy, 13,* 259–272.

Choquet, M., & Menke, H. (1990). Suicidal thoughts during early adolescence: Prevalence, associated troubles and help-seeking behavior. *Acta Psychiatrica Scandinavica, 81,* 170–177.

Chouinard, G., Annable, L., Ross-Chouinard, A., & Kropsky, M. L. (1979). Ethopropazine and benztropine in neuroleptic-induced parkinsonism. *Clinical Psychiatry, 40,* 147–152.

Christian, R. E., Frick, P. J., Hill, N. L., Tyler, L., & Frazer, D. R. (1997). Psychopathy and conduct problems in children: II. Implications for subtyping children with conduct problems. *Journal of the American Academy of Child and Adolescent Psychiatry, 36,* 233–242.

Chugani, D. C., Chugani, H. T., Nimura, K., & Muzik, O. (1997). Developmental differences in brain serotonin synthesis capacity in autistic and non-autistic children. *Society of Neuroscience Symposia, 23,* 859.

Cicchetti, D., & Cohen, D. J. (1995). Perspectives on developmental psychopathology. In D. Cicchetti & D. J. Cohen (Eds.), *Developmental psychopathology. Vol. 1: Theory and methods* (pp. 3–23). New York: Wiley.

Cicchetti, D., & Toth, S. L. (1995). A developmental psychopathology perspective on child abuse and neglect. *Journal of the American Academy of Child and Adolescent Psychiatry, 34,* 541–565.

Clark, A. F., & Lewis, S. W. (1998). Practitioner review: Treatment of schizophrenia in childhood and adolescence. *Journal of Child Psychology and Psychiatry, 39,* 1071–1081.

Clark, D. B., Smith, M. G., Neighbors, B. D., & Skerlec, L. M. (1994). Anxiety disorders in adolescence: Characteristics, prevalence, and comorbidities. *Clinical Psychology Review, 14,* 113–137.

Clark, H. B., Prange, M. E., Lee, B., Boyd, L. A., McDonald, B. A., & Steward, E. S. (1994). Improving adjustment outcomes for foster children with emotional and behavioral disorders: Early findings from a controlled study on individualized services. *Journal of Emotional and Behavioral Disorders, 2,* 207–218.

Clark, T., Feehan, C., Tinline, C., & Vostanis, P. (1999). Autistic symptoms in children with attention deficit-hyperactivity disorder. *European Child and Adolescent Psychiatry, 8,* 50–55.

Clarke, G. N., Rohde, P., Lewinsohn, P. M., Hops, H., & Seeley, J. R. (1999). Cognitive-behavioral treatment of adolescent depression: Efficacy of acute group treatment and booster sessions. *Journal of the American Academy of Child and Adolescent Psychiatry, 38,* 272–279.

Clarke, M., & Oxman, A. D. (1999). *Cochrane reviewers' handbook 4.0* [updated July 1999]; *Review manager* [Computer program]: Version 4.0. Oxford, UK: Cochrane Collaboration.

Clarkin, J. F., & Kendall, P. C. (1992). Comorbidity and treatment planning: Summary and future directions. *Journal of Consulting and Clinical Psychology, 60,* 904–908.

Clay, T. H., Gualtieri, C. T., Evans, R. W., & Guillion, C. M. (1988). Clinical and neuropsychological effects of the novel antidepressant buproprion. *Psychopharmacology Bulletin, 24*, 143–148.

Clegg, J., Hollis, C., & Rutter, M. (1999). Life sentence: What happens to children with developmental language disorders in later life? *Bulletin of the Royal College of Speech and Language Therapists, 571*, 16–18.

Cobham, V. E., Dadds, M. R., & Spence, S. H. (1998). The role of parental anxiety in the treatment of childhood anxiety. *Journal of Consulting and Clinical Psychology, 66*, 893–905.

Coffey, B., Frazier, J., & Chen, S. (1992). Comorbidity, Tourette sydrome and anxiety disorders. In T. N. Chase, A. J. Friedhoff., & D. J. Cohen (Eds.), *Advances in neurology* (pp. 341–362). New York: Raven.

Cohen, D. J. (1995). Psychosocial therapies for children and adolescents: Overview and future directions. *Journal of Abnormal Child Psychology, 23*, 141–156.

Cohen, D. J., Caparulo, B., & Shaywitz, B. (1976). Primary childhood aphasia and childhood autism: Clinical, biological, and conceptual observations. *Journal of the American Academy of Child Psychiatry, 15*, 604–645.

Cohen, D. J., Riddle, M. A., & Leckman, J. F. (1992). Pharmacotherapy of Tourette's syndrome and associated disorders. *Psychiatric Clinics of North America, 15*, 109–129.

Cohen, J. (1988). *Statistical power analysis for the behavioral sciences* (2nd ed.). Hillsdale, NJ: Erlbaum.

Cohen, L. G., & Biederman, J. (2000). *Treatment of risperidone-induced hyperprolactinemia with a dopamine agonist in children.* Paper presented at the 47th Annual Meeting of the American Academy of Adolescent Psychiatry, New York.

Cohen, L. H., Sargent, M. M., & Sechrest, L. B. (1986). Use of psychotherapy research by professional psychologists. *American Psychologist, 41*, 198–206.

Cohen, N. J., Barwick, M. A., Horodezky, N. B., Vallance, D. D., & Im, N. (1998a). Language, achievement, and cognitive processing in psychiatrically disturbed children with previously identified and unsuspected language impairments. *Journal of Child Psychology and Psychiatry, 39*, 865–877.

Cohen, N. J., Davine, M., Horodesky, N., Lipsett, L., & Isaacson, L. (1993a). Unsuspected language impairment in psychiatrically disturbed children: Prevalence and language and behavioral characteristics. *Journal of the American Academy of Child and Adolescent Psychiatry, 32*, 595–603.

Cohen, N. J., Menna, R., Vallance, D. D., Barwick, M. A., Im, N., & Horodezky, N. B. (1998b). Language, social cognitive processing, and behavioral characteristics of psychiatrically disturbed children with previously identified and unsuspected language impairments. *Journal of Child Psychology and Psychiatry, 39*, 853–864.

Cohen, N. J., Vallance, D. D., Barwick, M., Im, N., Menna, R., Horodezky, N. B., & Isaacson, L. (2000). The interface between ADHD and language impairment: An examination of language, achievement, and cognitive processing. *Journal of Child Psychology and Psychiatry, 41*, 353–362.

Cohen, P., Cohen, J., & Brook, J. (1993b). An epidemiological study of disorders in late childhood and adolescence: II. Persistence of disorders. *Journal of Child Psychology and Psychiatry, 34*, 869–877.

Cohen, P., Cohen, J., Kasen, S., Velez, C. N., Hartmark, C., Johnson, J., Rojas, M., Brook, J., & Struening, E. L. (1993c). An epidemiological study of disorders in late childhood and adolescence: I. Age- and gender-specific prevalence. *Journal of Child Psychology and Psychiatry, 34*, 851–867.

Cohen, P., Kasen, S., Brook, J. S., & Struening, E. L. (1991). Diagnostic predictors of treatment patterns in a cohort of adolescents. *Journal of the American Academy of Child and Adolescent Psychiatry, 30*, 989–993.

Cohen, P., Velez, C. N., Brook, J., & Smith, J. (1989). Mechanisms of the relation between perinatal problems, early childhood illness, and psychopathology in late childhood and adolescence. *Child Development, 60*, 701–709.

Coie, J. D., & Dodge, K. A. (1998). Aggression and antisocial behavior. In W. Damon (Ed.), *Hand-*

book of child psychology (5th ed.). *Vol. 3: Social, emotional, and personality development* (pp. 779–862). New York: Wiley.

Coie, J. D., Underwood, M., & Lochman, J. E. (1991). Programmatic intervention with aggressive children in the school setting. In D. J. Pepler & K. H. Rubin (Eds.), *The development and treatment of childhood aggression* (pp. 389–410). Hillsdale, NJ: Lawrence Erlbaum Associates.

Colder, C. R., & Chassin, L. (1999). The psychosocial characteristics of alcohol users versus problem users: Data from a study of adolescents at risk. *Development and Psychopathology, 11*, 321–348.

Cole, D. A., Peeke, L. G., Martin, J. M., Truglio, R., & Seroczynski, A. D. (1998). A longitudinal look at the relation between depression and anxiety in children and adolescents. *Journal of Consulting and Clinical Psychology, 66*, 451–460.

Coleman, M., Brubaker, J., Hunter, K., & Smith, G. (1988). Rett syndrome: A survey of North American patients. *Journal of Mental Deficiency Research, 32*, 117–124.

Coleman, M., & Gillberg, C. (1985). *The biology of the autistic syndromes.* New York: Praeger.

Colland, V. T. (1993). Learning to cope with asthma: A behavioral self-management program·for children. *Patient Education and Counseling, 22*, 141–152.

Collier, W. V., & Hill, R. H. (1993). *Family Ties Intensive Family Preservation Services Program: An evaluation report.* New York: New York City Department of Juvenile Justice.

Comings, D. E., & Comings, B. G. (1985). Tourette syndrome: Clinical and psychological aspects of 250 cases. *American Journal of Human Genetics, 37*, 435–450.

Comings, D. E., Comings, B. G., Devor, E. J., & Cloninger, C. R. (1984). Detection of major gene for Gilles de la Tourette syndrome. *American Journal of Human Genetics, 36*, 586–600.

Committee for the Study of Research on Child and Adolescent Mental Disorders. (1995). Report card on the National Plan for Research on Child and Adolescent Mental Disorders. *Archives of General Psychiatry, 52*, 715–723.

Committee on Child Health Financing and Committee on Substance Abuse. (1995). Financing of substance abuse treatment for children and adolescents. *Pediatrics, 95*, 308–310.

Connor, D. F., Barkley, R. A., & Davis, H. T. (in press). A pilot study of methylphenidate, clonidine, or the combination in ADHD comorbid with aggressive oppositional-defiant or conduct disorder. *Clinical Pediatrics.*

Connor, D. F., Fletcher, K. E., & Swanson, J. M. (1999). A meta-analysis of clonidine for symptoms of attention-deficit hyperactivity disorder. *Journal of the American Academy of Child and Adolescent Psychiatry, 38*, 151–159.

Connor, D. F., Ozbayrak, K. R., Benjamin, S., Ma, Y., & Fletcher, K. E. (1997a). A pilot study of nadolol for overt aggression in developmentally delayed individuals. *Journal of the American Academy of Child and Adolescent Psychiatry, 36*, 826–834.

Connor, D. F., Ozbayrak, K. R., Kusiak, K. A., Caponi, A. B., & Melloni, R. H. (1997b). Combined pharmacotherapy in children and adolescents in a residential treatment center. *Journal of the American Academy of Child and Adolescent Psychiatry, 36*, 248–254.

Connors, S. L., & Crowell, D. E. (1999). Secretin and autism: The role of cysteine (letter). *Journal of the American Academy of Child and Adolescent Psychiatry, 38*, 795–796.

Constantino, J. N., Liberman, M., & Kincaid, M. (1997). Effects of serotonin reuptake inhibitors on aggressive behavior in psychiatrically hospitalized adolescents: Results of an open trial. *Journal of Child and Adolescent Psychopharmacology, 7*, 31–44.

Coolidge, J. C., Brodie, R., & Feeney, B. (1964). A ten-year follow-up study of sixty-six school children. *American Journal of Orthopsychiatry, 34*, 675–684.

Coons, H. W., Klorman, R., & Borgstedt, A. D. (1987). Effects of methylphenidate on adolescents with a childhood history of attention deficit disorder: II. Information processing. *Journal of the American Academy of Child and Adolescent Psychiatry, 26*, 368–374.

Cooper, P. J., Charnock, D. J., & Taylor, M. J. (1987). The prevalence of bulimia nervosa: A replication study. *British Journal of Psychiatry, 151*, 684–686.

Coryell, W., Keller, M., Endicott, J., Andreasen, N., Clayton, P., & Hirschfeld, R. (1989). Bipolar II illness: Course and outcome over a five-year period. *Psychological Medicine, 19*, 129–141.

Costello, A. J., Edelbrock, C. S., & Dulcan, M. K. (1984). *Testing of the NIMH Diagnostic Interview for Children (DISC) in a clinical population.* Rockville, MD: NIMH Center for Epidemiological Studies.

Costello, D. F. (1990). Child psychiatric epidemiology: Implications for clinical research and practice. In B. B. Lahey & A. E. Kazdin (Eds.), *Advances in clinical child psychology* (Vol. 13, pp. 53–90). New York: Plenum Press.

Costello, E. J. (1989a). Child psychiatric disorders and their correlates: A primary care pediatric sample. *Journal of the American Academy for Child and Adolescent Psychiatry, 28,* 851–855.

Costello, E. J. (1989b). Developments in child psychiatric epidemiology. *Journal of the American Academy of Child and Adolescent Psychiatry, 28,* 836–841.

Costello, E. J., & Angold, A. (1995). Epidemiology. In J. S. March (Ed.), *Anxiety disorders in children and adolescents* (pp. 109–124). New York: Guilford Press.

Costello, E. J., Angold, A., Burns, B. J., Stangl, D. K., Tweed, D. L., Erkanli, A., & Worthman, C. M. (1996). The Great Smoky Mountains Study of Youth: Goals, design, methods, and the prevalence of DSM-III-R disorders. *Archives of General Psychiatry, 53,* 1129–1136.

Costello, E. J., Angold, A., & Keeler, G. P. (1999). Adolescent outcomes of childhood disorders: The consequences of severity and impairment. *Journal of the American Academy of Child and Adolescent Psychiatry, 38,* 121–128.

Costello, E. J., Costello, A. J., Edelbrock, C., Burns, B. J., Duncan, M. K., Brent, D., & Janiszewski, S. (1988). Psychiatric disorders in pediatric primary care: Prevalence and risk factors. *Archives of General Psychiatry, 45,* 1107–1116.

Cotgrove, A. J., Zirinsky, L., Black, D., & Weston, D. (1995). Secondary prevention of attempted suicide in adolescence. *Journal of Adolescence, 18,* 569–577.

Coupey, S. M., Bauman, L. J., Lauby, J. L., Koeber, C. R., & Stein, R. E. K. (1991). Mental health effects of a social skills intervention for adolescents with chronic illness. *Pediatric Research, 29,* 3A.

Courchesne, E., Yeung-Courchesne, R., Press, G. A., Hesselink, J., & Jernigan, T. L. (1988). Hypoplasia of cerebellar vermal lobules VI and VII in autism. *New England Journal of Medicine, 318,* 1349–1354.

Cousins, L. S., & Weiss, G. (1993). Parent training and social skills training for children with attention-deficit hyperactivity disorder. How can they be combined for greater effectiveness? *Canadian Journal of Psychiatry, 38,* 449–457.

Cox, S. M., Davidson, W. S., & Bynum, T. S. (1995). A meta-analytic assessment of delinquency-related outcomes of alternative education programs. *Crime and Delinquency, 41,* 219–234.

Crick, N. R. (1995). Relational aggression: The role of intent attributions, feeling of distress, and provocation type. *Development and Psychopathology, 7,* 313–322.

Crick, N. R., Bigbee, M. A., & Howes, C. (1996). Gender differences in children's normative beliefs about aggression: How do I hurt thee? Let me count the ways. *Child Development, 67,* 1003–1014.

Crisp, A. H., Burns, T., Drummond, L., Heavey, A., Lieberman, S., Norto, K., & Powell, A. S. (1987). *The learning of communication skills and psychotherapy by doctors training in psychiatry and preparing for entry into higher specialist training, and working in the South West Thames RHA London.* London: Division of Psychological Medicine, Department of Mental Health Sciences, St George's Hospital Medical School.

Crisp, A. H., Norton, K. R. W., Gowers, S. G., Halek, C., Levett, G., Yeldham, D., Bowyer, C., & Bhat, A. (1991). A controlled study of the effect of therapies aimed at adolescent and family psychopathology in anorexia nervosa. *British Journal of Psychiatry, 159,* 325–333.

Crisp, A. H., Palmer, R. L., & Kalucy, R. S. (1976). How common is anorexia nervosa? A prevalence study. *British Journal of Psychiatry, 128,* 549–554.

Crits-Christoph, P., Baranackie, K., Kurcias, J. S., Beck, A. T., Carroll, K., Perry, K., Luborsky, L., McLellan, A. T., Woody, G. E., Thompson, L., Gallagher, D., & Zitrin, C. (1991). Meta-analysis of therapist effects in psychotherapy outcome studies. *Psychotherapy Research, 1,* 81–91.

Cross Calvert, S., & McMahon, R. J. (1987). The treatment acceptability of a behavioral parent training programme and its components. *Behavior Therapy, 18,* 165–179.

Cueva, J. E., Overall, J. E., Small, A. M., Armenteros, J. L., Perry, R., & Campbell, M. (1996). Carbamazepine in aggressive children with conduct disorder: A double-blind and placebo-controlled study. *Journal of the American Academy of Child and Adolescent Psychiatry, 35,* 480–490.

Cuffe, S. P., Hall, W. S., & Rogers, K. (1999). *Mental health and juvenile justice: The South Carolina experience*. Paper presented at the 46th Annual Meeting of the American Academy of Child & Adolescent Psychiatry, Chicago.

Cunningham, C. E. (1990). A family systems approach to parent training. In R. A. Barkley (Ed.), *Attention deficit hyperactivity disorder: A handbook for diagnosis and treatment* (pp. 432–461). New York: Guilford Press.

Cunningham, C. E., Bremner, R., & Boyle, M. (1995). Large group community-based parenting programs for families of preschoolers at risk for disruptive behavior disorders: Utilization, cost-effectiveness and outcome. *Journal of Child Psychology and Psychiatry, 36*, 1141–1159.

Cunningham, C. E., Davis, J. R., Bremner, R., Rzasa, T., & Dunn, K. (1993). Coping modeling problem solving versus mastery modeling: Effects on adherence, in-session process, and skill acquisition in a residential parent training program. *Journal of Consulting and Clinical Psychology, 61*, 871–877.

Curran, P. J., Stice, E., & Chassin, L. (1997). The relation between adolescent alcohol use and peer alcohol use: A longitudinal random coefficients model. *Journal of Consulting and Clinical Psychology, 65*, 130–140.

Cyranowski, J. M., Frank, E., Young, E., & Shear, M. K. (2000). Adolescent onset of the gender difference in lifetime rates of major depression: A theoretical model. *Archives of General Psychiatry, 57*, 21–27.

Dadds, M. R., & McHugh, T. A. (1992). Social support and treatment outcome in behavioral family therapy for child conduct problems. *Journal of Consulting and Clinical Psychology, 60*, 252–259.

Dadds, M. R., Schwartz, S., & Sanders, M. R. (1987). Marital discord and treatment outcome in behavioral treatment of child conduct disorders. *Journal of Consulting and Clinical Psychology, 55*, 396–403.

Dadds, M. R., Spence, S. H., Holland, D. E., Barrett, P. M., & Laurens, K. R. (1997). Prevention and early intervention for anxiety disorders: A controlled trial. *Journal of Consulting and Clinical Psychology, 65*, 627–35.

Danziger, Y., Carcl, C. A., Varsono, I., Tyano, S., & Mimouni, M. (1988). Parental involvement in treatment of patients with anorexia nervosa in a pediatric day-care unit. *Pediatrics, 81*, 159–162.

Dare, C., Eisler, I., Russell, G., & Szmukler, G. (1990). The clinical and theoretical impact of a controlled trial of family therapy in anorexia nervosa. *Journal of Marital and Family Therapy, 16*, 39–57.

Dare, C., Le Grange, D., Eisler, I., & Rutherford, J. (1994). Redefining the psychosomatic family: Family process of 26 eating disorder families. *International Journal of Eating Disorder, 16*, 211–226.

Dare, C., & Szmukler, G. (1991). The family therapy of short history early onset anorexia nervosa. In D. B. Woodside & L. Shekter-Wolfson (Eds.), *Family approaches to eating disorders* (pp. 25–47). Washington, DC: American Psychiatric Press.

David, S. R., Taylor, C. C., Kinon, B. J., & Breier, A. (2000). The effects of olanzapine, risperidone, and haloperidol on plasma prolactin levels in patients with schizophrenia. *Clinical Therapeutics, 22*, 1085–1096.

Davis, H., Day, C., Cox, A., & Cutler, L. (2000). Child and adolescent mental health needs assessment and service: Implications in an inner city area. *Clinical Child Psychology and Psychiatry.*

de Haan, E., Hoogduin, K. A., Buitelaar, J. K., & Keijsers, G. P. (1998). Behavior therapy versus clomipramine for the treatment of obsessive–compulsive disorder in children and adolescents. *Journal of the American Academy of Child and Adolescent Psychiatry, 37*, 1022–1029.

Deitz, S. M. (1985). Good behavior game. In A. S. Bellack & M. Hersen (Eds.), *Dictionary of behavior therapy techniques* (pp. 131–132). New York: Pergamon Press.

Delamater, A. M., Bubb, J., Davis, S. G., Smith, J. A., Schmidt, L., White, N. H., & Santiago, J. V. (1990). Randomized prospective study of self-management training with newly diagnosed diabetic children. *Diabetes Care, 13*, 492–498.

DeLong, G. R. (1999). New data suggest a new hypothesis. *Neurology, 52*, 911–916.

DeLong, G. R., & Aldershof, A. L. (1987). Long-term experience with lithium treatment in childhood: Correlation with clinical diagnosis. *Journal of the American Academy of Child and Adolescent Psychiatry, 26*, 389–394.

DeLong, G. R., & Nieman, G. W. (1983). Lithium induced behavior changes in children with symptoms suggesting manic–depressive illness. *Psychopharmacology Bulletin, 19*, 258–265.

Demb, H. P., & Nguyen, K. T. (1999). Movement disorders in children with developmental disabilities taking risperidone (letter to the editor). *Journal of the American Academy of Child and Adolescent Psychiatry, 38*, 5–6.

DeMilio, L. (1989). Psychiatric syndromes in adolescent substance abusers. *American Journal of Psychiatry, 146*, 1212–1214.

DeMyer, M. K., Alpern, G. D., DeMyer, W. E., Churchill, D. W., Hingtgen, J. N., Bryson, C. K., Pontius, W., & Kimberlin, C. (1972). Imitation in autistic, early schizophrenic and nonpsychotic abnormal children. *Journal of Autism and Childhood Schizophrenia, 2*, 264–287.

Denckla, M. B. (1991). Academic and extracurricular aspects of nonverbal learning disabilities. *Psychiatric Annals, 21*, 717–724.

Denckla, M. B. (1993). The child with developmental disabilities grown up: Adult residua of childhood disorders. *Neurologic Clinics, 11*, 105–125.

Department of Health. (1999). *The National Service framework for mental health*. London: National Health Service Executive.

Department of Transport. (1993). *Road accidents in Great Britain*. London: Her Majesty's Stationery Office.

De Seixas Queiroz, L. O., Motta, M. A., Pinho Madi, M. B. B., Sossai, D. L., & Boren, J. J. (1981). A functional analysis of obsessive–compulsive problems with related therapeutic procedures. *Behaviour Research and Therapy, 19*, 377–388.

DeVane, L. C., & Sallee, F. R. (1996). Serotonin selective reuptake inhibitors in child and adolescent psychopharmacology: A review of published experience. *Journal of Clinical Psychiatry, 57*, 55–66.

DeVeaugh-Geiss, J., Moroz, G., Biederman, J., Cantwell, D. P., Fontaine, R., Greist, J. H., Reichler, R., Katz, R., & Landau, P. (1992). Clomipramine in child and adolescent obsessive–compulsive disorder: A multicenter trial. *Journal of the American Academy of Child and Adolescent Psychiatry, 31*, 45–49.

Dew, M. A., Bromet, E. J., Brent, D., & Greenhouse, J. B. (1987). A quantitative literature review of the effectiveness of suicide prevention centers. *Journal of Consulting and Clinical Psychology, 55*, 239–244.

Deykin, E. Y., Levy, J. C., & Wells, V. (1987). Adolescent depression, alcohol and drug abuse. *American Journal of Public Health, 77*, 178–182.

Diamond, G. S., Serrano, A. C., Dickey, M., & Sonis, W. A. (1996). Current status of family-based outcome and process research. *Journal of the American Academy of Child and Adolescent Psychiatry, 35*, 6–16.

Diamond, I. R., Tannock, R., & Schachar, R. J. (1999). Response to methylphenidate in children with ADHD and comorbid anxiety. *Journal of the American Academy of Child and Adolescent Psychiatry, 38*, 402–409.

Dickson, R. A., & Glazer, W. M. (1999). Neuroleptic-induced hyperprolactinemia. *Schizophrenia Research, 35*(Suppl.), 75S–86S.

Diekstra, R. F. W. (1982). Epidemiology of attempted suicide in the EEC. *Bibliotheca Psychiatrica, 162*, 1–16.

Diekstra, R. F. W. (1989). Suicidal behavior in adolescents and young adults: The international picture. *Crisis, 10*, 16–35.

Diekstra, R. F. W. (1993). The epidemiology of suicide and parasuicide. *Acta Psychiatrica Scandinavica Supplementum, 371*, 9–20.

Diekstra, R. F. W. (1995). Depression and suicidal behaviours in adolescence: Sociocultural and time trends. In M. Rutter (Ed.), *Psychosocial disturbances in young people* (pp. 212–243). Cambridge: Cambridge University Press.

Diekstra, R. F. W., de Heus, P., Garnefski, N., de Zwart, R., & Van Praag, B. M. S. (1991). *Monitoring the future: Behavior and health among high school students*. The Hague: National Institut voor Budgetvoorlichting.

Diekstra, R. F. W., Kienhorst, C. W. M., & de Wilde, E. J. (1995). Suicide and suicidal behaviour among adolescents. In M. Rutter & D. J. Smith (Eds.), *Psychosocial disorders in young people: Time trends and their causes* (pp. 686–761). Chichester: Wiley.

Dietch, J., & Jennings, R. (1988). Aggressive dyscontrol in patients treated with benzodiazepines. *Journal of Clinical Psychiatry, 49*, 184–188.

DiIulio, J. J., & Palubinsky, B. Z. (1997). How Philadelphia salvages teen criminals. *City Journal, 7*, 28–40.

Dijkers, M. (1999). Measuring quality of life: Methodological issues. *American Journal of Physical Medicine and Rehabilitation, 78*, 286–300.

Dillon, D. C., Salzman, I. J., & Schulsinger, D. A. (1985). The use of imipramine in Tourette's syndrome and attention deficit disorder: Case report. *Journal of Clinical Psychiatry, 46*, 348–349.

Dimigen, G., Del Priore, C., Butler, S., Evans, S., Ferguson, L., & Swan, M. (1999). Psychiatric disorder among children at the time of entering local authority care: A questionnaire survey. *British Medical Journal, 319*, 675–676.

Dishion, T. J., & Andrews, D. W. (1995). Preventing escalation in problem behaviors with high-risk young adolescents: Immediate and 1-year outcomes. *Journal of Consulting and Clinical Psychology, 63*, 538–548.

Dishion, T. J., & Patterson, G. R. (1992). Age effects in parent training outcome. *Behavior Therapy, 23*, 719–729.

Dishion, T. J., Patterson, G. R., & Kavanagh, K. A. (1992). An experimental test of the coercion model: Linking theory, measurement and intervention. In J. McCord & R. E. Tremblay (Eds.), *Preventing antisocial behavior: Intervention from birth through adolescence* (pp. 253–282). New York: Guilford Press.

Dishion, T. J., Patterson, G. R., Stoolmiller, M., & Skinner, M. L. (1991). Family, school, and behavioral antecedents to early adolescent involvement with antisocial peers. *Developmental Psychology, 27*, 172–180.

Dittmann, R. W., Czekalla, J., Hundemer, H. P., & Linden, M. (2000). Efficacy and safety findings from naturalistic fluoxetine drug treatment in adolescent and young adult patients. *Journal of Child and Adolescent Psychopharmacology, 10*, 91–102.

Doane, J. A., West, K. L., Goldstein, M. J., Rodnick, E. H., & Jones, J. E. (1981). Parental communication deviance and affective style: Predictors of subsequent schizophrenia spectrum disorders in vulnerable adolescents. *Archives of General Psychiatry, 38*, 697–685.

Dodge, E., Hodes, M., Eisler, I., & Dare, C. (1995). Family therapy for bulimia nervosa in adolescents: An exploratory study. *Journal of Family Therapy, 17*, 59–77.

Dodge, K. A. (1991). The structure and function of reactive and proactive aggression. In D. J. Pepler & K. H. Rubin (Eds.), *The development and treatment of childhood aggression* (pp. 201–218). Hillsdale, NJ: Erlbaum.

Dodge, K. A., Pettit, G. S., & Bates, J. E. (1994a). Socialization mediators of the relation between socioeconomic status and child conduct problems. *Child Development, 65*, 649–665.

Dodge, K. A., Pettit, G. S., & Bates, J. E. (1994b). Effects of physical maltreatment on the development of peer relations. *Development and Psychopathology, 6*, 43–55.

Doll, R. (1994). Summation of conference "Doing more good than harm: The evaluation of health care interventions." *American New York Academy of Science, 705*, 313.

Donovan, S. J., Stewart, J. W., Nunes, E. V., Quitkin, F. M., Parides, M., Daniel, W., Susser, E., & Klein, D. (2000). Divalproex treatment for youth with explosive temper and mood lability: A double-blind, placebo-controlled crossover design. *American Journal of Psychiatry, 157*, 818–820.

Donovan, S. J., Susser, E. S., Nunes, E. V., Stewart, J. W., Quitkin, F. M., & Klein, D. F. (1997). Divalproex treatment of disruptive adolescents: A report of 10 cases. *Journal of Clinical Psychiatry, 58*, 12–15.

Dorer, C., Feehan, C., Vostanis, P., & Winkley, L. (1999). The overdose process: Adolescents' experience of taking an overdose and their contact with services. *Journal of Adolescence, 22*, 413–417.

Drury, V., Birchwood, M., Cochrane, R., & MacMillan, F. (1996a). Cognitive therapy and recovery from acute psychosis: A controlled trial: I. Impact upon psychotic symptoms. *British Journal of Psychiatry, 169*, 593–601.

Drury, V., Birchwood, M., Cochrane, R., & MacMillan, F. (1996b). Cognitive therapy and recovery from acute psychosis: A controlled trial: II. Impact upon recovery time. *British Journal of Psychiatry, 169*, 602–607.

Dubow, E. F., Huesmann, L. R., & Eron, L. D. (1987). Mitigating aggression and promoting prosocial behavior in aggressive elementary schoolboys. *Behavior Research and Therapy, 25*, 527–531.

Dubow, E. F., Kausch, D. F., Blum, M. C., Reed, J., & Bush, E. (1989). Correlates of suicidal ideation and attempts in a community sample of junior high and high school students. *Journal of Clinical Child Psychology, 18*, 158–166.

Dubowitz, V., & Hersov, L. (1976). Management of children with non-organic (hysterical) disorders of motor function. *Developmental Medicine and Child Neurology, 18*, 358–368.

Ducharme, J. M., Atkinson, L., & Poulton, L. (2000). Success-based, noncoercive treatment of oppositional behavior in children from violent homes. *Journal of the American Academy of Child and Adolescent Psychiatry, 39*, 995–1004.

Duffy, J. C. (1991). *Trends in alcohol consumption patterns 1978–1989.* Henley-on-Thames: NTC Publications.

Dulcan, M. K. (1990). Using psychostimulants to treat behavioral disorders of children and adolescents. *Journal of Child and Adolescent Psychopharmacology, 1*, 7–20.

Dumas, J. E., & Albin, J. B. (1986). Parent training outcome: Does active parental involvement matter? *Behaviour Research and Therapy, 24*, 227–230.

Dumas, J. E., & Wahler, R. G. (1983). Predictors of treatment outcome in parent training: Mother insularity and socioeconomic disadvantage. *Behavioral Assessment, 5*, 301–313.

Dunlap, G., Koegel, R., Johnson, J., & O'Neill, R. (1987). Maintaining performance of autistic clients in community settings with delayed contingencies. *Journal of Applied Behavior Analysis, 20*, 185–191.

Dunn-Geier, B. J., McGrath, P. J., Rourke, B. P., Latter, J., & D'Astous, J. (1986). Adolescent chronic pain: The ability to cope. *Pain, 26*, 23–32.

DuPaul, G. J., Barkley, R. A., & McMurray, M. B. (1994). Response of children with ADHD to methylphenidate: Interaction with internalizing symptoms. *Journal of the American Academy of Child and Adolescent Psychiatry, 33*, 894–903.

DuPaul, G. J., Guevremont, D. C., & Barkley, R. A. (1992). Behavioural treatment of attention-deficit hyperactivity disorder in the classroom. *Behavior Modification, 16*, 204–225.

DuPaul, G. J., & Rapport, M. D. (1993). Does methylphenidate normalize the classroom performance of children with attention deficit disorder? *Journal of the American Academy of Child and Adolescent Psychiatry, 32*, 190–198.

Durlak, J. A., Fuhrman, T., & Lampman, C. (1991). Effectiveness of cognitive-behavior therapy for maladapting children: A meta-analysis. *Psychological Bulletin, 110*, 204–214.

Durlak, J. A., Wells, A. M., Cotten, J. K., & Johnson, S. (1995). Analysis of selected methodological issues in child psychotherapy research. *Journal of Clinical Child Psychology, 24*, 141–148.

Dush, D. M., Hirt, M. L., & Schroeder, H. E. (1989). Self statement modification in the treatment of child behavior disorders: A meta-analysis. *Psychological Bulletin, 106*, 97–106.

Dyche, G. M., & Johnson, D. A. (1991). Development and evaluation of CHIPASAT, an attention test for children: II. Test–retest reliability and practice effect for a normal sample. *Perceptual and Motor Skills, 72*, 563–572.

Dysken, M. W., Berecz, J. M., Samarza, A., & Davis, J. M. (1980). Clonidine in Tourette syndrome. *Lancet, 2*, 926–927.

Eaton, W. W., Bilker, W., Haro, J. M., Herrman, H., Mortensen, P. B., Freeman, H., & Burgess, P. (1992a). Long-term course of hospitalization for schizophrenia: Part II. Change with passage of time. *Schizophrenia Bulletin, 18*, 229–241.

Eaton, W. W., Mortensen, P. B., Herrman, H., Freeman, H., Bilker, W., Burgess, P., & Wooff, K. (1992b). Long-term course of hospitalization for schizophrenia: Part I. Risk for rehospitalization. *Schizophrenia Bulletin, 18*, 217–228.

Eaves, L. J., Silberg, J. L., Meyer, J. M., Maes, H. H., Simonoff, E., Pickles, A., Rutter, M., Neale, M. C., Reynolds, C. A., Erikson, M. T., Heath, A. C., Loeber, R., Truett, K. R., & Hewitt, J. K. (1997). Genetics and developmental psychopathology: 2. The main effects of genes and environment on behavioral problems in the Virginia Twin Study of Adolescent Behavioral Development. *Journal of Child Psychology and Psychiatry, 38,* 965–80.

Eckert, E. D., Goldberg, S. C., Halmi, K. A., Casper, R. C., & Davis, J. M. (1979). Behaviour therapy in anorexia nervosa. *British Journal of Psychiatry, 134,* 55–59.

Eckert, E. D., Goldberg, S. C., Halmi, K. A., Casper, R. C., & Davis, J. M. (1982). Depression in anorexia nervosa. *Psychological Medicine, 12,* 115–122.

Eckert, E. D., Halmi, K. A., Marchi, P., Grove, W., & Crosby, R. (1995). Ten-year follow-up of anorexia nervosa: Clinical course and outcome. *Psychological Medicine, 25,* 143–156.

Edeh, J. (1989). Volatile substance abuse in relation to alcohol and illicit drugs: Psychosocial perspectives. *Human Toxicology, 8,* 313–317.

Edelbrock, C., Costello, A., Dulcan, M., Conover, N., & Kala, R. (1986). Parent–child agreement on child psychiatric symptoms assessed via structured interview. *Journal of Child Psychology and Psychiatry, 27,* 181–190.

Egger, J., Carter, C. M., Graham, P. J., Gumley, D., & Soothill, J. F. (1985). Controlled trial of Oligo antigenic treatment in the hyperkinetic syndrome. *Lancet, 1,* 540–545.

Eggers, C. (1978). Course and prognosis in childhood schizophrenia. *Journal of Autism and Childhood Schizophrenia, 8,* 21–36.

Eggers, C. (1989). Schizo-affective psychoses in childhood: A follow-up study. *Journal of Autism and Childhood Schizophrenia, 19,* 327–342.

Ehlers, S., & Gillberg, C. (1989). The epidemiology of Asperger syndrome: A total population study. *Journal of Child Psychology and Psychiatry, 30,* 631–638.

Ehlers, S., Nyden, A., Gillberg, C., Sandberg, A. D., Dahlgren, S. O., Hjelmquist, E., & Oden, A. (1997). Asperger syndrome, autism and attention disorders: A comparative study of the cognitive profiles of 120 children. *Journal of Child Psychology and Psychiatry, 38,* 207–217.

Eiraldi, R. B., Power, T. J., & Nezu, C. M. (1997). Patterns of comorbidity associated with subtypes of attention-deficit/hyperactivity disorder among 6 to 12 year old children. *Journal of the American Academy of Child and Adolescent Psychiatry, 36,* 503–514.

Eisenberg, N., & Fabes, R. A. (1992). Emotion, regulation and the development of social competence. In M. Clarke (Ed.), *Review of personality and social psychology: Vol. 14: Emotion and social behavior* (pp. 119–150). Newbury Park, CA: Sage.

Eisler, I. (1988). Family therapy approaches to anorexia. In D. Scott (Ed.), *Anorexia and bulimia nervosa: Practical approaches* (pp. 95–107). New York: New York University Press.

Eisler, I., Dare, C., Hodes, M., Russell, G., Dodge, E., & Le Grange, D. (2000). Family therapy for adolescent anorexia nervosa: The results of a controlled comparison of two family interventions. *Journal of Child Psychology and Psychiatry, 41,* 727–736.

Eisler, I., Dare, C., Russell, G. F. M., Szmukler, G., le Grange, D., & Dodge, E. (1997). Family and individual therapy in anorexia nervosa: A 5-year follow-up. *Archives of General Psychiatry, 54,* 1025–1030.

Elkin, I., Shea, M. T., Watkins, J. T., Imber, S. D., Sotsky, S. M., Collins, J. F., Glass, D. R., Pilkonis, P. A., Lever, W. R., Docherty, J. P., Fiester, S. J., & Parloff, M. B. (1989). National Institute of Mental Health Treatment of Depression Collaborative Research Program: General effectiveness of treatment. *Archives of General Psychiatry, 46,* 971–982.

Elliott, D. S., Huizinga, D., & Menard, S. (1988). *Multiple problem youth: Delinquency, substance abuse, and mental health problems.* New York: Springer-Verlag.

Ellis, J. A., & Spanos, N. P. (1994). Cognitive-behavioural interventions for children's distress during bone marrow aspirations and lumbar punctures: A critical review. *Journal of Pain and Symptom Management, 9,* 96–108.

Emde, R. N., & Robinson, J. A. (2000). Guiding principles for a theory of early intervention: A developmental–psychoanalytic perspective. In S. J. Meisels & J. P. Shonkoff (Eds.), *Handbook of early childhood intervention* (2nd ed, pp. 160–178). New York: Cambridge University Press.

Eminson, M., Benjamin, S., Shortall, A., & Woods, T. (1996). Physical symptoms and illness attitudes in adolescents: An epidemiological study. *Journal of Child Psychology and Psychiatry and Allied Disciplines, 37,* 519–528.

Emslie, G. J., Rush, A. J., Weinberg, W. A., & Kowatch, R. A., Hughes, C. W., Carmody, T., &

Rintelmann, J. (1997). A double-blind randomized, placebo-controlled trial of fluoxetine in children and adolescents with depression. *Archives of General Psychiatry, 54,* 1031–1037.

Emslie, G. J., Rush, A. J., Weinberg, W. A., Rintelmann, J. W., & Roffwarg, H. P. (1990). Children with major depression show reduced rapid eye movement latencies. *Archives of General Psychiatry, 47,* 119–124.

Emslie, G. J., Walkup, J. T., Pliszka, S. R., & Ernst, M. (1999). Nontricyclic antidepressants: Current trends in children and adolescents. *Journal of the American Academy of Child and Adolescent Psychiatry, 38,* 517–528.

Ensminger, M. E., Kellam, S., & Rubin, B. R. (1983). School and family origins of delinquency: Comparisons by sex. In K. T. van Dusen & S. A. Mednick (Eds.), *Prospective studies of crime and delinquency* (pp. 73–97). Boston: Kluwer-Nijhoff.

Erenberg, G. (1992). Treatment of Tourette syndrome with neuroleptic drugs. *Advances in Neurology, 58,* 241–243.

Esbensen, F. A., & Osgood, D. W. (1999). Gang resistance education and training (GREAT): Results from the national evaluation. *Journal of Research in Crime and Delinquency, 36,* 194–225.

Esser, G., & Schmidt, M. H. (1987, May). *Antezedenten dissozialen Verhaltens.* Paper presented at the 20th Tagung der Deutschen Gesellschaft fur Kinder- und Jugendpsychiatrie, Feldkirch, Germany.

Esser, G., Schmidt, M. H., & Woerner, W. (1990). Epidemiology and course of psychiatric disorders in school-age children: Results of a longitudinal study. *Journal of Child Psychology and Psychiatry, 31,* 243–263.

Estrada, A. U., & Pinsof, W. M. (1995). The effectiveness of family therapies for selected behavioral disorders of childhood. *Journal of Marital and Family Therapy, 21,* 403–440.

Evans, D., & Mellins, R. B. (1991). Educational programs for children with asthma. *Pediatrician, 18,* 317–323.

Evans, R., Gergen, P., Mitchell, H., Kattan, M., Kercsmar, C., Crain, E., Anderson, J., Eggleston, P., Malveaux, J., & Wedner, H. (1999). A randomized clinical trial to reduce asthma morbidity among inner-city children: Results of the National Cooperative Inner-City Asthma Study. *Journal of Pediatrics, 135,* 332–338.

Evans, S., & Brown, R. (1993). Perception of need for child psychiatric services among parents and GPs. *Health Trends, 25,* 11.

Evans, S. W., & Pelham, W. E. (1991). Psychostimulant effects on academic and behavioral measures for ADHD junior high school students in a lecture format classroom. *Journal of Abnormal Child Psychology, 19,* 537–552.

Evans, S. W., Vallano, G., & Pelham, W. (1994). Treatment of parenting behavior with a psychostimulant: A case study of an adult with attention-deficit hyperactivity disorder. *Journal of Child and Adolescent Psychopharmacology, 4,* 63–69.

Evidence Based Care Resource Group. (1994). Evidence based care: 1. Setting priorities: How important is this problem? *Canadian Medical Association Journal, 150,* 1249–1254.

Eyberg, S. M., Boggs, S. R., & Algina, J. (1995). Parent–child interaction therapy: A psychosocial model for the treatment of young children with conduct problem behavior and their families. *Psychopharmacology Bulletin, 31,* 83–91.

Fagan, J. (1991). Community-based treatment for mentally disordered juvenile offenders. *Journal of Clinical Child Psychology, 20,* 42–50.

Fairburn, C. G. (1988). The current status of the psychological treatments for bulimia nervosa. *Journal of Psychosomatic Research, 32,* 635–646.

Fairburn, C. G. (1994). Interpersonal psychotherapy for bulimia nervosa. In G. L. Klerman & M. M. Weissman (Eds.), *New application of interpersonal psychotherapy* (pp. 353–378). New York: Guilford Press.

Fairburn, C. G., & Beglin, S. J. (1990). Studies in the epidemiology of bulimia nervosa. *American Journal of Psychiatry, 147,* 401–408.

Fairburn, C. G., Jones, R., Peveler, R. C., Carr, S. J., Solomon, R. A., O'Connor, M. E., Burton, J., & Hope, R. A. (1991). Three psychological treatments for bulimia nervosa: A comparative trial. *Archives of General Psychiatry, 48,* 463–469.

Fairburn, C. G., Jones, R., Peveler, R. C., Hope, R. A., & O'Connor, M. (1993a). Psychotherapy and bulimia nervosa: The longer-term effects of interpersonal psychotherapy, behaviour therapy, and cognitive behavior therapy. *Archives of General Psychiatry, 50,* 419–428.

Fairburn, C. G., Marcus, M. D., & Wilson, G. T. (1993b). Cognitive-behavioral therapy for binge eating and bulimia nervosa. *Behaviour Research and Therapy, 24,* 629–643.

Falik, L. H. (1995). Family patterns of reaction to a child with a learning disability: A mediational perspective. *Journal of Learning Disabilities, 28,* 335–341.

Falloon, I. R. H., Coverdale, J. H., Laidlaw, T. M., Merry, S., Kydd, R. R., & Morosini, P. (1998). Early intervention for schizophrenic disorders: Implementing optimal treatment strategies in routine clinical services. *British Journal of Psychiatry, 172*(Suppl. 33), 33–38.

Falloon, I. R. H., & Pederson, J. (1985). Family management in the prevention of morbidity of schizophrenia: The adjustment of the family unit. *British Journal of Psychiatry, 147,* 156–163.

Fankhauser, M. P., Karumanchi, V. C., German, M. L., Yates, A., & Karumanchi, S. D. (1992). A double-blind, placebo-controlled study of the efficacy of transdermal clonidine in autism. *Journal of Clinical Psychiatry, 53,* 77–82.

Farrell, A. D., & White, K. S. (1998). Peer influences and drug use among urban adolescents: Family structure and parent–adolescent relationship as protective factors. *Journal of Consulting and Clinical Psychology, 66,* 248–258.

Farrell, M. (1989). Ecstasy and the oxygen of publicity. *British Journal of Addiction, 84,* 943.

Farrell, M., & Taylor, E. (1994). Drug and alcohol use and misuse. In M. Rutter, E. Taylor, & L. Hersov (Eds.), *Child and adolescent psychiatry: Modern approaches* (3rd ed., pp. 529–545). Oxford, UK: Blackwell Scientific.

Farrington, D. P. (1992). Explaining the beginning, progress and ending of antisocial behavior from birth to adulthood. In J. McCord (Ed.), *Advances in criminological theory. Vol 3: Facts, frameworks and forecasts* (pp. 253–86). New Brunswick, NJ: Transaction Publishers.

Farrington, D. P. (1993). Understanding and preventing bullying. In M. Tonry (Ed.), *Crime and justice: A review of research* (Vol. 17, pp. 381–458). Chicago: University of Chicago Press.

Farrington, D. P. (1995). The Twelfth Jack Tizard Memorial Lecture: The development of offending and antisocial behaviour from childhood: Key findings from the Cambridge study in delinquent development. *Journal of Child Psychology and Psychiatry and Allied Disciplines, 36,* 929–964.

Farrington, D. P. (1996). *Understanding and preventing youth crime. Social policy research 93.* York, UK: Joseph Rowntree Foundation.

Farrington, D. P., Loeber, R., Stouthamer-Loeber, M., Van Kammen, W. B., & Schmidt, L. (1996). Self-reported delinquency and combined delinquency seriousness scale based on boys, others and teachers: Concurrent and predictive validity for African-Americans and Caucasians. *Criminology, 34,* 501–25.

Farwell, R. F., Lee, Y. Z., Hirtz, D. G., Sulzbacher, S. I., Ellenberg, J. H., & Nelson, J. B. (1990). Phenobarbital for febrile seizures: Effects on intelligence and on seizure recurrence. *New England Journal of Medicine, 322,* 364–369.

Faull, C., & Nicol, A. R. (1986). Abdominal pain in six-year-olds: An epidemiological study in a new town. *Journal of Child Psychology and Psychiatry and Allied Disciplines, 27,* 251–260.

Fava, M. (1996). Traditional and alternative research design and methods in clinical pediatric psychopharmacology. *Journal of the American Academy of Child and Adolescent Psychiatry, 35,* 1292–1303.

Fay, W. H., & Schular, A. L. (1980). *Emerging language in autistic children.* London: Arnold.

Federal Bureau of Investigation. (1996). *Uniform crime reports.* Washington, DC: U.S. Government Printing Office.

Feindler, E. L. (1990). Adolescent anger control: Review and critique. In M. Hersen, R. M. Eisler, & P. M. Miller (Eds.), *Progress in behavior modification* (Vol. 26, pp. 11–59). Newbury Park, CA: Sage.

Feindler, E. L. (1995). An ideal treatment package for children and adolescents with anger disorders. In H. Kassinove (Ed.), *Anger disorders: Definition, diagnosis, and treatment* (pp. 173–195). Washington, DC: Taylor & Francis.

Feindler, E. L., & Guttman, J. (1994). Cognitive-behavioral anger control training for groups of adolescents: A treatment manual. In C. W. LeCroy (Ed.), *Handbook of child and adolescent treatment* (pp. 170–199). New York: Free Press.

Feindler, E. L., Marriott, S. A., & Iwata, M. (1984). Group anger control training for junior high school delinquents. *Cognitive Therapy and Research, 8*, 299–311.

Feingold, B. F. (1975). Hyperkinesis and learning difficulties linked to artificial food colors and flavors. *American Journal of Nursing, 75*, 797–803.

Feldman, H., Crumrine, P., Handen, B. L., Alvin, R., & Teodori, J. (1989). Methylphenidate in children with seizures and attention deficit disorder. *American Journal of Disease in Childhood, 143*, 1081–1086.

Feldman, W., McGrath, P., Hodgson, C., Ritter, H., & Shipman, R. T. (1985). The use of dietary fiber in the management of simple, common, childhood, recurrent, abdominal pain. *American Journal of Disease in Children, 139*, 1216–1218.

Ferguson, C., La Via, M., Crossan, P., & Kaye, W. (1999). Are serotonin selective reuptake inhibitors effective in underweight anorexia nervosa? *International Journal of Eating Disorders, 25*, 11–17.

Fergusson, D. M., & Horwood, L. J. (1999). Prospective childhood predictors of deviant peer affiliations in adolescence. *Journal of Child Psychology and Psychiatry and Allied Disciplines, 40*, 581–592.

Fergusson, D. M., Horwood, L. J., & Lynskey, M. T. (1995). The stability of disruptive childhood behaviors. *Journal of Abnormal Child Psychology, 23*, 379–396.

Fergusson, D. M., Horwood, L. J., Shannon, F. T., & Lawton, J. M. (1989). The Christchurch child development study: A review of epidemiological findings. *Paediatric and Perinatal Epidemiology, 3*, 302–325.

Fergusson, D. M., & Lynskey, M. T. (1996). Adolescent resiliency to family adversity. *Journal of Child Psychology and Psychiatry, 37*, 281–292.

Ferro, T., Carlson, G. A., Grayson, P., & Klein, D. N. (1994). Depressive disorders: Distinctions in children. *Journal of the American Academy of Child and Adolescent Psychiatry, 33*, 664–670.

Field, T., Schanberg, S., Kuhn, C., Field, T., Fierro, K., Henteleff, T., Mueller, C., Yando, R., Shaw, S., & Burman, I. (1998). Bulimic adolescents benefit from massage therapy. *Adolescence, 33*, 556–563.

Fife, B. L. (1978). Reducing parental overprotection of the leukemic child. *Social Science and Medicine, 12*, 117–122.

Filipek, P. A. (1999). Neuroimaging in the developmental disorders: The state of the science. *Journal of Child Psychology and Psychiatry, 40*, 113–128.

Findling, R. L., McNamara, N. K., Branicky, L. A., Schluchter, M. D., Lemon, E., & Blumer, J. L. (2000). A double-blind pilot study of risperidone in the treatment of conduct disorder. *Journal of the American Academy of Child and Adolescent Psychiatry, 39*, 509–516.

Findling, R. L., Schulz, S. C., Reed, M. D., & Blumer, J. L. (1998). The antipsychotics: A pediatric perspective. *Pediatric Clinics of North America, 45*, 1205–1232.

Fine, P. (1993). *A developmental network approach to therapeutic foster care.* Washington, DC: Child Welfare League of America.

Fine, S., Forth, A., Gilbert, M., & Haley, G. (1991). Group therapy for adolescent depressive disorder: A comparison of social skills and therapeutic support. *Journal of the American Academy of Child and Adolescent Psychiatry, 30*, 79–85.

Firestone, P., Kelly, M. J., & Fike, S. (1980). Are fathers necessary in parent training groups? *Journal of Clinical Child Psychology, 9*, 44–47.

Fischer, K. W., & Ayoub, C. (1994). Affective splitting and dissociation in normal and maltreated children: Developmental pathways for self in relationships. In D. Cicchetti & S. L. Toth (Eds.), *Rochester Symposium on Developmental Psychopathology. Vol. 5: Disorders and dysfunctions of the self* (pp. 149–222). Rochester, NY: University of Rochester Press.

Fischer, M., Barkley, R. A., Fletcher, K. E., & Smallish, L. (1993a). The adolescent outcome of hyperactive children: Predictors of psychiatric, academic, social and emotional adjustment. *Journal of the American Academy of Child and Adolescent Psychiatry, 32*, 324–332.

Fischer, M., Barkley, R. A., Fletcher, K. E., & Smallish, L. (1993b). The stability of dimensions of behavior in ADHD and normal children over a 8-year follow-up. *Journal of Abnormal Child Psychology, 21*, 315–337.

Fisher, M. S., & Bentley, K. J. (1996). Two group therapy models for clients with a dual diagnosis of substance abuse and personality disorder. *Psychiatric Services, 47*, 1244–1250.

Fisher, S., & Greenberg, R. P. (1997). What are we to conclude about psychotropic drugs? Scanning the major findings. In S. Fisher & R. P. Greenberg (Eds.), *From placebo to panacea: Putting psychiatric drugs to the test* (pp. 359–384). New York: Wiley.

Fixsen, D. L., & Blase, K. A. (1993). Creating new realities: Programme development and dissemination. *Journal of Applied Behavior Analysis, 26*, 597–615.

Flakierska, N., Lindstrom, M., & Gillberg, C. (1988). School refusal: A 15–20 year follow-up study of 35 Swedish urban children. *British Journal of Psychiatry, 152*, 834–837.

Flament, M. F., Koby, E., Rapoport, J. L., Berg, C. J., Zahn, T., Cox, C., Denckla, M., & Lenane, M. (1990). Childhood compulsive disorder: A prospective follow-up study. *Journal of Child Psychology and Psychiatry, 31*, 363–380.

Flament, M. F., Rapoport, J. L., Berg, C. J., Sceery, W., Kilts, C., Mellström, B., & Linnoila, M. (1985). Clomipramine treatment of childhood obsessive–compulsive disorder: A double-blind controlled study. *Archives of General Psychiatry, 42*, 977–983.

Flament, M. F., & Vera, L. (1990). Treatment of childhood obsessive–compulsive disorder. A review in the light of recent findings. In J. G. Simeon & H. B. Ferguson (Eds.), *Treatment strategies in child adolescent psychiatry* (pp. 49–75). New York: Plenum Press.

Flament, M. F., Whitaker, A., & Rapoport, J. L. (1988). Obsessive compulsive disorder in adolescence: An epidemiological study. *Journal of the American Academy of Child and Adolescent Psychiatry, 27*, 764–771.

Flannery, D. J. (1997). *School violence: Risk, preventive intervention, and policy.* New York: ERIC Clearinghouse in Urban Education.

Flannery-Schroeder, E. C., & Kendall, P. C. (2000). Group and individual cognitive-behavioral treatments for youth with anxiety disorders: A randomized controlled trial. *Cognitive Therapy and Research, 24*, 251–2781.

Fleischman, M. J. (1981). A replication of Patterson's "Intervention for boys with conduct problems." *Journal of Consulting and Clinical Psychology, 49*, 342–351.

Fleischman, M. J., & Szykula, S. A. (1981). A community setting replication of a social learning treatment for aggressive children. *Behavior Therapy, 12*, 115–122.

Fleming, J. E., Offord, D. R., & Boyle, M. H. (1989). Prevalence of childhood and adolescent depression in the community: Ontario Child Health Study. *British Journal of Psychiatry, 155*, 647–654.

Flynn, J. M., & Rahbar, M. H. (1994). Prevalence of reading failure in boys compared with girls. *Psychology in the Schools, 31*, 66–71.

Foa, E., & Kozak, M. J. (1996). Obsessive–compulsive disorder: Long-term outcome of psychological treatment. In M. Mavissakalian & R. Prien (Eds.), *Long-term treatments of anxiety disorders: Psychological and pharmacological approaches* (pp. 285–310). Washington, DC: American Psychiatric Press.

Follansbee, D. J., La Greca, A. M., & Citrin, W. S. (1983). Coping skills training for adolescents with diabetes. *Diabetes, 32*, 147.

Folstein, S., & Rutter, M. (1988). Autism: Familial aggregation and genetic implications. *Journal of Autism and Developmental Disorders, 18*, 3–30.

Fombonne, E. (1994). The Chartres Study: I. Prevalence of psychiatric disorders among French school-aged children. *British Journal of Psychiatry, 164*, 69–79.

Fombonne, E. (1995). Eating disorders: Time trends and possible explanatory mechanisms. In M. Rutter & D. Smith (Eds.), *Psychosocial disorders in young people: Time trends and their causes* (pp. 544–685). Chichester: Wiley.

Fombonne, E. (1998). Epidemiology of autism and related conditions. In F. R. Volkmar (Ed.), *Autism and pervasive developmental disorders* (pp. 32–63). Cambridge: Cambridge University Press.

Fonagy, P., & Higgitt, A. (1989). Evaluating the performance of departments of psychiatry. *Psychoanalytic Psychotherapy, 4,* 121–153.

Fonagy, P., Moran, G. S., & Target, M. (1993). Aggression and the psychological self. *International Journal of Psycho-Analysis, 74,* 471–485.

Fonagy, P., & Target, M. (1994). The efficacy of psychoanalysis for children with disruptive disorders. *Journal of the American Academy of Child and Adolescent Psychiatry, 33,* 45–55.

Fonagy, P., & Target, M. (1996). A contemporary psychoanalytical perspective: Psychodynamic developmental therapy. In E. Hibbs & P. Jensen (Eds.), *Psychosocial treatments for child and adolescent disorders: Empirically based approaches* (pp. 619–638). Washington, DC: American Psychological Association and National Institutes of Health.

Fonagy, P., Target, M., Steele, M., Steele, H., Leigh, T., Levinson, A., & Kennedy, R. (1997). Morality, disruptive behavior, borderline personality disorder, crime, and their relationships to security of attachment. In L. Atkinson & K. J. Zucker (Eds.), *Attachment and psychopathology* (pp. 223–274). New York: Guilford Press.

Food and Drug Administration. (1994). Specific requirements on content and format of labeling for human prescription drugs: Revision of pediatric use subsection in the labeling. *Federal Register, 59,* 64240–64250.

Forehand, R., & Kotchick, B. A. (1996). Cultural diversity: A wake-up call for parent training. *Behavior Therapy, 27,* 187–206.

Forehand, R., & Long, N. (1988). Outpatient treatment of the acting out child: Procedures, long-term follow-up data, and clinical problems. *Advances in Behaviour Research and Therapy, 10,* 129–177.

Forehand, R., & McMahon, R. J. (1981). *Helping the noncompliant child: A clinician's guide to parent training.* New York: Guilford Press.

Forehand, R., Rogers, T., McMahon, R. J., Wells, K. C., & Griest, D. L. (1981). Teaching parents to modify child behavior problems: An examination of some follow-up data. *Journal of Pediatric Psychology, 6,* 313–322.

Forehand, R., Sturgis, E. T., McMahon, R. J., Aguar, D., Green, K., Wells, K., & Breiner, J. (1979). Parent behavioral training to modify child noncompliance: Treatment generalization across time and from home to school. *Behavior Modification, 3,* 3–25.

Forehand, R., Wells, K. C., & Griest, D. L. (1980). An examination of the social validity of a parent training program. *Behavior Therapy, 11,* 488–502.

Forgatch, M. S. (1991). The clinical science vortex: Developing a theory for antisocial behaviour. In D. Pepler & K. H. Rubin (Eds.), *The development and treatment of childhood aggression* (pp. 291–315). Hillsdale, NJ: Erlbaum.

Forgatch, M. S., & Patterson, G. R. (1989). *Parents and adolescents living together. Part 2: Family problem solving.* Eugene, OR: Castalia.

Forgatch, M. S., & Ramsey, E. (1994). Boosting homework: A videotape link between families and schools. *School Psychology Review, 23,* 472–484.

Forness, S. R., Cantwell, D. P., Swanson, J. M., Hanna, G. L., & Youpa, D. (1991). Differential effects of stimulant medication on reading performance of boys with hyperactivity with and without conduct disorder. *Journal of Learning Disabilities, 24,* 304–310.

Fosson, A., Knibbs, J., Bryant-Waugh, R., & Lask, B. (1987). Early-onset anorexia nervosa. *Archives of Disease in Childhood, 62,* 114–118.

Foster, K., Wilmot, A., & Dobbs, J. (1990). *General Household Survey, 1988.* London: Her Majesty's Stationery Office.

Frances, A., Docherty, J. P., & Kahn, D. A. (1996). The expert consensus guideline series. The treatment of schizophrenia. *Journal of Clinical Psychiatry, 57*(Suppl. 12B), 1–58.

Francis, G., Robbins, D. R., & Grapentine, W. L. (1992). Panic disorder in children and adolescents. *Rhode Island Medicine, 75,* 273–276.

Franklin, M. E., Kozak, M. J., Cashman, L. A., Coles, M. E., Rheingold, A. A., & Foa, E. B. (1998). Cognitive-behavioral treatment of pediatric obsessive–compulsive disorder: An open clinical trial. *Journal of the American Academy of Child and Adolescent Psychiatry, 37,* 412–419.

Fras, I., & Major, L. F. (1995). Clinical experience with risperidone. *Journal of the American Academy of Child and Adolescent Psychiatry, 34,* 833.

Frazier, F., & Matthes, W. A. (1975). Parent education: A comparison of Adlerian and behavioral approaches. *Elementary School Guidance and Counseling, 10,* 31–38.

Frazier, J. A., Gordon, C. T., & McKenna, K. (1994). An open trial of clozapine in 11 adolescents with childhood-onset schizophrenia. *Journal of the American Academy of Child and Adolescent Psychiatry, 33,* 658–663.

Freeman, L. N. P., Grossman, E. O., Pozanski, E., & Grossman, J. A. (1985). Psychotic and depressed children: A new entity. *Journal of the American Academy of Child and Adolescent Psychiatry, 24,* 95–102.

Freemantle, N., & Maynard, A. (1994). Something rotten in the state of clinical and economic evaluations? *Health Economics, 3,* 63–67.

Freud, A. (1965). *Normality and pathology in childhood.* Harmondsworth, UK: Penguin Books.

Frick, P. J., Kamphaus, R. W., Lahey, B. B., Loeber, R., Christ, M. A., Hart, E. L., & Tannenbaum, L. E. (1991). Academic underachievement and the disruptive behavior disorders. *Journal of Consulting and Clinical Psychology, 59,* 289–294.

Frick, P. J., Lahey, B. B., Loeber, R., Stouthammer-Loeber, M., Christ, M. A., & Hanson, K. (1992). Familial risk factors to oppositional defiant disorder and conduct disorder: Parental psychopathology and maternal parenting. *Journal of Consulting and Clinical Psychology, 60,* 49–55.

Frick, P. J., O'Brien, B. S., Wootton, J. M., & McBurnett, K. (1994). Psychopathy and conduct problems in children. *Journal of Abnormal Psychology, 103,* 700–707.

Frick, P. J., Van Horn, Y., Lahey, B. B., Christ, M. A. G., Loeber, R., Hart, E. A., Tannenbaum, L., & Hanson, K. (1993). Oppositional defiant disorder and conduct disorder: A meta-analytic review of factor analyses and cross-validation in a clinic sample. *Clinical Psychology Review, 13,* 319–340.

Friedmann, C. T. H., & Silvers, F. M. (1977). A multimodal approach to inpatient treatment of obsessive–compulsive disorder. *American Journal of Psychotherapy, 31,* 456–465.

Fritz, G. K., Fritsch, S., & Hagino, O. (1997). Somatoform disorders in children and adolescents: A review of the past 10 years. *Journal of the American Academy of Child and Adolescent Psychiatry, 36,* 1329–1338.

Fukuda, K., Straus, S., Hickie, I., Sharpe, M. C., Dobbins, J. G., & Komaroff, A. (1994). The chronic fatigue syndrome: A comprehensive approach to its defintion and study. *Annals of Internal Medicine, 121,* 953–959.

Fulcher, K. Y., & White, P. D. (1997). Randomised controlled trial of graded exercise in patients with the chronic fatigue syndrome. *British Medical Journal, 314,* 1647–1652.

Fuller, M. G. (1995). More is less: Increasing access as a strategy for managing health care costs. *Psychiatric Services, 46,* 1015–1017.

Funderburk, B. W., Eyberg, S. M., Newcomb, K., McNeil, C. B., Hembree-Kigin, T., & Capage, L. (1998). Parent–child interaction therapy with behavior problem children: Maintenance of treatment effects in the school setting. *Child and Family Behavior Therapy, 20,* 17–38.

Furnell, J. R. G., & Dutton, P. V. (1986). Alleviation of toddler's diarrhea by environmental management. *Journal of Psychosomatic Research, 30,* 283–288.

Gadow, K. D. (1992). Pediatric psychopharmacotherapy: A review of recent research. *Journal of Child Psychology and Psychiatry, 33,* 153–195.

Gadow, K. D., Nolan, E. E., Sverd, J., Sprafkin, J., & Paolicelli, L. (1990). Methylphenidate in aggressive–hyperactive boys: I. Effects on peer aggression in public school settings. *Journal of the American Academy of Child and Adolescent Psychiatry, 29,* 710–718.

Gadow, K. D., Sverd, J., Sprafkin, J., Nolan, E. E., & Ezor, S. N. (1995). Efficacy of methylphenidate for attention deficit hyperactivity disorder in children with tic disorder. *Archives of General Psychiatry, 52,* 444–455.

Gaffney, A., & Dunne, E. A. (1986). Developmental aspects of children's defintions of pain. *Pain, 26,* 105–117.

Gaffney, A., & Dunne, E. A. (1987). Children's understanding of the causality of pain. *Pain, 29,* 91–104.

Gaffney, G. R., Kuperman, S., Tsai, L. Y., & Minchin, S. (1988). Morphological evidence for brainstem involvement in infantile autism. *Biological Psychiatry, 24,* 578–586.

Garbarino, J. (1995). *Raising children in a socially toxic environment.* San Francisco: Jossey Bass.

Garber, J., Walker, L. S., & Zeman, J. (1991). Somatization symptoms in a community sample of children and adolescents: Further validation of the children's somatization inventory. *Journal of Consulting and Clinical Psychology, 3,* 588–595.

Garfield, S. L. (1996). Some problems associated with "validated" forms of psychotherapy. *Clinical Psychology: Science and Practice, 3,* 218–229.

Garfield, S. L., & Bergin, A. E. (1994). Introduction and historical overview. In A. E. Bergin & S. L. Garfield (Eds.), *Handbook of psychotherapy and behavior change.* New York: Wiley.

Garfinkel, M., Garfinkel, L., Himmelhoch, J., & McHugh, T. (1985). *Lithium carbonate and carbamazepine: An effective treatment for adolescent manic or mixed bipolar patients.* Paper presented at the 32nd annual meeting of the American Academy of Child and Adolescent Psychiatry, San Antonio, TX.

Garfinkel, P. R., & Garner, D. M. (1982). *Anorexia nervosa: A multidimensional perspective.* New York: Brunner/Mazel.

Garmezy, N., & Masten, A. (1994). Chronic adversities. In M. Rutter, E. Taylor, & L. Hersov (Eds.), *Child and adolescent psychiatry: Modern approaches* (pp. 191–208). Oxford: Blackwell Scientific.

Garner, D. M., & Garfinkel, P. E. (1979). The Eating Attitudes Test: An index of symptoms of anorexia nervosa. *Psychological Medicine, 9,* 273–279.

Garner, D. M., Olmsted, M. P., Bohr, Y., & Garfinkel, P. E. (1982). The Eating Attitudes Test: Psychometric features and clinical correlates. *Psychological Medicine, 12,* 871–878.

Garralda, M. E. (1992). A selective review of child psychiatric syndromes with a somatic presentation. *British Journal of Psychiatry, 161,* 759–773.

Garralda, M. E. (1996). Somatisation in children. *Journal of Child Psychology and Psychiatry, 37,* 13–33.

Garralda, M. E., & Bailey, D. (1986a). Children with psychiatric disorders in primary care. *Journal of Child Psychology and Psychiatry, 27,* 611–624.

Garralda, M. E., & Bailey, D. (1986b). Psychological deviance in children attending general practice. *Psychological Medicine, 16,* 423–429.

Garralda, M. E., & Bailey, D. (1987). Psychosomatic aspects of children's consultations in primary care. *Archives of Psychiatry and Neurological Sciences, 236,* 319–322.

Garralda, M. E., & Bailey, D. (1989). Psychiatric disorders in general paediatric referrals. *Archives of Disease in Childhood, 64,* 1727–1733.

Garralda, M. E., & Bailey, D. (1990a). Pediatric identification of psychological factors associated with general pediatric consultations. *Journal of Psychosomatic Research, 34,* 303–312.

Garrison, W., & McQuiston, S. (1989). *Chronic illness during childhood and adolescence: Psychological aspects.* Newbury Park, CA: Sage.

Gastfriend, D. R., Biederman, J., & Jellinek, M. S. (1985). Desipramine in the treatment of attention deficit disorder in adolescents. *Psychopharmacology Bulletin, 21,* 144–145.

Gaub, M., & Carlson, C. L. (1997). Gender differences in ADHD: A meta-analysis and critical review. *Journal of the American Academy of Child and Adolescent Psychiatry, 36,* 1036–1045.

Geist, R., Heinmaa, M., Stephens, D., Davis, R., & Katzman, D. (2000). Comparison of family therapy and family group psychoeducation in adolescents with anorexia nervosa. *Canadian Journal of Psychiatry, 45,* 173–178.

Geller, B., Cooper, T. B., Chestnut, E. C., Anker, J. A., & Schluchter, M. D. (1986). Preliminary data on the relationship between nortriptyline plasma level and response in depressed children. *American Journal of Psychiatry, 143,* 1283–1286.

Geller, B., Cooper, T. B., McCombs, H. G., Graham, D., & Wells, J. (1989). Double-blind, placebo-controlled study of nortriptyline in depressed children using a "fixed plasma level" design. *Psychopharmacology Bulletin, 25,* 101–108.

Geller, B., Cooper, T. B., Schluchter, M. D., Warham, J. E., & Carr, L. G. (1987). Child and adolescent nortriptyline single dose pharmacokinetics parameters: Final report. *Journal of Clinical Psychopharmacology, 7,* 321–323.

Geller, B., Cooper, T. B., Sun, K., Zimerman, B., Frazier, J., Williams, M., & Heath, J. (1998). Double-blind and placebo controlled study of lithium for adolescent bipolar disorders with secondary substance disorders. *Journal of the American Academy of Child and Adolescent Psychiatry, 37,* 171–178.

Geller, B., Cooper, T. B., Watts, H. E., Cosby, C. M., & Fox, L. W. (1992). Early findings from a pharmacokinetically designed double-blind placebo-controlled study of lithium for adolescents comorbid with bipolar and substance dependency disorders. *Progress in Neuropsychopharmacology and Biological Psychiatry, 16,* 281–299.

Geller, B., & Luby, J. (1997). Child and adolescent bipolar disorder: A review of the past 10 years. *Journal of the American Academy of Child and Adolescent Psychiatry, 36,* 1168–1176.

Geller, B., Reising, D., Leonard, H. L., Riddle, M. A., & Walsh, B. T. (1999). Critical review of tricyclic antidepressant use in children and adolescents. *Journal of the American Academy of Child and Adolescent Psychiatry, 38,* 513–516.

Geller, B., Sun, K., Zimerman, B., Luby, J., Frazier, J., & Williams, M. (1995a). Complex and rapid-cycling in bipolar children and adolescents: A preliminary study. *Journal of Affective Disorders, 34,* 259–268.

Geller, D. A., Biederman, J., Reed, E. D., Spencer, T., & Wilens, T. E. (1995b). Similarities in the response to fluoxetine in the treatment of children and adolescents with obsessive–compulsive disorder. *Journal of the American Academy of Child and Adolescent Psychiatry, 34,* 36–44.

Genius, M. L. (1995). The use of hypnosis in helping cancer patients control anxiety, pain and emesis: A review of recent empirical studies. *American Journal of Clinical Hypnosis, 37,* 316–325.

Ghaziuddin, N., & Alessi, N. E. (1992). An open clinical trial of trazodone in aggressive children. *Journal of Child and Adolescent Psychopharmacology, 2,* 291–297.

Ghodsian, M., & Power, C. (1987). Alcohol consumption between the ages of 16 and 23 in Britain: A longitudinal study. *British Journal of Addiction, 82,* 175–180.

Gibaldi, M., & Perrier, D. (1982). *Pharmacokinetics* (2nd ed.). New York: Marcel Dekker.

Gibbs, J. C., Arnold, K. D., Ahlborn, H. H., & Cheesman, F. L. (1984). Facilitation of sociomoral reasoning in delinquents. *Journal of Consulting and Clinical Psychology, 52,* 37–45.

Gibbs, J. C., Potter, G. B., Barriga, A. Q., & Liau, A. K. (1996). Developing the helping skills and prosocial motivation of aggressive adolescents in peer group programmes. *Aggression and Violent Behavior, 1,* 283–305.

Gilbert, D. L., Sethuraman, G., Sine, L., Peters, S., & Sallee, F. R. (2000). Tourette's syndrome improvement with pergolide in a randomized, double-blind, crossover trial. *Neurology, 54,* 1310–1315.

Gillberg, C. (1990a). Autism and pervasive developmental disorders. *Journal of Child Psychology and Psychiatry, 31,* 99–119.

Gillberg, C. (1990b). Infantile autism: Diagnosis and treatment. *Acta Psychiatrica Scandinavica, 81,* 209–215.

Gillberg, C. (1991). Outcome in autism and autistic-like conditions. *Journal of the American Academy of Child and Adolescent Psychiatry, 30,* 375–382.

Gillberg, C., Rasmussen, P., Carlstrom, G., Svenson, B., & Waldenstrom, E. (1982). Perceptual, motor, and attentional deficits in six year old children: Epidemiological aspects. *Journal of Child Psychology and Psychiatry, 23,* 131–144.

Gillberg, C., & Steffenberg, S. (1987). Outcome and prognostic factors in autism and similar conditions: A population based study of 46 cases followed through puberty. *Journal of Autism and Developmental Disorders, 17,* 273–287.

Gillberg, C., Steffenburg, S., & Schaumann, H. (1991). Is autism more common now than ten years ago? *British Journal of Psychiatry, 30,* 489–494.

Gillberg, I. C., & Gillberg, C. (1989). Asperger syndrome: Some epidemiological considerations. A research note. *Journal of Child Psychology and Psychiatry, 30,* 631–638.

Gillberg, I. C., Rastam, M., & Gillberg, C. (1994). Anorexia nervosa outcomes: Six-year controlled longitudinal study of 51 cases including a population cohort. *Journal of the American Academy of Child and Adolescent Psychiatry, 33,* 729–739.

Gittelman, R. (1983). Treatment of reading disorders. In M. Rutter (Ed.), *Developmental neuropsychiatry* (pp. 530–541). New York: Guilford Press.

Gittelman, R., & Klein, D. F. (1984). Relationship between separation anxiety and panic and agoraphobic disorders. *Psychopathology, 17*(Suppl.), 56–65.

Gittelman, R., Mannuzza, S., Shenker, R., & Bonagura, N. (1985). Hyperactive boys almost grown up: I. Psychiatric status. *Archives of General Psychiatry, 42,* 937–947.

Gittelman-Klein, R., & Klein, D. F. (1973). School phobia: Diagnostic considerations in the light of imipramine effects. *Journal of Nervous and Mental Disease, 156,* 199–215.

Glantz, L. H. (1996). Conducting research with children: Legal and ethical issues. *Journal of the American Academy of Child and Adolescent Psychiatry, 35,* 1283–1291.

Glisson, C. (1994). The effect of service coordination teams on outcomes for children in state custody. *Administration and Social Work, 18,* 1–23.

Glogowska, M., Roulstone, S., Enderby, P., & Peters, T. J. (2000). Randomised controlled trial of community based speech and language therapy in preschool children. *British Medical Journal, 321,* 923–926.

Goddard, E. (1996). *Teenage drinking in 1994.* London: Her Majesty's Stationery Office.

Goddard, E., & Iken, C. (1988). *Drinking in England and Wales in 1987.* London: Her Majesty's Stationery Office.

Goetz, C. G., Tanner, C. M., Wilson., R. S., Carroll, V. S., Como, P. G., & Shannon, K. M. (1987). Clonidine and Gilles de la Tourette syndrome: Double-blind study using objective rating methods. *Annals of Neurology, 21,* 307–310.

Goldacre, M., & Hawton, K. (1985). Repetition of self-poisoning and subsequent death in adolesents who take overdoses. *British Journal of Psychiatry, 146,* 395–398.

Goldfried, M. R. (1995). *From cognitive-behavior therapy to psychotherapy integration.* New York: Springer.

Goldfried, M. R., & Wolfe, B. E. (1996). Psychotherapy practice and research: Repairing a strained alliance. *American Psychologist, 51,* 1007–1016.

Goldstein, A. P., & Glick, B. (1994). Aggressive Replacement Training: Curriculum and evaluation. *Simulation and Gaming, 25,* 9–26.

Goldstein, A. P., Glick, B., Reiner, S., Zimmerman, D., & Coultry, T. (1986). *Aggression Replacement Training: A comprehensive intervention for aggressive youth.* Champaign, IL: Research Press.

Gonzales, A., & Michanie, C. (1992). Clozapine for refractory psychosis. *Journal of the American Academy of Child and Adolescent Psychiatry, 31,* 1169–1170.

Gonzalez, J. C., Routh, D. K., & Armstrong, F. D. (1993). Effects of maternal distraction versus reassurance on children's reactions to injections. *Journal of Pediatric Psychology, 18,* 593–604.

Gonzalez, N. M., Campbell, M., Small, A. M., Shay, J., Bluhm, L. D., Adams, P. B., & Foltz, R. L. (1994). Naltrexone plasma levels, clinical response and effect on weight in autistic children. *Psychopharmacology Bulletin, 30,* 203–208.

Goodman, R. (1997). The strengths and difficulties questionnaire: A research note. *Journal of Child Psychology and Psychiatry, 38,* 581–586.

Goodman, S. H., Schwab-Stone, M., Lahey, B. B., Shaffer, D., & Jensen, P. S. (2000). Major depression and dysthymia in children and adolescents: Discriminant validity and differential consequences in a community sample. *Journal of the American Academy of Child and Adolescent Psychiatry, 39,* 761–770.

Goodyer, I. (1981). Hysterical conversion reactions in childhood. *Journal of Child Psychology and Psychiatry and Allied Disciplines, 22,* 179–188.

Goodyer, I. M. (1989). *The Index of Friendships Interview for Young People* (2nd version). Unpublished manuscript.

Goodyer, I. M., Herbert, J., Secher, S., & Pearson, J. (1997). Short-term outcome of major depression: I. Comorbidity and severity at presentation as predictors of persistent disorder. *Journal of the American Academy of Child and Adolescent Psychiatry, 36,* 474–480.

Goodyer, I. M., & Mitchell, C. (1989). Somatic emotional disorders in childhood and adolescence. *Journal of Psychosomatic Research, 33,* 681–688.

Gordon, C. T., State, R. C., Nelson, J. E., Hamburger, S. D., & Rapoport, J. L. (1993). A double-blind comparison of clomipramine, desipramine, and placebo in the treatment of autistic disorder. *Archives of General Psychiatry, 50*, 441–447.

Gordon, D. A., & Arbuthnot, J. (1987). Individual, group, and family interventions. In H. C. Quay (Ed.), *Handbook of juvenile delinquency* (pp. 290–324). New York: Wiley.

Gordon, D. A., Arbuthnot, J., Gustafson, K. E., & McGreen, P. (1988). Home-based behavioral-systems family therapy with disadvantaged juvenile delinquents. *American Journal of Family Therapy, 16*, 243–255.

Gordon, D. A., Graves, K., & Arbuthnot, J. (1995). The effect of Functional Family Therapy for delinquents on adult criminal behavior. *Criminal Justice and Behaviour, 22*, 60–73.

Gottfredson, D. C., & Gottfredson, G. D. (1992). Theory-guided investigation: Three field experiments. In J. McCord & R. E. Tremblay (Eds.), *Preventing antisocial behavior: Interventions from birth through adolescence* (pp. 311–329). New York: Guilford Press.

Gottlieb, L., & Rowat, K. (1987). The McGill model of nursing: A practice derived model. *Advances in Nursing Science, 9*, 51–61.

Gottman, J. M., Katz, L. F., & Hooven, C. (1997). *Meta-emotion: How families communicate emotionally*. Mahwah, NJ: Erlbaum.

Gould, M. S., Bird, H. R., & Jaramillo, B. S. (1993). Correspondence between statistically derived behavior problem syndromes and child psychiatric diagnoses in a community sample. *Journal of Abnormal Child Psychology, 21*, 287–313.

Gould, M. S., Wallenstein, S., & Kleinman, M. (1990). Time–space clustering of teenage suicide. *American Journal of Epidemiology, 131*, 71–78.

Gould, M. S., Wunsch-Hitzig, R., & Dohrenwend, B. (1981). Estimating the prevalence of childhood psychopathology: A critical review. *Journal of the American Academy of Child and Adolescent Psychiatry, 20*, 462–476.

Gowers, S., Crisp, A., Joughin, N., & Bhat, A. (1991). Premenarchal anorexia nervosa. *Journal of Child Psychology and Psychiatry, 32*, 515–524.

Gowers, S., Norton, K., Halek, C., & Crisp, A. H. (1994). Outcome of outpatient psychotherapy in a random allocation treatment study of anorexia nervosa. *International Journal of Eating Disorders, 15*, 165–177.

Goyette, C. H., Conners, C. K., & Ulrich, R. F. (1978). Normative data for Revised Conners Parent and Teacher Rating Scales. *Journal of Abnormal Child Psychology, 6*, 221–236.

Graae, F., Milner, J., Rizzotto, L., & Klein, R. G. (1994). Clonazepam in childhood anxiety disorders. *Journal of the American Academy of Child and Adolescent Psychiatry, 33*, 372–376.

Grados, M. A., & Riddle, M. A. (2001). Pharmacological treatment of childhood obsessive–compulsive disorder: From theory to practice. *Journal of Clinical Child Psychology, 30*, 67–79.

Graham, P. J. (1986). Behavioural and intellectual development. *British Medical Bulletin, 42*, 155–162.

Grattan-Smith, P., Fairley, M., & Procopis, P. (1988). Clinical features of conversion disorder. *Archives of Disease in Childhood, 63*, 408–414.

Gray, G., Smith, A., & Rutter, M. (1980). School attendance and the first year of employment. In *Out of school: Modern perspectives in truancy and school refusal* (pp. 343–370). Chichester: Wiley.

Green, S. M., Loeber, R., & Lahey, B. B. (1991). Stability of mothers' recall of the age of onset of their child's attention and hyperactivity problems. *Journal of the American Academy of Child and Adolescent Psychiatry, 30*, 135–137.

Greenberg, R. P., Bornstein, R. F., Greenberg, M. D., & Fisher, S. (1992). A meta-analysis of antidepressant outcome under "blinder" conditions. *Journal of Consulting and Clinical Psychology, 60*, 664–669.

Greenhill, L. L. (1992). Pharmacologic treatment of attention deficit hyperactivity disorder. *Psychiatric Clinics of North America, 15*, 1–27.

Greenhill, L. L., Abikoff, H. B., Cantwell, D. P., Conners, C. K., Elliott, G., Hinshaw, S. P., Hoza, B., Jensen, P. S., March, J. S., Newcorn, J. H., Pelham, W. E., Severe, J. B., Swanson, J. M., Vitiello, B., & Wells, K. (1996). Medication treatment strategies in the MTA study: Relevance to clinicians and researchers. *Journal of the American Academy of Child and Adolescent Psychiatry, 35,* 1304–1313.

Greenhill, L. L., & Setterberg, S. (1992). Pharmacotherapy of disorders of adolescents. *Psychiatric Clinics of North America, 16,* 793–814.

Greenhill, L. L., Solomon, M., Pleak, R., & Ambrosini, P. (1985). Molindone hydrochloride treatment of hospitalized children with conduct disorder. *Journal of Clinical Psychiatry, 46,* 20–25.

Gregg, V., Gibbs, J. C., & Basinger, K. S. (1994). Patterns of developmental delay in moral judgment by male and female delinquents. *Merrill-Palmer Quarterly, 40,* 538–553.

Griest, D. L., Forehand, R., Rogers, T., Breiner, J. L., Furey, W., & Williams, C. A. (1982). Effects of Parent Enhancement Therapy on the treatment outcome and generalisation of a parent training programme. *Behaviour Research and Therapy, 20,* 429–436.

Griffiths, C. P. (1969). A follow-up study of children with disorders of speech. *British Journal of Disorders of Communication, 4,* 46–56.

Grizenko, N. (1997). Outcome of multimodal day treatment for children with severe behavior problems: A five-year follow-up. *Journal of the American Academy of Child and Adolescent Psychiatry, 36,* 989–997.

Grizenko, N., Papineau, D., & Sayegh, L. (1993). Effectiveness of a multimodal day treatment program for children with disruptive behavior problems. *Journal of the American Academy of Child and Adolescent Psychiatry, 32,* 127–134.

Guerra, N., & Slaby, R. G. (1990). Cognitive mediators of aggression in adolescent offenders: II. Intervention. *Developmental Psychology, 26,* 269–277.

Gunning, B. (1992). *A controlled trial of clonidine in hyperkinetic children.* Rotterdam: Department of Child and Adolescent Psychiatry, Academic Hospital.

Gustafsson, P. A., Kjellman, N.-I. M., & Cederblad, M. (1986). Family therapy in the treatment of severe childhood asthma. *Journal of Psychosomatic Research, 30,* 369–374.

Gustafsson, P. A., & Svedin, C. G. (1988). Cost effectiveness: Family therapy in a pediatric setting. *Family Systems Medicine, 6,* 162–175.

Gutgesell, H., Atkins, D., Barst, R., Buck, M., Franklin, W., Humes, R., Ringel, R., Shaddy, R., & Taubert, K. A. (1999). AHA Scientific Statement: Cardiovascular monitoring of children and adolescents receiving psychotropic drugs. *Journal of the American Academy of Child and Adolescent Psychiatry, 38,* 1047–1050.

Guthrie, D. W., Sargent, L., Speelman, D., & Parks, L. (1990). Effects of parental relaxation training on glycosylated hemoglobin of children with diabetes. *Patient Education and Counseling, 16,* 247–253.

Guy, W. (1976). *ECDEU assessment manual for psychopharmacology.* Washington, DC: U.S. Department of Health, Education, and Welfare.

Hagerman, R. J., Murphy, M. A., & Wittenberg, M. D. (1988). A controlled trial of stimulant medication in children with fragile X syndrome. *American Journal of Medical Genetics, 30,* 377–392.

Hagino, O. R., Weller, E. B., Weller, R. A., Washing, D., Fristad, M. A., & Kontras, S. B. (1995). Untoward effects of lithium treatment in children aged four through six years. *Journal of the American Academy of Child and Adolescent Psychiatry, 34,* 1584–1590.

Hahn, A., Leavitt, T., & Aaron, P. (1994). *Evaluation of the Quantum Opportunities Program: Did the program work?* Waltham, MA: Center for Human Resources, Brandeis University.

Hall, A. (1987). The place of family therapy in the treatment of anorexia nervosa. *Australian and New Zealand Journal of Psychiatry, 21,* 568–574.

Hall, A., & Crisp, A. H. (1983). Brief psychotherapy in the treatment of anorexia nervosa. In A. J. Krawkowski & C. P. Kimball (Eds.), *Psychosomatic medicine* (pp. 703–717). New York: Plenum Press.

Hallahan, D. P., Kauffman, J., & Lloyd, J. (1996). *Introduction to learning disabilities.* Needham Heights, MA: Allyn & Bacon.

Hallgren, L., Gillberg, C., Gillberg, J. C., & Enerskog, I. (1993). Children with deficits in attention, motor control and perception almost grown-up: General health at 16 years. *Developmental Medicine and Child Neurology, 35,* 881–892.

Halmi, K. A., Eckert, E., LaDu, T. J., & Cohen, J. (1986). Anorexia nervosa: Treatment efficacy of cyproheptadine and amitriptyline. *Archives of General Psychiatry, 43,* 177–181.

Hamilton, S. B., & MacQuiddy, S. L. (1984). Self-administered behavioral parent training: Enhancement of treatment efficacy using a time-out signal seat. *Journal of Clinical Child Psychology, 13,* 61–69.

Hammen, C., Rudolph, K., Weisz, J., Rao, U., & Burge, D. (1999). The context of depression in clinic-referred youth: Neglected areas in treatment. *Journal of the American Academy of Child and Adolescent Psychiatry, 38,* 64–71.

Hampe, E., Noble, H., Miller, L. C., & Barrett, C. L. (1973). Phobic children one and two years post-treatment. *Journal of Abnormal Psychology, 82,* 446–453.

Handen, B. L., Feldman, H. M., Lurier, A., & Huszar Murray, P. (1999). Efficacy of methylphenidate among preschool children with developmental disabilities and ADHD. *Journal of the American Academy of Child and Adolescent Psychiatry, 38,* 805–812.

Handen, B. L., McAuliffe, S., Janosky, J., Breaux, A. M., & Feldman, H. (1995). Methylphenidate in children with mental retardation and ADHD: Effects on independent play and academic functioning. *Journal of Developmental and Physical Disabilities, 7,* 91–103.

Harcherik, J. F., Leckman, J. F., Detlor, J., & Cohen, D. J. (1984). A new instrument for clinical studies of Tourette's syndrome. *Journal of the American Academy of Child and Adolescent Psychiatry, 23,* 153–160.

Hardy, J., & Streett, R. (1989). Family support and parenting education in the home: An effective extension of clinic-based preventive health care services for poor children. *Journal of Pediatrics, 115,* 927–931.

Harkavy-Friedman, J. M., Asnis, G. M., Boeck, M., & DiFiore, J. (1987). Prevalence of specific suicidal behaviors in a high school sample. *American Journal of Psychiatry, 144,* 1203–1206.

Harrington, R. (1992). The natural history and treatment of child and adolescent affective disorders. *Journal of Child Psychology and Psychiatry, 33,* 1287–1302.

Harrington, R. (1993). *Depressive disorder in childhood and adolescence.* Chichester: Wiley.

Harrington, R. (2001). Childhood depression and conduct disorder: Different routes to the same outcome? *Archives of General Psychiatry, 58,* 237–238.

Harrington, R., Bredenkamp, D., Groothues, C., Rutter, M., Fudge, H., & Pickles, A. (1994). Adult outcomes of childhood and adolescent depression: III. Links with suicidal behaviours. *Journal of Child Psychology and Psychiatry, 35,* 1309–1319.

Harrington, R., Fudge, H., Rutter, M., Pickles, A., & Hill, J. (1990). Adult outcomes of childhood and adolescent depression: I. Psychiatric status. *Archives of General Psychiatry, 47,* 465–473.

Harrington, R., Fudge, H., Rutter, M., Pickles, A., & Hill, J. (1991). Adult outcomes of childhood and adolescent depression: II. Links with antisocial disorders. *Journal of the American Academy of Child and Adolescent Psychiatry, 30,* 434–439.

Harrington, R., Kerfoot, M., Dyer, E., McNiven, F., Gill, J., Harrington, V., & Woodham, A. (2000a). Deliberate self-poisoning in adolescence: Why does a brief family intervention work in some cases and not others? *Journal of Adolescnce, 23,* 13–20.

Harrington, R., Kerfoot, M., Dyer, E., McNiven, F., Gill, J., Harrington, V., Woodham, A., & Byford, S. (1998a). Randomized trial of a home-based family intervention for children who have deliberately poisoned themselves. *Journal of the American Academy of Child and Adolescent Psychiatry, 37,* 512–518.

Harrington, R., Peters, S., Green, J., Byford, S., Woods, J., & McGowan, R. (2000b). Randomised comparison of the effectiveness and costs of community and hospital based mental health services for children with behavioural disorders. *British Medical Journal, 321,* 1047–1050.

Harrington, R., Whittaker, J., & Shoebridge, P. (1998b). Psychological treatment of depression in children and adolescents: A review of treatment research. *British Journal of Psychiatry, 173,* 291–298.

Harrington, R., Whittaker, J., Shoebridge, P., & Campbell, F. (1998c). Systematic review of efficacy of cognitive behaviour therapies in childhood and adolescent depressive disorder. *British Medical Journal, 316*, 1559–1563.

Harris, J. R. (1998). *The nurture assumption: Why children turn out the way they do: Parents matter less than you think and peers matter more.* New York: Free Press.

Harris, P. L. (1989). *Children and emotion: The development of psychological understanding.* Oxford: Blackwell.

Harris, P. L. (1994). The child's understanding of emotion: Developmental change and the family environment. *Journal of Child Psychology and Psychiatry, 35*, 3–28.

Harris, S. L., Handleman, J. S., Kristoff, B., Bass, L., & Gordon, R. (1990). Changes in language development among autistic and peer children in segregated and integrated preschool settings. *Journal of Autism and Developmental Disorders, 20*, 23–31.

Harter, S. (1988). Issues in the assessment of the self-concept of children and adolescents. In A. M. La Greca (Ed.), *Through the eyes of the child: Obtaining self-reports from children and adolescents* (pp. 292–325). Needham Heights, MA: Allyn & Bacon.

Hauser, S. T., Powers, S. I., Noan, G. G., & Jacobson, A. M. (1984). Familial contexts of adolescent ego development. *Child Development, 55*, 195–213.

Hawkins, J. D., Catalano, R. F., & Miller, Y. (1992). Risk and protective factors for alcohol and other drug problems in adolescence and early adulthood: Implications for substance abuse prevention. *Psychological Bulletin, 112*, 64–105.

Hawkins, J. D., Jenson, J. M., Catalano, R. F., & Lishner, D. M. (1988). Delinquency and drug abuse: Implications for social services. *Social Service Review, 62*, 258–264.

Hawkins, J. D., Jenson, J. M., Catalano, R. F., & Wells, E. A. (1991). Effects of a skills training intervention with juvenile delinquents. *Research in Social Work and Practice, 1*, 107–121.

Hawley, R. M. (1985). The outcome of anorexia nervosa in younger subjects. *British Journal of Psychiatry, 146*, 657–660.

Hawton, K. (1996). Suicide and attempted suicide in young people. In A. Macfarlane (Ed.), *Adolescent medicine* (pp. 117–130). London: Royal College of Physicians.

Hawton, K., & Fagg, J. (1992a). Deliberate self-poisoning and self-injury in adolescents: A study of characteristics and trends in Oxford, 1976–89. *British Journal of Psychiatry, 161*, 816–823.

Hawton, K., & Fagg, J. (1992b). Trends in deliberate self poisoning and self-injury in Oxford, 1976–90. *British Medical Journal, 304*, 1409–1411.

Hawton, K., Fagg, J., Simkin, S., Bale, E., & Bond, A. (2000). Deliberate self-harm in adolescents in Oxford, 1985–1995. *Journal of Adolescence, 23*, 47–55.

Hawton, K., Kingsbury, S., Steinhardt, K., James, A., & Fagg, J. (1999). Repetition of deliberate self-harm by adolescents: The role of psychological factors. *Journal of Adolescence, 22*, 369–378.

Hawton, K., O'Grady, J., Osborn, M., & Cole, D. (1982). Adolescents who take overdoses: Their characteristics, problems and contacts with helping agencies. *British Journal of Psychiatry, 140*, 118–123.

Haynes, C., & Naidoo, S. (1991). *Children with specific speech and language impairment.* London: MacKeith Press.

Hayward, C., Killen, J. D., Hammer, L. D., Litt, I. F., Wilson, D. M., Simmonds, B., & Taylor, C. B. (1992). Pubertal stage and panic attack history in sixth- and seventh-grade girls. *American Journal of Psychiatry, 149*, 1239–1243.

Hayward, C., Varady, S., Albano, A. M., Thienemann, M., Henderson, L., & Schatzberg, A. F. (2000). Cognitive-behavioral group therapy for social phobia in female adolescents: Results of a pilot study. *Journal of the American Academy of Child and Adolescent Psychiatry, 39*, 721–726.

Hazelrigg, M. D., Cooper, H. M., & Borduin, C. M. (1987). Evaluating the effectiveness of family therapies: An integrative review and analysis. *Psychological Bulletin, 101*, 428–442.

Health Education Authority. (1992). *Tomorrow's young adults: 9–15 year-olds look at alcohol, drugs, exercise and smoking.* London: Author.

Heath, G. A., Hardesty, V. A., Goldfine, P. E., & Walker, A. M. (1983). Childhood firesetting: An empirical study. *Journal of the American Academy of Child Psychiatry, 22*, 370–374.

Hechtman, L. (1985). Adolescent outcome of hyperactive children treated with stimulants in childhood: A review. *Psychopharmacology Bulletin, 21,* 178–191.

Hechtman, L., & Greenfield, B. (1997). Juvenile onset bipolar disorder. *Current Opinion in Pediatrics, 9,* 346–353.

Hechtman, L., Weiss, G., & Perlman, T. (1984). Hyperactive as young adults: Initial predictors of adult outcome. *Journal of the American Academy of Child and Adolescent Psychiatry, 23,* 250–260.

Heimann, M., Nelson, K. E., Tjus, T., & Gillberg, C. (1995). Increasing reading and communication skills in children with autism through an interactive multimedia computer program. *Journal of Autism and Developmental Disorders, 25,* 459–480.

Heinicke, C. M. (1965). Frequency of psychotherapeutic session as a factor affecting the child's developmental status. *The Psychoanalytic Study of the Child, 20,* 42–98.

Heinicke, C. M., & Ramsey-Klee, D. M. (1986). Outcome of child psychotherapy as a function of frequency of sessions. *Journal of the American Academy of Child Psychiatry, 25,* 247–253.

Hembree-Kigin, T. L., & McNeil, C. B. (1995). *Parent–child interaction therapy: A step-by-step guide for clinicans.* New York: Plenum Press.

Henggeler, S. W., Borduin, C. M., Melton, G. G., Mann, B. J., Smith, L., Hall, J. A., Cone, L., & Fuccie, B. R. (1991). Effects of multisystemic therapy on drug use and abuse in serious juvenile offenders: A progress report from two outcome studies. *Family Dynamics of Addiction Quarterly, 1,* 40–51.

Henggeler, S. W., Cunningham, P. B., Pickrel, S. G., Schoenwald, S. K., & Brondino, M. J. (1996a). Multisystemic therapy: An effective violence prevention approach for serious juvenile offenders. *Journal of Adolescence, 19,* 47–61.

Henggeler, S. W., Melton, G. B., Brondino, M. J., Scherer, D. G., & Hanley, J. H. (1997). Multisystemic therapy with violent and chronic juvenile offenders and their families: The role of treatment fidelity in successful dissemination. *Journal of Consulting and Clinical Psychology, 65,* 821–833.

Henggeler, S. W., Melton, G. B., & Smith, L. A. (1992). Family preservation using multisystemic therapy: An effective alternative to incarcerating serious juvenile offenders. *Journal of Consulting and Clinical Psychology, 60,* 953–961.

Henggeler, S. W., Melton, G. B., Smith, L. A., Schoenwald, S. K., & Hanley, J. H. (1993). Family preservation using multisystemic treatment: Long-term follow-up to a clinical trial with serious juvenile offenders. *Journal of Child and Family Studies, 2,* 283–293.

Henggeler, S. W., Pickrel, S. G., Brondino, M. J., & Crouch, J. L. (1996b). Eliminating (almost) treatment dropout of substance abusing or dependent delinquents through home-based multisystemic therapy. *American Journal of Psychiatry, 153,* 427–428.

Henggeler, S. W., Rodick, J., Borduin, C. M., Hanson, C., Watson, S., & Urey, J. (1986). Multisystemic treatment of juvenile offenders: Effects on adolescent behavior and family interaction. *Developmental Psychology, 22,* 132–141.

Henggeler, S. W., Schoenwald, S. K., Borduin, C. M., Rowland, M. D., & Cunningham, P. B. (1998). *Multisystemic treatment of antisocial behavior in children and adolescents.* New York: Guilford Press.

Henggeler, S. W., Schoenwald, S. K., & Pickrel, S. G. (1995). Multisystemic therapy: Bridging the gap between university and community-based treatment. *Journal of Consulting and Clinical Psychology, 63,* 709–717.

Henggeler, S. W., Schoenwald, S. K., Pickrel, S. G., Brondino, S. J., Borduin, C. M., & Hall, J. A. (1994). *Treatment manual for family preservation using multisystemic therapy.* Charleston: South Carolina Health and Human Services Finance Commission.

Henggeler, S. W., Schoenwald, S., Rowland, M., & Ward, D. (1999). *MST versus psychiatric hospitalization: Placement outcomes post-treatment.* Paper presented at the 46th Annual Meeting of the American Academy of Child and Adolescent Psychiatry, Chicago.

Herbert, M. (1995). A collaborative model of training for parents of children with disruptive behaviour disorders. *British Journal of Clinical Psychology, 34,* 325–342.

Hermann, C., Kim, M., & Blanchard, E. B. (1995). Behavioral and prophylactic pharmacological intervention studies of pediatric migraine: An exploratory meta-analysis. *Pain, 60,* 239–256.

Herpertz-Dahlmann, B. M., & Remschmidt, H. (1993). Depression and psychosocial adjustment in adolescent anorexia nervosa. A controlled 3-year follow-up study. *European Child and Adolescent Psychiatry, 2,* 146–154.

Herpertz-Dahlmann, B. M., Wewetzer, C., & Remschmidt, H. (1995). The predictive value of depression in anorexia nervosa: Results of a 7-year follow-up study. *Acta Paediatrica Scandinavica, 91,* 114–119.

Herpertz-Dahlmann, B. M., Wewetzer, C., Schulz, E., & Remschmidt, H. (1996). Course and outcome in adolescent anorexia nervosa. *International Journal of Eating Disorders, 19,* 335–345.

Herzog, D. B. (1995). Psychodynamic psychotherapy. In C. G. Fairburn & G. T. Wilson (Eds.), *Binge eating: Nature, assessment, and treatment* (pp. 330–335). New York: Guilford Press.

Herzog, D. B., Keller, M. B., Lavori, P. W., & Sacks, N. R. (1991). The course and outcome of bulimia nervosa. *Journal of Clinical Psychiatry, 52,* 4–8.

Higgs, J., Goodyer, I., & Birch, J. (1989). Anorexia nervosa and food avoidance emotional disorder. *Archives of Disease in Childhood, 64,* 346–351.

Himmelhoch, J. M., & Garfinkel, M. E. (1986). Mixed mania: Diagnosis and treatment. *Psychopharmacology Bulletin, 22,* 613–620.

Hinshaw, S. P. (1991). Stimulant medication in the treatment of aggression in children with attentional deficits. *Journal of Clinical Child Psychology, 12,* 301– 312.

Hinshaw, S. P. (1992a). Academic underachievement, attention deficits, and aggression: Comorbidity and implications for intervention. *Journal of Consulting and Clinical Psychology, 60,* 893–903.

Hinshaw, S. P. (1992b). Externalizing behavior problems and academic under-achievement in childhood and adolescence: Causal relationships and underlying mechanisms. *Psychological Bulletin, 111,* 127–155.

Hinshaw, S. P. (1994). *Attention deficits and hyperactivity in children.* Thousand Oaks, CA: Sage.

Hinshaw, S. P., Buhrmester, D., & Heller, T. (1989a). Anger control in response to verbal provocation: Effects of stimulant medication for boys with ADHD. *Journal of Abnormal Child Psychology, 17,* 393–407.

Hinshaw, S. P., Heller, T., & McHale, J. P. (1992). Covert antisocial behavior in boys with attention-deficit hyperactivity disorder: External validation and effects of methylphenidate. *Journal of Consulting and Clinical Psychology, 60,* 274–281.

Hinshaw, S. P., Henker, B., & Whalen, C. K. (1984a). Cognitive-behavioral and pharmacologic interventions for hyperactive boys: Comparative and combined effects. *Journal of Consulting and Clinical Psychology, 52,* 739–749.

Hinshaw, S. P., Henker, B., & Whalen, C. K. (1984b). Self-control in anger-inducing situations: Effects of cognitive-behavioral training and methylphenidate. *Journal of Abnormal Child Psychology, 12,* 55–77.

Hinshaw, S. P., Henker, B., Whalen, C. K., Erhardt, D., & Dunnington, R. E. (1989b). Aggressive, prosocial, and nonsocial behavior in hyperactive boys: Dose effects of methylphenidate in naturalistic settings. *Journal of Consulting and Clinical Psychology, 57,* 636–643.

H. M. Government Statistical Service. (1994). *Statistics of drug addicts notified to the Home Office, United Kingdom, 1993.* Home Office Statistical Bulletin 10/94. London: Her Majesty's Stationery Office.

Hoagwood, K., Hibbs, E., Brent, D., & Jensen, P. (1995). Introduction to the special section: Efficacy and effectiveness in studies of child and adolescent psychotherapy. *Journal of Consulting and Clinical Psychology, 63,* 683–687.

Hoagwood, K., Jensen, P. S., Petti, T., & Burns, B. J. (1996). Outcomes of mental health care for children and adolescents: I. A comprehensive conceptual model. *Journal of the American Academy of Child and Adolescent Psychiatry, 35,* 1055–1063.

Hoagwood, K., & Rupp, A. (1995, March). Mental health services needs, use and costs for children and adolescents with mental disorders and their families: Preliminary evidence. *Psychiatric Times, 12,* 62–63.

Hodges, K. (1995). *The Child and Adolescent Functioning Assessment Scale* (unpublished manuscript).

Hodges, K., Bickman, L., Ring-Kurtz, S., & Rieter, M. (1991). Multi-dimensional measure of level of functioning for children and adolescents. In A. Algarian & R. Friedman (Eds.), *A system of care for children's mental health: Expanding the research base* (pp. 149–154). Tampa, FL: Research and Training Center for Children's Mental Health.

Hogarty, G. E., Anderson, C. M., Reiss, D. J., Kornblith, S. J., Greenwald, D. P., Javna, C. D., & Madonia, M. J. (1986). Family psychoeducation, social skills training, and maintenance chemotherapy in the aftercare treatment of schizophrenia: I. One-year effects of a controlled study on relapse and expressed emotion. *Archives of General Psychiatry, 43*, 633–642.

Holden, G. W., Lavigne, V. V., & Cameron, A. M. (1990). Probing the continuum of effectiveness in parent training: Characteristics of parents and preschoolers. *Journal of Clinical Child Psychology, 19*, 2–8.

Holford, L. E., Van der Walt, A., & Peter, E. (2000). *Risperidone for behavior disorders in children with mental retardation.* Paper presented at the 47th Annual Meeting of the American Academy of Child and Adolescent Psychiatry, New York.

Holland, R., Moretti, M. M., Verlaan, V., & Peterson, S. (1993). Attachment and conduct disorder: The response programme. *Canadian Journal of Psychiatry, 38*, 420–431.

Holmes, T. H., & Rahe, R. H. (1967). The social readjustment rating scale. *Journal of Psychosomatic Research, 11*, 213–218.

Hooper, S. R., Murphy, J., Devaney, A., & Hultman, T. (2000). Ecological outcomes of adolescents in a psychoeducational residential treatment facility. *American Journal of Orthopsychiatry, 70*, 491–500.

Hops, H., & Walker, H. M. (1988). *CLASS: Contingencies for Learning Academic and Social Skills.* Seattle, WA: Educational Achievement Systems.

Horn, W. F., Ialongo, N. S., Pascoe, J. M., Greenberg, G., Packard, T., Lopez, M., Wagner, A., & Puttler, L. (1991). Additive effects of psychostimulants, parent training, and self-control therapy with ADHD children. *Journal of the American Academy of Child and Adolescent Psychiatry, 30*, 233–240.

Horne, A. M., & Van Dyke, B. (1983). Treatment and maintenance of social learning family therapy. *Behavior Therapy, 14*, 606–613.

Horowitz, H. A. (1977). Lithium and the treatment of adolescent manic depressive illness. *Diseases of the Nervous System, 38*, 480–483.

Horton, L. (1984). The father's role in behavioral parent training: A review. *Journal of Clinical Child Psychology, 13*, 274–279.

House of Commons Health Committee. (1997). *The specific health needs of children and young people* (Vol. 1). London: Her Majesty's Stationery Office.

Hovens, J. G. F. M., Cantwell, D. P., & Kiriakos, R. (1994). Psychiatric comorbidity in hospitalized adolescent substance abusers. *Journal of the American Academy of Child and Adolescent Psychiatry, 33*, 476–483.

Howard, B. L., & Kendall, P. C. (1996a). *Cognitive-behavioral family therapy for anxious children: Therapist manual.* Ardmore, PA: Workbook.

Howard, B. L., & Kendall, P. C. (1996b). Cognitive-behavioral family therapy for anxiety-disordered children: A multiple-baseline evaluation. *Cognitive Therapy and Research, 20*, 423–443.

Howard, K. I., Orlinsky, D. E., & Lueger, R. J. (1995). The design of clinically relevant outcome research: Some considerations and an example. In M. Aveline & D. A. Shapiro (Eds.), *Research foundations for psychotherapy practice* (pp. 3–47). Chichester: Wiley.

Howell, J. C. (Ed.). (1995). *Guide for implementing the comprehensive strategy for serious, violent and chronic juvenile offenders.* Washington, DC: Office of Juvenile Justice and Delinquency Prevention.

Howlin, P., Mawhood, L., & Rutter, M. (2000). Autism and developmental receptive language disorder—A follow-up comparison in early adult life. II: Social, behavioural, and psychiatric outcomes. *Journal of Child Psychology and Psychiatry, 41*, 561–578.

Howlin, P., & Rutter, M. (1987). *Treatment of autistic children.* Chichester: Wiley.

Hsu, L. K. G. (1986a). Lithium resistant adolescent mania. *Journal of the American Academy of Child and Adolescent Psychiatry, 25*, 280–283.

Hsu, L. K. G. (1986b). The treatment of anorexia nervosa. *American Journal of Psychiatry, 143*, 573–581.

Hsu, L. K. G. (1988). The outcome of anorexia nervosa: A reappraisal. *Psychological Medicine, 18*, 807–812.

Hsu, L. K. G. (1990). *Eating disorders.* New York: Guilford Press.

Hudson, J., Nutter, R. W., & Galaway, B. (1994). Treatment foster care program: A review of evaluation research and suggested directions. *Social Work Research, 18*, 198–210.

Huesmann, L. R., Leonard, D. E., & Monroe, M. L. (1984). Stability of aggression over time and generations. *Developmental Psychology, 20*, 1120–1134.

Huey, W. C., & Rank, R. C. (1984). Effects of counselor and peer-led group assertiveness training on black adolescent aggression. *Journal of Counseling Psychology, 31*, 95–98.

Hughes, C. W., Preskorn, S. H., Weller, E., Weller, R., Hassanein, R., & Tucker, S. (1990). The effect of concomitant disorders in childhood depression on predicting treatment response. *Psychopharmacology Bulletin, 26*, 235–238.

Humphrey, G. B., Boon, C. M. J., Linden Van den Heuvell, G. F. E. C., & Van de Wiel, H. B. M. (1992). The occurrence of high levels of acute behavioral distress in children and adolescents undergoing routine venepuncture. *Pediatrics, 90*, 87–91.

Humphreys, L., Forehand, R., McMahon, R., & Roberts, M. (1978). Parent behavioral training to modify child noncompliance: Effects on untreated siblings. *Journal of Behavior Therapy and Experimental Psychiatry, 9*, 235–238.

Hunsley, J., & Rumstein-McKean, O. (1999). Improving psychotherapeutic services via randomized clinical trials, treatment manuals, and component analysis designs. *Journal of Clinical Psychology, 55*, 1507–1517.

Hunt, A., & Shepherd, C. (1993). A prevalence study of autism in tuberous sclerosis. *Journal of Autism and Developmental Disorders, 23*, 329–339.

Hunt, R. D. (1987). Treatment effects of oral and transdermal clonidine in relation to methylphenidate: An open pilot study in ADHD. *Psychopharmacology Bulletin, 23*, 111–114.

Hunt, R. D., Arnstein, A., & Asbell, M. (1995). An open label trial of guanfacine in the treatment of attention deficit hyperactivity disorder. *Journal of the American Academy of Child and Adolescent Psychiatry, 34*, 50–54.

Hunt, R. D., Capper, L., & O' Donnell, P. (1990). Clonidine in child and adolescent psychiatry. *Journal of Child and Adolescent Psychopharmacology, 1*, 87–102.

Hunt, R. D., Minderaa, R. B., & Cohen, D. (1985). Clonidine benefits children with attention deficit disorder and hyperactivity: Report of a double-blind placebo-crossover trial. *Journal of the American Academy of Child and Adolescent Psychiatry, 24*, 617–629.

Hunt, R. D., Minderaa, R. B., & Cohen, D. J. (1986). The therapeutic effect of clonidine in attention deficit disorder with hyperactivity: A comparison with placebo and methylphenidate. *Psychopharmacology Bulletin, 22*, 229–236.

Ialongo, N. S., Edelsohn, G., Werthamer-Larsson, L., Crockett, L., & Kellam, S. (1994). The significance of self-reported anxious symptoms in first-grade children. *Journal of Abnormal Child Psychology, 22*, 441–455.

Ialongo, N. S., Edelsohn, G., Werthamer-Larsson, L., Crockett, L., & Kellam, S. (1995). The significance of self-reported anxious symptoms in first-grade children: Prediction to anxious symptoms and adaptive functioning in fifth grade. *Journal of Child Psychology and Psychiatry, 36*, 427–437.

Ingenmey, R., & Van Houten, R. (1991). Using time delay to promote spontaneous speech in an autistic child. *Journal of Applied Behavior Analysis, 24*, 591–596.

Ioannidis, J. P., Haidich, A. B., & Lau, J. (2001). Any casualties in the clash of randomised and observational evidence? *British Medical Journal, 322*, 879–880.

Ireys, H. T., Chernoff, R., DeVet, K. A., & Kim, Y. (2001). Maternal outcomes of a randomized controlled trial of a community-based support program for families of children with chronic illnesses. *Archives of Pediatrics and Adolescent Medicine, 155*(7), 771–777.

Ireys, H. T., Sills, E. M., Kolodner, K. B., & Walsh, B. B. (1996). A social support intervention for parents of children with juvenile rheumatoid arthritis: Results of a randomized trial. *Journal of Pediatric Psychology, 21*, 633–641.

Ireys, H. T., Silver, E. J., Stein, R. E. K., Bencivenga, K., & Koeber, C. (1991). Evaluating a parent support program for mothers of chronically ill children. *American Journal of Disease in Children*, 145, 397.

Iwamasa, G. Y. (1996). Introduction to the special series: Ethnic and cultural diversity in cognitive and behavioral practice. *Cognitive and Behavioral Practice*, 3, 209–213.

Iwata, B. A., Pace, G. M., & Willis, K. D. (1986). Operant studies of self-injurious hand-biting in the Rett syndrome. *American Journal of Medical Genetics*, 24, 157–166.

Jacknow, D. S., Tschann, J. M., Link, M. P., & Boyce, W. T. (1994). Hypnosis in the prevention of chemotherapy-related nausea and vomiting in children: A prospective study. *Developmental and Behavioral Pediatrics*, 15, 258–264.

Jacobson, N., & Truax, P. (1991). Clinical significance: A statistical approach to defining meaningful change in psychotherapy research. *Journal of Consulting and Clinical Psychology*, 59, 12–19.

Jacobson, N. S., & Christensen, A. (1996). *Integrative couple therapy: Promoting acceptance and change.* New York: Norton.

Jacobson, N. S., & Revenstorf, D. (1988). Statistics for assessing the clinical significance of psychotherapy techniques: Issues, problems, and new developments. *Behavioral Assessment*, 10, 133–145.

Jacobvitz, D., Sroufe, L. A., Stewart, M., & Leffert, N. (1990). Treatment of attentional and hyperactivity problems in children with sympathomimetic drugs: A comprehensive review. *Journal of the American Academy of Child and Adolescent Psychiatry*, 29, 677–688.

Jaffa, T. (1995). Adolescent psychiatry services. *British Journal of Psychiatry*, 166, 306–310.

Jankovic, J. (1993). Deprenyl in attention deficit associated with Tourette's syndrome. *Archives of Neurology*, 50, 286–288.

Jaselskis, C. A., Cook, E. H., Fletcher, K. E., & Leventhal, B. L. (1992). Clonidine treatment of hyperactive and impulsive children with autistic disorder. *Journal of Clinical Psychopharmacology*, 12, 322–327.

Jay, S. M., Elliott, C. H., Fitzgibbons, I., Woody, P., & Siegel, S. E. (1995). A comparative study of cognitive behavior therapy versus general anesthesia for painful medical procedures in children. *Pain*, 62, 3–9.

Jay, S. M., Elliott, C. H., Katz, E., & Siegel, S. E. (1987). Cognitive-behavioral and pharmacologic interventions for children's distress during painful medical procedures. *Journal of Consulting and Clinical Psychology*, 55, 860–865.

Jay, S. M., Elliott, C. H., Ozolins, M., Olson, R. A., & Pruitt, S. D. (1985). Behavioural management of children's distress during painful medical procedures. *Behaviour Research and Therapy*, 23, 513–520.

Jaycox, L. H., Reivich, K. J., Gillham, J. E., & Seligman, M. E. P. (1994). Prevention of depressive symptoms in schoolchildren. *Behavioral Research and Therapy*, 32, 801–816.

Jayson, D., Wood, A., Kroll, L., Fraser, J., & Harrington, R. (1998). Which depressed patients respond to cognitive-behavioral treatment? *Journal of the American Academy of Child and Adolescent Psychiatry*, 37, 35–39.

Jenike, M. A. (1990). Predictors of treatment failure. In M. A. Jenike, L. Baer, & W. E. Minichiello (Eds.), *Obsessive–compulsive disorders: Theory and management* (pp. 76–93). Chicago: Year Book Medical Publishers.

Jensen, P. S. (1999). Fact versus fancy concerning the Multimodal Treatment Study for attention deficit hyperactivity disorder. *Canadian Journal of Psychiatry*, 44, 975–980.

Jensen, P. S., Hoagwood, K., & Petti, T. (1996). Outcomes of mental health care for children and adolescents: II. Literature review and application of a comprehensive model. *Journal of the American Academy of Child and Adolescent Psychiatry*, 35, 1064–1077.

Jensen, P. S., Kettle, L., Roper, M. T., Sloan, M. T., Dulcan, M. K., Hoven, C., Bird, H. R., Bauermeister, J. J., & Payne, J. D. (1999). Are stimulants overprescribed? Treatment of ADHD in four U.S. communities. *Journal of the American Academy of Child and Adolescent Psychiatry*, 38, 797–804.

Jensen, P. S., Ryan, N. D., & Prien, R. (1994). Psychopharmacology of child and adolescent major depression. *Journal of Child and Adolescent Psychopharmacology*, 2, 31–45.

Jensen, P. S., Vitiello, B., Leonard, H., & Laughren, T. (1992). Child and adolescent psychopharmacology: Expanding the research base. *Psychopharmacology Bulletin, 30*, 3–8.

Jenson, J. M., & Howard, M. O. (1998). Youth crime, public policy, and practice in the juvenile justice system: Recent trends and needed reforms. *Social Work, 43*, 324–334.

Jessop, D. J., Reissman, C. K., & Stein, R. E. (1988). Chronic childhood illness and maternal mental health. *Journal of Developmental Behavioral Pediatrics, 9*, 147–156.

Jessor, T., & Jessor, S. L. (1977). *Problem behavior and psychosocial development: A longitudinal study of youth.* San Diego, CA: Academic Press.

Joanning, H., Quinn, T. F., & Mullen, R. (1992). Treating adolescent drug abuse: A comparison of family systems therapy, group therapy, and family drug education. *Journal of Marital and Family Therapy, 18*, 345–356.

John, K., Gammon, G. D., Prusoff, B. A., & Warner, V. (1987). The Social Adjustment Inventory for Children and Adolescents (SAICA): Testing of a new semi-structured interview. *Journal of the American Academy of Child and Adolescent Psychiatry, 26*, 898–911.

Johnson, C. J., Beitchman, J. H., Young, A., Escobar, M., Atkinson, L., Wilson, B., Brownlie, E. B., Douglas, L., Taback, N., Lam, I., & Wang, M. (1999). Fourteen-year follow-up of children with and without speech/language impairments: Speech/language stability and outcomes. *Journal of Speech Language, and Hearing Research, 42*, 744–760.

Johnson, C. L., Tobin, D. L., & Lipkin, J. (1989). Epidemiologic changes in bulimia behavior among female adolescents over a five-year period. *International Journal of Eating Disorders, 8*, 647–656.

Johnson, S. B., & Rodrigue, J. R. (1997). Health-related disorders. In E. J. Mash & L. G. Terdal (Eds.), *Assessment of childhood disorders* (3rd ed., pp. 481–519). New York: Guilford Press.

Johnston, C. (1996). Addressing parent cognitions in interventions with families of disruptive children. In K. S. Dobson & K. D. Craig (Eds.), *Advances in cognitive-behavior therapy* (pp. 193–209). Thousand Oaks, CA: Sage.

Johnston, C., & Mash, E. J. (1989). A measure of parenting satisfaction and efficacy. *Journal of Clinical Child Psychology, 18*, 167–175.

Joint Working Group of the Colleges of Physicians, Psychiatrists and General Practitioners. (1996). *Chronic fatigue syndrome.* London: Royal College of Physicians.

Jones, D. I. (1977). Self-poisoning with drugs: The past 20 years in Sheffield. *British Medical Journal, 1* (6052), 28–29.

Jouriles, E. N., Murphy, C. M., Farris, A. M., Smith, D. A., Richter, J. E., & Waters, E. (1991). Marital adjustment, parental disagreements about childrearing, and behavior problems in boys: Increasing the specificity of the marital assessment. *Child Development, 62*, 1424–1433.

Joyce, P. R. (1984). Age of onset of bipolar affective disorder and misdiagnosis as schizophrenia. *Psychological Medicine, 14*, 145–149.

Kafantaris, V. (1995). Treatment of bipolar disorder in children and adolescents. *Journal of the American Academy of Child and Adolescent Psychiatry, 34*, 732–741.

Kafantaris, V., Campbell, M., Padron-Gayol, M. V., Small, A. M., Locascio, J. J., & Rosenberg, C. R. (1992). Carbamazepine in hospitalized aggressive conduct disorder children: An open pilot study. *Psychopharmacology Bulletin, 28*, 193–199.

Kahle, A. L., & Kelley, M. L. (1994). Children's homework problems: A comparison of goal setting and parent training. *Behavior Therapy, 25*, 275–290.

Kaminer, Y., Tarter, R. E., Bukstein, O. G., & Kabene, M. (1992). Comparison between treatment completers and noncompleters among dually diagnosed substance-abusing adolescents. *Journal of the American Academy of Child and Adolescent Psychiatry, 31*, 1046–1049.

Kandel, D. B., & Faust, R. (1975). Sequence and stages in patterns of adolescent drug use. *Archives of General Psychiatry, 32*, 923–932.

Kane, M., & Kendall, P. (1989). Anxiety disorders in children: Evaluation of a cognitive-behavioral treatment. *Behavior Therapy, 20*, 499–508.

Kanner, L. (1943). Autistic disturbance of affective contact. *Nervous Child, 2*, 217–250.

Kaplan, B. J., McNicol, J., Conte, R. A., & Moghadam, H. K. (1989). Dietary replacement in preschool aged hyperactive boys. *Pediatrics, 83*, 7–17.

Kaplan, R. M., Chadwick, M. W., & Schimmel, L. E. (1985). Social learning intervention to promote metabolic control in type I diabetes mellitus: Pilot experiment results. *Diabetes Care, 8,* 152–155.

Kaplan, S., Busner, J., Kupietz, S., Wassermann, E., & Segal, B. (1990). Effects of methylphenidate on adolescents with aggressive conduct disorder and ADDH: A preliminary report. *Journal of the American Academy of Child and Adolescent Psychiatry, 60,* 274–281.

Kaplan, S. L., Simms, R. M., & Busner, J. (1994). Prescribing practices of outpatient child psychiatrists. *Journal of the American Academy of Child and Adolescent Psychiatry, 33,* 35–44.

Kashani, J. H., Beck, N. C., Hoeper, E. W., Fallah, C., Corcoran, C. M., McAllister, J. A., Rosenberg, T. K., & Reid, J. C. (1987). Psychiatric disorders in a community sample of adolescents. *American Journal of Psychiatry, 144,* 584–589.

Kashani, J. H., & Orvaschel, H. (1990). A community study of anxiety in children and adolescents. *American Journal of Psychiatry, 147,* 313–318.

Kaslow, N. J., & Thompson, M. P. (1998). Applying the criteria for empirically supported treatments to studies of psychosocial interventions for child and adolescent depression. *Journal of Clinical Child Psychology, 27,* 146–155.

Kauffman, J. M. (1997). *Characteristics of emotional and behavioral disorders of children and youth* (6th ed.). Englewood Cliffs, NJ: Prentice-Hall.

Kaur, B., Anderson, H. R., Austin, J., Burr, M., Harkins, L. S., & Strachan, D. P. (1998). Prevalence of asthma symptoms, diagnosis, and treatment in 12–14 year old children across Great Britain (international study of asthma and allergies in childhood, ISAAC UK). *British Medical Journal, 316,* 118–124.

Kavale, K. (1982). The efficacy of stimulant drug treatment for hyperactivity: A meta-analysis. *Journal of Learning Disabilities, 15,* 280–289.

Kavale, K. A., & Forness, S. R. (1995). *The nature of learning disabilities: Critical elements of diagnosis and classification.* Mahwah, NJ: Erlbaum.

Kavanagh, C. (1983). Psychological intervention with the severely burned child: Report of an experimental comparison of two approaches and their effects on psychological sequelae. *Journal of American Academy of Child Psychiatry, 22,* 145–156.

Kazak, A. E., Penati, B., Boyer, B. A., Himelstein, B., Brophy, P., Waibel, M. K., Blackall, G. F., Daller, R., & Johnson, K. (1996). A randomized controlled prospective outcome study of a psychological and pharmacological intervention protocol for procedural distress in pediatric leukemia. *Journal of Pediatric Psychology, 21,* 615–631.

Kazdin, A. E. (1990a). Childhood depression. *Journal of Child Psychology and Psychiatry, 31,* 121–160.

Kazdin, A. E. (1990b). Premature termination from treatment among children referred for antisocial behavior. *Journal of Child Psychology and Psychiatry, 31,* 415–425.

Kazdin, A. E. (1992). Overt and covert antisocial behavior: Child and family characteristics among psychiatric inpatient children. *Journal of Child and Family Studies, 1,* 3–20.

Kazdin, A. E. (1994). Psychotherapy for children and adolescents. In A. E. Bergin & S. L. Garfield (Eds.), *Handbook of psychotherapy and behavior change* (4th ed., pp. 543–594). New York: Wiley.

Kazdin, A. E. (1995a). Child, parent, and family dysfunction as predictors of outcome in cognitive-behavioural treatment of antisocial children. *Behaviour Research and Therapy, 33,* 271–281.

Kazdin, A. E. (1995b). *Conduct disorder in childhood and adolescence* (2nd ed.). Thousand Oaks, CA: Sage.

Kazdin, A. (1996a). Combined and multimodal treatments in child and adolescent psychotherapy: Issues, challenges and research directions. *Clinical Psychology: Science and Practice, 3,* 69–100.

Kazdin, A. E. (1996b). Problem solving and parent management in treating aggressive and antisocial behavior. In E. D. Hibbs & P. S. Jensen (Eds.), *Psychosocial treatments for child and adolescent disorders: Empirically based strategies for clinical practice* (pp. 377–408). Washington, DC: American Psychological Association.

Kazdin, A. E. (1996c). Developing effective treatments for children and adolescents. In E. D. Hibbs & P. S. Jensen (Eds.), *Psychosocial treatments for child and adolescent disorders: Empirically based strategies for clinical practice* (pp. 9–18). Washington, DC: American Psychological Association.

Kazdin, A. E. (1996d). Dropping out of child psychotherapy: Issues for research and implications for practice. *Clinical Child Psychology and Psychiatry, 1*, 133–156.

Kazdin, A. E. (1997a). A model for developing effective treatments: Progression and interplay of theory, research, and practice. *Journal of Clinical Child Psychology, 26*, 114–129.

Kazdin, A. E. (1997b). Parent management training: Evidence, outcomes, and issues. *Journal of the American Academy of Child and Adolescent Psychiatry, 36*, 1349–1356.

Kazdin, A. E. (1997c). Practitioner review: Psychosocial treatments for conduct disorder in children. *Journal of Child Psychology and Psychiatry and Allied Disciplines, 38*, 161–178.

Kazdin, A. E. (1998). *Research design in clinical psychology.* Needham Heights, MA: Allyn & Bacon.

Kazdin, A. E. (2000a). Developing a research agenda for child and adolescent psychotherapy. *Archives of General Psychiatry, 57*, 829–835.

Kazdin, A. E. (2000b). *Psychotherapy for children and adolescents: Directions for research and practice.* Oxford: Oxford University Press.

Kazdin, A. E. (2000c). *Psychotherapy for children and adolescents: Directions for research and practice.* New York: Oxford University Press.

Kazdin, A. E. (in press). Treatment of conduct disorders. *Cambridge Monographs in Child and Adolescent Psychiatry: Conduct Disorders.*

Kazdin, A. E., Bass, D., Ayers, W. A., & Rodgers, A. (1990a). Empirical and clinical focus of child and adolescent psychotherapy research. *Journal of Consulting and Clinical Psychology, 58*, 729–740.

Kazdin, A. E., Bass, D., Ayers, W. A., & Rodgers, A. (1990b). Empirical and clinical focus of child and adolescent psychotherapy research. *Journal of Consulting and Clinical Psychology, 58*, 729–740.

Kazdin, A. E., Bass, D., Siegel, T. C., & Thomas, C. (1989). Cognitive-behavioral therapy and relationship therapy in the treatment of children referred for antisocial behavior. *Journal of Consulting and Clinical Psychology, 57*, 522–535.

Kazdin, A. E., & Crowley, M. (1997). Moderators of treatment outcome in cognitively based treatment of antisocial children. *Cognitive Therapy and Research, 21*, 185–207.

Kazdin, A. E., Esveldt-Dawson, K., French, N. H., & Unis, A. S. (1987a). Effects of parent management training and problem-solving skills training combined in the treatment of antisocial child behavior. *Journal of the American Academy of Child and Adolescent Psychiatry, 26*, 416–424.

Kazdin, A. E., Esveldt-Dawson, K., French, N. H., & Unis, A. S. (1987b). Problem-solving skills training and relationship therapy in the treatment of antisocial child behavior. *Journal of Consulting and Clinical Psychology, 55*, 76–85.

Kazdin, A. E., Holland, L., & Breton, S. (1991). *Barriers to participation in treatment scale: Patient and therapist.* New Haven, CT: Yale University Press.

Kazdin, A. E., Holland, L., & Crowley, M. (1997). Family experience of barriers to treatment and premature termination from child therapy. *Journal of Consulting and Clinical Psychology, 65*, 453–463.

Kazdin, A. E., & Kendall, P. C. (1998). Current progress and future plans for developing effective treatments: Comments and perspectives. *Journal of Clinical Child Psychology, 27*, 217–226.

Kazdin, A. E., & Marciano, P. L. (1998). Childhood and adolescent depression. In E. J. Mash & R. A. Barkley (Eds.), *Treatment of childhood disorders* (pp. 211–248). New York: Guilford Press.

Kazdin, A. E., Mazurick, J. L., & Siegel, T. C. (1994). Treatment outcome among children with externalizing disorder who terminate prematurely versus those who complete psychotherapy. *Journal of the American Academy of Child and Adolescent Psychiatry, 33*, 549–557.

Kazdin, A. E., Siegel, T. C., & Bass, D. (1990). Drawing upon clinical practice to inform research on child and adolescent psychotherapy: A survey of practitioners. *Professional Psychology: Research and Practice, 21*, 189–198.

Kazdin, A. E., Siegel, T. C., & Bass, D. (1992). Cognitive problem-solving skills training and parent management training in the treatment of antisocial behavior in children. *Journal of Consulting and Clinical Psychology, 60*, 733–747.

Kazdin, A. E., & Wasser, G. (2000). Therapeutic changes in children, parents and families resulting from treatment of children with conduct problems. *Journal of the American Academy of Child and Adolescent Psychiatry, 39,* 414–420.

Kearney, C. A., & Silverman, W. K. (1990). Treatment of an adolescent with obsessive–compulsive disorder by alternating response prevention and cognitive therapy: An empirical analysis. *Journal of Behaviour Therapy and Experimental Psychiatry, 21,* 39–47.

Kearney, C. A., & Silverman, W. K. (1999). Functionally based prescriptive and nonprescriptive treatment for children and adolescents with school refusal behavior. *Behavior Therapy, 30,* 673–693.

Keller, M. B., Lavori, P. W., Mueller, T. I., Endicott, J., Coryell, W., Hirschfeld, R. M., & Shea, T. (1992a). Time to recovery, chronicity, and levels of psychopathology in major depression: A 5-year prospective follow-up of 431 subjects. *Archives of General Psychiatry, 49,* 809–816.

Keller, M. B., Lavori, P. W., Wunder, J., Beardslee, W. R., Schwartz, C. E., & Roth, J. (1992b). Chronic course of anxiety disorders in children and adolescents. *Journal of the American Academy of Child and Adolescent Psychiatry, 31,* 595–599.

Kemph, J. P., DeVane, C. L., Levin, G. M., Jarecke, R., & Miller, R. L. (1993). Treatment of aggressive children with clonidine: Results of an open pilot study. *Journal of the American Academy of Child and Adolescent Psychiatry, 32,* 577–581.

Kempton, S., Vance, A., Maruff, P., Luk, E., Costin, J., & Pantelis, C. (1999). Executive function and attention deficit hyperactivity disorder: Stimulant medication and better executive function performance in children. *Psychological Medicine, 29,* 527–538.

Kendall, P. C. (1993). Cognitive-behavioral therapies with youth: Guiding theory, current status and emerging developments. *Journal of Consulting and Clinical Psychology, 61,* 235–247.

Kendall, P. C. (1994). Treating anxiety disorders in children: Results of a randomized clinical trial. *Journal of Consulting and Clinical Psychology, 62,* 100–110.

Kendall, P. C. (2000). Round of applause for an agenda and regular report cards for child and adolescent psychotherapy research. *Archives of General Psychiatry, 57,* 839–840.

Kendall, P. C., & Braswell, L. (1985). *Cognitive-behavioral therapy for impulsive children.* New York: Guilford Press.

Kendall, P. C., & Braswell, L. (1993). *Cognitive-behavioral therapy for impulsive children* (2nd ed.). New York: Guilford Press.

Kendall, P. C., & Flannery-Schroeder, E. (1998). Methodological issues in treatment research for anxiety disorders in youth. *Journal of Abnormal Child Psychology, 26,* 27–38.

Kendall, P. C., Flannery-Schroeder, E., Panichelli-Mindel, S. M., Southam-Gerow, M. A., Henin, A., & Warman, M. (1997). Therapy for youths with anxiety disorders: A second randomized clinical trial. *Journal of Consulting and Clinical Psychology, 65,* 366–380.

Kendall, P. C., & MacDonald, J. P. (1993). Cognition in the psychopathology of youth and implications for treatment. In K. S. Dobson & P. C. Kendall (Eds.), *Psychopathology and cognition* (pp. 387–426). San Diego, CA: Academic Press.

Kendall, P. C., Reber, M., McLeer, S., Epps, J., & Ronan, K. R. (1990). Cognitive-behavioral treatment of conduct-disordered children. *Cognitive Therapy and Research, 14,* 279–297.

Kendall, P. C., & Southam-Gerow, M. A. (1995). Issues in the transportability of treatment: The case of anxiety disorders in youths. *Journal of Consulting and Clinical Psychology, 63,* 702–708.

Kendall, P. C., & Southam-Gerow, M. A. (1996). Long-term follow-up of a cognitive-behavioral therapy for anxiety-disordered youths. *Journal of Consulting and Clinical Psychology, 64,* 724–730.

Kendler, K. S. (1995). Genetic epidemiology in psychiatry: Taking both genes and environment seriously. *Archives of General Psychiatry, 52,* 895–899.

Kendler, K. S., Maclean, C., Neale, M., Kessler, R., Heath, A., & Eaves, L. (1991). The genetic epidemiology of bulimia nervosa. *American Journal of Psychiatry, 148,* 1627–1637.

Kendler, K. S., & Tsuang, M. T. (1988). Outcome and familial psychopathology in schizophrenia. *Archives of General Psychiatry, 45,* 338–346.

Kent, M. A., Camfield, C. S., & Camfield, P. R. (1999). Double-blind methylphenidate trials. *Archive of Pediatrics and Adolescent Medicine, 153,* 1292–1296.

Kerfoot, M. (1988). Deliberate self-poisoning in childhood and early adolescence. *Journal of Child Psychology and Psychiatry, 29,* 335–343.

Kerfoot, M., & Huxley, P. (1995). Suicide and deliberate self-harm in young people. *Current Opinion in Psychiatry, 8,* 214–217.

Kernberg, P., & Chazan, S. E. (1991). *Children with conduct disorders: A psychotherapy manual.* New York: Basic Books.

Kerr, A. H., & Stephenson, J. B. P. (1985). Rett's syndrome in the West of Scotland. *British Medical Journal, 291,* 579–582.

Kerr, A. M. (1986). Report on the Rett syndrome workshop: Glasgow, Scotland, 24–25 May. *Journal of Mental Deficiency Research, 31,* 93–113.

Kerr, M., Tremblay, R. E., Pagani, L., & Vitaro, F. (1997). Boys' behavioral inhibition and the risk of later delinquency. *Archives of General Psychiatry, 54,* 809–816.

Kessler, R. C., McGonagle, K. A., Zhao, S., Nelson, C. B., Hughes, M., Eshleman, S., Wittchen, H. U., & Kendler, K. S. (1994). Lifetime and 12–month prevalence of DSM-III-R psychiatric disorders in the United States: Results from the National Comorbidity Study. *Archives of General Psychiatry, 51,* 8–19.

Kessler, R. C., Nelson, C. B., McGonagle, K. A., Edlund, M. J., Frank, R. G., & Leaf, P. J. (1996). The epidemiology of co-occurring addictive and mental disorders: Implications for prevention and service utilization. *American Journal of Orthopsychiatry, 66,* 17–31.

Ketterlinus, R. D., & Lamb, M. E. (Eds.). (1994). *Adolescent problem behaviors: Issues and research.* Hillsdale, NJ: Erlbaum.

Kibby, M., Tyc, V., & Mulhern, R. (1998). Effectiveness of psychological intervention for children and adolescents with chronic medical illness: A meta analysis. *Clinical Psychology Review, 18,* 103–117.

Kienhorst, C. W., De Wilde, E. J., Van den Bout, J., Diekstra, R. F., & Wolters, W. H. (1990). Characteristics of suicide attempters in a population-based sample of Dutch adolescents. *British Journal of Psychiatry, 156,* 243–248.

Kilian, J. G., Kerr, K., & Lawrence, C. (1999). Myocarditis and cardiomyopathy associated with clozapine. *Lancet, 354,* 1841–1845.

King, C. A., Hovey, J. D., Brand, E., Wilson, R., & Ghaziuddin, N. (1997). Suicidal adolescents after hospitalization: Parent and family impacts on treatment follow-through. *Journal of the American Academy of Child and Adolescent Psychiatry, 36,* 85–93.

King, C. A., & Kirschenbaum, D. S. (1990). An experimental evaluation of a school-based program for children-at-risk: Wisconsin early intervention. *Journal of Community Psychology, 18,* 167–177.

King, N. J., Cranstoun, F., & Josephs, A. (1989). Emotive imagery and children's nighttime fears: A multiple baseline design evaluation. *Journal of Behavior Therapy and Experimental Psychiatry, 20,* 125–135.

King, N. J., & Ollendick, T. H. (1997). Annotation: Treatment of childhood phobias. *Journal of Child Psychology and Psychiatry, 38,* 389–400.

King, N. J., Tonge, B. J., Heyne, D., Pritchard, M., Rollings, S., Young, D., Myerson, N., & Ollendick, T. H. (1998). Cognitive-behavioral treatment of school-refusing children: A controlled evaluation. *Journal of the American Academy of Child and Adolescent Psychiatry, 37,* 395–403.

Kirigin, K. A. (1996). Teaching-Family Model of group home treatment of children with severe behavior problems. In M. C. Roberts (Ed.), *Model programs in child and family mental health* (pp. 231–247). Mahwah, NJ: Erlbaum.

Kirigin, K. A., Braukmann, C. J., Atwater, J. D., & Wolf, M. M. (1982). An evaluation of Teaching-Family (Achievement Place) group homes for juvenile offenders. *Journal of Applied Behavior Analysis, 15,* 1–16.

Kirkley, B. G., Schneider, J. A., Agras, W. S., & Bachman, J. A. (1985). Comparison of two group treatments for bulimia. *Journal of Consulting and Clinical Psychology, 53,* 43–48.

Kiser, L. J., Millsap, P. A., & Hickerson, S. (1996). Results of treatment one year later: Child and adolescent partial hospitalization. *Journal of the American Academy of Child and Adolescent Psychiatry, 35,* 81–90.

Klein, D. F. (1996). Preventing hung juries about therapy studies. *Journal of Consulting and Clinical Psychology, 64,* 81–87.

Klein, D. F., Mannuzza, S., Chapman, T., & Fyer, A. J. (1992a). Child panic revisited. *Journal of the American Academy of Child and Adolescent Psychiatry, 31,* 112–114; discussion 114–116.

Klein, D. N., Lewinsohn, P. M., & Seeley, J. R. (1997). Psychosocial characteristics of adolescents with a past history of dysthymic disorder: Comparison with adolescents with past histories of major depressive and non-affective disorders, and never mentally ill controls. *Journal of Affective Disorder, 42,* 127–135.

Klein, N. C., Alexander, J. F., & Parsons, B. V. (1977). Impact of family systems intervention on recidivism and sibling delinquency: A model of primary prevention and program evaluation. *Journal of Consulting and Clinical Psychology, 45,* 469–474.

Klein, R. (1991). *Preliminary results: Lithium effects in conduct disorders.* Paper presented at the CME Syllabus and Proceedings Summary, 144th Annual Meeting of the American Psychiatric Association, New Orleans.

Klein, R. G., Abikoff, H., Klass, E., Ganeles, D., Seese, L. M., & Pollack, S. (1997). Clinical efficacy of methylphenidate in conduct disorder with and without attention deficit hyperactivity disorder. *Archives of General Psychiatry, 54,* 1073–1079.

Klein, R. G., Abikoff, H., Klass, E., Shah, M., & Seese, L. (1994). *Controlled trial of methylphenidate, lithium, and placebo in children and adolescents with conduct disorders.* Paper presented at the Meeting of the Society for Research in Child and Adolescent Psychopathology, London.

Klein, R. G., Koplewicz, H. S., & Kanner, A. (1992b). Imipramine treatment of children with separation anxiety disorder. *Journal of the American Academy of Child and Adolescent Psychiatry, 31,* 21–28.

Klein, R. G., Landa, B., Mattes, J. A., & Klein, D. F. (1988). Methylphenidate and growth in hyperactive children: A controlled withdrawal study. *Archives of General Psychiatry, 45,* 1127–1130.

Kleinberg, D. L., Davis, J. M., de Coster, R., Van Baelen, B., & Brecher, M. (1999). Prolactin levels and adverse events in patients treated with risperidone. *Journal of Clinical Psychopharmacology, 19,* 57–61.

Kleinman, A. (1977). Depression, somatization and the new "cross-cultural psychiatry." *Social Science and Medicine, 11,* 3–10.

Klerman, G. L., Weissman, M. M., Rounsaville, B. J., & Chevron, E. S. (1984). *Interpersonal psychotherapy of depression.* New York: Basic Books.

Klin, A. (1994). Asperger syndrome. *Child and Adolescent Psychiatric Clinics of North America, 3,* 131–148.

Klin, A., & Volkmar, F. R. (1995). Autism and the pervasive developmental disorders. *Child and Adolescent Psychiatric Clinics of North America, 4,* 617–630.

Klorman, R., Brumaghim, J. T., Fitzpatrick, P. A., & Borgstedt, A. D. (1990). Clinical effects of a controlled trial of methylphenidate on adolescents with attention deficit disorder. *Journal of the American Academy of Child and Adolescent Psychiatry, 29,* 702–709.

Knapp, M. R. J. (1997). Economic evaluations and interventions for children and adolescents with mental health problems. *Journal of Child Psychology and Psychiatry, 38,* 3–25.

Knox, M., King, C., Hanna, G., Logan, D., & Ghaziuddin, N. (2000). Aggressive behavior in clinically depressed adolescents. *Journal of the American Academy of Child and Adolescent Psychiatry, 39,* 611–618.

Kohler, F. W., Strain, P. S., Hoyson, M., Davis, L., Donina, W. M., & Rapp, N. (1995). Using a group-oriented contingency to increase social interactions between children with autism and their peers. *Behavior Modification, 19,* 10–32.

Kolko, D. J. (1996). Education and counseling for child firesetters: A comparison of skills training programs with standard practice. In E. D. Hibbs & P. S. Jensen (Eds.), *Psychosocial treatments for child and adolescent disorders: Empirically based strategies for clinical practice* (pp. 409–433). Washington, DC: American Psychological Association.

Kolko, D. J., Bukstein, O. G., & Barron, J. (1999). Methylphenidate and behavior modification in children with ADHD and comorbid ODD or CD: Main and incremental effects across settings. *Journal of the American Academy of Child and Adolescent Psychiatry, 38,* 578–586.

Kolko, D. J., & Kazdin, A. E. (1988). Prevalence of firesetting and related behaviors among child psychiatric inpatients. *Journal of Consulting and Clinical Psychology, 56,* 628–630.

Kolko, D. J., & Kazdin, A. E. (1993). Emotional/behavioral problems in clinic and nonclinic children: Correspondence among child, parent and teacher reports. *Journal of Child Psychology and Psychiatry, 34,* 991–1006.

Kolmen, B. K., Feldman, H. M., Handen, B. L., & Janosky, J. E. (1995). Naltrexone in young autistic children: A double-blind placebo-controlled crossover study. *Journal of the American Academy of Child and Adolescent Psychiatry, 34,* 223–231.

Kolmen, B. K., Feldman, H. M., Handen, B. L., & Janosky, J. E. (1997). Naltrexone in young autistic children: Replication study and learning measures. *Journal of the American Academy of Child and Adolescent Psychiatry, 35,* 1570–1578.

Kolvin, I., Garside, R. F., Nicol, A. R., Leitch, I., & Macmillan, A. (1977). Screening schoolchildren for high risk of emotional and educational disorder. *British Journal of Psychiatry, 131,* 192–206.

Kolvin, I., Garside, R. F., Nicol, A. R., MacMillan, A., Wolstenholme, F., & Leitch, I. M. (1981). *Help starts here: The maladjusted child in the ordinary school.* London: Tavistock.

Kolvin, I., Miller, F. J. W., Fleeting, M., & Kolvin, P. A. K. (1988). Risk/protective factors for offending with particular reference to deprivation. In M. Rutter (Ed.), *Studies of psychosocial risk: The power of longitudinal data* (pp. 77–95). Cambridge: Cambridge University Press.

Kondas, O. (1967). Reduction of examination anxiety and "stage fright" by group desensitization and relaxation. *Behaviour Research and Therapy, 5,* 275–281.

Kopta, S. M., Lueger, R. J., Saunders, S. M., & Howard, K. I. (1999). Individual psychotherapy outcome and process research: Challenges leading to greater turmoil or a positive transition? *Annual Review of Psychology, 50,* 441–469.

Kotses, H., Harver, A., Segreto, J., Glaus, K. D., Creer, T. L., & Young, G. A. (1991). Long-term effects of biofeedback-induced facial relaxation on measures of asthma severity in children. *Biofeedback and Self-Regulation, 16,* 1–21.

Kotsopoulos, S., Walker, S., Beggs, K., & Jones, B. (1996). A clinical and academic outcome study of children attending a day treatment program. *Canadian Journal of Psychiatry, 41,* 371–378.

Kovacs, M. (1985). The Children's Depression Inventory (CDI). *Psychopharmacology Bulletin, 21,* 995–998.

Kovacs, M. (1996). Presentation and course of major depressive disorder during childhood and later years of the lifespan. *Journal of the American Academy of Child and Adolescent Psychiatry, 35,* 705–715.

Kovacs, M. (1997). Depressive disorders in childhood: An impressionistic landscape. *Journal of Child Psychology and Psychiatry, 38,* 287–298.

Kovacs, M., Akiskal, H. S., Gatsonis, C., & Parrone, P. L. (1994). Childhood-onset dysthymic disorder. Clinical features and prospective naturalistic outcome. *Archives of General Psychiatry, 51,* 365–374.

Kovacs, M., & Devlin, B. (1998). Internalizing disorders in childhood. *Journal of Child Psychology and Psychiatry, 39,* 47–63.

Kovacs, M., & Gatsonis, C. (1989). Stability and change in childhood-onset depressive disorders: Longitudinal course as a diagnostic validator. In L. N. Robins & J. E. Barrett (Eds.), *The validity of psychiatric diagnosis* (pp. 57–73). New York: Raven.

Kovacs, M., Iyengar, S., Goldston, D., Obrosky, D. S., Stewart, J., & Marsh, J. (1990). Psychological functioning among mothers of children with insulin dependent diabetes mellitus: A longitudinal study. *Journal of Consulting and Clinical Psychology, 58,* 189–195.

Kovacs, M., Obrosky, S., Gatsonis, C., & Richards, C. (1997). First episode of major depressive and dysthymic disorder in childhood: Clinical and socio-demographic factors in recovery. *Journal of the American Academy of Child and Adolescent Psychiatry, 36,* 777–784.

Kovacs, M., Paulauskas, S., Gatsonis, C., & Richards, C. (1988). Depressive disorders in childhood: III. A longitudinal study of comorbidity with and risk for conduct disorders. *Journal of Affective Disorders, 15,* 205–217.

Kowatch, R. A., & Bucci, J. P. (1998). Mood stabilizers and anticonvulsants. *Pediatric Clinics of North America, 45,* 1173–1186.

Kowatch, R. A., Suppes, T., Carmody, T. J., Bucci, J. P., Hume, J. H., Kromelis, M. R., Emslie, G. J., Weinberg, W. A., & Rush, A. J. (2000). Effect size of lithium, divalproex sodium and carbamazepine in children and adolescents with bipolar disorder. *Journal of the American Academy of Child and Adolescent Psychiatry, 39*, 713–720.

Kreipe, R. E., Churchill, B. H., & Strauss, J. (1989). Long-term outcome of adolescents with anorexia nervosa. *American Journal of Diseases of Children, 143*, 1322–1327.

Kreitman, N. (1977). *Parasuicide*. London: Wiley.

Kroll, L., Harrington, R., Jayson, D., Fraser, J., & Gowers, S. (1996). Pilot study of continuation cognitive-behavioral therapy for major depression in adolescent psychiatric patients. *Journal of the American Academy of Child and Adolescent Psychiatry, 35*, 1156–1161.

Kruesi, M. J. P., & Lelio, D. F. (1996). Disorders of conduct and behavior. In J. M. Wiener (Ed.), *Diagnosis and psychopharmacology of childhood and adolescent disorders* (2nd ed., pp. 401–447). New York: Wiley.

Krupinski, J., Baikie, A. G., Stoller, A., Graves, J., O'Day, D. M., & Polke, P. (1967). A community health survey of Hayfield, Victoria. *Medical Journal of Australia, 1*, 1204–1211.

Kugler, B. (1998). The differentiation between autism and Asperger's syndrome. *Autism, 2*, 11–32.

Kuhne, M., Schachar, R., & Tannock, R. (1997). Impact of comorbid oppositional or conduct problems on attention-deficit hyperactivity disorder. *Journal of the American Academy of Child and Adolescent Psychiatry, 36*, 1715–1725.

Kuipers, E., Fowler, D., Garety, P., Chisholm, D., Freeman, D., Dunn, G., Bebbington, P., & Hadley, C. (1998). London-East Anglia randomised controlled trial of cognitive-behavioural therapy for psychosis: III. Follow-up evaluation at 18 months. *British Journal of Psychiatry, 173*, 61–68.

Kumpfer, K. L., Molgaard, V., & Spoth, R. (1996). The Strengthening Families Program for the prevention of delinquency and drug use. In R. D. Peters & R. J. McMahon (Eds.), *Preventing childhood disorders, substance abuse, and delinquency* (pp. 241–267). Thousand Oaks, CA: Sage.

Kumpfer, K. L., & Szapocznik, J. (1998). *Preventing substance abuse among children and adolescents: Family-centered approaches* (DHHS 3228–FY98). Rockville, MD: Substance Abuse and Mental Health Services Administration.

Kumra, S., Frazier, J. A., Jacobsen, L. K., McKenna, K., Gordon, C. T., Lenane, M. C., Hamburger, S. D., Smith, A. K., Albus, K. E., Alaghband-Rad, J., & Rapoport, J. L. (1996). Childhood schizophrenia: A double-blind clozapine haloperidol comparison. *Archives of General Psychiatry, 53*, 1090–1097.

Kupietz, S. S., Winsberg, B. G., Richardson, E., Maitinsky, S., & Mendell, N. (1988). Effects of methylphenidate dosage in hyperactive reading-disabled children: I. Behavior and cognitive performance effects. *Journal of the American Academy of Child and Adolescent Psychiatry, 27*, 70–77.

Kurlan, R., Como, P. G., Deeley, C., McDermott, M., & McDermott, M. P. (1993). A pilot controlled study of fluoxetine for obsessive–compulsive symptoms in children with Tourette's syndrome. *Clinical Neuropharmacology, 16*, 167–172.

Kuroda, J. (1969). Elimination of children's fears of animals by the method of experimental desensitization: An application of learning theory to child psychology. *Psychologia, 12*, 161–165.

Kurtz, Z., Thornes, R., & Bailey, S. (1998). Children in the criminal justice and secure care systems: How their mental health needs are met. *Journal of Adolescence, 21*, 543–553.

Kurtz, Z., Thornes, R., & Wolkind, S. (1994). *Services for the mental health of children and young people in England*. London: Maudsley Hospital and South Thames Regional Health Authority.

Kutcher, S. P. (1997). *Child and adolescent psychopharmacology*. Philadephia: Saunders.

Kutcher, S. P., & Mackenzie, S. (1988). Successful clonazepam treatment of adolescents with panic disorder. *Journal of Clinical Psychopharmacology, 8*, 299–301.

Kye, C. H., Waterman, G. S., Ryan, N. D., Birmaher, B., Williamson, D. E., Iyengar, S., & Dachille, S. (1996). Randomized, controlled trial of amitriptyline in the acute treatment of adolescent major depression. *Journal of the American Academy of Child and Adolescent Psychiatry, 35*, 1139–1144.

Lacey, J. H. (1983). Bulimia nervosa, binge eating and psychogenic vomiting: A controlled treatment study and long-term outcome. *British Medical Journal, 286*, 1609–1613.

Ladd, G. W., & Burgess, K. B. (1999). Charting the relationship trajectories of aggressive, withdrawn, and aggressive/withdrawn children during early grade school. *Child Development, 70*, 910–929.

Lahey, B. B., Applegate, B., Barkley, R. A., Garfinkel, B., McBurnett, K., Kerdyck, L., Greenhill, L., Hynd, G. W., Frick, P. J., Newcorn, J., Biederman, J., Ollendick, T., Hart, E. L., Perez, D., Waldman, I., & Shaffer, D. (1994). DSM-IV field trials for oppositional defiant disorder and conduct disorder in children and adolescents. *American Journal of Psychiatry, 151*, 1163–1171.

Lahey, B. B., & Carlson, C. (1992). Validity of the diagnostic category of attention deficit disorder without hyperactivity: A review of the literature. In S. E. Shaywitz & B. A. Shaywitz (Eds.), *Attention deficit disorder comes of age: Toward the twenty-first century* (pp. 119–144.). Austin, TX: Pro-ed.

Lahey, B. B., Goodman, S. H., Waldman, I. D., Bird, H., Canino, G., Jensen, P. S., Regier, D., Leaf, P. J., Rathouz, P., Gordon, R., & Applegate, B. (1998). Relation of age of onset to the type and severity of child and adolescent conduct problems. *Journal of Abnormal Child Psychology, 27*, 247–260.

Lahey, B. B., Loeber, R., & Burke, J. (1999). *Recovery from childhood-onset conduct disorder*. Paper presented at the 46th annual meeting of the American Academy of Child and Adolescent Psychiatry, Chicago.

Lahey, B. B., Loeber, R., Hart, E. L., Frick, P. J., Applegate, B., Zhang, Q., Green, S. M., & Russo, M. F. (1995). Four-year longitudinal study of conduct disorder in boys: Patterns and predictors of persistence. *Journal of Abnormal Psychology, 104*, 83–93.

Lahey, B. B., Loeber, R., Quay, H., Applegate, B., Shaffer, D., Waldman, I., Hart, E. L., McBurnett, K., Frick, P. J., Jensen, P. S., Dulcan, M. K., Canino, G., & Bird, H. R. (1998). Validity of DSM-IV subtypes of conduct disorder based on age of onset. *Journal of the American Academy of Child and Adolescent Psychiatry, 37*, 435–442.

Lahey, B. B., McBurnett, K., & Loeber, R. (2000). Are attention-deficit/hyperactivity disorder and oppositional defiant disorder developmental precursors to conduct disorder? In A. Sameroff, M. Lewis, & S. M. Miller (Eds.), *Handbook of developmental psychopathology* (pp. 431–446). New York: Plenum Press.

Lahey, B. B., Miller, T. L., Gordon, R. A., & Riley, A. W. (1999a). Developmental epidemiology of the disruptive behavior disorders. In H. C. Quay & A. Hogan (Eds.), *Handbook of the disruptive behavior disorders* (pp. 23–48). New York: Plenum Press.

Lahey, B. B., Waldman, I. D., & McBurnett, K. (1999b). Annotation: The development of antisocial behaviour: An integrative causal model. *Journal of Child Psychology and Psychiatry, 40*, 669–682.

Lainhart, J. E., & Folstein, S. E. (1994). Affective disorders in people with autism: A review of published cases. *Journal of Autism and Developmental Disorders, 24*, 587–601.

Lansdown, R., & Sokel, B. (1993). Approaches to pain management in children. *ACPP Review and Newsletter, 15(3)*, 105–111.

Lapouse, R. (1965a). The relationship of behavior to adjustment in a representative sample of children. *American Journal of Public Health, 55*, 1130–1141.

Lapouse, R., & Monk, M. A. (1958). An epidemiologic study of behavior characteristics in children. *American Journal of Public Health, 48*, 1134–1144.

Lapouse, R., & Monk, M. A. (1959). Fears and worries in a representative sample of children. *American Journal of Orthopsychiatry, 29*, 803–818.

Lapouse, R., & Monk, M. A. (1964). Behavior deviations in a representative sample of children: Variation by sex, age, race, social class and family size. *American Journal of Orthopsychiatry, 34*, 426–446.

Lapouse, R. (1965b). Who is sick? *American Journal of Orthopsychiatry, 35*, 138–144.

Larsson, B., Daleflod, B., Hakansson, L., & Melin, L. (1987). Therapist-assisted versus self-help relaxation treatment of chronic headaches in adolescents: A school-based intervention. *Journal of Child Psychology and Psychiatry, 28*, 127–136.

Larsson, B., & Melin, L. (1988). The psychological treatment of recurrent headache in adolescents: Short-term outcome and its prediction. *Headache, 28*, 187–195.

Lasch, C. (1978). *The culture of narcissism: American life in an age of diminishing expectations.* New York: Norton.

Lask, B., & Fosson, A. (1989). *Childhood illness. The psychosomatic approach.* Chichester: Wiley.

Lask, B., & Matthew, D. (1979). Childhood asthma: A controlled trial of family psychotherapy. *Archives of Disease in Childhood, 54,* 116–119.

Last, C. G., Hansen, C., & Franco, N. (1998). Cognitive-behavioral treatment of school phobia. *Journal of the American Academy of Child and Adolescent Psychiatry, 37,* 404–411.

Last, C. G., Hersen, M., Kazdin, A. E., Finkelstein, R., & Strauss, C. C. (1987a). Comparison of DSM-III separation anxiety and overanxious disorders: Demographic characteristics and patterns of comorbidity. *Journal of the American Academy of Child and Adolescent Psychiatry, 26,* 527–531.

Last, C. G., Hersen, M., Kazdin, A. E., Orvaschel, H., & Perrin, S. (1991). Anxiety disorders in children and their families. *Archives of General Psychiatry, 48,* 928–934.

Last, C. G., Perrin, S., Hersen, M., & Kazdin, A. E. (1992). DSM-III-R anxiety disorders in children: Sociodemographic and clinical characteristics. *Journal of the American Academy of Child and Adolescent Psychiatry, 31,* 1070–1076.

Last, C. G., Perrin, S., Hersen, M., & Kazdin, A. E. (1996). A prospective study of childhood anxiety disorders. *Journal of the American Academy of Child and Adolescent Psychiatry, 35,* 1502–1510.

Last, C. G., Phillips, J. E., & Statfeld, A. (1987b). Childhood anxiety disorders in mothers and their children. *Child Psychiatry and Human Development, 18,* 103–117.

Lavigne, J. V., & Faier-Routman, J. (1992). Psychological adjustment to pediatric physical disorders: A meta-analytic review. *Journal of Pediatric Psychology, 17,* 133–157.

Lavigne, J. V., Ross, C. K., Berry, S. L., Hayford, J. R., & Pachman, L. M. (1992). Evaluation of a psychological treatment package for treating pain in juvenile rheumatoid arthritis. *Arthritis Care and Research, 5,* 101–110.

Lavik, N., Clausen, S., & Pedersen, W. (1991). Eating behaviour, drug use psychopathology and parental bonding in adolescents in Norway. *Acta Psychiatrica Scandanavica, 84,* 387–390.

Lavin, M., & Rifkin, A. (1993). Diagnosis and pharmacotherapy of conduct disorder. *Progress in Neuro-psychopharmacology and Biological Psychiatry, 17,* 875–885.

Law, J., Boyle, J., Harris, F., Harkness, A., & Nye, C. (1998). Screening for speech and language delay: A systematic review of the literature. *Health Technology Assessment, 2,* 1–81.

Law, S. F., & Schachar, R. J. (1999). Do typical doses of methylphenidate cause tics in children treated for attention deficit hyperactivity disorder? *Journal of the American Academy of Child and Adolescent Psychiatry, 38,* 944–951.

Leaf, P. J., Alegria, M., Cohen, P., Goodman, S. H., Horwitz, S. M., Hoven, C. W., Narrow, W. E., Vaden-Kiernan, M., & Regier, D. A. (1996). Mental health service use in the community and schools: Results from the Four-Community MECA Study. *Journal of the American Academy of Child and Adolescent Psychiatry, 35,* 889–897.

Lebow, J. L., & Gurman, A. S. (1995). Research assessing couple and family therapy. *Annual Review of Psychology, 46,* 27–57.

Leckman, J. F., & Cohen, D. J. (1994). Tic disorders. In M. Rutter, E. Taylor, & L. Hersov (Eds.), *Child and adolescent psychiatry: Modern approaches* (pp. 455–466). Oxford: Blackwell Scientific Publications.

Leckman, J. F., Dolnansky, E. S., Hardin, M. T., Clubb, M., Walkup, J. T., Stevenson, J., & Pauls, D. L. (1990). Perinatal factors in the expression of Tourette's syndrome: An exploration study. *Journal of the American Academy of Child and Adolescent Psychiatry, 29,* 220–226.

Leckman, J. F., Hardin, M. T., Riddle, M. A., Stevenson, J., Ort, S. I., & Cohen, D. J. (1991). Clonidine treatment of Gilles de la Tourette syndrome. *Archives of General Psychiatry, 48,* 324–328.

Leckman, J. F., Towbin, K. E., Ort, S. I., & Cohen, D. J. (1988). Clinical assessment of tic disorder severity. In D. J. Cohen & R. D. Bruun (Eds.), *Tourette's syndrome and tic disorders: Clinical understanding and treatment* (pp. 55–78). New York: Wiley.

Le Couteur, A., Rutter, M., Lord, C., Rios, P., Robertson, S., Holdgrafer, M., & Mclennon, J. D. (1989). Autism diagnostic interview: A semi-structured interview for parents and caregivers of autistic persons. *Journal of Autism and Developmental Disorders, 19,* 363–387.

Lee, N. F., & Rush, A. J. (1986). Cognitive-behavioral group therapy for bulimia. *International Journal of Eating Disorders, 5*, 599–615.

Leeman, L. W., Gibbs, J. C., & Fuller, D. (1993). Evaluation of a multicomponent group treatment program for juvenile delinquents. *Aggressive Behavior, 19*, 281–292.

Lees, A. J. (1985). *Tics and related disorders.* Edinburgh: Churchill Livingstone.

Leff, J., Kuipers, L., Berkowitz, R., Eberlein-Vries, R., & Sturgeon, D. (1982). A controlled trial of social intervention in the families of schizophrenia patients. *British Journal of Psychiatry, 141*, 121–134.

Leff, J., Kuipers, L., Berkowitz, R., & Sturgeon, D. (1985). A controlled trial of social intervention in the families of schizophrenic patients: Two year follow up. *British Journal of Psychiatry, 146*, 594–600.

Lehrer, P. M., Sargunaraj, D., & Hochron, S. (1992). Psychological approaches to the treatment of asthma. *Journal of Consulting and Clinical Psychology, 60*, 639–643.

Leonard, H. L., Lenane, M. C., Swedo, S. E., Rettew, D. C., Gershon, E. S., & Rapaport, J. L. (1992). Tics and Tourette's disorder: A 2- to 7-year follow-up of 54 obsessive–compulsive children. *American Journal of Psychiatry, 149*, 1244–1251.

Leonard, H. L., March, J., Rickler, K. C., & Allen, A. J. (1997). Review of the pharmacology of the selective serotonin reuptake inhibitors in children and adolescents. *Journal of the American Academy of Child and Adolescent Psychiatry, 36*, 725–736.

Leonard, H. L., Swedo, S. E., Lenane, M. C., Rettew, D. C., Cheslow, D. L., Hamburger, S. D., & Rapoport, J. L. (1991). A double-blind desipramine substitution during long-term clomipramine treatment in children and adolescents with obsessive–compulsive disorder. *Archives of General Psychiatry, 48*, 922–927.

Leonard, H. L., Swedo, S. E., Rapoport, J. L., Koby, E. V., Lenane, M., Cheslow, D. L., & Hamburger, S. D. (1989). Treatment of obsessive–compulsive disorder with clomipramine and desipramine in children and adolescents. *Archives of General Psychiatry, 46*, 1088–1092.

Leslie, S. A. (1974). Psychiatric disorder in the young adolescents of an industrial town. *British Journal of Psychiatry, 125*, 113–124.

Leslie, S. A. (1988). Diagnosis and treatment of hysterical conversion reactions. *Archives of Disease in Childhood, 63*, 506–511.

Lester, D. (1974). Effect of suicide prevention centers on suicide rates in the United States. *Health Services Reports, 89*, 37–39.

Leventhal, B. L., Cook, E. H., Morford, M., Ravitz, A. J., Heller, W., & Freedman, D. X. (1993). Clinical and neurochemical effects of fenfluramine in children with autism. *Journal of Neuropsychiatry and Clinical Neurosciences, 5*, 307–315.

Levy, T., & Orlans, M. (1995). *Intensive short-term therapy with attachment disordered children.* Unpublished manuscript.

Lewandowski, L. M., Gebing, T. A., Anthony, J. L., & O'Brien, W. H. (1997). Meta-analysis of cognitive-behavioral treatment studies for bulimia. *Clinical Psychology Review, 17*, 703–718.

Lewinsohn, P. M., Antonuccio, D. O., Steinmetz-Breckenridge, J., & Teri, L. (1984). *The Coping with Depression Course: A psychoeducational intervention for unipolar depression.* Eugene, OR: Castalia Press.

Lewinsohn, P. M., & Clarke, G. N. (1999). Psychosocial treatments for adolescent depression. *Clinical Psychology Review, 19*, 329–342.

Lewinsohn, P. M., Clarke, G. N., Hops, H., & Andrews, J. (1990). Cognitive-behavioral treatment for depressed adolescents. *Behavior Therapy, 21*, 385–401.

Lewinsohn, P. M., Clarke, G. N., & Rohde, P. (1994). Psychological approaches to the treatment of depression in adolescents. In W. M. Reynolds & H. F. Johnston (Eds.), *Handbook of depression in children and adolescents* (pp. 309–344). New York: Plenum Press.

Lewinsohn, P. M., Clarke, G. N., Rohde, P., Hops, H., & Seeley, J. R. (1996a). A course in coping: A cognitive-behavioral approach to the treatment of adolescent depression. In E. D. Hibbs & P. S. Jensen (Eds.), *Psychosocial treatments for child and adolescent disorders: Empirically based strategies for clinical practice* (pp. 109–135). Washington, DC: American Psychological Association.

Lewinsohn, P. M., Hops, H., Roberts, R. E., Seeley, J. R., & Andrews, J. A. (1993). Adolescent psychopathology: I. Prevalence and incidence of depression and other DSM-III-R disorders in high school students [published erratum appears in *Journal of Abnormal Psychology* (1993), *102*, 517]. *Journal of Abnormal Psychology, 102*, 133–144.

Lewinsohn, P. M., Rohde, P., Klein, D., & Seeley, J. R. (1999). Natural course of adolescent major depressive disorder: I. Continuity into young adulthood. *Journal of the American Academy of Child and Adolescent Psychiatry, 38*, 56–63.

Lewinsohn, P. M., Rohde, P., & Seeley, J. R. (1995). Adolescent psychopathology: III. The clinical consequences of comorbidity. *Journal of the American Academy of Child and Adolescent Psychiatry, 34*, 510–519.

Lewinsohn, P. M., Rohde, P., & Seeley, J. R. (1998). Treatment of adolescent depression: Frequency of services and impact on functioning in young adulthood. *Depression and Anxiety, 7*, 47–52.

Lewinsohn, P. M., Seeley, J. R., Hibbard, J., Rhode, P., & Sack, W. H. (1996b). Cross-sectional and prospective relationships between physical morbidity and depression in older adolescents. *Journal of the American Academy of Child and Adolescent Psychiatry, 35*, 1120–1129.

Lewinsohn, P. M., Zinbarg, R., Seeley, J. R., Lewinsohn, M., & Sack, W. H. (1997). Lifetime comorbidity among anxiety disorders and between anxiety disorders and other mental disorders in adolescents. *Journal of Anxiety Disorders, 11*, 377–394.

Lewis, C., Hitch, G. J., & Walker, P. (1994). The prevalence of specific arithmetic difficulties and specific reading difficulties in 9- to 10-year-old boys and girls. *Journal of Child Psychology and Psychiatry, 35*, 283–92.

Lewis, C. E., Rachelefsky, G., Lewis, M. A., de la Sota, A., & Kaplan, M. (1984). A randomized trial of A.C.T. (Asthma Care Training) for kids. *Pediatrics, 74*, 478–486.

Lewis, R. A., Piercy, F., Sprenkle, D., & Trepper, T. (1990). Family-based interventions and community networking for helping drug abusing adolescents: The impact of near and far environments. *Journal of Adolescent Research, 5*, 82–95.

Liddle, B., & Spence, S. H. (1990). Cognitive-behavioural therapy with depressed primary school children: A cautionary note. *Behavioural Psychotherapy, 18*, 85–102.

Liebman, R., Minuchin, S., & Baker, L. (1974). The use of structural family therapy in the treatment of intractable asthma. *American Journal of Psychiatry, 131*, 535–540.

Lifrak, P. D., McKay, J. R., Rostain, A., Alterman, A. I., & O'Brien, C. P. (1997). Relationship of perceived competencies, perceived social support, and gender to substance use in young adolescents. *Journal of the American Academy of Child and Adolescent Psychiatry, 36*, 933–940.

Lilford, R., & Jackson, J. (1995). Equipoise and the ethics of randomizations. *Journal of Research in Social Medicine, 88*, 552–559.

Lilienfeld, S. O. (1992). The association between antisocial personality and somatization disorders: A review and integration of theoretical models. *Clinical Psychology Review, 12*, 641–662.

Lindgren, S. D., & Lyons, D. A. (1984). *Pediatric assessment of cognitive efficiency (PACE)*. Iowa City: University of Iowa Department of Pediatrics.

Lipsey, M. (1995). What do we learn from 400 research studies on the effectiveness of treatment with juvenile delinquents? In J. McGuire (Ed.), *What works: Reducing reoffending: Guidelines from research and practice* (pp. 63–78). Chichester: Wiley.

Lipsey, M., & Wilson, D. B. (1998). Effective intervention for serious juvenile offenders: A synthesis of research. In R. L. Loeber & D. P. Farrington (Eds.), *Serious and violent juvenile offenders: Risk factors and successful interventions* (pp. 313–45). Thousand Oaks, CA: Sage.

Lipsey, M. W., & Wilson, D. B. (1993). The efficacy of psychological, educational, and behavioral treatment: Confirmation from meta-analysis. *American Psychologist, 48*, 1181–1209.

Little, E., & Hudson, A. (1998). Conduct problems and treatment across home and school: A review of the literature. *Behavior Change, 15*, 213–227.

Littlewood, R. (1990). From categories to contexts: A decade of the "new cross-cultural psychiatry." *British Journal of Psychiatry, 56*, 308–327.

Locascio, J. L., Malone, R. P., Small, A. M., Kafantaris, V., Ernst, M., Lynch, N. S., Overall, J. E., & Campbell, M. (1991). Factors related to haloperidol response and dyskinesias in autistic children. *Psychopharmacology Bulletin, 27*, 119–126.

Lochman, J. E. (1992). Cognitive-behavioural interventions with aggressive boys: Three year follow-up and preventive effects. *Journal of Consulting and Clinical Psychology, 60*, 426–432.

Lochman, J. E., Burch, P. R., Curry, J. F., & Lampron, L. B. (1984). Treatment and generalization effects of cognitive-behavioral and goal-setting interventions with aggressive boys. *Journal of Consulting and Clinical Psychology, 52*, 915–916.

Lochman, J. E., & Lampron, L. B. (1988). Cognitive behavioral interventions for aggressive boys: Seven months follow-up effects. *Journal of Child and Adolescent Psychotherapy, 5*, 15–23.

Lochman, J. E., Lampron, L. B., Gemmer, T. C., & Harris, S. R. (1989). Teacher consultation and cognitive-behavioral interventions with aggressive boys. *Psychology in the Schools, 26*, 179–188.

Lochman, J. E., & Wells, K. C. (1996). A social–cognitive intervention with aggressive children: Prevention effects and contextual implementation issues. In R. D. Peters & R. J. McMahon (Eds.), *Preventing childhood disorders, substance abuse, and delinquency* (pp. 111–143). Thousand Oaks, CA: Sage.

Loeber, R. (1988). Natural histories of conduct problems, delinquency, and associated substance use: Evidence for developmental progressions. In B. B. Lahey & A. E. Kazdin (Eds.), *Advances in clinical child psychology* (Vol. 11, pp. 73–124). New York: Plenum Press.

Loeber, R., Burke, J. D., Lahey, B. B., Winters, A., & Zera, M. (2000). Oppositional defiant and conduct disorder: A review of the past 10 years. Part I. *Journal of the American Academy of Child and Adolescent Psychiatry, 39*, 1468–1484.

Loeber, R., Farrington, D. P., Stouthamer-Loeber, M., & Van Kammen, W. B. (1998a). *Antisocial behavior and mental health problems: Explanatory factors in childhood and adolescence.* Mahwah, NJ: Erlbaum.

Loeber, R., Farrington, D. P., & Waschbusch, D. A. (1998b). Serious and violent juvenile offenders. In R. Loeber & D. P. Farrington (Eds.), *Serious and violent juvenile offenders: Risk factors and successful interventions* (pp. 13–29). Thousand Oaks, CA: Sage.

Loeber, R., Green, S. M., & Lahey, B. B. (1990). Mental health professionals' perception of the utility of children, mothers and teachers as informants on childhood psychopathology. *Journal of Clinical Child Psychology, 19*, 136–143.

Loeber, R., & Keenan, K. (1994). Interaction between conduct disorder and its comorbid conditions: Effects of age and gender. *Clinical Psychology Review, 14*, 497–523.

Loeber, R., Russo, M., Stouthamer-Loeber, M., & Lahey, B. (1994). Internalizing problems and their relation to the development of disruptive behaviors in adolescence. *Journal of Research on Adolescence, 4*, 615–637.

Loeber, R., & Schmaling, K. B. (1985a). Empirical evidence for overt and covert patterns of antisocial conduct problems: A meta-analysis. *Journal of Abnormal Child Psychology, 13*, 337–352.

Loeber, R., & Schmaling, K. B. (1985b). The utility of differentiating between mixed and pure forms of antisocial child behavior. *Journal of Abnormal Child Psychology, 13*, 315–336.

Loeber, R., & Stouthamer-Loeber, M. (1986). Family factors as correlates and predictors of juvenile conduct problems and delinquency. In M. Tonry & N. Morris (Eds.), *Crime and justice: An annual review of research* (Vol. 7, pp. 29–150). Chicago: University of Chicago Press.

Loeber, R., Stouthamer-Loeber, M., Van Kammen, W., & Farrington, D. P. (1991). Initiation, escalation and desistance in juvenile offending and their correlates. *Journal of Criminal Law and Criminology, 82*, 36–82.

Logan, G. D., & Cowan, W. B. (1984). On the ability to inhibit thought and action: A theory of an act of control. *Psychological Review, 91*, 295–327.

Lombroso, P. J., Scahill, L., King, R. A., Lynch, K. A., Chappell, P. B., Peterson, B. S., McDougle, C. J., & Leckman, J. F. (1995). Risperidone treatment of children and adolescents with chronic tic disorders: A preliminary report. *Journal of the American Academy of Child and Adolescent Psychiatry, 34*, 1147–1152.

Loney, B. R., Frick, P. J., Ellis, M., & McCoy, M. G. (1998). Intelligence, callous–unemotional traits, and antisocial behavior. *Journal of Psychopathology and Behavioral Assessment, 20*, 231–247.

Loney, J. (1988). Substance abuse in adolescents: Diagnostic issues derived from studies of attention deficit disorder with hyperactivity. *NIDA Research Monograph, 77*, 19–26.

Long, P., Forehand, R., Wierson, M., & Morgan, A. (1994). Moving into adulthood: Does parent training with young noncompliant children have long-term effects? *Behaviour Research and Therapy, 32,* 101–107.

Lonigan, C. J., Elbert, J. C., & Johnson, S. B. (1998). Empirically supported psychosocial interventions for children: An overview. *Journal of Clinical Child Psychology, 27,* 138–145.

Lord, C., & Rutter, M. (1994). Autism and pervasive developmental disorders. In M. Rutter, E. Taylor, & L. Hersov (Eds.), *Child and adolescent psychiatry: Modern approaches* (3rd ed., pp. 569–593). Oxford: Blackwell Scientific.

Lösel, F. (1995a). The efficacy of correctional treatment: A review and synthesis of meta-evaluations. In J. McGuire (Ed.), *What works: Reducing reoffending* (pp. 57–82). Chichester: Wiley.

Lösel, F. (1995b). Increasing consensus in the evaluation of offender rehabilitation? Lessons from recent research synthesis. *Psychology, Crime and the Law, 2,* 19–39.

Losse, A., Henderson, S. E., Elliman, D., Hall, D., Knight, E., & Jongmans, M. (1991). Clumsiness in children—Do they grow out of it?: A 10-year follow-up study. *Developmental Medicine and Child Neurology, 33,* 55–68.

Lotter, V. (1974). Factors related to outcome in autistic children. *Journal of Autism and Childhood Schizophrenia, 4,* 263–277.

Lotter, V. (1978). Follow-up studies. In M. Rutter & E. Schopler (Eds.), *Autism: A reappraisal of concepts and treatment* (pp. 475–495). New York: Plenum Press.

Lovaas, O. L. (1987). Behavioral treatment and normal educational and intellectual functioning in young autistic children. *Journal of Consulting and Clinical Psychology, 55,* 3–9.

Love, A. J., & Thompson, M. G. (1988). Language disorders and attention deficit disorders in young children referred for psychiatric services: Analysis of prevalence and a conceptual synthesis. *American Journal of Orthopsychiatry, 58,* 52–64.

Luborsky, L., & Bachrach, H. (1974). Health Sickness Rating Scale. *Archives of General Psychiatry, 31,* 292–299.

Luborsky, L., Diguer, L., Seligman, D. A., Rosenthal, R., Krause, E. D., Johnson, S., Halperin, G., Bishop, M., Berman, J. S., & Schweizer, E. (1999). The researcher's own therapy allegiances: A "wild card" in comparisons of treatment efficacy. *Clinical Psychology: Science and Practice, 6,* 95–106.

Lundy, M., Pfohl, B., & Kuperman, S. (1993). Adult criminality among formerly hospitalized child psychiatric patients. *Journal of the American Academy of Child and Adolescent Psychiatry, 32,* 568–576.

Lutzker, J. R. (1996). Timeout from emotion, time for science: A response to Kemp. *Child and Family Behavior Therapy, 18,* 29–34.

Lynam, D. R. (1998). Early identification of the fledgling psychopath: Locating the psychopathic child in the current nomenclature. *Journal of Abnormal Psychology, 107,* 566–575.

Lynskey, M. T., Fergusson, D. M., & Horwood, L. J. (1998). Origins of the correlations between tobacco, alcohol, and cannabis use during adolescence. *Journal of Child Psychology and Psychiatry, 39,* 995–1005.

Lyon, G. R., & Cutting, L. E. (1998). Learning disabilities. In E. J. Mash & R. A. Barkley (Eds.), *Treatment of childhood disorders* (pp. 468–498). New York: Guilford Press.

Lyons, J. S. (2000). A call for outcomes data: Psychopharmacology with children. *Outcomes and Accountability Alert, 5,* 12.

MacEwan, T. H., & Morton, M. J. S. (1996). Use of clozapine in a child with treatment resistant schizophrenia. *British Journal of Psychiatry, 168,* 376–378.

MacLean, W. E., Perrin, J. M., Gortmaker, S. L., & Pierre, C. B. (1992). Psychological adjustment of children with asthma: Effects of illness severity and recent life events. *Journal of Pediatric Psychology, 17,* 159–171.

Maddocks, S., Kaplan, A. S., Woodside, D. B., Langdon, L., & Piran, N. (1992). Two-year follow-up of bulimia nervosa: The importance of abstinence as the criterion of outcome. *International Journal of Eating Disorders, 12,* 133–141.

Madge, N., & Harvey, J. G. (1999). Suicide among the young: The size of the problem. *Journal of Adolescence, 22,* 145–155.

Mahler, M. S. (1971). A study of separation–individuation process and its possible application to borderline phenomena in the psychoanalytic situation. *The Psychoanalytic Study of the Child, 26,* 403–424.

Malone, M. A., & Swanson, J. M. (1993). Effects of methylphenidate on impulsive responding in children with attention-deficit hyperactivity disorder. *Journal of Child Neurology, 8,* 157–163.

Malone, R. P., Bennett, D. S., Luebbert, J. F., Rowan, A. B., Biesecker, K. A., Blaney, B. L., & Delaney, M. A. (1998). Aggression classification and treatment response. *Psychopharmacology Bulletin, 34,* 41–45.

Malone, R. P., Delaney, M. A., Luebbert, J. F., Cater, J., & Campbell, M. (2000). A double-blind placebo-controlled study of lithium in hospitalized aggressive children and adolescents with conduct disorder. *Archives of General Psychiatry, 57,* 649–654.

Malone, R. P., Luebbert, J. F., Delaney, M. A., Biesecker, K. A., Blaney, B. L., Rowan, A. B., & Campbell, M. (1997). Nonpharmacological response in hospitalized children with conduct disorder. *Journal of the American Academy of Child and Adolescent Psychiatry, 36,* 242–247.

Maloney, M. J., McGuire, J., Daniels, S. R., & Specker, B. (1989). Dieting behavior and eating attitudes in children. *Pediatrics, 84,* 482–489.

Mann, B. J., Borduin, C. M., Henggeler, S. W., & Blaske, D. M. (1990). An investigation of systemic conceptualizations of parent–child coalitions and symptom change. *Journal of Consulting and Clinical Psychology, 58,* 336–344.

Mann, E. M., Ikeda, Y., Mueller, C. W., Takahashi, A., Tai Tao, K., Humris, E., Ling Li, B., & Chin, D. (1992). Cross-cultural differences in rating hyperactive–disruptive behaviors in children. *American Journal of Psychiatry, 149,* 1539–1542.

Mann, J., & Rosenthal, T. L. (1969). Vicarious and direct counter-conditioning of test anxiety through individual and group desensitisation. *Behaviour Research and Therapy, 7,* 359–367.

Manne, S. L., Bakeman, R., Jacobsen, P. B., Gorfinkle, K., & Redd, W. H. (1994). An analysis of a behavioral intervention for children undergoing venipuncture. *Health Psychology, 13,* 556–566.

Mannuzza, S., Klein, R. G., Bonagura, N., Malloy, P., Giampino, T., & Addalli, K. A. (1991). Hyperactive boys almost grown up: V. Replication of psychiatric status. *Archives of General Psychiatry, 48,* 77–83.

Manos, M. J., Short, E. J., & Findling, R. L. (1999). Differential effectiveness of methylphenidate and Adderall in school-age youths with attention-deficit/hyperactivity disorder. *Journal of the American Academy of Child and Adolescent Psychiatry, 38,* 813–819.

Marans, S., Berkowitz, S. J., & Cohen, D. J. (1998). Police and mental health professionals: Collaborative responses to the impact of violence on children and families. *Child and Adolescent Psychiatric Clinics of North America, 7,* 635–651.

March, J. S. (1995). Cognitive-behavioral psychotherapy for children and adolescents with OCD: A review and recommendations for treatment. *Journal of the American Academy Child and Adolescent Psychiatry, 34,* 7–18.

March, J. S. (1999). *Psychopharmacological management of pediatric obsessive–compulsive disorder (OCD).* Paper presented at the 46th Annual Meeting of the American Academy of Child and Adolescent Psychiatry, Chicago.

March, J. S., Biederman, J., Wolkow, R., Safferman, A., Mardekian, J., Cook, E. H., Cutler, N. R., Dominguez, R., Ferguson, J., Muller, B., Riesenberg, R., Rosenthal, M., Sallee, F. R., Wagner, K. D., & Steiner, H. (1998). Sertraline in children and adolescents with obsessive–compulsive disorder: A multicenter randomized controlled trial. *Journal of the American Medical Association, 280,* 1752–1756.

March, J. S., Franklin, M., Nelson, A., & Foa, E. (2001). Cognitive-behavioral psychotherapy for pediatric obsessive–compulsive disorder. *Journal of Clinical Child Psychology, 30,* 8–18.

March, J. S., & Leonard, H. L. (1996). Obsessive–compulsive disorder in children and adolescents: A review of the past 10 years. *Journal of the American Academy of Child and Adolescent Psychiatry, 35,* 1265–1273.

March, J. S., & Mulle, K. (1995). Behavioral psychotherapy for obsessive–compulsive disorder: A preliminary single-case study. *Journal of Anxiety Disorders, 9,* 175–184.

March, J. S., Mulle, K., & Herbel, B. (1994). Behavioral psychotherapy for children and adolescents with obsessive–compulsive disorder: An open trial of a new protocol-driven treatment package. *Journal of the American Academy of Child and Adolescent Psychiatry, 33,* 333–341.

March, J. S., Swanson, J. M., Arnold, L. E., Hoza, B., Conners, K., Hinshaw, S. P., Hechtman, L., Kraemer, H. C., Greenhill, L. L., Abikoff, H. B., Elliott, L. G., Jensen, P. S., Newcorn, J. F., Vitiello, B., Severe, J., Wells, K. C., & Pelham, W. E. (2000). Anxiety as a predictor and outcome variable in the multimodal treatment study of children with ADHD (MTA). *Journal of Abnormal Child Psychology, 28,* 527–541.

Marcotte, D., & Baron, P. (1993). L'efficacité d'une strategie d'intervention emotio-rationelle aupres d'adolescents depressifs du milieu scolaire [The efficacy of a school-based rational–emotive intervention strategy with depressive adolescents]. *Canadian Journal of Counselling, 27,* 77–92.

Marcovitch, H. (1997). Managing chronic fatigue syndrome in children. *British Medical Journal, 314,* 1635–1636.

Marteau, T. M., Gillespie, C., & Swift, P. G. F. (1987). Evaluation of a weekend group for parents of children with diabetes. *Diabetic Medicine, 4,* 488–490.

Martens, B. K., & Hiralall, A. S. (1997). Scripted sequences of teacher interaction: A versatile, low-impact procedure for increasing appropriate behaviour in a nursery school. *Behavior Modification, 21,* 308–323.

Martin, B. (1977). Brief family intervention: Effectiveness and the importance of including the father. *Journal of Consulting and Clinical Psychology, 45,* 1002–1010.

Martin, F. E. (1985). The treatment and outcome of anorexia nervosa in adolescents: A prospective study and 5 year follow-up. *Journal of Psychiatric Research, 19,* 509–514.

Marton, P., Korenblum, M., Kutcher, S. P., Stein, B., Kennedy, B., & Pakes, J. (1989). Personality dysfunction in depressed adolescents. *Canadian Journal of Psychiatry, 34,* 810–813.

Marttunen, M. J., Aro, H. M., Henriksson, M. M., & Lonnqvist, J. K. (1991). Mental disorders in adolescent suicide. *Archives of General Psychiatry, 48,* 834–839.

Mas, C. H., Alexander, J. F., & Barton, C. W. (1985). Modes of expression in family therapy: A process study of roles and gender. *Journal of Marital and Family Therapy, 11,* 411–415.

Mash, E. J. (1998). Treatment of child and family disturbance: A behavioral-systems perspective. In E. J. Mash & R. A. Barkley (Eds.), *Treatment of childhood disorders* (2nd ed., pp. 3–54). New York: Guilford Press.

Matson, J. L. (1989). *Treating depression in children and adolescents.* New York: Pergamon Press.

Matson, J. L., Sevin, J. A., Box, M. L., & Francis, K. L. (1993). An evaluation of two methods for increasing self-initiated verbalizations in autistic children. *Journal of Applied Behavior Analysis, 26,* 389–398.

Matson, J. L., Sevin, J. A., Fridley, D., & Love, S. R. (1990). Increasing spontaneous language in three autistic children. *Journal of Applied Behavior Analysis, 23,* 227–234.

Matson, J. L., & Swiezy, N. (1994). Social skills training with autistic children. In J. L. Matson (Ed.), *Autism in children and adults: Etiology assessment and intervention* (pp. 241–260). Pacific Grove, CA: Brooks/Cole.

Matsuura, M., Okubo, Y., Kojima, T., Takahashi, R., Wang, Y.-F., Shen, Y.-C., & Lee, C. K. (1993). A cross-national prevalence study of children with emotional and behavioural problems: A WHO collaborative study in the Western Pacific region. *Journal of Child Psychology and Psychiatry and Allied Disciplines, 34,* 307–315.

Mattes, J. A. (1990). Comparative effectiveness of carbamazepine and propranolol for rage outbursts. *Journal of Neuropsychiatry and Clinical Neurosciences, 2,* 159–164.

Mattes, J. A., & Gittleman, R. (1981). Effects of artificial food colourings in children with hyperactive symptoms. *Archives of General Psychiatry, 38,* 714–718.

Maughan, B. (1994). School influences. In M. Rutter & D. Hay (Eds.), *Development through life: A handbook for clinicians* (pp. 134–58). Oxford: Blackwell Scientific.

Maughan, B. (1995). Annotation: Long-term outcomes of developmental reading problems. *Journal of Child Psychology and Psychiatry, 36,* 357–371.

Maughan, B., Pickles, A., Hagell, A., Rutter, M., & Yule, W. (1996). Reading problems and antisocial behaviour: Developmental trends in comorbidity. *Journal of Child Psychology and Psychiatry, 37*, 405–418.

Maughan, B., & Yule, W. (1994). Reading and other learning disabilities. In M. Rutter, E. Taylor, & L. Hersov (Eds.), *Child and adolescent psychiatry: Modern approaches* (pp. 647–665). Oxford: Blackwell Scientific.

Mawhood, L., Howlin, P., & Rutter, M. (2000). Autism and developmental receptive language disorder—A comparative follow-up in early adult life: I. Cognitive and language outcomes. *Journal of Child Psychology and Psychiatry, 41*, 547–559.

Mayes, S., Crites, D., Bixler, E., Humphrey, F., & Mattison, R. (1994). Methylphenidate and ADHD: Influence of age, IQ, neurodevelopmental status. *Developmental Medicine and Child Neurology, 36*, 1099–1107.

Mayou, R., & Sharpe, M. (1997). Treating medically unexplained physical symptoms. *British Medical Journal, 315*, 561–562.

McBride, M. (1988). An individual double-blind crossover trial for assessing methylphenidate response in children with attention deficit disorders. *Journal of Pediatrics, 113*, 137–145.

McCann, J. B., James, A., Wilson, S., & Dunn, G. (1996). Prevalence of psychiatric disorders in young people in the care system. *British Medical Journal, 313*, 1529–1530.

McClellan, J., & Werry, J. S. (1997). Practice parameters for the assessment and treatment of children and adolescents with schizophrenia. *Journal of the American Academy of Child and Adolescent Psychiatry, 36*(Suppl. 10), 177S–193S.

McClellan, J. M., Rubert, M. P., Reichler, R. J., & Sylvester, C. E. (1990). Attention deficit disorder in children at risk for anxiety and depression. *Journal of the American Academy of Child and Adolescent Psychiatry, 29*, 534–539.

McClellan, J. M., Werry, J. S., & Ham, M. (1993). A follow-up study of early onset psychosis: Comparison between outcome diagnosis of schizophrenia, mood disorders and personality disorders. *Journal of Autism and Developmental Disorders, 23*, 243–262.

McClure, G. (2000). Analysis of suicide data from the Office for National Statistics. *British Journal of Psychiatry, 176*, 64–67.

McConville, B. J., Arvanitis, L. A., Thyrum, P. T., Yeh, C., Wilkinson, L. A., Chaney, R. O., Foster, K. D., Sorter, M. T., Friedman, L. M., Brown, K. L., & Heubi, J. E. (2000). Pharmacokinetics, tolerability, and clinical effectiveness of quetiapine fumarate: An open-label trial in adolescents with psychotic disorders. *Journal of Clinical Psychiatry, 61*, 252–260.

McCord, J. (1988). Identifying developmental paradigms leading to alcoholism. *Journal of Studies on Alcohol, 49*, 357–362.

McCord, J., Tremblay, R. E., Vitaro, F., & Desmarais-Gervais, L. (1994). Boys' disruptive behavior, school adjustmnet, and delinquency: The Montreal prevention experiement. *International Journal of Behavioral Development, 17*, 739–752.

McCulloc, J. W., Henderson, A., & Philip, A. E. (1966). Psychiatric illness in Edinburgh teenagers. *Scottish Medical Journal, 11*, 277–281.

McDermott, P. A. (1996). A nationwide study of developmental and gender prevalence for psychopathology in childhood and adolescence. *Journal of Abnormal Child Psychology, 24*, 53–65.

McEachin, J. J., Smith, T., & Lovaas, O. I. (1993). Long-term outcome for children with autism who received early intensive behavioral treatment. *American Journal on Mental Retardation, 97*, 359–372.

McGee, B., Feehan, M., Williams, S., Partridge, F., Silva, P., & Kelly, J. (1990). DSM-III disorders in a large sample of adolescents. *Journal of the American Academy of Child and Adolescent Psychiatry, 29*, 611–619.

McGee, R., Feehan, M., Williams, S., & Anderson, J. (1992). DSM-III disorders from age 11 to age 15 years. *Journal of the American Academy of Child and Adolescent Psychiatry, 31*, 50–59.

McGee, R., Partridge, F., Williams, S., & Silva, P. A. (1991). A twelve-year follow-up of pre-school hyperactive children. *Journal of the American Academy of Child and Adolescent Psychiatry, 30*, 224–232.

McGrath, P. (1995). Annotation: Aspects of pain in children and adolescents. *Journal of Child Psychology and Psychiatry and Allied Disciplines, 36*, 717–730.

McGrath, P. J., Humphreys, P., Goodman, J. T., Keene, D., Firestone, P., Jacob, P., & Cunningham, S. J. (1988). Relaxation prophylaxis for childhood migraine: A randomised placebo-controlled trial. *Developmental Medicine and Child Neurology, 30,* 626–631.

McGrath, P. J., Humphreys, P., Keene, D., Goodman, J. T., Lascelles, M. A., Cunningham, S. J., & Firestone, P. (1992). The efficacy and efficiency of a self-administered treatment for adolescent migraine. *Pain, 49,* 321–324.

McGuire, J., & Priestley, P. (1995). Reviewing "what works": Past, present and future. In J. McGuire (Ed.), *What works: Reducing reoffending: Guidlines from research and practice* (pp. 3–34). Chichester: Wiley.

McKeith, I. G., Williams, A., & Nicol, A. R. (1981). Clonidine in Tourette's syndrome. *Lancet, 1,* 270–271.

McKnew, D. H., Cytryn, L., Buchsbaum, M. D., Hammovit, J., Lamour, M., Rapoport, J. L., & Gershon, E. S. (1981). Lithium in the children of lithium responding parents. *Psychiatry Research, 4,* 171–180.

McLellan, J. M., Rubert, M. P., Reichler, R. J., & Sylvester, C. E. (1990). Attention deficit-disorder in children at risk for anxiety and depression. *Journal of the American Academy of Child and Adolescent Psychiatry, 29,* 534–539.

McMahon, R. J., & Estes, A. M. (1997). Conduct problems. In E. J. Mash & L. G. Terdal (Eds.), *Assessment of childhood disorders* (3rd ed., pp. 130–193). New York: Guilford Press.

McMahon, R. J., Forehand, R., Griest, D. L., & Wells, K. C. (1981). Who drops out of treatment during parent behavioural training? *Behavioural Counselling Quarterly, 1,* 79–95.

McNeil, C. B., Eyberg, S., Eisenstadt, T. H., Newcomb, K., & Funderburk, B. (1991). Parent–child interaction therapy with behavior problem children: Generalization of treatment effects to the school setting. *Journal of Clinical Child Psychology, 20,* 140–151.

Mehr, M., Zeltzer, L. K., & Robinson, R. (1981). Continued self-destructive behaviors in adolescent suicide attemptors: Part I. *Journal of Adolescent Health Care, 1,* 269–274.

Mehr, M., Zeltzer, L. K., & Robinson, R. (1982). Continued self-destructive behaviors in adolescent suicide attemptors: II. A pilot study. *Journal of Adolescent Health Care, 2,* 183–187.

Meichenbaum, D. (1997). The evolution of a cognitive-behavior therapist. In J. K. Zeig (Ed.), *The evolution of psychotherapy: The third conference* (pp. 95–104). New York: Brunner/Mazel.

Meltzer, H., Gatward, R., Goodman, R., & Ford, T. (2000). *Mental health of children and adolescents in Great Britain.* London: Her Majesty's Stationery Office.

Mendel, R. A. (2000). *Less hype, more help: Reducing juvenile crime, what works—and what doesn't.* Washington, DC: American Youth Policy Forum.

Mendlowitz, S. L., Manassis, K., Bradley, S., Scalpillato, D., Miezitis, S., & Shaw, B. F. (1999). Cognitive-behavioral group treatments in childhood anxiety disorders: The role of parental involvement. *Journal of the American Academy of Child and Adolescent Psychiatry, 38,* 1223–1229.

Menzies, R. G., & Clarke, J. C. (1993). A comparison of in vivo and vicarious exposure in the treatment of childhood water phobia. *Behaviour Research and Therapy, 31,* 9–15.

Mesibov, G. B. (1986). A cognitive program for teaching social behaviors in verbal autistic adolescents and adults. In E. Schopler & G. B. Mesibov (Eds.), *Social behavior and autism* (pp. 265–283). New York: Plenum Press.

Mezzacappa, E., Steingard, R., Kindlon, D., Saul, J. P., & Earls, F. (1998). Tricyclic antidepressants and cardiac autonomic control in children and adolescents. *Journal of the American Academy of Child and Adolescent Psychiatry, 37,* 52–59.

Michelson, L., Mannarino, A. P., Marchione, K. E., Stern, M., Figueroa, J., & Beck, S. (1983). A comparative outcome study of behavioural social-skills training, interpersonal-problem-solving and nondirective control treatments with child psychiatric outpatients. *Behaviour Research and Therapy, 21,* 545–556.

Michielutte, R., Patterson, R. B., & Herndon, A. (1981). Evaluation of a home visitation program for familes of children with cancer. *American Journal of Pediatric Hematology/Oncology, 3,* 239–245.

Miklowitz, D. J., Goldstein, M. J., Neuchterlein, K. H., Snyder, K. S., & Mintz, J. (1988). Family factors and the course of bipolar affective disorder. *Archives of General Psychiatry, 45,* 225–231.

Milich, R., & Dodge, K. A. (1984). Social information processing in child psychiatric populations. *Journal of Abnormal Child Psychology, 12*, 471–490.

Milin, R., Simeon, J., & Spenst, W. (1999). *Double-blind study of paroxetine in adolescents with unipolar major depression.* Paper presented at the 46th Annual Meeting of the American Academy of Child and Adolescent Psychiatry, Chicago.

Miller, A., & Glinski, J. (2000). Youth suicidal behavior: Assessment and intervention. *Journal of Clinical Psychology, 56*, 1131–1152.

Miller, G. E., & Prinz, R. J. (1990). Enhancement of social learning family interventions for childhood conduct disorder. *Psychological Bulletin, 108*, 291–307.

Miller, H. L., Coombs, D. W., Leeper, J. D., & Barton, S. N. (1984). An analysis of the effects of suicide prevention facilities on suicide rates in the United States. *American Journal of Public Health, 74*, 340–343.

Miller, L. C., Barrett, C. L., Hampe, E., & Noble, H. (1972). Comparison of reciprocal inhibition psychotherapy and waiting list control of phobic children. *Journal of Abnormal Psychology, 79*, 269–279.

Miller, P., & Plant, M. (1996). Drinking, smoking and illicit drug use among 15 and 16 year-olds in the United Kingdom. *British Medical Journal, 313*, 394–397.

Mitchell, J. E., Pyle, R. L., Eckert, E. D., Hatsukami, D., Pomeroy, C., & Zimmerman, R. (1990). A comparison study of antidepressants and structured intensive group psychotherapy in the treatment of bulimia nervosa. *Archives of General Psychiatry, 47*, 149–157.

Moens, G. F. (1990). *Aspects of the epidemiology and prevention of suicide.* Leuven: Leuven University Press.

Moffitt, T. E. (1993). "Adolescence-limited" and "life-course-persistent" antisocial behavior: A developmental taxonomy. *Psychological Review, 100*, 674–701.

Moffitt, T. E., Caspi, A., Dickson, N., Silva, P., & Stanton, W. (1996). Childhood-onset versus adolescent-onset antisocial problems in males: Natural history from ages 3 to 18 years. *Developmental Psychopathology, 9*, 399–424.

Moncrieff, J., Wessley, S., & Hardy, R. (1998). Meta-analysis of trials comparing antidepressants with active placebos. *British Journal of Psychiatry, 172*, 227–231.

Moore, D., Chamberlain, P., & Mukai, L. (1979). Children at risk for delinquency: A follow-up comparison of aggressive children and children who steal. *Journal of Abnormal Child Psychology, 7*, 345–355.

Moore, K. E., Geffken, G. R., & Royal, G. P. (1995). Behavioral intervention to reduce child distress during self- injection. *Clinical Pediatrics, 34*, 530–534.

Moran, G., Fonagy, P., Kurtz, A., Bolton, A., & Brook, C. (1991). A controlled study of the psychoanalytic treatment of brittle diabetes. *Journal of the American Academy of Child and Adolescent Psychiatry, 30*, 926–935.

Moreau, D., Mufson, L., Weissman, M. M., & Klerman, G. L. (1991). Interpersonal psychotherapy for adolescent depression: Description of modification and preliminary application. *Journal of the American Academy of Child and Adolescent Psychiatry, 30*, 642–651.

Moretti, M. M., Holland, R., & Peterson, S. (1994). Long-term outcome of an attachment-based program for conduct disorder. *Canadian Journal of Psychiatry, 39*, 360–369.

Morgan, H. G., & Russell, G. F. (1975). Value of family background and clinical features as predictors of long-term outcome in anorexia nervosa: Four-year follow-up study of 41 patients. *Psychological Medicine, 5*, 355–371.

Morris, R. J., & Kratochwill, T. R. (Eds.). (1991). *The practice of child therapy* (2nd ed.). Elmsford, NY: Pergamon.

Morrow-Bradley, C., & Elliott, R. (1986). Utilization of psychotherapy research by practicing psychotherapists. *American Psychologist, 41*, 188–197.

Mortimore, P. (1995). The positive effects of schooling. In M. Rutter (Ed.), *Psychosocial disturbances in young people: Challenges for prevention* (pp. 333–363). Cambridge: Cambridge University Press.

Mortimore, P., Sammons, P., Stoll, L., Lewis, D., & Ecob, R. (1988). *School matters: The junior years.* Wells, Somerset, UK: Open Books.

Mott, J. (1985). Self-reported cannabis use in Great Britain in 1981. *British Journal of Addiction, 80,* 37–43.

Mozes, T., Toren, P., Chernauzan, N., Mester, R., Yoran-Hegesh, R., Blumensohn, R., & Weizman, A. (1994). Clozapine treatment in very early onset schizophrenia. *Journal of the American Academy of Child and Adolescent Psychiatry, 33,* 65–70.

The MTA Cooperative Group. (1999a). A 14–month randomised clinical trial of treatment strategies for attention deficit hyperactivity disorder. *Archives of General Psychiatry, 56,* 1073–1085.

The MTA Cooperative Group. (1999b). Moderators and mediators of treatment response for children with attention-deficit/hyperactivity disorder. *Archives of General Psychiatry, 56,* 1088–1096.

Mufson, L., Moreau, D., & Weissman, M. M. (1996). Focus on relationships: Interpersonal psychotherapy for adolescent depression. In E. D. Hibbs & P. S. Jensen (Eds.), *Psychosocial treatments for child and adolescent disorders: Empirically based strategies for clinical practice* (pp. 137–155). Washington, DC: American Psychological Association.

Mufson, L., Moreau, D., Weissman, M. M., Wickramaratne, P., Martin, J., & Samoilov, A. (1994). Modification of interpersonal psychotherapy with depressed adolescents (IPT-A): Phase I and II studies. *Journal of the American Academy of Child and Adolescent Psychiatry, 33,* 695–705.

Mufson, L., Weissman, M. M., Moreau, D., & Garfinkel, R. (1999). Efficacy of interpersonal psychotherapy for depressed adolescents. *Archives of General Psychiatry, 56,* 573–579.

Multimodal Treatment Study of Children with ADHD Cooperative Group. (1999). Moderators and mediators of treatment response for children with attention deficit hyperactivity disorder: The multimodal treatment study of children with attention deficit hyperactivity disorder. *Archives of General Psychiatry, 56,* 1088–1096.

Muratori, F., Picchi, L., Casella, C., Tancredi, R., Milone, A., & Patarnello, M. G. (2002). Efficacy of brief dynamic psychotherapy for children with emotional disorders. *Psychotherapy and Psychosomatics, 71,* 2838.

Muris, P., Meesters, C., Merckelbach, H., Sermon, A., & Zwakhalen, S. (1998). Worry in normal children. *Journal of the American Academy of Child and Adolescent Psychiatry, 37,* 703–710.

Musten, L. M., Firestone, P., Pisterman, S., Bennett, S., & Mercer, J. (1997). Effects of methylphenidate on pre-school children with ADHD: Cognitive and behavioral functions. *Journal of the American Academy of Child and Adolescent Psychiatry, 36,* 1407–1415.

Myers, M. G., & Brown, S. A. (1990). Coping and appraisal in relapse risk situations among adolescent substance abusers following treatment. *Journal of Adolescent Chemical Dependency, 1,* 95–115.

Myers, M. G., Brown, S. A., & Mott, M. A. (1993). Coping as a predictor of adolescent substance abuse treatment outcome. *Journal of Substance Abuse, 5,* 15–29.

Myers, P. I., & Hammill, D. D. (1992). *Learning disabilities: Basic concepts, assessment practices, and instructional strategies* (4th ed.). Austin, TX: PRO-ED.

Nagin, D. S., & Tremblay, R. E. (2001). Parental and early childhood predictors of persistent physical aggression in boys from kindergarten to high school. *Archives of General Psychiatry, 58,* 389–394.

National Criminal Justice Reference Service. (1996). *Youth violence: A community based response— One city's success.* Washington, DC: U.S. Department of Justice.

National Institute for Clinical Excellence. (2000). *Guidance on the use of methylphenidate for ADHD.* London: National Institute for Clinical Excellence.

National Institute on Drug Abuse. (1996). *National survey results on drug use from the Monitoring the Future Study, 1975–1995: Vol. 1. Secondary school students.* Bethesda, MD: Author.

Neighbors, B., Kempton, T., & Forehand, R. (1992). Co-occurrence of substance abuse with conduct, anxiety, and depression disorders in juvenile delinquents. *Addictive Behaviors, 17,* 379–386.

Nelson, J. R., Smith, D. J., & Dodd, J. (1990). The moral reasoning of juvenile delinquents: A meta-analysis. *Journal of Abnormal Child Psychology, 18,* 231–239.

Nelson, K. E., Camarata, S. M., Welsh, J., Butkovsky, L., & Camarata, M. (1996). Effects of imitative and conversational recasting treatment on the acquisition of grammar in children with specific language impairment and younger language-normal children. *Journal of Speech and Hearing Research, 39,* 850–859.

Netten, A., & Dennett, J. H. (1996). *Unit costs of health and social care 1996.* University of Kent, Canterbury: Personal Social Services Research Unit.

Newcorn, J. H., Sharma, V., Matier, K., Hall, S., & Halperin, J. M. (1992). *Differential effect of oppositional/conduct and anxiety disorders on individual symptom domains.* Paper presented at the Annual meeting of the Society for Research in Child and Adolescent Psychopathology, Sarasota, FL.

Newman, D. L., Moffitt, T. E., Silva, P. A., Caspi, A., Magdol, L., & Stanton, W. R. (1996). Psychiatric disorder in a birth cohort of young adults: Prevalence, comorbidity, clinical significance, and new case incidence from ages 11 to 21. *Journal of Consulting and Clinical Psychology, 64,* 552–562.

Newsom, C., & Rincover, A. (1989). Autism. In E. J. Mash & R. A. Barkley (Eds.), *Treatment of childhood disorders* (pp. 286–346). New York: Guilford Press.

Neziroglu, F., Yaryura-Tobias, J. A., Walz, J., & McKay, D. (2000). The effect of fluvoxamine and behavior therapy on children and adolescents with obsessive–compulsive disorder. *Journal of Child and Adolescent Psychopharmacology, 10,* 295–306.

Nicolson, R. (2000). *Prolactin elevations in pediatric patients on antipsychotics.* Paper presented at the American Academy of Child and Adolescent Psychiatry Annual Meeting, New York.

Nolan, E. E., & Gadow, K. D. (1997). Children with ADHD and tic disorder and their classmates: Behavioral normalization with methylphenidate. *Journal of the American Academy of Child and Adolescent Psychiatry, 36,* 597–604.

Nolan, T., Zvagulis, I., & Pless, B. (1987). Controlled trial of social work in childhood chronic illness. *Lancet, 2*(8556), 411–415.

Nordin, V., Gillberg, C., & Nyden, A. (1998). The Swedish version of the Childhood Autism Rating Scale in a clinical setting. *Journal of Autism and Developmental Disorders, 28,* 69–75.

North, C., & Gowers, S. (1999). Anorexia nervosa, psychopathology, and outcome. *International Journal of Eating Disorders, 26,* 386–391.

Novins, D. K., Beals, J., Shore, J. H., & Manson, S. M. (1996). Substance abuse treatment of American Indian adolescents: Comorbid symptomatology, gender differences, and treatment patterns. *Journal of the American Academy of Child and Adolescent Psychiatry, 35,* 1593–1601.

Nugent, W. R., Carpenter, D., & Parks, J. (1993). A statewide evaluation of family preservation and family reunification services. *Research on Social Work Practice, 3,* 40–65.

Nye, C. L., Zucker, R. A., & Fitzgerald, H. E. (1995). Early intervention in the path to alcohol problems through conduct problems: Treatment involvement and child behavior change. *Journal of Consulting and Clinical Psychology, 63,* 831–840.

O'Connor, S. C., & Spreen, O. (1988). The relationship between parents' socioeconomic status and education level, and adult occupational and educational achievement of children with learning disabilities. *Journal of Learning Disabilities, 21,* 148–153.

O'Dell, S. L. (1974). Training parents in behavior modification: A review. *Psychological Bulletin, 81,* 418–433.

O'Dell, S. L. (1985). Progress in parent training. In M. Hersen, R. M. Eisler, & P. M. Miller (Eds.), *Progress in behavior modification* (Vol. 9, pp. 57–108). New York: Academic Press.

Office of Technology Assessment. (1980). *The efficacy and cost-effectiveness of psychotherapy. Background Paper No. 3: The implications of cost-effectiveness analysis of medical technology.* Washington, DC: U.S. Government Printing Office.

Offord, D. R., Alder, R. J., & Boyle, M. H. (1986). Prevalence and sociodemographic correlates of conduct disorder. *American Journal of Social Psychiatry, 6,* 272–278.

Offord, D. R., Boyle, M., Szatmari, P., Rae-Grant, N. I., Links, P. S., Cadman, D. T., Byles, J. A., Crawford, J. W., Munroe Blum, H., Byrne, C., Thomas, H., & Woodward, C. A. (1987). Ontario Child Health Study: II. Six month prevalence of disorder and rates of service utilization. *Archives of General Psychiatry, 44,* 832–836.

Offord, D. R., Boyle, M. H., Racine, Y. A., Fleming, J. E., Cadman, D. T., Blum, H. M., Byrne, C.,

Links, P. S., Lipman, E. L., MacMillan, H. L., Rae Grant, N. I., Sanford, M. N., Szatmari, P., Thomas, H., & Woodward, C. A. (1992). Outcome, prognosis and risk in a longitudinal follow-up study. *Journal of the American Academy of Child and Adolescent Psychiatry, 31*, 916–923.

Oldehinkel, A. J., Wittchen, H. U., & Schuster, P. (1999). Prevalence, 20–month incidence and outcome of unipolar depressive disorders in a community sample of adolescents. *Psychological Medicine, 29*, 655–668.

Olds, D., & Kitzman, H. (1993). Review of research on home visiting for pregnant women and parents of young children. *Future of Children, 3*, 53–92.

Olds, D. L., Henderson, C. R., Chamberlin, R., & Tatelbaum, R. (1986). Preventing child abuse and neglect: A randomized trial of nurse home visitation. *Pediatrics, 78*, 65–78.

Olds, J., Nixon, M. K., & Votta, E. (1999). *Group anger management for internalizing symptomatology in adolescent day hospitalization.* Paper presented at the 46th annual meeting of the American Academy of Child and Adolescent Psychiatry, Chicago.

Olfson, M. (1999). Emerging methods in mental health outcomes research. *Journal of Practical Psychiatry and Behavioral Health, 5*, 20–24.

Ollendick, T. H. (1995). Cognitive behavioral treatment of panic disorder with agoraphobia in adolescents: A multiple baseline design analysis. *Behavior Therapy, 26*, 517–531.

Ollendick, T. H., & King, N. J. (1998). Empirically supported treatments for children with phobic and anxiety disorders. *Journal of Clinical Child Psychology, 27*, 156–167.

Olsson, I., Steffenberg, S., & Gillberg, C. (1988). Epilepsy in autism and autistic-like conditions: A population-based study. *Archives of Neurology, 45*, 666–668.

Olweus, D. (1991). Bully/victim problems among schoolchildren: Basic facts and effects of a school-based intervention program. In D. J. Pepler & K. H. Rubin (Eds.), *The development and treatment of childhood aggression* (pp. 411–448). Hillsdale, NJ: Erlbaum.

Olweus, D. (1992). Bullying among schoolchildren: Intervention and prevention. In R. D. Peters, R. J. McMahon, & V. L. Quinsey (Eds.), *Aggression and violence throughout the lifespan* (pp. 100–125). Newbury Park, CA: Sage.

Olweus, D. (1993). Victimization by peers: Antecedents and long-term outcomes. In K. H. Rubin & J. B. Asendorpf (Eds.), *Social withdrawal, inhibition, and shyness in childhood* (pp. 315–341). Hillsdale, NJ: Erlbaum.

Olweus, D. (1996). Bullying at school: Knowledge base and an effective intervention program. *Annals of the New York Academy of Sciences, 794*, 265–276.

Ornitz, E. M., Guthrie, D., & Farley, A. H. (1977). The early development of autistic children. *Journal of Autism and Childhood Schizophrenia, 7*, 207–229.

Osborne, R. B., Hatcher, J. W., & Richtsmeier, A. J. (1989). The role of social modeling in unexplained pediatric pain. *Journal of Pediatric Psychology, 14*, 43–61.

Osterhaus, S. O. L., Passchier, J., Van der Helm-Hylkema, H., de Jong, K. T., Orlebeke, J. F., de Grauw, A. J. C., & Dekker, P. H. (1993). Effects of behavioral psychophysiological treatment on school children with migraine in a nonclinical setting: Predictors and process variables. *Journal of Pediatric Psychology, 18*, 697–715.

Otto, U. (1972). Suicidal acts by children and adolescents: A follow-up study. *Acta Psychiatrica Scandinavica, 233*(Suppl.), 7–123.

Overall, J. E., & Gorman, D. R. (1962). The Brief Psychiatric Rating Scale. *Psychological Reports, 10*, 799–812.

Ozonoff, S., & Miller, J. N. (1995). Teaching theory of mind: A new approach to social skills training for individuals with autism. *Journal of Autism and Developmental Disorders, 25*, 415–433.

Ozonoff, S. J., Rogers, S. J., & Pennington, B. F. (1991). Asperger's syndrome: Evidence of an empirical distinction from high-functioning autism. *Journal of Child Psychology and Psychiatry, 32*, 1107–1122.

Papatheodorou, G., & Kutcher, S. P. (1993). Divalproex sodium treatment in late adolescent and young adult acute mania. *Psychopharmacology Bulletin, 29*, 213–219.

Papatheodorou, T. (2000). Management approaches employed by teachers to deal with children's behavior problems in nursery classes. *School Psychology International, 21*, 415–440.

Papay, J. P., & Spielberger, C. D. (1986). Assessment of anxiety and achievement in kindergarten and first- and second-grade children. *Journal of Abnormal Child Psychology, 14*, 279–286.

Park, S., Como, P. G., Cui, L., & Kurlan, R. (1993). The early course of the Tourette's syndrome clinical spectrum. *Neurology, 43*, 1712–1715.

Parry-Jones, W. L. (1995). The future of adolescent psychiatry. *British Journal of Psychiatry, 166*, 299–305.

Patterson, G. R. (1976). *Living with children: New methods for parents and teachers* (rev. ed.). Champaign, IL: Research Press.

Patterson, G. R. (1982). *Coercive family processes.*, Eugene, OR: Castalia.

Patterson, G. R., & Chamberlain, P. (1988). Treatment process: A problem at three levels. In L. C. Wynne (Ed.), *The state of the art in family therapy research: Controversies and recommendations* (pp. 189–223). New York: Family Process Press.

Patterson, G. R., & Chamberlain, P. (1994). A functional analysis of resistance during parent training therapy. *Clinical Psychology: Science and Practice, 1*, 53–70.

Patterson, G. R., Chamberlain, P., & Reid, J. B. (1982). A comparative evaluation of a parent training program. *Behavior Therapy, 13*, 638–650.

Patterson, G. R., Cobb, J. A., & Ray, R. S. (1973). A social engineering technology for retraining the families of aggressive boys. In H. E. Adams & I. P. Unikel (Eds.), *Issues and trends in behavior therapy* (Vol. III, pp. 139–210). Springfield, IL: Charles C. Thomas.

Patterson, G. R., & Forgatch, M. S. (1987). *Parents and adolescents living together: Part 1. The basics.* Eugene, OR: Castalia.

Patterson, G. R., & Forgatch, M. S. (1995). Predicting future clinical adjustment from treatment outcome and process variables. *Psychological Assessment, 7*, 275–285.

Patterson, G. R., Reid, J. B., & Dishion, T. J. (1992). *Antisocial boys.* Eugene, OR: Castalia.

Patterson, G. R., Reid, J. B., Jones, R. R., & Conger, R. E. (1975). *A social learning approach to family intervention. Vol. 1: Families with aggressive children.* Eugene, OR: Castalia.

Patterson, J., & Blum, R. W. (1996). Risk and resilience among children and youth with disabilities. *Archives of Pediatric and Adolescent Medicine, 150*, 692–698.

Pauls, D. L., Raymond, C. L., Stevenson, J. M., & Leckman, J. F. (1991). A family study of Gilles de la Tourette syndrome. *Human Genetics, 48*, 154–163.

Pauls, D. L., Towbin, K. E., Leckman, J. F., Zahner, G. E. P., & Cohen, D. J. (1986). Gilles de la Tourette's syndrome and obsessive–compulsive disorder: Evidence supporting a genetic relationship. *Archives of General Psychiatry, 43*, 1180–1182.

Pavuluri, M. N., Luk, S., & McGee, R. (1996). Help-seeking for behavior problems by parents of preschool children: A community study. *Journal of the American Academy of Child and Adolescent Psychiatry, 35*, 215–223.

Payton, J. B., Burkhart, J. E., Hersen, M., & Helsen, W. J. (1989). Treatment of ADDH in mentally retarded children: A preliminary study. *Journal of the American Academy of Child and Adolescent Psychiatry, 28*, 761–767.

Pearson, G., Ditton, J., Newcombe, R., & Gilman, M. (1991). *Drug misuse in Britain: National Audit of Drug Misuse Statistics.* London: Institute for the Study of Drug Dependency (ISDD).

Peed, S., Roberts, M., & Forehand, R. (1977). Evaluation of the effectiveness of a standardized parent training program in altering the interaction of mothers and their noncompliant children. *Behavior Modification, 1*, 323–350.

Pelham, W. E. (1999). The NIMH Multimodal Treatment Study for Attention Deficit Hyperactivity Disorder: Just say yes to drugs alone? *Canadian Journal of Psychiatry, 44*, 981–990.

Pelham, W. E., Aronoff, H. R., Midlam, J. K., Shapiro, C. J., Gnagy, E. M., Chronis, A. M., Onyango, A. N., Forehand, G., Nguyen, A., & Waxmonsky, J. (1999a). A comparison of Ritalin and Adderall: Efficacy and time-course in children with attention-deficit/hyperactivity disorder. *Pediatrics, 103*, e43.

Pelham, W. E., Burrows-Maclean, L., & Gnagy, E. M. (1999b). *Once-a-day Concerta (methylphenidate HCl) extended release tablets versus t.i.d. methylphenidate in natural settings: Safety and efficacy.* Buffalo: State University of New York.

Pelham, W. E., Carlson, C., Sams, S. E., Vallano, G., Dixon, J., & Hoza, B. (1993). Separate and combined effects of methylphenidate and behavior modification on boys with attention deficit-hyperactivity disorder in the classroom. *Journal of Consulting and Clinical Psychology, 61,* 506–515.

Pelham, W. E., Gnagy, E. M., Burrows-Maclean, L., Williams, A., & Fabiano, G. A. (1999c). *Once-a-day Concerta (methylphenidate HCI) extended release tablets versus t.i.d. methylphenidate in a laboratory setting.* Buffalo: State University of New York.

Pelham, W. E., Gnagy, E. M., Greiner, A. R., Hoza, B., Hinshaw, S. P., Swanson, J. M., Simpson, S., Shapiro, C., Bukstein, O., Baron-Myak, C., & McBurnett, K. (2000). Behavioral versus behavioral and pharmacological treatment in ADHD children attending a summer treatment program. *Journal of Abnormal Child Psychology, 28,* 507–525.

Pelham, W. E., Greenslade, K. E., Vodde-Hamilton, M., Murphy, D. A., Greenstein, J. J., Gnagy, E. M., Guthrie, K. J., Hoover, M. D., & Dahl, R. E. (1990a). Relative efficacy of long-acting stimulants on children with attention deficit-hyperactivity disorder: A comparison of standard methylphenidate, sustained-release methylphenidate, sustained-release dextroamphetamine, and pemoline. *Pediatrics, 86,* 226–237.

Pelham, W. E., & Hoza, B. (1996a). Comprehensive treatment for ADHD: A proposal for intensive summer treatment programs and outpatient follow-up. In E. D. Hibbs & P. S. Jensen (Eds.), *Psychosocial treatment research of child and adolescent disorders* (pp. 311–340). Washington, DC: American Psychiatric Assocation.

Pelham, W. E., & Hoza, B. (1996b). Intensive treatment: A summer treatment program for children with ADHD. In E. D. Hibbs & P. S. Jensen (Eds.), *Psychosocial treatments for child and adolescent disorders: Empirically based strategies for clinical practice* (pp. 311–340). Washington, DC: American Psychological Association.

Pelham, W. E., McBurnett, K., Harper, G. W., Milich, R., Murphy, D. A., Clinton, J., & Thiele, C. (1990b). Methylphenidate and baseball playing in ADHD children: Who's on first? *Journal of Consulting and Clinical Psychology, 58,* 130–133.

Pelham, W. E., Milich, R., & Walker, J. L. (1986). Effects of continuous and partial reinforcement and methylphenidate on learning in children with attention deficit disorder. *Journal of Abnormal Psychology, 95,* 319–325.

Pelham, W. E., & Murphy, H. A. (1986). Behavioral and pharmacological treatments of hyperactivity and attention deficit disorders. In M. Herson & S. Brewing (Eds.), *Pharmacological and behavioral treatment: An integrative approach* (pp. 108–147). New York: Wiley.

Pelham, W. E., & Waschbusch, D. (1999). Behavioral intervention in ADHD. In H. P. Quay & A. E. Hogan (Eds.), *Handbook of disruptive behavior disorders* (pp. 255–278). New York: Plenum.

Penn, D. L., & Mueser, K. T. (1996). Research update on the psychosocial treatment of schizophrenia. *American Journal of Psychiatry, 153,* 607–617.

Pennington, B. F., Van-Orden, G. C., Smith, S. D., Green, P. A., & Haith, M. M. (1990). Phonological processing skills and deficits in adult dyslexics. *Child Development, 61,* 1753–1778.

Pepler, D. J., Craig, W. M., Ziegler, S., & Charach, A. (1993). A school-based antibullying intervention: Preliminary evaluation. In D. Tattum (Ed.), *Understanding and managing bullying* (pp. 76–91). Oxford: Heinemann.

Pepler, D. J., Craig, W. M., Ziegler, S., & Charach, A. (1994). An evaluation of an anti-bullying intervention in Toronto schools. *Canadian Journal of Community Mental Health, 13,* 95–110.

Perrin, J. M., Maclean, W. E., Gortmaker, S. L., & Asher, K. N. (1992). Improving the psychological status of children with asthma: A randomized controlled trial. *Developmental and Behavioral Pediatrics, 13,* 241–247.

Perry, A. (1991). Rett syndrome: A comprehensive review of the literature. *American Journal of Mental Retardation, 96,* 275–290.

Petersen, A. C., & Leffert, N. (1995). Developmental issues influencing guidelines for adolescent health research: A review. *Journal of Adolescent Health, 17(5),* 298–305.

Peterson, C. B., & Mitchell, J. E. (1999). Psychosocial and pharmacological treatment of eating disorders: A review of research findings. *Journal of Clinical Psychology, 55,* 685–697.

Pfeffer, C. R., Jiang, H., & Domeshek, L. J. (1997). Buspirone treatment of psychiatrically hospitalized prepubertal children with symptoms of anxiety and moderately severe aggression. *Journal of Child and Adolescent Psychopharmacology, 7,* 145–155.

Pfeffer, C. R., Klerman, G. L., Hurt, S. W., Lesser, M., Peskin, J. R., & Siefker, C. A. (1991). Suicidal children grow up: Demographic and clinical risk factors for adolescent suicide attempts. *Journal of the American Acadamy of Child and Adolescent Psychiatry, 30,* 609–616.

Pfiffner, L., Jouriles, E., Brown, M., Etscheidt, M., & Kelly, J. (1990). Effects of problem-solving therapy on outcomes of parent training for single-parent families. *Child and Family Behavior Therapy, 12,* 1–11.

Pfiffner, L. J., & Barkley, R. A. (1990). Educational placement and classroom management. In R. A. Barkley (Ed.), *Attention deficit hyperactivity disorder: A handbook for diagnosis and treatment.* (pp. 498–539). New York: Guilford Press.

Pfiffner, L. J., & O'Leary, S. G. (1987). The efficacy of all-positive management as a function of the prior use of negative consequences. *Journal of Applied Behavior Analysis, 20,* 265–271.

Phillipart, M. (1986). Clinical recognition of Rett syndrome. *American Journal of Medical Genetics, 24,* 111–118.

Piacentini, J., & Graae, F. (1997). Childhood OCD. In E. Hollander & D. Stein (Eds.), *Obsessive–compulsive disorders: Diagnosis, etiology, treatment* (pp. 23–46). New York: Marcel Dekker.

Piacentini, J., Rotheram-Borus, M. J., & Cantwell, C. (1995). Brief cognitive-behavioral family therapy for suicidal adolescents. In L. VandeCreek, S. Knapp, & T. Jackson (Eds.), *Innovations in clinical practice: A source book* (Vol. 14, pp. 151–168). Sarasota, FL: Professional Resource Press.

Pigott, H. E., & Heggie, D. L. (1986). Interpreting the conflicting results of individual versus group contingencies in classrooms: The targeted behavior as a mediating variable. *Child and Family Behavior Therapy, 7,* 1–15.

Pisterman, S., Firestone, P., McGrath, P., Goodman, J. T., Webster, I., Mallory, R., & Goffin, B. (1992). The role of parent training in treatment of preschoolers with ADDH. *American Journal of Orthopsychiatry, 62,* 397–408.

Pisterman, S., McGrath, P., Firestone, P., Goodman, J. T., Webster, I., & Mallory, R. (1989). Outcome of parent-mediated treatment of preschoolers with attention deficit disorder with hyperactivity. *Journal of Consulting and Clinical Psychology, 57,* 628–635.

Piven, L., Nehme, H., Simon, J., Barta, P., Pearlson, G., & Folstein, S. E. (1992). Magnetic resonance imaging in autism: Measurement of the cerebellum, pons and fourth ventricle. *Biological Psychiatry, 31,* 491–504.

Plant, M. A., Peck, D. F., & Samuel, E. (1985). *Alcohol, drugs and school-leavers.* London: Tavistock.

Platt, S., Hawton, K., Kreitman, N., Fagg, J., & Foster, J. (1988). Recent clinical and epidemiological trends in parasuicide in Edinburgh and Oxford: A tale of two cities. *Psychological Medicine, 18,* 405–418.

Platt, S., Bille-Brahe, U., Kerkhof, A., Schmidtke, A., Bjerke, T., Crepet, P., De-Leo, D., Haring, C., Lonnqvist, J., & Michel, K. (1992). Parasuicide in Europe: The WHO/EURO multicentre study on parasuicide: I. Introduction and preliminary analysis for 1989. *Acta Psychiatrica Scandinavica, 85,* 97–104.

Pless, I. B., Cripps, H. A., Davies, J. M. C., & Wadsworth, M. E. J. (1989). Chronic physical illness in childhood: Psychological and social effects in adolescence and adult life. *Developmental Medicine and Child Neurology, 31,* 746–755.

Pless, I. B., Feeley, N., Gottlieb, L., Rowat, K., Dougherty, G., & Willard, B. (1994). A randomized trial of a nursing intervention to promote the adjustment of children with chronic physical disorders. *Pediatrics, 94,* 70–75.

Pless, I. B., & Nolan, T. (1991). Revision, replication and neglect: Research on maladjustment in chronic illness. *Journal of Child Psychology and Psychiatry, 32,* 347–365.

Pless, I. B., Power, C., & Peckham, C. S. (1993). Long-term psychosocial sequelae of chronic physical disorders in childhood. *Pediatrics, 91,* 1131–1136.

Pless, I. B., & Satterwhite, B. (1972). Chronic illness in childhood: Selection, activities, and evaluation of nonprofessional family counselors. *Clinical Pediatrics, 11,* 403–410.

Pliszka, S. R. (1989). Effect of anxiety on cognition, behavior and stimulant response in ADHD. *Journal of the American Academy of Child and Adolescent Psychiatry, 28*, 882–887.

Pliszka, S. R. (1992). Comorbidity of attention-deficit hyperactivity disorder and overanxious disorders. *Journal of the American Academy of Child and Adolescent Psychiatry, 31*, 197–203.

Pliszka, S. R., Browne, R. G., Olvera, R. L., & Wynne, S. K. (2000). A double-blind, placebo-controlled study of Adderall and methylphenidate in the treatment of attention deficit hyperactivity disorder. *Journal of the American Academy of Child and Adolescent Psychiatry, 39*, 619–626.

Plomin, R. (1994). *Genetics and experience: The interplay between nature and nurture.* Thousand Oaks, CA: Sage.

Pollack, M. H., Otto, M. W., Sabatino, S., Majcher, D., Worthington, J. J., McArdle, E. t., & Rosenbaum, J. F. (1996). Relationship of childhood anxiety to adult panic disorder: Correlates and influence on course. *American Journal of Psychiatry, 153*, 376–381.

Pool, D., Bloom, W., Mielke, D. H., Roniger, J. J., & Gallant, D. M. (1976). A controlled evaluation of loxitane in seventy-five adolescent schizophrenic patients. *Current Therapeutic Research, 19*, 99–104.

Porrino, L. J., Rapoport, J. L., Behar, D., Ismond, D. R., & Bunney, W. E. J. (1983). A naturalistic assessment of the motor activity of hyperactive boys: II. Stimulant drug effects. *Archives of General Psychiatry, 40*, 688–693.

Power, C., Higgins, A., & Kohlberg, L. (1989). *Lawrence Kohlberg's approach to moral education.* New York: Columbia University Press.

Powers, S. W., & Roberts, M. W. (1995). Simulation training with parents of oppositional children: Preliminary findings. *Journal of Clinical Child Psychology, 24*, 89–97.

Prendergast, M., Taylor, E., Rapaport, J. L., Bartko, J., Donnelly, M., Zametkin, A., Ahearn, M. B., Dunn, G., & Wieselberg, H. M. (1988). The diagnosis of childhood hyperactivity: A US-UK cross-sectional study of DSM-III and ICD-9. *Journal of Child Psychology and Psychiatry, 29*, 289–300.

Preskorn, S. H., Weller, E. B., Hughes, C. W., Weller, R. A., & Bolte, K. (1987). Depression in prepubertal children: Dexamethasone nonsuppression predicts differential response to imipramine vs. placebo. *Psychopharmacology Bulletin, 23*, 128–133.

Prien, R. R., & Potter, W. Z. (1990). NIMH Workshop on Treatment of Bipolar Disorders. *Psychopharmacology Bulletin, 26*, 409–427.

Prinz, R. J., Blechman, E. A., & Dumas, J. E. (1994). An evaluation of peer coping-skills training for childhood aggression. *Journal of Clinical Child Psychology, 23*, 193–203.

Prinz, R. J., & Miller, G. E. (1994). Family-based treatment for childhood antisocial behavior: Experimental influences on dropout and engagement. *Journal of Consulting and Clinical Psychology, 52*, 645–650.

Prior, M., Smart, D., Sanson, A., & Oberklaid, F. (1999). Relationships between learning difficulties and psychological problems in preadolescent children from a longitudinal sample. *Journal of the American Academy of Child and Adolescent Psychiatry, 38*, 429–436.

Pronovost, J., Cote, L., & Ross, C. (1990). Epidemiological study of suicidal behaviour among secondary-school students. *Canada's Mental Health, 38*, 9–14.

Pryor, T., McGilley, B., & Roach, N. E. (1990). Psychopharmacology and eating disorders: Dawning of a new age. *Psychiatric Annals, 20*, 711–722.

Puig-Antich, J., Perel, J. M., Lupatkin, W., Chambers, W. J., Tabrizi, M. A., King, J., Goetz, R., Davies, M., & Stiller, R. L. (1987). Imipramine in prepubertal major depressive disorders. *Archives of General Psychiatry, 44*, 81–89.

Pulkkinen, L. (1996). Proactive and reactive aggression in early adolescence as precursors to anti- and prosocial behaviors in young adults. *Aggressive Behavior, 22*, 241–257.

Puura, K., Almqvist, F., Tamminen, T., Piha, J., Kumpulainen, K., Rasanen, E., Moilanen, I., & Koivisto, A.-M. (1998). Children with symptoms of depression: What do adults see? *Journal of Child Psychology and Psychiatry, 39*, 577–585.

Pyle, R. L., Halvorson, P. A., Neuman, P. A., & Mitchell, J. E. (1986). The increasing prevalence of bulimia in freshman college students. *International Journal of Eating Disorders, 5*, 631–647.

Quay, H. C., & LaGreca, A. M. (1986). Disorders of anxiety, withdrawal, and dysphoria. In H. C. Quay & J. S. Werry (Eds.), *Psychopathological disorders of childhood* (3rd ed., pp. 111–155). New York: Wiley.

Quiason, N., Ward, D., & Kitchen, T. (1991). Buspirone for aggression. *Journal of the American Academy of Child and Adolescent Psychiatry, 30*, 1026.

Quintana, H., Birmaher, B., Stedge, D., Lennon, S., Freed, J., Bridge, J., & Greenhill, L. (1995). Use of methylphenidate in the treatment of children with autistic disorder. *Journal of Autism and Developmental Disorders, 25*, 283–294.

Quinton, D., Gulliver, L., & Rutter, M. (1995). A 15–20-year follow-up of adult psychiatric patients: Psychiatric disorder and social functioning. *British Journal of Psychiatry, 167*, 315–323.

Rahim, S. I. A., & Cederblad, M. (1984). Effects of rapid urbanization on child behaviour and health in a part of Khartoum, Sudan. *Journal of Child Psychology and Psychiatry, 24*, 629–641.

Rainwater, N., Sweet, A. A., Elliott, L., & Bowers, M. (1988). Systematic desensitization in the treatment of needle phobias for children with diabetes. *Child and Family Behavior Therapy, 10*, 19–31.

Rao, U., Hammen, C., & Daley, S. E. (1999). Continuity of depression during the transition to adulthood: A 5-year longitudinal study of young women. *Journal of the American Academy of Child and Adolescent Psychiatry, 38*, 908–915.

Rao, U., Ryan, N. D., Birmaher, B., Dahl, R. E., Williamson, D. E., Kaufman, J., Rao, R., & Nelson, B. (1995). Unipolar depression in adolescents: Clinical outcome in adulthood. *Journal of the American Academy of Child and Adolescent Psychiatry, 34*, 566–578.

Rapport, M. D., Carlson, G. A., Kelly, K. L., & Pataki, C. (1993). Methylphenidate and desipramine in hospitalized children: I. Separate and combined effects on cognitive function. *Journal of the American Acadamy of Child and Adolescent Psychiatry, 32*, 333.

Rapport, M. D., Denney, C., DuPaul, G. J., & Gardner, M. J. (1994). Attention deficit disorder and methylphenidate: Normalization rates, clinical effectiveness, and response prediction in 76 children. *Journal of the American Academy of Child and Adolescent Psychiatry, 33*, 882–893.

Rastam, M. (1992). Anorexia nervosa in 51 Swedish adolescents: Premorbid problems and comorbidity. *Journal of the American Academy of Child and Adolescent Psychiatry, 31*, 819–829.

Rastam, M., & Gillberg, C. (1992). Background factors in anorexia nervosa: A controlled study of 51 teenage cases including a population sample. *European Child and Adolescent Psychiatry, 1*, 54–65.

Ratey, J., Sovner, R., Parks, A., & Rogentine, K. (1991). Buspirone treatment of aggression and anxiety in mentally retarded patients: A multiple baseline, placebo lead-in study. *Journal of Clinical Psychology, 52*, 159–162.

Realmuto, G. M., Erickson, W. D., Yellin, A. M., Hopwod, J. H., & Greenberg, L. M. (1984). Clinical comparison of thiothixene and thioridazine in schizophrenic adolescents. *American Journal of Psychiatry, 141*, 440–442.

Reddy, L. A., & Pfeiffer, S. I. (1997). Effectiveness of treatment foster care with children and adolescents: A review of outcome studies. *Journal of the American Academy of Child and Adolescent Psychiatry, 36*, 581–588.

Rehm, L. P., Kaslow, N. J., Rabin, A. S., & Willard, R. (1984). *Outcome of self-control behavior therapy programs for depression with cognitive, behavioral and combined targets.* Unpublished manuscript.

Reid, J. B. (1993). Prevention of conduct disorder before and after school entry: Relating interventions to developmental findings. *Development and Psychopathology, 5*, 243–262.

Reid, J. G., Hinojosa Rivera, G., & Lorber, R. (1980). *A social learning approach to the outpatient treatment of children who steal.* Unpublished manuscript, Oregon Social Learning Center, Eugene, OR.

Reinecke, M. A., Ryan, N. E., & DuBois, D. L. (1998). Cognitive-behavioral therapy of depression and depressive symptoms during adolescence: A review and meta-analysis. *Journal of the American Academy of Child and Adolescent Psychiatry, 37*, 26–34.

Reiss, D., Hetherington, E. M., Plomin, R., Howe, G. W., Simmens, S. J., Henderson, S. H., O'Connor, T. J., Bussell, D. A., Anderson, E. R., & Law, T. (1995). Genetic questions for environmental studies: Differential parenting and psychopathology in adolescence. *Archives of General Psychiatry, 52*, 925–936.

Reitman, D., Hummel, R., Franz, D. Z., & Gross, A. M. (1998). A review of methods and instruments for assessing externalizing disorders: Theoretical and practical considerations in rendering a diagnosis. *Clinical Psychology Review, 18*, 555–584.

Remshmidt, H., Schulze, E., & Martin, M. (1994). An open trial of clozapine in thirty-six adolescents with schizophrenia. *Journal of Child and Adolescent Psychopharmacology, 4*, 31–41.

Renaud, J., Birmaher, B., Wassick, S. C., & Bridge, J. (1999a). Use of selective serotonin reuptake inhibitors for the treatment of childhood panic disorder: A pilot study. *Journal of Child and Adolescent Psychopharmacology, 9*, 73–83.

Renaud, J., Brent, D. A., Baugher, M., Birmaher, B., Kolko, D., & Bridge, J. (1998). Rapid response to psychosocial treatments for adolescent depression: A two-year follow-up. *Journal of the American Academy of Child and Adolescent Psychiatry, 37*, 1184–1190.

Renaud, J., Brent, D. A., Birmaher, B., Chiappetta, L., & Bridge, J. (1999b). Suicide in adolescents with disruptive disorders. *Journal of the American Academy of Child and Adolescent Psychiatry, 38*, 846–851.

Renik, O. (1993). Analytic interaction: Conceptualizing technique in the light of the analyst's irreducible subjectivity. *Psychoanalytic Quarterly, 62*, 553–571.

Renouf, A. G., & Kovacs, M. (1994). Concordance between mothers' reports and children's self-reports of depressive symptoms: A longitudinal study. *Journal of the American Academy of Child and Adolescent Psychiatry, 33*, 208–216.

Rescorla, L., & Schwartz, E. (1990). Outcome of toddlers with specific expressive language delay. *Applied Psycholinguistics, 11*, 393–407.

Rey, J. M., Denshire, E., Wever, C., & Apollonov, I. (1998). Three-year outcome of disruptive adolescents treated in a day programme. *European Child and Adolescent Psychiatry, 7*, 42–48.

Rey, J. M., Singh, M., Hung, S., Dossetor, D. R., Newman, L., Plapp, J. M., & Bird, K. D. (1997). A global scale to measure the quality of the family environment. *Archives of General Psychiatry, 54*, 817–822.

Reynolds, D., Sammons, P., Stoll, L., Barber, M., & Hillman, J. (1996). School effectiveness and school improvement in the United Kingdom. *School Effectiveness and School Improvement, 7*, 133–158.

Reynolds, W. M., & Coats, K. I. (1986). A comparison of cognitive-behavioral therapy and relaxation training for the treatment of depression in adolescents. *Journal of Consulting and Clinical Psychology, 54*, 653–660.

Ribner, S. (1978). The effects of special class placement on the self-concept of exceptional children. *Journal of Learning Disabilities, 11*, 319–323.

Richardson, E., Kupietz, S. S., Winsberg, B. G., Maitinsky, S., & Mendell, N. (1988). Effects of methylphenidate dosage in hyperactive reading-disabled children: II. Reading achievement. *Journal of the American Academy of Child and Adolescent Psychiatry, 27*, 78–87.

Richardson, M. A., Haugland, G., & Craig, T. J. (1991). Neuroleptic use, parkinsonian symptoms, tardive dyskinesia and associated factors in child and adolescent psychiatric patients. *American Journal of Psychiatry, 148*, 1322–1328.

Richer, J., & Zappella, M. (1989). Changing social behavior: The plus of holding. *Communication, 23*, 35–39.

Richman, L. C., & Eliason, M. J. (1992). Disorders of communications: Developmental language disorders and cleft palate. In C. E. Walker & M. C. Roberts (Eds.), *Handbook of clinical child psychology* (pp. 537–552). New York: Wiley.

Richman, N., Stevenson, J., & Graham, P. J. (1982). *Pre-school to school: A behavioural study.* London: Academic Press.

Richman, N., Stevenson, J. E., & Graham, P. J. (1975). Prevalence of behaviour problems in 3 year old children: An epidemiological study in a London borough. *Journal of Child Psychology and Psychiatry, 16*, 277–287.

Richters, J. E., Arnold, L. E., Jensen, P. S., Abikoff, H., Conners, K., Greenhill, L. L., Hechtman, L., Hinshaw, S. P., W.E., P., & Swanson, J. M. (1995). NIMH Collaborative Multisite Multimodal Treatment Study of Children with ADHD: I. Background and rationale. *Journal of the American Academy of Child and Adolescent Psychiatry, 34*, 987–1000.

Riddle, M. A., Bernstein, G. A., Cook, E. H., Leonard, H. L., March, J. S., & Swanson, J. M. (1999). Anxiolytics, adrenergic agents and naltrexone. *Journal of the American Academy of Child and Adolescent Psychiatry, 38,* 546–556.

Riddle, M. A., Hardin, M., Cho, S. C., Woolston, J. L., & Leckman, J. F. (1988a). Desipramine treatment of boys with attention deficit disorder and tics: Preliminary clinical experience. *Journal of the American Academy of Child and Adolescent Psychiatry, 27,* 811–814.

Riddle, M. A., Hardin, M. T., & King, R. A. (1990). Fluoxetine treatment of children and adolescents with Tourette's and obsessive compulsive disorders: Preliminary clinical experience. *Journal of the American Academy of Child and Adolescent Psychiatry, 29,* 45–48.

Riddle, M. A., Hardin, M. T., Towbin, K. E., Leckman, J. F., & Cohen, D. J. (1987). Tardive dyskinesia following haloperidol treatment for Tourette's syndrome [letter]. *Archives of General Psychiatry, 44,* 98–99.

Riddle, M. A., King, R., Hardin, M., & Scahill, L. (1990/91). Behavioral side effects of fluoxetine in children and adolescents. *Journal of Child and Adolescent Psychopharmacology, 1,* 193–198.

Riddle, M. A., Leckman, J. F., Hardin, M. T., Anderson, G. M., & Cohen, D. J. (1988b). Fluoxetine treatment of obsessions and compulsions in patients with Tourette's syndrome [letter]. *American Journal of Psychiatry, 145,* 1173–1174.

Riddle, M. A., Reeve, E. A., Yaryura-Tobias, J. A., Yang, H. M., Claghorn, J. L., Gaffney, G., Greist, J. H., Holland, D., McConville, B. J., Pigott, T., & Walkup, J. T. (2001). Fluvoxamine for children and adolescents with obsessive–compulsive disorder: A randomized, controlled, multicenter trial. *Journal of the American Academy of Child and Adolescent Psychiatry, 40,* 222–229.

Riddle, M. A., Scahill, L., King, R. A., Hardin, M. T., Anderson, G. M., Ort, S. I., Smith, J. C., Leckman, J. F., & Cohen, D. J. (1992). Double-blind cross-over trial of fluoxetine and placebo in children and adolescents with obsessive–compulsive disorder. *Journal of the American Academy of Child and Adolescent Psychiatry, 31,* 1062–1069.

Rifkin, A., Doddi, S., & Dicker, R. (1989, May). *Lithium in adolescence with conduct disorder.* Paper presented at the Annual New Clinical Drug Evaluation Unit Meeting, Key Biscayne, FL.

Rifkin, A., Karajgi, B., Dicker, R., Perl, E., Boppana, V., Hasan, N., & Pollack, S. (1997). Lithium treatment of conduct disorders in adolescents. *American Journal of Psychiatry, 154,* 554–555.

Riggs, P. D., Leon, S. L., Mikulich, S. K., & Pottle, L. C. (1998). An open trial of bupropion for ADHD in adolescents with substance use disorders and conduct disorder. *Journal of the American Academy of Child and Adolescent Psychiatry, 37,* 1271–1278.

Rimland, B., & Edelson, S. M. (1995). Brief report: A pilot study of auditory integration training in autism. *Journal of Autism and Developmental Disorders, 25,* 61–70.

Ritter, B. (1968). The group desensitisation of children's snake phobias using vicarious and contact desensitisation procedures. *Behaviour Research and Therapy, 6,* 1–6.

Ritvo, E. R., Freeman, B. J., Geller, E., & Yuwiler, A. (1983). Effects of fenfluramine on 14 outpatients with the syndrome of autism. *Journal of the American Academy of Child Psychiatry, 22,* 549–558.

Ritvo, E. R., Freeman, B. J., Yuwiler, A., Geller, E., Schroth, P., Yokota, A., Mason-Brothers, A., August, G. J., Klykylo, W., & Leventhal, B. (1986). Fenfluramine treatment of autism: UCLA collaborative study of 81 patients at nine medical centers. *Psychopharmacology Bulletin, 22,* 133–140.

Ritvo, E. R., Yuwiler, A., Geller, E., Kales, A., Rashkis, S., Schicor, A., Plotkin, S., Axelrod, R., & Howard, C. (1971). Effects of L-dopa in autism. *Journal of Autism and Childhood Schizophrenia, 1,* 190–205.

Rivinus, T. M., Jamison, D. L., & Graham, P. J. (1975). Childhood organic neurological disease presenting as psychiatric disorder. *Archives of Disease in Childhood, 50,* 115–119.

Robbins, M. S., Alexander, J. F., Newell, R. M., & Turner, C. W. (1996). The immediate effect of reframing on client attitude in family therapy. *Journal of Family Psychology, 10,* 28–34.

Robbins, M. S., Alexander, J. F., & Turner, C. W. (2000). Disrupting defensive family interactions in family therapy with delinquent adolescents. *Journal of Family Psychology, 14,* 688–701.

Robertson, M. (1989). The Gilles de la Tourette syndrome: The current status. *British Journal of Psychiatry, 154,* 147–169.

Robertson, M., & Eapen, V. (1992). Pharmacologic controversy of CNS stimulants in Gilles de la Tourette's syndrome. *Clinical Neuropharmacology, 15,* 408–425.

Robin, A. L., Bedway, M., Siegel, P. T., & Gilroy, M. (1996). Therapy for adolescent anorexia nervosa: Addressing cognitions, feelings, and the family's role. In E. D. Hibbs & P. S. Jensen (Eds.), *Psychosocial treatments for child and adolescent disorders: Empirically based strategies for clinical practice* (pp. 239–259). Washington, DC: American Psychological Association.

Robin, A. L., Gilroy, M., & Dennis, A. B. (1998). Treatment of eating disorders in children and adolescents. *Clinical Psychology Review, 18,* 421–446.

Robin, A. L., Siegel, P. T., Koepke, T., Moye, A., & Tice, S. (1994). Family therapy versus individual therapy for adolescent females with anorexia nervosa. *Journal of Developmental and Behavioral Pediatrics, 15,* 111–116.

Robin, A. L., Siegel, P. T., & Moye, A. (1995). Family versus individual therapy for anorexia: Impact on family conflict. *International Journal of Eating Disorders, 17,* 313–322.

Robin, A. L., Siegel, P. T., Moye, A. W., Gilroy, M., Baker-Dennis, A., & Sikard, A. (1999). A controlled comparison of family versus individual therapy for adolescents with anorexia nervosa. *Journal of the American Academy of Child and Adolescent Psychiatry, 38,* 1482–1489.

Robins, L. N., Locke, B. Z., & Regier, D. A. (1991). An overview of psychiatric disorders in America. In L. N. Robins & D. A. Regier (Eds.), *Psychiatric disorders in America: The Epidemiologic Catchment Area study* (pp. 328–366). New York: Free Press.

Robins, L. N., & Price, R. K. (1991). Adult disorders predicted by childhood conduct problems: Results from the NIMH Epidemiologic Catchment Area project. *Psychiatry, 54,* 116–132.

Robinson, L. A., Berman, J. S., & Neimeyer, R. A. (1990). Psychotherapy for the treatment of depression: A comprehensive review of controlled outcome research. *Psychological Bulletin, 108,* 30–49.

Robinson, T. R., Smith, S. W., Miller, M. D., & Brownell, M. T. (1999). Cognitive behavior modification of hyperactivity–impulsivity and aggression: A meta-analysis of school-based studies. *Journal of Educational Psychology, 91,* 195–203.

Robson, P. (1996). Young people and illegal drugs. In A. Macfarlane (Ed.), *Adolescent medicine* (pp. 131–138). London: Royal College of Physicians.

Rogler, L. H. (1989). The meaning of culturally sensitive research in mental health. *American Journal of Psychiatry, 146,* 296–303.

Rohde, P., Lewinsohn, P. M., & Seeley, J. R. (1994). Are adolescents changed by an episode of major depression? *Journal of the American Academy of Child and Adolescent Psychiatry, 33,* 1289–1298.

Roker, D. (1995). *Young people and drugs in Surrey.* Brighton: Trust for the Study of Adolescence.

Rosen, H. S., & Rosen, L. A. (1983). Eliminating stealing: Use of stimulus control with an elementary student. *Behavior Modification, 7,* 56–63.

Rosen, J., & Leitenberg, H. (1982). Bulimia nervosa: Treatment with exposure and response prevention. *Behavior Therapy, 13,* 117–124.

Rosen, L. A., Gabardi, L., Miller, C. D., & Miller, L. (1990). Home-based treatment of disruptive junior high school students: An analysis of the differential effects of positive and negative consequences. *Behavioral Disorders, 15,* 227–232.

Rosen, L. N., Rosenthal, N. E., Van Dusen, P. H., Dunner, D. L., & Fieve, R. R. (1983). Age at onset and number of psychotic symptoms in bipolar I and schizoaffective disorder. *American Journal of Psychiatry, 140,* 1523–1524.

Rosenberg, D. R., Stewart, C. M., Fitzgerald, K. D., Tawile, V., & Carroll, E. (1999). Paroxetine open-label treatment of pediatric outpatients with obsessive–compulsive disorder. *Journal of the American Academy of Child and Adolescent Psychiatry, 38,* 1180–1185.

Rosenthal, M. (1989). The therapeutic community: Exploring the boundaries. *British Journal of Addiction, 84,* 141–150.

Rosenthal, R. (1995). Writing meta-analytic reviews. *Psychological Bulletin, 118,* 183–192.

Rosenthal, R. (1996). Progress in clinical psychology: Is there any? *Clinical Psychology: Science and Practice, 2,* 133–150.

Ross, M. S., & Muldofsky, H. (1978). A comparison of pimozide and haloperidol in the treatment of Gilles de la Tourette's syndrome. *American Journal of Psychiatry, 1,* 107–111.

Rosselló, J., & Bernal, G. (1999). The efficacy of cognitive-behavioral and interpersonal treatments for depression in Puerto Rican adolescents. *Journal of Consulting and Clinical Psychology, 67,* 734–745.

Roth, A., & Fonagy, P. (1996). *What works for whom? A critical review of psychotherapy research.* New York: Guilford Press.

Roth, A., Fonagy, P., & Parry, G. (1996). Psychotherapy research, funding, and evidence-based practice. In A. Roth & P. Fonagy (Eds.), *What works for whom? A critical review of psychotherapy research* (pp. 37–56). New York: Guilford Press.

Rotheram-Borus, M., Piacentini, J., Van Rossem, R., Graae, F., Cantwell, C., Castro-Blanco, D., & Feldman, J. (1999). Treatment adherence among Latina female adolescent suicide attempters. *Suicide and Life-Threatening Behavior, 29,* 319–331.

Rotheram-Borus, M. J., Piacentini, J., Van Rossem, R., Graae, F., Cantwell, C., Castro-Blanco, D., Miller, S., & Feldman, J. (1996). Enhancing treatment adherence with a specialized emergency room program for adolescent suicide attempters. *Journal of the American Academy of Child and Adolescent Psychiatry, 35,* 654–663.

Rourke, B. P., & Del Dotto, J. E. (1992). Learning disabilities: A neuropsychological perspective. In C. E. Walker & M. C. Roberts (Eds.), *Handbook of clinical child psychology* (pp. 511–536). New York: Wiley.

Routh, C. P., Hill, J. W., Steele, H., Elliott, C. E., & Dewey, M. E. (1995). Maternal attachment status, psychosocial stressor and problem behaviour: Follow-up after parent training course for conduct disorder. *Journal of Child Psychology and Psychiatry, 36,* 1179–1198.

Rowe, K. S., & Rowe, K. J. (1994). Synthetic food coloring and behavior: A dose response effect in a double-blind, placebo-controlled, repeated-measures study. *Journal of Pediatrics, 125,* 691–698.

Rowland, M. D., Henggeler, S., Pickrel, S., & Edwards, J. (1999). *MST versus psychiatric hospitalization: Clinical outcomes post-treatment.* Paper presented at the 46th Annual Meeting of the American Academy of Child and Adolescent Psychiatry, Chicago.

Rubin, D. H., Leventhal, J. M., Sadock, R. T., Letovsky, E., Schottland, P., Clemente, I., & McCarthy, P. (1986). Educational intervention by computer in childhood asthma: A randomized clinical trial testing the use of a new teaching intervention in childhood asthma. *Pediatrics, 77,* 1–10.

Rubin, K. H., & Mills, R. S. L. (1988). The many faces of social isolation in childhood. *Journal of Consulting and Clinical Psychology, 6,* 916–924.

Ruma, P. R., Burke, R. V., & Thompson, R. W. (1996). Group parent training: Is it effective for children of all ages? *Behavior Therapy, 27,* 159–169.

Rund, B. R., Moe, L., Sollien, T., Fjell, A., Borchgrevink, T., Hallert, M., & Naess, P. O. (1994). The Psychosis Project: Outcome and cost-effectiveness of a psychoeducational programme for schizophrenic adolescents. *Acta Psychiatrica Scandinavica, 89,* 211–218.

Russell, A., Bott, L., & Sammons, C. (1989). The phenomenology of schizophrenia occurring in childhood. *Journal of the American Academy of Child and Adolescent Psychiatry, 28,* 399–407.

Russell, G. F. M. (1979). Bulimia nervosa: An ominous variant of anorexia nervosa. *Psychological Medicine, 9,* 429–448.

Russell, G. F. M., Szmukler, G., Dare, C., & Eisler, I. (1987). An evaluation of family therapy in anorexia nervosa and bulimia nervosa. *Archives of General Psychiatry, 44,* 1047–1056.

Russo, M. F., & Beidel, D. C. (1994). Comorbidity of childhood anxiety and externalizing disorders: Prevalence, associated characteristics, and validation issues. *Clinical Psychology Review, 14,* 199–221.

Rutter, M. (1967). A child's behaviour questionnaire for completion by teachers: preliminary findings. *Journal of Child Psychology and Psychiatry, 8,* 1–11.

Rutter, M. (1978a). Diagnosis and definition. In M. Rutter & E. Schopler (Eds.), *Autism: A reappraisal of concepts and treatment* (pp. 1–25). New York: Plenum Press.

Rutter, M. (1978b). Diagnosis and definitions of childhood autism. *Journal of Autism and Childhood Schizophrenia, 8,* 139–161.

Rutter, M. (1979). Protective factors in children's responses to stress and disadvantage. In M. W.

Kent & J. E. Rolf (Eds.), *Primary prevention of psychopathology: Vol.3: Social competence in children* (pp. 49–74). Hanover, NH: University Press of New England.

Rutter, M. (1981). Epidemiological/longitudinal strategies and causal research in child psychiatry. *Journal of the American Academy of Child Psychiatry, 20,* 513–544.

Rutter, M. (1985a). Family and school influences on behavioral development. *Journal of Child Psychology and Psychiatry, 26,* 349–368.

Rutter, M. (1985b). The treatment of autistic children. *Journal of Child Psychology and Psychiatry, 26,* 193–214.

Rutter, M. (1989). Isle of Wight revisited: Twenty-five years of child psychiatric epidemiology. *Journal of the American Academy of Child and Adolescent Psychiatry, 28,* 633–653.

Rutter, M. (1994). Beyond longitudinal data: Causes, consequences, changes, and continuity. *Journal of Consulting and Clinical Psychology, 62,* 928–940.

Rutter, M. (1997). Child psychiatric disorder: Measures, causal mechanisms, and interventions. *Archives of General Psychiatry, 54,* 785–789.

Rutter, M. (1998). Routes from research to clinical practice in child psychiatry: Retrospect and prospect. *Journal of Child Psychology and Psychiatry, 39,* 805–816.

Rutter, M. (1999). Psychosocial adversity and child psychopathology. *British Journal of Psychiatry, 174,* 480–493.

Rutter, M., Cox, A., Tupling, C., Berger, M., & Yule, W. (1975). Attainment and adjustment in two geographical areas: 1. The prevalence of psychiatric disorder. *British Journal of Psychiatry, 126,* 493–509.

Rutter, M., & Garmezy, N. (1983). Developmental psychopathology. In P. Mussen (Ed.), *Handbook of child psychology* (4th ed., pp. 775–911). New York: Wiley.

Rutter, M., & Giller, H. (1983). *Juvenile delinquency: Trends and perspectives.* Harmondsworth, Middlesex: Penguin.

Rutter, M., Giller, H., & Hagell, A. (1998). *Antisocial behaviour by young people.* Cambridge: Cambridge University Press.

Rutter, M., & Graham, P. (1968). The reliability and validity of the psychiatric assessment of the child: I. Interview with the child. *British Journal of Psychiatry, 114,* 563–579.

Rutter, M., Graham, P., & Yule, W. (1970a). *A neuropsychiatric study in childhood.* London: Heinemann/SIMP.

Rutter, M., Maughan, B., Mortimore, P., & Ouston, J. (with Smith, A.). (1979). *Fifteen thousand hours: Secondary schools and their effects on children.* London: Open Books.

Rutter, M., & Sandberg, S. (1985). Epidemiology of child psychiatric disorder: Methodological issues and some substantive findings. *Child Psychiatry and Human Development, 15,* 209–233.

Rutter, M., & Smith, D. J. (Eds.). (1995a). *Psychosocial disorders in young people. Time trends and their causes.* Chichester, UK: Wiley.

Rutter, M., & Smith, D. J. (1995b). Towards causal explanations of time trends in psychosocial disorders of young people. In D. J. Smith & M. Rutter (Eds.), *Psychosocial disorders in young people. Time trends and their causes* (pp. 782–808). Chichester: Wiley.

Rutter, M., Tizard, J., & Whitmore, K. (Eds.). (1970b). *Education, health and behaviour.* London: Longmans.

Rutter, M., Tizard, J., Yule, W., Graham, P., & Whitmore, K. (1976). Isle of Wight Studies 1964–1974. *Psychological Medicine, 6,* 313–332.

Ryan, N. D., Puig-Antich, J., Ambrosini, P., Rabinovich, H., Robinson, D., Nelson, B., Iyengar, S., & Twomey, J. (1987). The clinical picture of major depression in children and adolescents. *Archives of General Psychiatry, 44,* 854–861.

Sabbeth, B., & Leventhal, J. (1984). Marital adjustment to chronic childhood illness: A critique of the literature. *Pediatrics, 73,* 762–767.

Saccomani, L., Rizzo, P., & Nobili, L. (2000). Combined treatment with haloperidol and trazadone in patients with tic disorders. *Journal of Child and Adolescent Psychopharmacology, 10,* 307–310.

Sackett, D. L., Rosenberg, W. M., Gray, J. A. M., Haynes, R. B., & Richardson, W. S. (1996). Evidence based medicine: What it is and what it isn't. *British Medical Journal, 312,* 71–72.

Safer, D., & Krager, J. M. (1994). The increased rate of stimulant treatment for hyperactive/inattentive students in secondary schools. *Pediatrics, 94*, 462–464.

Safran, J. D., & Muran, J. C. (2000). *Negotiating the therapeutic alliance.* New York: Guilford Press.

Sallee, F. R. (1999, October). *Targets of pharmacotherapy in tic and obsessive–compulsive (OCD) disorder.* Paper presented at the 46th annual meeting of the American Academy of Child and Adolescent Psychiatry, Chicago.

Sallee, F. R., Kurlan, R., Goetz, C. G., Singer, H., Scahill, L., Law, G., Dittman, V. M., & Chappell, P. B. (2000). Ziprasidone treatment of children and adolescents with Tourette's syndrome: A pilot study. *Journal of the American Academy of Child and Adolescent Psychiatry, 39*, 292–299.

Sallee, R. F., Nesbitt, L., Jackson, C., Sine, L., & Sethuraman, G. (1997). Relative efficacy of haloperidol and pimozide in children and adolescents with Tourette's disorder. *American Journal of Psychiatry, 154*, 1057–1062.

Sallee, F. R., Sethuraman, G., & Rock, C. M. (1994). Effects of pimozide on cognition in children with Tourette syndrome: Interaction with comorbid attention deficit hyperactivity disorder. *Acta Psychiatrica Scandinavica, 90*, 4–9.

Sameroff, A. J. (1995). General systems theories and developmental psychopathology. In J. Cicchetti & D. J. Cohen (Eds.), *Developmental psychopathology: Vol 1. Theory and methods* (pp. 659–695). New York: Wiley.

Sameroff, A. J. (1998). Understanding the social context of early psychopathology. In J. Noshpitz (Ed.), *Handbook of child and adolescent psychiatry* (pp. 285–324). New York: Basic Books.

Sandberg, S. T. (1982). The overinclusiveness of the diagnosis of hyperkinetic syndrome. In M. Gittleman (Ed.), *Strategic interventions for hyperactive children* (pp. 8–38). Armonk, NY: M. E. Sharpe.

Sandberg, S. T., Rutter, M., & Taylor, E. (1978). Hyperkinetic disorder in psychiatric clinic attenders. *Developmental Medicine and Child Neurology, 20*, 279–299.

Sanders, A. F. (1983). Toward a model of stress and human performance. *Acta Psychologica, 53*, 61–97.

Sanders, M. R. (1982). The generalisation of parent responding to community settings: The effects of instructions, plus feedback, and self-management training. *Behavioural Psychotherapy, 10*, 273–287.

Sanders, M. R., & Glynn, T. (1981). Training parents in behavioral self-management: An analysis of generalisation and maintenance. *Journal of Applied Behavior Analysis, 14*, 223–237.

Sanders, M. R., Rebgetz, M., Morrison, M., Bor, W., Gordon, A., Dadds, M., & Shepherd, R. (1989). Cognitive-behavioral treatment of recurrent nonspecific abdominal pain in children: An analysis of generalization, maintenance, and side effects. *Journal of Consulting and Clinical Psychology, 57*, 294–300.

Sanders, M. R., Shepherd, R. W., Cleghorn, G., & Woolford, H. (1994). The treatment of recurrent abdominal pain in children: A controlled comparison of cognitive-behavioral family intervention and standard pediatric care. *Journal of Consulting and Clinical Psychology, 62*, 306–314.

Sandor, P., Musisi, S., Muldofsky, H., & Lang, A. (1990). Tourette syndrome: A follow-up study. *Journal of Clinical Psychopharmacology, 10*, 197–199.

Sanford, M., Szatmari, P., Spinner, M., Munroe-Blum, H., Jamieson, E., Walsh, C., & Jones, D. (1995). Predicting the one-year course of adolescent major depression. *Journal of the American Academy of Child and Adolescent Psychiatry, 34*, 1618–1628.

Sanford, M. N., Offord, D. R., Boyle, M. H., Peace, A., & Racine, Y. (1992). Ontario Child Health Study: Social and school impairments in children aged 6–16 years. *Journal of the American Academy of Child and Adolescent Psychiatry, 31*, 60–67.

Santiseban, D. A., Szapocznik, J., Perez-Vidal, A., Kurtines, W. M., Coatsworth, J. D., & LaPierre, A. (in preparation). *The efficacy of brief strategic/structural family therapy in modifying behavior problems and an exploration of the role that family functioning plays in behavior change.* Miami: University of Miami, Center of Family Studies.

Santor, D. A., & Kusumakar, V. (2001). Open trial of interpersonal therapy in adolescents with moderate to severe major depression: Effectiveness of novice IPT therapists. *Journal of the American Academy of Child and Adolescent Psychiatry, 40*, 236–240.

Satin, W., la-Greca, A. M., Zigo, M. A., & Skyler, J. S. (1989). Diabetes in adolescence: Effects of multifamily group intervention and parent simulation of diabetes. *Journal of Pediatric Psychology, 14*, 259–275.

Satterfield, J. H., Satterfield, B. T., & Cantwell, D. P. (1981). Three-year multimodality treatment study of 100 hyperactive boys. *Journal of Pediatrics, 98*, 650–655.

Satterfield, J. H., Satterfield, B. T., & Schell, A. M. (1987). Therapeutic interventions to prevent delinquency in hyperactive boys. *Journal of the American Academy of Child and Adolescent Psychiatry, 26*, 56–64.

Saunderson, T., Haynes, R., & Langford, I. H. (1998). Urban–rural variations in suicides and undetermined deaths in England and Wales. *Journal of Public Health Medicine, 20*, 261–267.

Sayger, T. V., Horne, A. M., & Glaser, B. A. (1993). Marital satisfaction and social learning family therapy for child conduct problems: Generalization of treatment effects. *Journal of Marital and Family Therapy, 19*, 393–402.

Sayger, T. V., Horne, A. M., Walker, J. M., & Passmore, J. L. (1988). Social learning family therapy with aggressive children: Treatment outcome and maintenance. *Journal of Family Psychology, 1*, 261–285.

Scarborough, H. S. (1984). Continuity between childhood dyslexia and adult reading. *British Journal of Psychology, 75*(3), 329–48.

Schachar, R. J., Rutter, M., & Smith, A. (1981). The characteristics of situationally and pervasively hyperactive children: Implications for syndrome definition. *Journal of Child Psychology and Psychiatry, 22*, 375–392.

Schachar, R. J., Tannock, R., & Logan, G. (1993). Inhibitory control, impulsiveness, and attention deficit hyperactivity disorder. *Clinical Psychology Review, 13*, 721–739.

Schachar, R. J., Taylor, E., Wieselberg, M., Thorley, G., & Rutter, M. (1987). Changes in family function and relationships in children who respond to methylphenidate. *Journal of the American Academy of Child and Adolescent Psychiatry, 26*, 728–732.

Schinke, P. P., Orlandi, M. A., & Cole, K. C. (1992). Boys and girls clubs in public housing developments: Prevention services for youth at risk. *Journal of Community Psychology, 1992*, 118–128.

Schleien, S. J., Mustonen, T., & Rynders, J. E. (1995). Participation of children with autism and nondisabled peers in a cooperatively structured community art program. *Journal of Autism and Developmental Disorders, 25*, 397–413.

Schleifer, N., Weiss, G., Cohen, N., Elmen, M., Cvejic, H., & Kruger, E. (1975). Hyperactivity in preschoolers and the effect of methylphenidate. *American Journal of Orthopsychiatry, 45*, 38–50.

Schlichter, K. J., & Horan, J. J. (1981). Effects of stress inoculation on the anger and aggression management skills of institutionalized juvenile delinquents. *Cognitive Therapy and Research, 5*, 359–365.

Schmidt, M., Trott, G., & Blanz, B. (1990). Psychiatry: A world perspective. In C. Stefanis, A. Rabavilas, & R. Soldatos (Eds.), *Psychiatry: A world perspective* (pp. 1100–1104). Amsterdam: Excerpta Medica.

Schmidt, S. E., Liddle, H. A., & Dakof, G. A. (1996). Changes in parenting practices and adolescent drug abuse during multidimensional family therapy. *Journal of Family Psychology, 10*, 12–27.

Schmidt, U., Hodes, M., & Treasure, J. (1992). Early onset bulimia nervosa—Who is at risk? *Psychological Medicine, 22*, 623–628.

Schmidtke, A., Bille-Brahe, U., DeLeo, D., Kerkhof, A., Bjerke, T., Crepet, P., Haring, C., Hawton, K., Lonnqvist, J., Michel, K., Pommereau, X., Querejeta, I., Phillipe, I., Salander-Renberg, E., Temesvary, B., Wasserman, D., Fricke, S., Weinacker, B., & Sampaio-Faria, J. G. (1996). Attempted suicide in Europe: Rates, trends and sociodemographic characteristics of suicide attempters during the period 1989–1992. Results of the WHO/EURO Multicentre Study on Parasuicide. *Acta Psychiatrica Scandinavica, 93*, 327–338.

Schneider, T. (1999). *Measuring adaptation in middle childhood: The development of the Hampstead Child Adaptation Measure*. London: UCL.

Schools Health Education Unit. (1994). *Young people and illegal drugs 1989–1995: Facts and predictions*. Exeter: University of Exeter.

Schopler, E., Mesibov, G. B., & Hearsey, K. (1995). Structured teaching in the TEACCH system. In E. Schopler & G. B. Mesibov (Eds.), *Learning and cognition in autism: Current issues in autism* (pp. 243–268). New York: Plenum Press.

Schreier, H. A. (1998). Risperidone for young children with mood disorders and aggressive behavior. *Journal of Child and Adolescent Psychopharmacology, 8,* 49–59.

Schroeder, C. S., & Gordon, B. N. (1991). *Assessment and treatment of childhood problems: A clinician's guide.* New York: Guilford Press.

Schuhmann, E. M., Foote, R. C., Eyberg, S. M., Boggs, S. R., & Algina, J. (1998). Efficacy of parent–child interaction therapy: Interim report of a randomized trial with short-term maintenance. *Journal of Clinical Child Psychology, 27,* 34–45.

Schumacher, M., & Kurz, G. A. (2000). *The 8% solution: Preventing serious, repeat juvenile crime.* Thousand Oaks, CA: Sage.

Schvela, T. T., Mandoki, M. W., & Sumner, G. S. (1994). Clonidine therapy for comorbid attention deficit hyperactivity disorder and conduct disorder: Preliminary findings in a children's inpatient unit. *Southern Medical Journal, 87,* 692–695.

Schwartz, R. C., Barrett, M. J., & Saba, G. (1985). Family therapy for bulimia. In D. M. Garner & P. E. Garfinkel (Eds.), *Handbook of psychotherapy for anorexia nervosa and bulimia* (pp. 280–307). New York: Guilford Press.

Scott, S., Spender, Q., Doolan, M., Jacobs, B., & Aspland, H. (2001). Multicentre controlled trial of parenting groups for child antisocial behaviour in clinical practice. *British Medical Journal, 323*(7306), 194–198.

Seeger, T. F., Seymour, P. A., Schmidt, A. W., Zorn, S. H., Schulz, D. W., Lebel, L. A., McLean, S., Guanowsky, V., Howard, H. R., Lowe, J. A., & Heym, J. (1995). Ziprasidone (CP-88,059): A new antipsychotic with combined dopamine and serotonin receptor antagonist activity. *Journal of Pharmacology and Experimental Therapeutics, 275,* 101–113.

Sellar, C., Hawton, K., & Goldacre, M. J. (1990). Self-poisoning in adolescents: Hospital admissions and deaths in the Oxford region 1980–85. *British Journal of Psychiatry, 156,* 866–870.

Semrud-Clikeman, M., & Hynd, G. W. (1990). Right hemispheric dysfunction in nonverbal learning disabilities: Social, academic, and adaptive functioning in adults and children. *Psychological Bulletin, 107,* 196–209.

Serbin, L. A., Peters, P. L., McAffer, V., & Schwartzman, A. E. (1991). Childhood aggression and withdrawal as predictors of adolescent pregnancy, early parenthood, and environmental risk for the next generation. *Canadian Journal of Behavioural Science, 23,* 318–331.

Serketich, W. J., & Dumas, J. E. (1996). The effectiveness of behavioral parent training to modify antisocial behavior in children: A meta-analysis. *Behavior Therapy, 27,* 171–186.

Seymour, F. W., & Epston, D. (1989). An approach to childhood stealing with evaluation of 45 cases. *Australian and New Zealand Journal of Family Therapy, 10,* 137–143.

Shadish, W. R., Montgomery, L. M., Wilson, P., Wilson, M. R., Bright, I., & Okwumabua, T. (1993). Effects of family and marital psychotherapies: A meta-analysis. *Journal of Consulting and Clinical Psychology, 61,* 992–1002.

Shadish, W. R. J., & Sweeney, R. B. (1991). Mediators and moderators in meta-analysis: There's a reason we don't let dodo birds tell us which psychotherapies should have prizes. *Journal of Consulting and Clinical Psychology, 59,* 883–893.

Shaffer, D. (1974). Suicide in childhood and early adolescence. *Journal of Child Psychology and Psychiatry, 15,* 275–291.

Shaffer, D., Fisher, P., Duclan, M., Davies, M., Piacentini, J., Schwab-Stone, M., Lahey, B. B., Bourdon, K., Jensen, P., Bird, H., Canino, G., & Regier, D. (1996). The NIMH Diagnostic Interview Schedule for Children Version 2.3 (DISC 2.3): Description, acceptability, prevalence rates, and performances in the MECA study. *Journal of American Academy of Child and Adolescent Psychiatry, 35,* 865–877.

Shaffer, D., Garland, A., Gould, M., Fisher, P., & Trautman, P. (1988). Preventing teenage suicide: A critical review. *Journal of the American Academy of Child and Adolescent Psychiatry, 27,* 675–687.

Shaffer, D., Gould, M. S., & Brasic, J. A. (1983). Children's Global Assessment Scale (CGAS). *Archives of General Psychiatry, 40,* 1228–1231.

Shaffer, D., & Piacentini, J. (1994). Suicide and attempted suicide. In M. Rutter, E. Taylor, & L. Herzov (Eds.), *Child and adolescent psychiatry: Modern approaches* (3 ed., pp. 407–440). Oxford: Blackwell Scientific.

Shafii, M., Carrigan, S., Whittinghill, J. R., & Derrick, A. M. (1985). Psychological autopsy of completed suicide of children and adolescents. *American Journal of Psychiatry, 142,* 1061–1064.

Shafii, M., Steltz-Lenarsky, J., Derrick, A. M., Beckner, C., & Whittinghill, J. R. (1988). Comorbidity of mental disorders in the post-mortem diagnosis of completed suicide in children and adolescents. *Journal of Affective Disorders, 15,* 227–233.

Shapiro, A. K., & Shapiro, E. (1982a). Clinical efficacy of haloperidol, pimozide, penfluridol and clonidine in the treatment of Tourette syndrome. In A. J. Friedhoff & T. N. Chase (Eds.), *Gilles de la Tourette syndrome: Advances in neurology, 35* (pp. 383–386). New York: Raven Press.

Shapiro, A. K., & Shapiro, E. (1984). Controlled study of pimozide vs. placebo in Tourette's syndrome. *Journal of the American Academy of Child and Adolescent Psychiatry, 23,* 161–173.

Shapiro, A. K., Shapiro, E. S., Young, J. G., & Feinberg, T. E. (1988). *Gilles de la Tourette syndrome* (2nd ed.). New York: Raven Press.

Shapiro, D., & Shapiro, D. (1982b). Meta-analysis of comparative outcome studies: A replication and refinement. *Psychological Bulletin, 92,* 581–604.

Shapiro, E., Shapiro, A. K., Fulop, G. K., Hubbard, M., Mandeli, J., Nordlie, J., & Phillips, R. A. (1989). Controlled study of haloperidol, pimozide and placebo for the treatment of Gilles de la Tourette's syndrome. *Archives of General Psychiatry, 46,* 722–730.

Sharfstein, S. S., & Clark, H. W. (1978). Economics and the chronic mental patient. *Schizophrenia Bulletin, 4,* 399–414.

Sharpe, M., Archard, L., Banatvala, J., Borysiewicz, L. K., Clare, A. W., David, A., Edwards, R. H., Hawton, K. E., Lambert, H. P., & Lane, R. J. (1991). Chronic fatigue syndrome: Guidelines for research. *Journal of the Royal Society of Medicine, 84,* 118–121.

Sharpe, M., Hawton, K., Simkin, S., Surawy, C., Hackmann, A., Klimes, I., Peto, T., Warrell, D., & Seagroatt, V. (1996). Cognitive behaviour therapy for the chronic fatigue syndrome: A randomised controlled trial. *British Medical Journal, 312,* 22–26.

Shaw, D. S., Gilliom, M., Ingoldsby, E. M., & Schonberg, M. A. (2001, April 19–22). *Developmental trajectories of early conduct problems from ages 2 to 10: Symposium on developmental trajectories in antisocial behavior from infancy to adolescence.* Paper presented at the biennial meeting of the Society for Research in Child Development, Minneapolis, MN.

Shaywitz, B. A., Fletcher, J. M., Holahan, J. M., & Shaywitz, S. E. (1992a). Discrepancy compared to low achievement definitions of reading disability: Results from the Connecticut Longitudinal Study. *Journal of Learning Disabilities, 25,* 639–648.

Shaywitz, S. E., Escobar, M. D., Shaywitz, B. A., Fletcher, J. M., & Makuch, R. (1992b). Evidence that dyslexia may represent the lower tail of a normal distribution of reading ability. *New England Journal of Medicine, 326,* 145–150.

Shaywitz, S. E., Shaywitz, B. A., Fletcher, J. M., & Escobar, M. D. (1990). Prevalence of reading disability in boys and girls. Results of the Connecticut Longitudinal Study. *Journal of the American Medical Association, 264,* 998–1002.

Shedler, J., & Block, J. (1990). Adolescent drug use and psychological health: A longitudinal inquiry. *The American Psychologist, 45,* 612–630.

Sheeber, L. B., & Johnson, J. H. (1994). Evaluation of a temperament-focused, parent-training program. *Journal of Clinical Child Psychology, 23,* 249–259.

Shelden, R. G. (1999). *Detention diversion adequacy: An evaluation.* Washington, DC: Office of Juvenile Justice and Delinquency Prevention.

Sheldon, T. A., Song, F., & Davey-Smith, G. (1993). Critical appraisal of the medical literature: How to assess whether health care interventions do more good than harm. In M. F. Drummond & A. Maynard (Eds.), *Purchasing and providing cost effective health care* (pp. 31–48). London: Churchill Livingstone.

Shelton, T. L., Barkley, R. A., Crosswait, C., Moorehouse, M., Fletcher, K., Barrett, S., Jenkins, L., & Metevia, L. (1998). Psychiatric and psychological morbidity as a function of adaptive disability in preschool children with aggressive and hyperactive- impulsive-inattentive behavior. *Journal of Abnormal Child Psychology, 26,* 475–94.

Shelton, T. L., Barkley, R. A., Crosswait, C., Moorehouse, M., Fletcher, K., Barrett, S., Jenkins, L., & Metevia, L. (2000). Multimethod psychoeducational intervention for preschool children with disruptive behavior: Two-year post-treatment follow-up. *Journal of Abnormal Child Psychology, 28,* 253–266.

Shirk, S. (1998, November). *Adult versus child psychodynamic outcomes: Why the disparity?* Paper presented at the meeting of the Research Committee on Psychodynamic Treatment Techniques, Athens, Greece.

Shirk, S. R., & Russell, R. L. (1992). A reevaluation of estimates of child therapy effectiveness. *Journal of the American Academy of Child and Adolescent Psychiatry, 31,* 703–709.

Sholevar, G. P., & Sholevar, E. H. (1995). Overview. In G. P. Sholevar (Ed.), *Conduct disorders in children and adolescents* (pp. 3–26). Washington, DC: American Psychiatric Press.

Siefen, G., & Remschmidt, H. (1986). Results of treatment with clozapine in schizophrenic adolescents. *Zeitschrift für Kinder und Jugendpsychiatrie, 14,* 245–257.

Siegel, B., Pliner, C., Eschler, J., & Elliott, G. R. (1988). How children with autism are diagnosed: Difficulties in identification of children with multiple developmental delays. *Journal of Developmental and Behavioral Pediatrics, 9,* 199–204.

Sikich, L., Williamson, K., Malekpour, A., Bashford, R., Hooper, S., Sheitman, G., & Lieberman, J. (1999, October). *Double-blind comparison of haloperidol, risperidone, and olanzapine in psychotic youth.* Paper presented at the 46th annual meeting of the American Academy of Child and Adolescent Psychiatry, Chicago.

Silbereisen, R. K., Robins, L., & Rutter, M. (1995). Secular trends in substance abuse: Concepts and data on the impact of social change on alcohol and drug abuse. In M. Rutter & D. J. Smith (Eds.), *Psychosocial disorders in young people: Time trends and their causes* (pp. 490–543). Chichester: Wiley.

Silva, P. A. (1990). The Dunedin Multidisciplinary Health and Development Study: A 15 year longitudinal study. *Paediatric and Perinatal Epidemiology, 4,* 96–127.

Silva, R. R., Campbell, M., Golden, R. R., Small, A. M., Pataki, C. S., & Rosenberg, C. R. (1992). Side effects associated with lithium and placebo administration in aggressive children. *Psychopharmacology Bulletin, 28,* 319–326.

Silva, R. R., Dinohra, M. D., Munoz, M. D., & Alpert, M. (1996). Carbamazepine use in children and adolescents with features of attention-deficit hyperactivity disorder: A meta-analysis. *Journal of the American Academy of Child and Adolescent Psychiatry, 35,* 352–358.

Silva, R. R., Munoz, D. M., Barickman, J., & Friedhoff, A. J. (1995). Environmental factors and related fluctuations in children and adolescents with Tourette's disorder. *Journal of Child Psychology and Psychiatry, 36,* 305–312.

Silverman, W. K., Cerny, J. A., Nelles, W. B., & Burke, A. E. (1988). Behavior problems in children of parents with anxiety disorders. *Journal of the American Academy of Child and Adolescent Psychiatry, 27,* 779–784.

Silverman, W. K., Kurtines, W. M., Ginsburg, G. S., Weems, C. F., Lumpkin, P. W., & Carmichael, D. H. (1999a). Treating anxiety disorders in children with group cognitive-behaviorial therapy: A randomized clinical trial. *Journal of Consulting and Clinical Psychology, 67,* 995–1003.

Silverman, W. K., Kurtines, W. M., Ginsburg, G. S., Weems, C. F., Rabian, B., & Serafini, L. T. (1999b). Contingency management, self-control, and education support in the treatment of childhood phobic disorders: A randomized clinical trial. *Journal of Consulting and Clinical Psychology, 67,* 675–687.

Simeon, J. G., Dinicola, V. F., Ferguson, H., & Copping, W. (1990). Adolescent depression: A placebo controlled fluoxetine treatment study and follow-up. *Progress in Neuropsychopharmacology and Biological Psychiatry, 14,* 791–795.

Simeon, J. G., Ferguson, H. B., Knott, V., Roberts, N., Gauthier, B., Dubois, C., & Wiggins, D. (1992). Clinical, cognitive and neurophysiological effects of alprazolam in children and adolescents with overanxious and avoidant disorders. *Journal of the American Academy of Child and Adolescent Psychiatry, 31*, 29–33.

Simeon, J. G., & Wiggins, D. M. (1993). Pharmacotherapy of attention deficit hyperactivity disorder. *Canadian Journal of Psychiatry, 38*, 443–448.

Simeonsson, R. J., Olley, J. G., & Rosenthal, S. L. (1987). Early intervention for children with autism. In M. J. Guralnick & F. C. Bennett (Eds.), *The effectiveness of early intervention for at-risk and handicapped children* (pp. 275–296). New York: Academic Press.

Simonoff, E., Pickles, A., Meyer, J., Silberg, J. L., Maes, H. H., Loeber, R., Rutter, M., Hewitt, J. K., & Eaves, L. J. (1997). The Virginia Twin Study of Adolescent Behavioral Development: Influences of age, sex and impairment on rates of disorder. *Archives of General Psychiatry, 54*, 801–808.

Singer, H. S., Brown, J., Quaskey, S. W., Mellits, E. D., Denckla, M. B., & Rosenberg, L. A. (1995). The treatment of attention-deficit hyperactivity disorder in Tourette syndrome: A double-blind placebo-controlled study with clonidine and desipramine. *Pediatrics, 95*, 74–80.

Singer, H. S., & Rosenberg, L. A. (1989). Development of behavioral and emotional problems in Tourette syndrome. *Pediatric Neurology, 5*, 41–44.

Singer, H. S., Schuerholz, I. J., & Denckla, M. B. (1995). Learning difficulties in children with Tourette syndrome. *Journal of Child Neurology, 10*(Suppl.), 58S–61S.

Singer, M. I., Petchers, M. K., & Hussey, D. (1989). The relationship between sexual abuse and substance abuse among psychiatrically hospitalised patients. *Child Abuse and Neglect, 13*, 319–325.

Smith, D. J. (1995). Youth crime and conduct disorders: Trends, patterns and causal explanations. In M. Rutter & D. J. Smith (Eds.), *Psychosocial disorders in young people: Time trends and their causes* (pp. 389–489). Chichester, UK: Wiley.

Smith, K., & Crawford, S. (1986). Suicidal behavior among "normal" high school students. *Suicide and Life Threatening Behavior, 16*, 313–325.

Smith, M. L., & Glass, G. V. (1977). Meta-analysis of psychotherapy outcome studies. *American Psychologist, 32*, 752–760.

Smith, P. K., & Sharp, S. (Eds.). (1994a). *School bullying: Insights and perspectives*. London: Routledge.

Smith, P. K., & Sharp, S. (Eds.). (1994b). *Tackling bullying in your school: A practical handbook for teachers*. London: Routledge.

Snyder, H. (1994). *Juvenile violent crime arrest rates 1972–1992*. U.S. Office of Juvenile Justice and Delinquency Prevention, Fact Sheet 14.

Snyder, H. N., & Sickmund, M. (1995). *Juvenile offenders and victims: A national report*. Washington, DC: Office of Juvenile Justice and Delinquency Prevention.

Snyder, J. J., Suarez, M., & Brooker, M. C. (2001, April 19–22). *Growth, continuity, and correlates of direct and relational aggression in 5 to 7 year old boys and girls. Symposium on developmental trajectories in antisocial behavior from infancy to adolescence*. Paper presented at the biennial meeting of the Society for Research in Child Development, Minneapolis, MN.

Snyder, K. V., Kymissis, P., & Kessler, K. (1999). Anger management for adolescents: Efficacy of brief group therapy. *Journal of the American Academy of Child and Adolescent Psychiatry, 38*, 1409–1416.

Sohn, D. (1996). Publication bias and the evaluation of psychotherapy efficacy in reviews of the research literature. *Clinical Psychology Review, 16*, 147–156.

Solanto, M. V., Jacobson, M. S., Heller, L., Golden, N. H., & Hertz, S. (1994). Rate of weight gain of inpatients with anorexia nervosa under two behavioral contracts. *Pediatrics, 93*, 989–991.

Soni, P., & Weintraub, A. (1992). Buspirone-associated mental status changes. *Journal of the American Academy of Child and Adolescent Psychiatry, 31*, 1098–1099.

Sourander, A., Helenius, H., & Piha, J. (1996). Child psychiatric short-term inpatient treatment: CGAS as follow-up measure. *Child Psychiatry and Human Development, 27*, 93–104.

Spaccarelli, S. (1992). Problem-solving skills training as a supplement to behavioral parent training. *Cognitive Therapy and Research, 16*, 1–17.

Spence, S. H., & Marzillier, J. S. (1981). Social skills training with adolescent male offenders: II. Short-term, long-term, and generalised effects. *Behaviour Research and Therapy, 19*, 349–368.

Spencer, E. K., & Campbell, M. (1994). Children with schizophrenia: Diagnosis, phenomenology, and pharmacotherapy. *Schizophrenia Bulletin, 20*, 713–725.

Spencer, E. K., Kafantaris, V., Padron-Gayol, M. V., Rosenberg, C., & Campbell, M. (1992). Haloperidol in schizophrenic children: Early findings from a study in progress. *Psychopharmacology Bulletin, 28*, 183–186.

Spencer, T., Biederman, J., Harding, M., Wilens, T., & Faraone, S. (1995a). The relationship detween tic disorders and Tourette's syndrome revisited. *Journal of the American Academy of Child and Adolescent Psychiatry, 34*, 1133–1139.

Spencer, T., Biederman, J., Wilens, T., Harding, M., O'Donnell, D., & Griffin, S. (1996). Pharmacotherapy of attention deficit hyperactivity disorder across the life cycle. *Journal of the American Academy of Child and Adolescent Psychiatry, 35*, 409–432.

Spencer, T., Biederman, J., Wilens, T., Steingard, R., & Geist, D. (1993). Nortriptyline in the treatment of children with attention deficit hyperactivity disorder and tic disorder or Tourette's syndrome. *Journal of the American Academy of Child and Adolescent Psychiatry, 32*, 205–210.

Spencer, T., Wilens, T., & Biederman, J. (1995b). Psychotropic medication for children and adolescents. *Child and Adolescent Psychiatric Clinics of North America, 4*, 97–122.

Spieker, S. J., Larson, N. C., Lewis, S. M., Keller, T. E., & Gilchrist, L. (1999). Developmental trajectories of disruptive behavior problems in preschool children of adolescent mothers. *Child Development, 70*, 443–468.

Spielberger, C. D., Gorsuch, R. L., & Lushene, R. E. (1970). *The State-Trait Anxiety Inventory (Self-Evaluation Questionnaire)*. Palo Alto, CA: Consulting Psychologists Press.

Spirito, A., Brown, L., Overholser, J., & Fritz, G. (1989). Attempted suicide in adolescence: Review and critique of the literature. *Clinical Psychology Review, 9*, 335–363.

Spitzer, R. L., Endicott, J., & Robins, E. (1978). Research diagnostic criteria: Rationale and reliability. *Archives of General Psychiatry, 35*, 778–782.

Spitzer, R. L., Williams, J. B. W., & Gibbon, M. (1987). *Structured Clinical Interview for DSM-III (SCID)*. New York: New York Psychiatric Institute, Biometrics Research.

Spivak, G., & Shure, M. B. (1974). *Social adjustment of young children*. San Francisco: Jossey-Bass.

Spivak, G., & Shure, M. B. (1976). *The problem-solving approach to adjustment*. San Francisco: Jossey-Bass.

Spivak, G., & Shure, M. B. (1978). *Problem solving techniques in child-rearing*. San Francisco: Jossey-Bass.

Spoth, R. L., Redmond, C., & Shin, C. (2000). Reducing adolescents' aggressive and hostile behaviors: Randomized trial effects of a brief family intervention 4 years past baseline. *Archives of Pediatrics and Adolescent Medicine, 154*, 1248–1257.

Spreen, O. (1987). *Learning disabled children growing up: A follow-up into adulthood*. Lisse, Netherlands: Swets & Zeitlinger.

Stanger, C., Achenbach, T. M., & Verhulst, F. C. (1997). Accelerated longitudinal comparisons of aggressive versus delinquent syndromes. *Development and Psychopathology, 9*, 43–58.

Stanton, M. D., & Shadish, W. R. (1997). Outcome, attrition and family/couples treatment for drug abuse: A meta-analysis and review of the controlled and comparative studies. *Psychological Bulletin, 122*, 170–191.

Stark, K. D. (1990). *Childhood depression: School-based intervention*. New York: Guilford Press.

Stark, K. D., Reynolds, W. M., & Kaslow, N. J. (1987). A comparison of the relative efficacy of self-control therapy and a behavioral problem-solving therapy for depression in children. *Journal of Abnormal Child Psychology, 15*, 91–113.

St. Claire, L., & Osborn, A. F. (1987). The ability and behaviour of children who have been "in care" or separated from their parents. Report for the Economic and Social Research Council. *Early Child Development and Care, 28*, 187–354.

Stein, R. E. K., & Jessop, D. J. (1984). Does pediatric home care make a difference for children with chronic illness? Findings from the Pediatric Ambulatory Care Treatment Study. *Pediatrics, 73*, 845–853.

Stein, R. E. K., & Jessop, D. J. (1991). Long-term mental health effects of a pediatric home care program. *Pediatrics, 88,* 490–496.

Steinberg, L., Darling, N., Fletcher, A. C., Brown, B. B., & Dornbush, S. M. (1995). Authoritative parenting and adolescent adjustment: An ecological journey. In P. Moen, G. H. Elder, & K. Luscher (Eds.), *Examining lives in context* (pp. 423–466). Washington, DC: American Psychological Association.

Steiner, H., Garcia, I., & Mattews, Z. (1997). PRSD in incarcerated juvenile delinquents. *Journal of the American Academy of Child and Adolescent Psychiatry, 36,* 357–365.

Steiner, H., Mazer, C., & Litt, I. F. (1990). Compliance and outcome in anorexia nervosa. *Western Journal of Medicine, 153,* 133–139.

Steiner, H., & Stone, L. A. (1999). Introduction: Violence and related psychopathology. *Journal of the American Academy of Child and Adolescent Psychiatry, 38,* 232–234.

Steingard, R., Biederman, J., Spencer, T., & Gonzalez, A. (1993). Comparison of clonidine response in the treatment of attention deficit hyperactivity disorder with and without comorbid tic disorders. *Journal of the American Academy of Child and Adolescent Psychiatry, 32,* 350–353.

Steinhausen, H. C. (1985). Evaluation of inpatient treatment of adolescent anorexic patients. *Journal of Psychiatric Research, 19,* 371–375.

Steinhausen, H. C. (1987). Global assessment of child psychopathology. *Journal of the American Academy of Child and Adolescent Psychiatry, 26,* 203–206.

Steinhausen, H. C. (1995). Treatment and outcome of adolescent anorexia nervosa. *Hormone Research, 43,* 168–170.

Steinhausen, H. C. (1997). Annotation: Outcome of anorexia nervosa in the younger patient. *Journal of Child Psychology and Psychiatry, 38,* 271–276.

Steinhausen, H. C. (2000). Eating disorders. In H. C. Steinhausen & F. Verhulst (Eds.), *Risks and outcomes in developmental psychopathology* (pp. 210–230). Oxford: Oxford University Press.

Steinhausen, H. C., & Glanville, K. (1983). A long-term follow-up of adolescent anorexia nervosa. *Acta Psychiatrica Scandinavica, 68,* 1–10.

Steinhausen, H. C., Rauss-Mason, C., & Seidel, R. (1991). Follow-up studies of anorexia nervosa: A review of four decades of outcome research. *Psychological Medicine, 21,* 447–454.

Steinhausen, H. C., & Seidel, R. (1992). A prospective follow-up study in early-onset eating disorders. In W. Herzog, H. Deter, & W. Vandereycken (Eds.), *The course of eating disorders* (pp. 108–117). London: Springer-Verlag.

Steinhausen, H. C., & Seidel, R. (1993). Outcome in adolescent eating disorders. *International Journal of Eating Disorders, 14,* 487–496.

Steinhausen, H.-C., Seidel, R., & Metzke, C.-W. (2000). Evaluation of treatment and intermediate and long-term outcome of adolescent eating disorders. *Psychological Medicine, 30,* 1089–1098.

Sterling, T. D. (1959). Publication decisions and their possible effects on inferences drawn from tests of significance—Or vice versa. *Journal of the American Statistical Association, 54,* 30–34.

Stern, L. M., Walker, M. K., Sawyer, M. G., Oades, R. D., & Badcock, N. R. (1990). A controlled crossover trial of fenfluramine in autism. *Journal of Child Psychology and Psychiatry, 31,* 569–585.

Stevens, V., Van Oost, P., & de Bourdeaudhuij, I. (2000). The effects of an anti-bullying intervention program on peers' attitudes and behavior. *Journal of Adolescence, 23,* 21–34.

Stiller, C. A. (1994). Centralised treatment, entry to trials, and survival. *British Journal of Cancer, 70,* 352–362.

Stoewe, J. K., Kruesi, M. J. P., & Lelio, D. F. (1995). Psychopharmacology of aggressive states and features of conduct disorder. *Child and Adolescent Psychiatric Clinics of North America, 4,* 359–379.

Stoff, D. M., & Cairns, R. B. (Eds.). (1996). *Aggression and violence: Genetic, neurobiological and biosocial perspectives.* Mahwah, NJ: Erlbaum.

Stothard, S. E., Snowling, M. J., Bishop, D. V., Chipchase, B. B., & Kaplan, C. A. (1998). Language-impaired preschoolers: A follow-up into adolescence. *Journal of Speech, Language and Hearing Research, 41,* 407–418.

Stouthamer-Loeber, M., & Loeber, R. (1986). Boys who lie. *Journal of Abnormal Child Psychology, 14,* 551–564.

Strain, P. S., Steele, P., Ellis, T., & Timm, M. A. (1982). Long-term effects of oppositional child treatment with mothers as therapists and therapist trainers. *Journal of Applied Behavior Analysis, 15,* 163–169.

Straus, M. A. (1990). The Conflict Tactics Scales and its critics: An evaluation and new data on validity and reliability. In M. A. Straus & R. J. Gelles (Eds.), *Physical violence in American families: Risk factors and adaptations to violence in 8,145 families* (pp. 49–73). New Brunswick, NJ: Transaction Press.

Strauss, C. C., & Last, C. G. (1993). Social and simple phobias in children. *Journal of Anxiety Disorders, 7,* 141–152.

Strauss, C. C., Last, C. G., Hersen, M., & Kazdin, A. E. (1988a). Association between anxiety and depression in children and adolescents with anxiety disorders. *Journal of Abnormal Child Psychology, 16,* 57–68.

Strauss, C. C., Lease, C. A., Last, C. G., & Francis, G. (1988b). Overanxious disorder: Examination of developmental difference. *Journal of Abnormal Child Psychology, 16,* 433–443.

Strayhorn, J. M., & Weidman, C. S. (1989). Reduction of attention deficit and internalizing symptoms in preschoolers through parent–child interaction training. *Journal of the American Academy of Child and Adolescent Psychiatry, 28,* 888–896.

Strober, M., Freeman, R., DeAntonio, M., Lampert, C., & Diamond, J. (1997a). Does adjunctive fluoxetine influence the post-hospital course of restrictor-type anorexia nervosa? A 24–month prospective, longitudinal follow-up and comparison with historical controls. *Psychopharmacology Bulletin, 33,* 425–431.

Strober, M., Freeman, R., & Morrell, W. (1997b). The long-term course of severe anorexia nervosa in adolescents: Survival analysis of recovery, relapse and outcome predictors over 10–15 years in a prospective study. *International Journal of Eating Disorders, 22,* 339–360.

Strober, M., Morrell, W., & Burroughs, J. (1990). Relapse following discontinuation of lithium maintenance therapy in adolescents with bipolar I illness: A naturalistic study. *American Journal of Psychiatry, 147,* 457–461.

Strober, M., Morrell, W., Burroughs, J., Lampert, C., Danforth, H., & Freeman, R. (1988). A family study of bipolar I disorder in adolescence. *Journal of Affective Disorders, 15,* 255–268.

Strober, M., Schmidt-Lackner, S., Freeman, R., Bower, S., Lampert, C., & De Antonio, M. (1995). Recovery and relapse in adolescents with bipolar affective illness: A five year naturalistic, prospective follow-up study. *Journal of the American Academy of Child and Adolescent Psychiatry, 34,* 724–731.

Strober, M. C., & Carlson, G. (1982). Bipolar illness in adolescents with major depression. *Archives of General Psychiatry, 39,* 549–555.

Subotsky, F. (1992). Psychiatric treatment for children—The organization of services. *Archives of the Disabled Child, 67,* 971–975.

Suzuki, M., Morita, H., & Kamoshita, S. (1990). Epidemiological survey of psychiatric disorders in Japanese school children: Part III. Prevalence of psychiatric disorders in junior high school children. *Nippon Koshu Eisei Zasshi, 37,* 991–1000.

Sverd, J., Curley, A., Jandorf, L., & Volkersz, L. (1988). Behavior disorder and attention deficits in children with Tourette syndrome. *Journal of the American Academy of Child and Adolescent Psychiatry, 27,* 413–417.

Swadi, H. (1988). Drug and substance use among 3,333 London adolescents. *British Journal of Addictions, 83,* 935–942.

Swanson, J., Cantwell, D., Lerner, M., McBurnett, K., & Hanna, G. (1991). Effects of stimulant medication on learning in children with ADHD. *Learning Disabilities, 24,* 219–229.

Swanson, J., Wigal, S., Greenhill, L., Browne, R., Waslick, B., Lerner, M., Williams, L., Flynn, D., Agler, D., Crowley, K. L., Fineberg, E., Regino, R., Baren, M., & Cantwell, D. (1998). Objective and subjective measures of the pharmacodynamic effects of Adderall in the treatment of children with ADHD in a controlled laboratory classroom setting. *Psychopharmacology Bulletin, 34,* 55–60.

Swanson, J. M. (1992). *School-based assessments and interventions for ADD students.* Irvine, CA: KC Publications.

Swanson, J. M., Flockhart, D., Udrea, D., Cantwell, D., Connor, D., & Williams, L. (1996). Clonidine in the treatment of ADHD: Questions about safety and efficacy. *Journal of Child and Adolescent Psychopharmacology, 5,* 301–304.

Swanson, J. M., Lerner, M., & Williams, L. (1995a). More frequent diagnosis of ADHD. *New England Journal of Medicine, 333,* 944.

Swanson, J. M., McBurnett, K., Christian, D. L., & Wigal, T. (1995b). Stimulant medications and the treatment of children with ADHD. In T. H. Ollendick & R. J. Prinz (Eds.), *Advances in clinical child psychology* (pp. 265–322). New York: Plenum Press.

Swanson, J. M., McBurnett, K., & Wiwal, T. (1993). Effect of stimulant medication on children with attention deficit disorder: A "review of reviews." *Exceptional Children, 60,* 154–162.

Swedo, S. C., Rapoport, J. L., Leonard, H. I., & Lenane, M. (1989). Obsessive–compulsive disorder in children and adolescents: Clinical phenomonology of 70 consecutive cases. *Archives of General Psychiatry, 46,* 335–341.

Switzer, E. G., Deal, T. E., & Bailey, J. S. (1977). The reduction of stealing in second graders using a group contingency. *Journal of Applied Behavior Analysis, 10,* 267–272.

Szapocznik, J., & Kurtines, W. (1989). *Breakthroughs in family therapy with drug-abusing and problem youth.* New York: Springer.

Szapocznik, J., Kurtines, W., Santisteban, D. A., & Rio, A. (1990). Interplay of advances between theory, research, and application in treatment interventions aimed at behavior problem children and adolescents. *Journal of Consulting and Clinical Psychology, 58,* 696–703.

Szapocznik, J., Perez-Vidal, A., Brickman, A. L., Foote, F. H., Santisteban, D., Hervis, O., & Kurtines, W. M. (1988). Engaging adolescent drug abusers and their families in treatment: A strategic structural systems approach. *Journal of Consulting and Clinical Psychology, 56,* 552–557.

Szapocznik, J., Rio, A., Murray, E., Cohen, R., Scopetta, M., Rivas-Valquez, A., Hervis, O., Posada, V., & Kurtines, W. (1989). Structural family versus psychodynamic child therapy for problematic Hispanic boys. *Journal of Consulting and Clinical Psychology, 57,* 571–578.

Szapocznik, J., & Williams, R. A. (2000). Brief strategic family therapy: Twenty-five years of interplay among theory, research and practice in adolescent behavior problems and drug abuse. *Clinical Child and Family Psychology Review, 3,* 117–134.

Szatmari, P. (1991). Asperger's syndrome, diagnosis, treatment and outcome. *Psychiatric Clinics of North America, 14,* 81–93.

Szatmari, P., Offord, D. R., & Boyle, M. H. (1989). Ontario Child Health Study: Prevalence of attention deficit disorder with hyperactivity. *Journal of Child Psychology and Psychiatry and Allied Disciplines, 30,* 219–230.

Szmukler, G. I. (1983). Weight and food preoccupation in a population of English schoolgirls. In G. J. Bargman (Ed.), *Understanding anorexia nervosa and bulimia* (pp. 21–27). Columbus, OH: Ross Laboratories.

Tager-Flusberg, H. C. (1981). Sentence comprehension in autistic children. *Applied Psycholinguistics, 2,* 5–24.

Taggart, V. S., Zuckerman, A. E., Sly, R. M., Steinmueller, C., Newman, G., O'Brien, R. W., Schneider, S., & Bellanti, J. A. (1991). You can control asthma: Evaluation of an asthma education program for hospitalized inner-city children. *Patient Education and Counseling, 17,* 35–47.

Tannock, R., Ickowicz, A., & Schachar, R. (1995a). Differential effects of methylphenidate on working memory in ADHD children with and without comorbid anxiety. *Journal of the American Academy of Child and Adolescent Psychiatry, 34,* 886–896.

Tannock, R., Schachar, R., & Logan, G. (1995b). Methylphenidate and cognitive flexibility: Dissociated dose effects in hyperactive children. *Journal of Abnormal Child Psychology, 23,* 234–266.

Tantum, D. (1988). Annotation: Asperger's syndrome. *Journal of Child Psychology and Psychiatry, 29,* 245–255.

Target, M., & Fonagy, P. (1992). *Raters' manual for the Hampstead Child Adaptation Measure (HCAM).* London: UCL.

Target, M., & Fonagy, P. (1994a). The efficacy of psychoanalysis for children with emotional disorders. *Journal of the American Academy of Child and Adolescent Psychiatry, 33,* 361–371.

Target, M., & Fonagy, P. (1994b). The efficacy of psychoanalysis for children: Developmental considerations. *Journal of the American Academy of Child and Adolescent Psychiatry, 33,* 1134–1144.

Tate, D. C., Reppucci, N. D., & Mulvey, E. P. (1995). Violent juvenile delinquents: Treatment effectiveness and implications for future action. *American Psychologist, 50,* 777–781.

Taylor, E. (1986). Childhood hyperactivity. *British Journal of Psychiatry, 149,* 562–573.

Taylor, E. (1994). Syndromes of attention deficit and overactivity. In M. Rutter, E. Taylor, & L. Hersov (Eds.), *Adolescent psychiatry: Modern approaches* (pp. 285–307). Oxford: Blackwell Scientific.

Taylor, E. (1999). Development of clinical services for attention deficit hyperactivity disorder. *Archives of General Psychiatry, 56,* 1097–1099.

Taylor, E., Sandberg, S., Thorley, G., & Giles, S. (1991). *The epidemiology of childhood hyperactivity. Maudsley Monographs, No. 33.* London: Institute of Psychiatry.

Taylor, E., Schachar, R., Thorley, G., Wieselberg, M., Everitt, B., & Rutter, M. (1987). Which boys respond to stimulant medication? A controlled trial of methylphenidate in boys with disruptive behaviour. *Psychological Medicine, 17,* 121–143.

Thal, D. J. (1991). Language and cognition in normal and late-talking toddlers. *Topics in Language Disorders, 11,* 33–42.

Thien, V., Thomas, A., Markin, D., & Birmingham, C. (2000). Pilot study of a graded exercise program for the treatment of anorexia nervosa. *International Journal of Eating Disorders, 28,* 101–106.

Thomas, C., Holzer, C., & Enriquez, J. (1999). *Collaborative, community based truancy program.* Paper presented at the 46th annual meeting of the American Academy of Child and Adolescent Psychiatry, Chicago.

Thomas, C. S., & Lewis, S. (1998). Which atypical antipsychotic? *British Journal of Psychiatry, 172,* 106–109.

Thompson, E., Eggert, L., & Herting, J. (2000). Mediating effects of an indicated prevention program for reducing youth depression and suicide risk behaviors. *Suicide and Life-Threatening Behavior, 30,* 252–271.

Thompson, R. W., Ruma, P. R., Schuchmann, L. F., & Burke, R. V. (1996). A cost-effectiveness evaluation of parent training. *Journal of Child and Family Studies, 5,* 415–429.

Thomsen, P. H. (1995). Obsessive–compulsive disorder in children and adolescents. A 6–22-year follow-up study of social outcome. *European Child and Adolescent Psychiatry, 4,* 112–122.

Thomsen, P. H., & Mikkelsen, H. U. (1995). Course of obsessive–compulsive disorder in children and adolescents: A prospective follow-up study of 23 Danish cases. *Journal of the American Academy of Child and Adolescent Psychiatry, 34,* 1432–1440.

Thomson, A. P. J., & Sills, J. A. (1988). Diagnosis of functional illness presenting with gait disorder. *Archives of Disease in Childhood, 63,* 148–153.

Thomson, R. (1982). Side effects and placebo amplification. *British Journal of Psychiatry, 140,* 64–68.

Thorley, G. (1984). Hyperkinetic syndrome of childhood: Clinical characteristics. *British Journal of Psychiatry, 144,* 16–24.

Tierney, J. P., Grossman, J. B., & Resch, N. L. (1995). *Making a difference: An impact study of big brothers/big sisters.* Philadelphia: Public/Private Ventures.

Tissue, R., & Korz, A. C. (1993). When emotionally troubled children grow up: Adjustment in young adults who attended a psycho-educational treatment center. *Child Psychiatry and Human Development, 23,* 175–182.

Todd, T. C. (1985). Anorexia and bulimia—Expanding the structural model. In M. P. Mirkin (Ed.), *Handbook of adolescent and family therapy* (pp. 223–244). New York: Gardner Press.

Tolbert, H. A. (1996). Psychoses in children and adolescents: A review. *Journal of Clinical Psychiatry, 57*(Suppl. 3), 4–8.

Tomblin, J. B., & Buckwalter, P. R. (1994). Studies of genetics of specific language impairment. In R. V. Watkins & M. L. Rice (Eds.), *Communication and language intervention series: Vol. 4. Specific language impairments in children* (pp. 17–34). Baltimore: Paul H. Brookes.

Tomblin, J. B., Records, N. L., Buckwalter, P., Zhang, X., Smith, E., & O'Brien, M. (1997). Prevalence of specific language impairment in kindergarten children. *Journal of Speech, Language and Hearing Research, 40*, 1245–1260.

Toppelberg, C. O., & Shapiro, T. (2000). Language disorders: A 10-year research update review. *Journal of the American Academy of Child and Adolescent Psychiatry, 39*, 143–152.

Toren, P., Wolmer, L., Rosental, B., Eldar, S., Koren, S., Lask, M., Weizman, R., & Laor, N. (2000). Case series: Brief parent–child group therapy for childhood anxiety disorders using a manual-based cognitive-behavioral technique. *Journal of the American Academy of Child and Adolescent Psychiatry, 39*, 1309–1312.

Torgesen, J. K., Wagner, R. K., & Rashotte, C. A. (1994). Longitudinal studies of phonological processing and reading. *Journal of Learning Disabilities, 27*, 276–286.

Torrey, E. F. (1987). Prevalence studies in schizophrenia. *British Journal of Psychiatry, 150*, 598–608.

Toth, S. L., & Cicchetti, D. (1999). Developmental psychotherapy and child psychotherapy. In S. W. Russ & T. H. Ollendick (Eds.), *Handbook of psychotherapies with children and families* (pp. 15–44). New York: Kluwer Academic/Plenum.

Tracey, S. A., Patterson, M., Mattis, S. G., Chorpita, B. F., Albano, A. M., Heimberg, R. G., & Barlow, D. H. (1999). *Cognitive behavioral group treatment of social phobia in adolescents: Preliminary examination of the contribution of parental involvement.* Paper presented at the annual meeting of the Anxiety Disorders Association of America, San Diego.

Trautman, P. D., Stewart, N., & Morishima, A. (1993). Are adolescent suicide attempters noncompliant with outpatient care? *Journal of the American Academy of Child and Adolescent Psychiatry, 32*, 89–94.

Treasure, J., & Holland, A. (1990). Genetic vulnerability to eating disorders: Evidence from twin and family studies. In H. Remschmidt & M. Schmidt (Eds.), *Anorexia nervosa* (pp. 59–68). Toronto: Hogrefe and Huber.

Tremblay, R. E., Masse, L. C., Pagani, L., & Vitaro, F. (1996). From childhood physical aggression to adolescent maladjustment: The Montreal prevention experiment. In R. D. Peters & R. J. McMahon (Eds.), *Preventing childhood disorders, substance abuse, and delinquency* (pp. 268–299). Thousand Oaks, CA: Sage.

Tremblay, R. E., Pagani-Kurtz, L., Masse, L. C., Vitaro, F., & Pihl, R. O. (1995). A bimodal preventive intervention for disruptive kindergarten boys: Its impact through mid-adolescence. *Journal of Consulting and Clinical Psychology, 63*, 560–568.

Tremblay, R. E., Pihl, R. O., Vitaro, F., & Dobkin, P. L. (1994). Predicting early onset of male antisocial behavior from preschool behavior: A test of two personality theories. *Archives of General Psychiatry, 51*, 732–738.

Tremblay, R. E., Vitaro, F., Bertrand, L., LeBlanc, M., Beauchesne, H., Boileau, H., & Lucille, D. (1992). Parent and child training to prevent early onset of delinquency: The Montreal longitudinal experimental study. In J. McCord & R. E. Tremblay (Eds.), *Preventing antisocial behavior: Interventions from birth through adolescence* (pp. 117–138). New York: Guilford Press.

Trevathan, E., & Adams, M. J. (1988). The epidemiology and public health significance of Rett syndrome. *Journal of Child Neurology, 3*(Suppl.), 17S–20S.

Trevathan, E., & Naidu, S. (1988). The clinical recognition and differential diagnosis of Rett syndrome. *Journal of Child Neurology, 3*(Suppl.), 6S–16S.

Trott, G. E., Friese, H. J., Menzel, M., & Nissen, G. (1991). Use of moclobemide in children with attention deficit hyperactivity disorder. *Jugendpsychiatrie, 19*, 248–253.

Turecki, S., & Tonner, L. (1985). *The difficult child.* New York: Bantam.

Turk, J. (1993). Cognitive approaches. In B. Lask & R. Bryant-Waugh (Eds.), *Chilhood onset anorexia and related eating disorders* (pp. 177–190). Hillsdale, NJ: Erlbaum.

Twemlow, S. W., Fonagy, P., & Sacco, F. C. (2001). An innovative psychodynamically influenced approach to reduce school violence. *Journal of the American Academy of Child and Adolescent Psychiatry, 40*, 377–379.

Twemlow, S. W., Sacco, F. C., Giess, M. L., Ewbank, R., & Fonagy, P. (2001). Creating a peaceful school learning environment. A controlled study of an elementary school intervention to reduce violence. *American Journal of Psychiatry, 158*, 808–810.

Ultee, C. A., Griffiaen, D., & Schellekens, J. (1982). The reduction of anxiety in children: A comparison of the effects of systematic desensitisation in vitro and systematic desensitisation in vivo. *Behaviour Research and Therapy, 20*, 61–67.

Unis, A. S., Cook, E. H., Vincent, J. G., Gjerde, D. K., Perry, B. D., Mason, C., & Mitchell, J. (1997). Platelet serotonin measures in adolescents with conduct disorder. *Biological Psychiatry, 42*, 553–559.

U.S. Department of Education. (1995). *Seventeenth annual report of Congress on the implementation of the Individuals with Disabilities Education Act.* Washington, DC: U.S. Office of Special Education Program.

U.S. Department of Transportation. (1993). *Traffic safety facts 1992.* Washington DC: National Center for Statistics and Analysis.

VandenBos, G. R. (1996). Special issue: Outcome assessment of psychotherapy. *American Psychologist, 51*, 1005–1079.

Vandereycken, W. (1984). Neuroleptics in the short-term treatment of anorexia nervosa: A double-blind placebo-controlled study with sulpiride. *British Journal of Psychiatry, 144*, 288–292.

Vandereycken, W. (1987). The constructive family approach to eating disorders: Critical remarks on the use of family therapy in anorexia nervosa and bulimia. *International Journal of Eating Disorders, 6*, 455–468.

Vandereycken, W., & Pierloot, R. (1982). Pimozide combined with behavior therapy in the short-term treatment of anorexia nervosa: A double-blind placebo-controlled cross-over study. *Acta Psychiatrica Scandinavica, 66*, 445–450.

Van der Ham, T., Van Strien, D. C., & Van Engeland, H. (1994). A four-year prospective follow-up study of 49 eating-disordered adolescents: Differences in course of illness. *Acta Psychiatrica Scandinavica, 90*, 229–235.

Van der Helm-Hylkema, H., Orlebeke, J. F., Enting, L. A., Thijssen, J. H. H., & Van Ree, J. (1990). Effects of behavior therapy on migraine and plasma beta-endorphin in young migraine patients. *Psychoneuroendocrinology, 15*, 39–45.

Van der Meere, J. J., Gunning, B., & Stemerdink, B. A. (1996). Changing a response set in normal development and in ADHD children with and without tics. *Journal of Abnormal Child Psychology, 24*, 767–785.

Van der Meere, J. J., Gunning, B., & Stemerdink, N. (1999). The effect of methylphenidate and clonidine on response inhibition and state regulation in children with ADHD. *Journal of Child Psychology and Psychiatry, 40*, 291–298.

Van der Meere, J. J., Stemerdink, N., & Gunning, B. (1995). Effects of presentation rate of stimuli on response inhibition in ADHD with and without tics. *Journal of Perceptual and Motor Skills, 81*, 259–262.

Van Goozen, S. H., Matthys, W., Cohen-Kettenis, P. T., Gispen-de Wied, C., Wiegant, V. M., & Van Engeland, H. (1998). Salivary cortisol and cardiovascular activity during stress in oppositional-defiant disorder boys and normal controls. *Biological Psychiatry, 43*, 531–539.

Van Goozen, S. H. M., Van den Ban, E., Matthys, W., Cohen-Kettenis, P. T., Thijssen, J. H. H., & Van Engeland, H. (2000). Increased adrenal androgen functioning in children with oppositional defiant disorder: A comparison with psychiatric and normal controls. *Journal of the American Academy of Child and Adolescent Psychiatry, 39*, 1446–1451.

Varanka, T. M., Weller, R. A., & Weller, E. B. (1988). Lithium treatment of manic episodes with psychotic features in prepubertal children. *American Journal of Psychiatry, 145*, 1557–1559.

Varley, C. K., & Trupin, E. W. (1983). Double-blind assessment of stimulant medication for attention deficit disorder: A model for clinical application. *American Journal of Orthopsychiatry, 53*, 542–547.

Varni, J. W., Katz, E. R., Colegrove, R., & Dolgin, M. (1993). The impact of social skills training on the adjustment of children with newly diagnosed cancer. *Journal of Pediatric Psychology, 18*, 751–767.

Vasquez, M. I., & Buceta, J. M. (1993a). Effectiveness of self-management programs and relaxation training in the treatment of bronchial asthma: Relationships with trait anxiety and emotional attack triggers. *Journal of Psychosomatic Research, 37*, 71–81.

Vasquez, M. I., & Buceta, J. M. (1993b). Psychological treatment of asthma: Effectiveness of a self-management program with and without relaxation training. *Journal of Asthma, 30,* 171–183.

Vasquez, M. I., & Buceta, J. M. (1993c). Relaxation therapy in the treatment of bronchial asthma: Effects on basal spirometric values. *Psychotherapy and Psychosomatics, 60,* 106–112.

Vaughn, C. E., & Leff, J. P. (1981). Patterns of emotional response in relatives of schizophrenic patients. *Schizophrenia Bulletin, 7,* 43–44.

Vaughn, S., Hogan, A., Kouzekani, K., & Shapiro, S. (1990). Peer acceptance, self-perceptions, and social skills of learning disabled students prior to identification. *Journal of Educational Psychology, 82,* 101–106.

Velez, C. N., Johnson, J., & Cohen, P. (1989). Longitudinal analyses of selected risk factors for childhood psychopathology. *Journal of the American Academy of Child and Adolescent Psychiatry, 28,* 861–864.

Velting, O. N., & Albano, A. M. (2001). Current trends in the understanding and treatment of social phobia in youth. *Journal of Child Psychology and Psychiatry, 42,* 127–140.

Vennard, J., Sugg, D., & Hedderman, C. (1997). Part I: The use of cognitive-behavioural approaches with offenders: Messages from the research; *Changing offenders' attitudes and behaviour: What works?* (Home Office Research Study No.171) (pp. 1–35). London: Her Majesty's Stationery Office.

Venter, A., Lord, C., & Schopler, E. (1992). A follow-up study of high-functioning autistic children. *Journal of Child Psychology and Psychiatry, 33,* 489–507.

Vereker, M. I. (1992). Chronic fatigue syndrome: A joint paediatric–psychiatric approach. *Archives of Disease in Childhood, 67,* 550–555.

Verhulst, F. C., & Achenbach, T. M. (1995). Empirically based assessment and taxonomy of psychopathology: Cross-cultural applications. *European Child and Adolescent Psychiatry, 4,* 61–76.

Verhulst, F. C., Achenbach, T. M., Ferdinand, R. F., & Kasius, M. C. (1993). Epidemiological comparisons of Dutch adolescents' self-reports. *Journal of the American Academy of Child and Adolescent Psychiatry, 32,* 1135–1144.

Verhulst, F. C., & Koot, H. M. (1992). *Child psychiatric epidemiology: Concepts, methods, and findings.* Newbury Park, CA: Sage.

Vessey, J. A., Carlson, K. L., & McGill, J. (1994). Use of distraction with children during an acute pain experience. *Nursing Research, 43,* 369–372.

Vincent, J., Unis, A., & Hardy, J. (1990). Pharmacotherapy of aggression. *Journal of the American Academy of Child and Adolescent Psychiatry, 29,* 839–840.

Vitaro, F., Gendreau, P. L., Tremblay, R. E., & Oligny, P. (1998). Reactive and proactive aggression differentially predict later conduct problems. *Journal of Child Psychology and Psychiatry, 39,* 377–385.

Vitaro, F., & Tremblay, R. E. (1994). Impact of a prevention program on aggressive children's friendships and social adjustment. *Journal of Abnormal Child Psychology, 22,* 457–475.

Vitiello, B., Behar, D., & Malone, R. (1988). Pharmacokinetics of lithium carbonate in children. *Journal of Clinical Psychopharmacology, 8,* 355–359.

Vitiello, B., Hill, J., Elia, J., Cunningham, E., McLeer, S. V., & Behar, D. (1991). PRN medication in child psychiatric patients: A placebo-controlled study. *Journal of Clinical Psychiatry, 52,* 499–501.

Vitiello, B., & Jensen, P. (1997). Medication development and testing in children and adolescents: Current problems, future directions. *Archives of General Psychiatry, 54,* 871–876.

Vitiello, B., & Jensen, P. S. (1995). Developmental perspectives in pediatric psychopharmacology. *Psychopharmacology Bulletin, 31,* 75–81.

Vitiello, B., & Stoff, D. M. (1997). Subtypes of aggression and their relevance to child psychiatry. *Journal of the American Academy of Child and Adolescent Psychiatry, 36,* 307–315.

Vitousek, K., Watson, S., & Wilson, G. T. (1998). Enhancing motivation for change in treatment-resistant eating disorders. *Clinical Psychology Review, 18,* 391–420.

Volkmar, F. R. (1996a). Childhood and adolescent psychosis: A review of the last 10 years. *Journal of the American Academy of Child and Adolescent Psychiatry, 35,* 843–851.

Volkmar, F. R. (1996b). The disintegrative disorders: Childhood disintegrative disorder and Rett's disorder. In F. R. Volkmar (Ed.), *Psychoses and pervasive developmental disorders in childhood and adolescence* (pp. 223–248). Washington DC: American Psychiatric Press.

Volkmar, F. R., Cohen, D. J., Hoshino, Y., Rende, R. D., & Paul, R. (1988). Phenomenology and classification of the childhood psychoses. *Psychological Medicine, 18*, 191–201.

Volkmar, F. R., & Nelson, D. S. (1990). Seizure disorders in autism. *Journal of the American Academy of Child and Adolescent Psychiatry, 29*, 127–129.

Von Knorring, A., Andersson, O., & Magnusson, D. (1987). Psychiatric care and course of psychiatric disorders from childhood to early adulthood in a representative sample. *Journal of Child Psychology and Psychiatry, 28*, 329–341.

Vostanis, P., Feehan, C., Grattan, E., & Bickerton, W. L. (1996a). A randomized controlled out-patient trial of cognitive-behavioural treatment for children and adolescents with depression: 9–month follow-up. *Journal of Affective Disorders, 40*, 105–116.

Vostanis, P., Feehan, C., Grattan, E., & Bickerton, W. L. (1996b). Treatment for children and adolescents with depression: Lessons from a controlled trial. *Clinical Child Psychology and Psychiatry, 1*, 199–212.

Wachtel, P. L. (1977). *Psychoanalysis and behavior therapy: Toward an integration.* New York: Basic Books.

Wachtel, P. L. (1987). *Action and insight.* New York: Guilford Press.

Wade, W. A., Treat, T., & Stuart, G. L. (1998). Transporting an empirically supported treatment for panic disorder to a service clinic setting: A benchmarking strategy. *Journal of Consulting and Clinical Psychology, 66*, 231–239.

Wagner, K. D., & Ambrosini, P. J. (2001). Childhood depression: Pharmacological therapy/treatment (pharmacotherapy of childhood depression). *Journal of Clinical Child Psychology, 30*, 88–97.

Wahler, R. G., Cartor, P. G., Fleischman, J., & Lambert, W. (1993). The impact of synthesis teaching and parent training with mothers of conduct disordered children. *Journal of Abnormal Child Psychology, 21*, 425–440.

Wakefield, A. J., Anthony, A., & Schepelmann, S. (1998). Autistic enteropathy: A new inflammatory bowel disease? *Gut, 42*(Suppl. 1), 340.

Waldman, I. D., & Lahey, B. B. (1994). Design of the DSM-IV disruptive behavior disorder field trials. *Child and Adolescent Psychiatric Clinics of North America, 3*, 195–208.

Walker, H. M., Colvin, G., & Ramsey, E. (1995). *Antisocial behavior in school: Strategies and best practices.* Pacific Grove, CA: Brooks/Cole.

Walker, H. M., Hops, H., & Greenwood, C. R. (1981). RECESS: Research and development of a behavior management package for remediating social aggression in the school setting. In P. S. Strain (Ed.), *The utilization of classroom peers as behavior change agents* (pp. 261–303). New York: Plenum Press.

Walker, H. M., Hops, H., & Greenwood, C. R. (1984). The CORBEH research and development model: Programmatic issues and strategies. In S. C. Paine, G. T. Bellamy, & B. Wilcox (Eds.), *Human services that work: From innovation to clinical practice* (pp. 57–77). Baltimore: Paul H. Brookes.

Walker, H. M., Hops, H., & Johnson, S. M. (1975). Generalisation and maintenance of classroom treatment effects. *Behavior Therapy, 6*, 188–200.

Walker, H. M., & Walker, J. E. (1991). *Coping with noncompliance in the classroom: A positive approach for teachers.* Austin, TX: PRO-ED.

Walker, J. L., Lahey, B. B., Russo, M. F., Frick, P. J., Christ, M. A., McBurnett, K., Loeber, R., Stouthamer-Loeber, M., & Green, S. M. (1991). Anxiety, inhibition, and conduct disorder in children: I. Relations to social impairment. *Journal of the American Academy of Child and Adolescent Psychiatry, 30*, 187–191.

Walkup, J. T. (1995). Clinical decision making in child and adolescent psychopharmacology. *Child and Adolescent Psychiatric Clinics of North America, 4*, 23–40.

Walkup, J. T., Rosenberg, L. A., Brown, J., & Singer, H. S. (1992). The validity of instruments measuring tic severity in Tourette's syndrome. *Journal of the American Academy of Child and Adolescent Psychiatry, 31*, 472–477.

Wall, V., & Womack, W. (1989). Hypnotic versus active cognitive strategies for alleviation of procedural distress in pediatric oncology patients. *American Journal of Clinical Hypnosis, 31,* 181–191.

Wallach, G. P., & Butler, K. G. (1994). *Language learning disabilities in school-age children and adolescents: Some principles and applications.* Paramus, NJ: Prentice-Hall.

Walsh, B. T. (1999, October). *Time and the response of eating disorders to pharmacotherapy.* Paper presented at the 46th annual meeting of the American Academy of Child and Adolescent Psychiatry, Chicago.

Wampold, B. E., Mondin, G. W., Moody, M., Stich, F., Benson, K., & Ahn, H. (1997). A meta-analysis of outcome studies comparing bona fide psychotherapies: Empirically, "all must have prizes." *Psychological Bulletin, 122,* 203–215.

Weber, K. S., Frankenberger, W., & Heilman, K. (1992). The effects of Ritalin on the academic achievement of children diagnosed with attention-deficit hyperactivity disorder. *Developmental Disabilities Bulletin, 20,* 49–68.

Webster-Stratton, C. (1985). The effects of father involvement in parent training for conduct problem children. *Journal of Child Psychology and Psychiatry, 26,* 801–810.

Webster-Stratton, C. (1989). Systematic comparison of consumer satisfaction of three cost-effective parent training programs for conduct problem children. *Behavior Therapy, 20,* 103–115.

Webster-Stratton, C. (1990a). Enhancing the effectiveness of self-administered videotape parent training for families with conduct-problem children. *Journal of Abnormal Child Psychology, 18,* 479–492.

Webster-Stratton, C. (1990b). Long-term follow-up of families with young conduct problem children: From preschool to grade school. *Journal of Clinical Child Psychology, 19,* 144–149.

Webster-Stratton, C. (1992). Individually administered videotape parent training: "Who benefits?" *Cognitive Therapy and Research, 16,* 31–35.

Webster-Stratton, C. (1994). Advancing videotape parent training: A comparison study. *Journal of Consulting and Clinical Psychology, 62,* 583–593.

Webster-Stratton, C. (1996a). Early intervention with videotape modeling: Programs for families of children with oppositional defiant disorder or conduct disorder. In E. S. Hibbs & P. S. Jensen (Eds.), *Psychosocial treatments for child and adolescent disorders: Empirically based strategies for clinical practice* (pp. 435–474). Washington, DC: American Psychological Association.

Webster-Stratton, C. (1996b). Early-onset conduct problems: Does gender make a difference? *Journal of Consulting and Clinical Psychology, 64,* 540–551.

Webster-Stratton, C. (1996c). *Preventing conduct problems in Head Start children: Strengthening parenting competencies.* Paper presented at the meeting of the American Public Health Association, New York.

Webster-Stratton, C. (1998). Preventing conduct problems in Head Start children: Strengthening parenting competencies. *Journal of Consulting and Clinical Psychology, 66,* 715–730.

Webster-Stratton, C., & Hammond, M. (1988). Maternal depression and its relationship to life stress, perceptions of child behavior problems, parenting behaviors, and child conduct problems. *Journal of Abnormal Child Psychology, 16,* 299–315.

Webster-Stratton, C., & Hammond, M. (1997). Treating children with early-onset conduct problems: A comparison of child and parent training interventions. *Journal of Consulting and Clinical Psychology, 65,* 93–109.

Webster-Stratton, C., & Herbert, M. (1993). What really happens in parent training? *Behavior Modification, 17,* 407–456.

Webster-Stratton, C., & Herbert, M. (1994). *Troubled families: Problem children. Working with parents: A collaborative process.* Chichester: Wiley.

Webster-Stratton, C., Hollinsworth, T., & Kolpacoff, M. (1989). The long-term cost-effectiveness and clinical significance of three cost-effective training programs for families with conduct problem children. *Journal of Consulting and Clinical Psychology, 57,* 550–553.

Webster-Stratton, C., Kolpacoff, M., & Hollinsworth, T. (1988). Self-administered videotape therapy for families with conduct problem children: Comparison of two cost-effective treatments and a control group. *Journal of Consulting and Clinical Psychology, 57,* 550–553.

Webster-Stratton, S., & Spitzer, A. (1996). Parenting a young child with conduct problems: New insights using qualitative methods. In T. H. Ollendick & R. J. Prinz (Eds.), *Advances in clinical child psychology* (Vol. 18, pp. 1–62). New York: Plenum Press.

Weinberg, N. Z., Rahdert, E., Colliver, J. D., & Glantz, M. D. (1998). Adolescent substance abuse: A review of the past 10 years. *Journal of the American Academy of Child and Adolescent Psychiatry, 37*, 252–261.

Weinrott, M. R., Bauske, B. W., & Patterson, G. R. (1979). Systematic replication of a social learning approach to parent training. In P. O. Sjoden (Ed.), *Trends in behavior therapy* (pp. 331–351). New York: Academic Press.

Weinrott, M. R., Jones, R. R., & Howard, J. R. (1982). Cost-effectiveness of teaching family programs for delinquents: Results of a national evaluation. *Evaluation Review, 6*, 173–201.

Weiss, B., Catron, T., Harris, V., & Phung, T. M. (1999). The effectiveness of traditional child psychotherapy. *Journal of Consulting and Clinical Psychology, 67*, 82–94.

Weiss, G., & Hechtman, L. T. (1993). *Hyperactive children grown up*. New York: Guilford Press.

Weissman, M. M., Warner, V., Wickramaratne, P., Moreau, D., & Olfson, M. (1997). Offspring of depressed parents: 10 years later. *Archives of General Psychiatry, 54*, 932–940.

Weissman, M. M., Wolk, S., Wickramaratne, P., Goldstein, R. B., Adams, P., Greenwald, S., Ryan, N. D., Dahl, R. E., & Steinberg, D. (1999). Children with prepubertal-onset major depressive disorder and anxiety grown up. *Archives of General Psychiatry, 56*, 794–801.

Weisz, J. R. (2000). Agenda for child and adolescent psychotherapy research. *Archives of General Psychiatry, 57*, 837–838.

Weisz, J. R., Donenberg, G. R., Han, S. S., & Weiss, B. (1995a). Bridging the gap between laboratory and clinic in child and adolescent psychotherapy. *Journal of Consulting and Clinical Psychology, 63*, 688–701.

Weisz, J. R., Eastman, K. L., Donenberg, G. R., Granger, D. A., Han, S., Yeh, M., Thurber, C. A., Huey, S., Weersing, V. R., McCarty, C., & Valeri, S. (1998a). *Studying clinic-based child mental health care*. Unpublished raw data.

Weisz, J. R., Han, S. S., & Valeri, S. M. (1997a). More of what? Issues raised by Fort Bragg. *American Psychologist, 52*, 541–545.

Weisz, J. R., & Hawley, K. M. (1998). Finding, evaluating, refining and applying empirically supported treatments for children and adolescents. *Journal of Clinical Child Psychology, 27*, 206–216.

Weisz, J. R., Huey, S. J., & Weersing, V. R. (1998b). Psychotherapy outcome research with children and adolescents: The state of the art. In T. H. Ollendick & R. J. Prinz (Eds.), *Advances in clinical child psychology* (Vol. 20, pp. 49–91). New York: Plenum Press.

Weisz, J. R., Thurber, C. A., Sweeney, L., Proffitt, V. D., & LeGagnoux, G. L. (1997b). Brief treatment of mild-to-moderate child depression using primary and secondary control enhancement training. *Journal of Consulting and Clinical Psychology, 65*, 703–707.

Weisz, J. R., Valeri, S. M., McCarty, C. A., & Moore, P. S. (1999). Interventions for child and adolescent depression: Features, effects, and future directions. In C. A. Essau & F. Petermann (Eds.), *Depressive disorders in children and adolescents: Epidemiology, risk factors and treatment* (pp. 383–435). Northvale, NJ: Jason Aronson.

Weisz, J. R., Walter, B. R., Weiss, B., Fernandez, G. A., & Mikow, V. A. (1990). Arrests among emotionally disturbed violent and assaultive individuals following minimal versus lengthy intervention through North Carolina's Willie M Program. *Journal of Consulting and Clinical Psychology, 58*, 720–728.

Weisz, J. R., & Weiss, B. (1989). Assessing the effects of clinic-based psychotherapy with children and adolescents. *Journal of Consulting and Clinical Psychology, 57*, 741–746.

Weisz, J. R., & Weiss, B. (1993). *Effects of psychotherapy with children and adolescents*. Newbury Park, CA: Sage.

Weisz, J. R., Weiss, B., Alicke, M. D., & Klotz, M. L. (1987). Effectiveness of psychotherapy with children and adolescents: Meta-analytic findings for clinicians. *Journal of Consulting and Clinical Psychology, 55*, 542–549.

Weisz, J. R., Weiss, B., & Donenberg, G. R. (1992). The lab versus the clinic: Effects of child and adolescent psychotherapy. *American Psychologist, 47*, 1578–1585.

Weisz, J. R., Weiss, B., Han, S. S., Granger, D. A., & Morton, T. (1995b). Effects of psychotherapy with children and adolescents revisited: A meta-analysis of treatment outcome studies. *Psychological Bulletin, 117*, 450–468.

Wells, K. B. (1999). Treatment research at the crossroads: The scientific interface of clinical trials and effectiveness research. *American Journal of Psychiatry, 156*, 5–10.

Wells, K. C. (1985). Behavioral family therapy. In A. S. Bellack & M. Hersen (Eds.), *Dictionary of behavior therapy techniques* (pp. 25–30). New York: Pergamon Press.

Wells, K. C., & Egan, J. (1988). Social learning and systems family therapy for childhood oppositional disorder: Comparative treatment outcome. *Comprehensive Psychiatry, 29*, 138–146.

Wells, K. C., Epstein, J. N., Hinshaw, S. P., Conners, C. K., Klaric, J., Abikoff, H. B., Abramowitz, A., Arnold, L. E., Elliott, G., Greenhill, L. L., Hechtman, L., Hoza, B., Jensen, P. S., March, J. S., Pelham, W., Pfiffner, L., Severe, J., Swanson, J. M., Vitiello, B., & Wigal, T. (2000). Parenting and family stress treatment outcomes in attention-deficit/hyperactivity disorder (ADHD): An empirical analysis in the MTA Study. *Journal of Abnormal Child Psychology, 28*, 543–553.

Wells, K. C., Griest, D. L., & Forehand, R. (1980). The use of a self-control package to enhance temporal generality of a parent training programme. *Behaviour Research and Therapy, 18*, 347–353.

Wells, K. C., Pelham, W. E., Kotkin, R. A., Hoza, B., Abikoff, H. B., Abramowitz, A., Arnold, L. E., Cantwell, D. P., Conners, C. K., Carmen, R. D., Elliott, G., Greenhill, L. L., Hechtman, L., Hibbs, E., Hinshaw, S. P., Jensen, P. S., March, J. S., Swanson, J. M., & Schiller, E. (2000). Psychosocial treatment strategies in the MTA study: Rationale, methods, and critical issues in design and implementation. *Journal of Abnormal Child Psychology, 28*, 483–505.

Wender, E. H. (1986). The food-additive-free diet in the treatment of behavior disorders: A review. *Journal of Developmental and Behavioral Pediatrics, 7*, 35–42.

Werkman, S. (1987). Anxiety disorders. In H. I. Kaplan, A. M. Freedman, & B. J. Sadock (Eds.), *Comprehensive textbook of psychiatry* (Vol. III, pp. 2620–2631). Baltimore: Williams & Wilkins.

Werry, J. S. (1994). Pharmacotherapy of disruptive behavior disorders. *Child and Adolescent Psychiatric Clinics of North America, 3*, 321–341.

Werry, J. S., & McClellan, J. M. (1992). Predicting outcome in child and adolescent (early onset) schizophrenia and bipolar disorder. *Journal of the American Academy of Child and Adolescent Psychiatry, 31*, 147–150.

Werry, J. S., McClellan, J. M., & Chard, L. (1991). Childhood and adolescent schizophrenia, bipolar and affective disorders: A clinical and outcome study. *Journal of the American Academy of Child and Adolescent Psychiatry, 30*, 457–465.

Werry, J. S., & Taylor, E. (1994). Schizophrenia and allied disorders. In M. Rutter, E. Taylor, & L. Hersov (Eds.), *Child and adolescent psychiatry: Modern approaches* (3rd ed., pp. 594–615). Oxford: Blackwell Scientific.

West, S. A., Keck, P. E., & McElroy, S. L. (1994). Open trial of valproate in the treatment of adolescent mania. *Journal of Child and Adolescent Psychopharmacology, 4*, 263–267.

Westen, D., & Morrison, K. (in press). How empirically valid are empirically validated therapies? A critical appraisal. *Journal of Consulting and Clinical Psychology.*

Westenberg, P. M., Siebelink, B. M., Warmenhoven, N. J. C., & Treffers, P. D. A. (1999). Separation anxiety and overanxious disorders: Relations to age and level of psychosocial maturity. *Journal of the American Academy of Child and Adolescent Psychiatry, 38*, 1000–1007.

Whalen, C. K., & Henker, B. (1985). The social worlds of hyperactive (ADDH) children. *Clinical Psychology Review, 5*, 447–478.

Whalen, C. K., & Henker, B. (1991). Social impact of stimulant treatment for hyperactive children. *Journal of Learning Disability, 24*, 231–241.

Whalen, C. K., Henker, B., Buhrmester, D., Hinshaw, S. P., Huber, A., & Laski, K. (1989). Does stimulant medication improve the peer status of hyperactive children? *Journal of Consulting and Clinical Psychology, 57*, 545–549.

Whitaker, A., Johnson, J., Shaffer, D., Rapoport, J., Kalikow, K., Walsh, B. T., Davies, M., Braiman, S., & Dolinsky, A. (1990). Uncommon troubles in young people: Prevalence estimates of selected psychiatric disorders in a non-referred adolescent population. *Archives of General Psychiatry, 47*, 487–496.

White, J. L., Moffitt, T. E., Caspi, A., Bartusch, D. J., Needles, D., & Stouthamer-Loeber, M. (1994). Measuring impulsivity and examining its relationship to delinquency. *Journal of Abnormal Psychology, 103,* 1922–1205.

Whitehurst, G. J., Fischel, J. E., & Lonigan, C. J. (1991). Treatment of early expressive language delay: If, when, and how. *Topics in Language Disorders, 11,* 55–68.

Wilens, T. E., & Biederman, J. (1992). The stimulants. *Psychiatric Clinics of North America, 15,* 191–208.

Wilens, T. E., Biederman, J., Abrantes, A. M., & Spencer, T. J. (1997). Clinical characteristics of psychiatrically referred adolescent outpatients with substance use disorder. *Journal of the American Academy of Child and Adolescent Psychiatry, 36,* 941–947.

Wilens, T. E., Biederman, J., Geist, D. E., Steingard, R., & Spencer, T. (1993). Nortriptyline in the treatment of attention deficit hyperactivity disorder: A chart review of 58 cases. *Journal of the American Academy of Child and Adolescent Psychiatry, 32,* 343–349.

Wilkison, P. C., Kircher, J. C., McMahon, W. M., & Sloane, H. N. (1995). Effects of methylphenidate on reward strength in boys with attention-deficit hyperactivity disorder. *Journal of the American Academy of Child and Adolescent Psychiatry, 34,* 897–901.

Williams, R., & Morgan, H. G. (1994). *Suicide prevention—The challenge confronted. NHS Health Advisory Service.* London: Her Majesty's Stationery Office.

Williams, R. A., Hollis, H. M., & Benoit, K. (1998). Attitudes toward psychiatric medications among incarcerated female adolescents. *Journal of the American Academy of Child and Adolescent Psychiatry, 37,* 1301–1307.

Williamson, D. A., Baker, J. D., & Cubic, B. A. (1993). Advances in pediatric headache research. In T. H. Ollendick & R. J. Prinz (Eds.), *Advances in clinical child psychology* (Vol. 15, pp. 275–304). New York: Plenum Press.

Williamson, D. A., Prather, R. C., Bennett, S. M., Davis, C. J., Watkins, P. C., & Grenier, C. E. (1989). An uncontrolled evaluation of inpatient and outpatient cognitive-behavior therapy for bulimia nervosa. *Behavior Modification, 13,* 340–360.

Wilsher, C. R. (1991). Is medicinal treatment of dyslexia advisable? In M. Snowling & M. Thomson (Eds.), *Dyslexia: Integrating theory and practice* (pp. 204–212). London: Whurr.

Wilson, P. H., & McKenzie, B. E. (1998). Information processing deficits associated with developmental coordination disorder: A meta-analysis of research findings. *Journal of Child Psychology and Psychiatry, 39,* 829–840.

Wiltz, N. A. (1974). An evaluation of parent training procedures designed to alter inappropriate aggressive behavior of boys. *Behavior Therapy, 5,* 215–221.

Wimpory, D., & Cochrane, V. (1991). Criteria for evaluative research—With special reference to holding therapy. *Communication, 25,* 15–17.

Wing, L. (1989). The diagnosis of autism. In C. Gillberg (Ed.), *Diagnosis and treatment of autism.* New York: Plenum Press.

Wing, L. (1996). Wing schedule for handicaps, behaviour and skills (HBS). In I. Rabin (Ed.), *Preschool children with inadequate communication* (pp. 268–296). London: MacKeith Press.

Winokur, G., Zimmerman, M., & Cadoret, R. (1988). 'Cause the Bible tells me so. *Archives of General Psychiatry, 45,* 683–684.

Wodrich, D. I., Benjamin, E., & Lachar, D. (1997). Tourette's syndrome and psychopathology in a child psychiatry setting. *Journal of the American Academy of Child and Adolescent Psychiatry, 36,* 1618–1624.

Wolchik, S. A., Weiss, L., & Katzman, M. A. (1986). An empirically validated, short term psychoeducational group treatment program for bulimia. *International Journal of Eating Disorders, 5,* 21–34.

Wolf, M. M., Braukmann, C. J., & Ramp, K. A. (1987). Serious delinquent behavior as part of a siginificantly handicapping condition: Cures and suppportive environments. *Journal of Applied Behavior Analysis, 20,* 347–359.

Wolf, M. M., Kirigin, K. A., Fixsen, D. L., Blase, K. A., & Braukmann, C. J. (1995). The Teaching Family Model: A case study in data-based program development and refinement (and dragon wrestling). *Journal of Organizational Behavior Management, 15,* 11–68.

Wolfberg, P. J., & Schuler, A. L. (1993). Integrated play groups: A model for promoting the social and cognitive dimensions of play in children with autism. *Journal of Autism and Developmental Disorders, 23*, 467–489.

Wolfe, K. D., Weller, R. A., Fristad, M. A., & Mac, D. (1993). *Treating children with attention deficit disorder: A double-blind buproprion trial.* Paper presented at the 40th annual meeting of the American Academy of Child and Adolescent Psychiatry, San Antonio, TX.

Wolff, S. (1961). Symptomatology and outcome of pre-school children with behaviour disorders attending a child guidance clinic. *Journal of Child Psychology and Psychiatry, 2*, 269–276.

Wolraich, M. L., Hannah, J. N., Baumgaertel, A., & Feurer, I. D. (1998). Examination of DSM-IV criteria for attention deficit/hyperactivity disorder in a county-wide sample. *Journal of Developmental and Behavioural Pediatrics, 19*, 162–168.

Wolraich, M. L., Hannah, J. N., Pinnock, T. Y., Baumgaertel, A., & Brown, J. (1996). Comparison of diagnostic criteria for attention deficit hyperactivity disorder in a country-wide sample. *Journal of the American Academy of Child and Adolescent Psychiatry, 35*, 319–324.

Wood, A. J., Harrington, R. C., & Moore, A. (1996). Controlled trial of a brief cognitive-behavioural intervention in adolescent patients with depressive disorders. *Journal of Child Psychology and Psychiatry, 37*, 737–46.

Woolf, S. H., Battista, R. N., Anderson, G. M., Logan, A. G., Wang, E., & the Canadian Task Force on the Periodic Health Examination. (1990). Assessing the effectiveness of preventive maneuvers: Analytic principles and systematic methods in reviewing evidence and developing clinical practice recommendations. *Journal of Clinical Epidemiology, 43*, 891–905.

Wootton, J. M., Frick, P. J., Shelton, K. K., & Silverthorn, P. (1997). Ineffective parenting and childhood conduct problems: The moderating role of callous-unemotional traits. *Journal of Consulting and Clinical Psychology, 65*, 301–308.

World Health Organization. (1967). *International classification of diseases: Manual of the international statistical classication of diseases, injuries and causes of death* (8th ed.). Geneva: Author.

World Health Organization. (1981). *Document on nomenclature and classification.* Geneva: Author.

World Health Organization. (1992a). *International statistical classification of diseases and related health problems.* (10th ed.). Geneva: Author.

World Health Organisation. (1992b). *World health statistics annual.* Geneva: Author.

World Health Organization. (1993). *The ICD-10 classification of mental and behavioral disorders. Diagnostic criteria for research.* Geneva: Author.

Wright, J., & Pearl, L. (1995). Knowledge and experience of young people regarding drug misuse, 1969–1994. *British Medical Journal, 310*, 20–24.

Wu, P., Hoven, C. W., Bird, H. R., Morre, R. E., Cohen, P., Alegria, M., Dulcan, M. K., Goodman, S. H., McCue Horowitz, S., Lichtman, J. H., Narrow, W. E., Rae, D. S., Regier, D. A., & Roper, M. T. (1999). Depressive and disruptive disorders and mental health service utilization in children and adolescents. *Journal of the American Academy of Child and Adolescent Psychiatry, 38*, 1081–1090.

Wudarsky, M., Nicolson, R., Hamburger, S. D., Spechler, L., Gochman, P., Bedwell, J., Lenane, M. C., & Rapoport, J. L. (1999). Elevated prolactin in pediatric patients on typical and atypical antipsychotics. *Journal of Child and Adolescent Psychopharmacology, 9*, 239–245.

Wysocki, T., Harris, M., Greco, P., Bubb, J., Danda, C., Harvey, L., McDonell, K., Taylor, A., & White, N. (2000). Randomized, controlled trial of behavior therapy for families of adolescent with insulin dependent diabetes mellitus. *Journal of Pediatric Psychology, 25*, 23–33.

Yates, B. T. (1994). Toward the incorporation of costs, cost-effectiveness analysis and cost-benefit analysis into clinical research. *Journal of Consulting and Clinical Psychology, 62*, 729–736.

Youngerman, J., & Canino, I. A. (1978). Lithium carbonate use in children and adolescents: A survey of the literature. *Archives of General Psychiatry, 35*, 216–224.

Zabin, L. S., Hardy, J. B., Smith, E. A., & Hirsch, M. B. (1986). Substance use and its relation to sexual activity among inner-city adolescents. *Journal of Adolescent Healthcare, 7*(5), 320—331.

Zahn-Waxler, C. (1993). Warriors and worriers: Gender and psychopathology. *Development and Psychopathology, 5*, 79–89.

Zahn-Waxler, C., Cole, C. M., Welsh, J. D., & Fox, N. A. (1995). Psychophysiological correlates of empathy and prosocial behaviours in preschool children with behavior problems. *Development and Psychopathology, 7*, 27–48.

Zametkin, A., Rapaport, J. L., Murphy, D. L., Linnoila, M., & Ismond, D. (1985). Treatment of hyperactive children with monoamine oxidase inhibitors: I. Clinical efficacy. *Archives of General Psychiatry, 42*, 962–966.

Zangwill, W. M. (1983). An evaluation of a parent training program. *Child and Family Behavior Therapy, 5*, 1–16.

Zeltzer, L. K., Altman, A., Cohen, D., LeBaron, S., Munuksela, E. L., & Schecter, N. L. (1990). Report of the subcommittee on the management of pain associated with procedures in children with cancer. *Pediatrics, 86*, 826–831.

Zeltzer, L. K., Dolgin, M. J., LeBaron, S., & LeBaron, C. (1991). A randomized controlled study of behavioral intervention for chemotherapy distress in children with cancer. *Pediatrics, 88*, 34–42.

Zeltzer, L. K., & LeBaron, S. (1982). Hypnosis and nonhypnotic techniques for reduction of pain and anxiety during painful procedures in children and adolescents with cancer. *Behavioral Pediatrics, 101*, 1032–1035.

Zentall, S., & Ferkis, A. (1993). Mathematical problem solving for youth with ADHD, with and without learning disabilities. *Learning Disability Quarterly, 16*, 6–18.

Zigler, E., & Levine, J. (1981). Age of first hospitalization of schizophrenia. *Journal of Abnormal Psychology, 90*, 458–467.

Zito, J. M., Craig, T. J., & Wanderling, J. (1994). Pharmacoepidemiology of 330 child/adolescent psychiatric patients. *Journal of Pharmacoepidemiology, 3*, 47–62.

Zito, J. M., & Riddle, M. A. (1995). Psychiatric pharmacoepidemiology for children and adolescents. *Child and Adolescent Psychiatric Clinics of North America, 4*, 77–95.

Zoccolillo, M. (1992). Co-occurrence of conduct disorder and its adult outcomes with depressive and anxiety disorders: A review. *Journal of the American Academy of Child and Adolescent Psychiatry, 31*, 547–556.

Zoccolillo, M., Pickles, A., Quinton, D., & Rutter, M. (1992). The outcome of childhood conduct disorder: Implications for defining adult personality disorder and conduct disorder. *Psychological Medicine, 22*, 971–986.

Zoccolillo, M., Vitaro, F., & Tremblay, R. E. (1999). Problem drug and alcohol use in a community sample of adolescents. *Journal of the American Academy of Child and Adolescent Psychiatry, 38*, 900–907.

Zubieta, J., & Alessi, N. (1992). Acute and chronic administration of trazodone in the treatment of disruptive behavior disorders in children. *Journal of Clinical Psychopharmacology, 12*, 346–351.

Index

Abdominal pain, 331–333
Academic performance
  ADHD and, 198
  in alternative school settings, 169–170
  comorbidity and, 56
  delinquency and, 169–170, 171
  disturbances of conduct and, 110
  psychostimulant effects, 208–210
  and risk of psychiatric disorders, 60
Adaptation
  measures of, 8
  as outcome measure, 7–9
  psychostimulant effects, 207–210
Adderall, 200
ADHD. *See* Attention-deficit/hyperactivity disorder
Adherence/compliance, 310–311
Affective functioning
  autism manifestations, 266
  capacity for change, 9
  expressed emotion in schizophrenia, 250
  in schizoaffective disorders, 250–251
Age variables
  in anxiety disorder presentation, 67–68
  in methylphenidate effects, 203–204
  in prevalence of mental disorders, 50, 64
Aggression Replacement Training, 168–169
Aggressive behavior
  classification, 112
  comorbid ADHD, 205–206
  disturbances of conduct and, 112–113
  neurobiological disorders in, 112
  parent training intervention to manage, 124–126
Alcohol consumption
  drug abuse and, 316
  extent, 315–316, 324
  mortality/morbidity, 318–319
  See also Substance misuse
Alprazolam, 71
Amitriptyline, 94, 294
Anger management training, 138
  for disturbances of conduct, 144, 181–182
  juvenile delinquency interventions, 166–167
Anorexia nervosa. *See* Eating disorders
Anticonvulsants, 408–409
  bipolar disorder treatment, 259
  conduct problem treatment, 188
Antidepressant medications
  eating disorder treatment, 294–295
  See also specific drug; specific drug type
Antipsychotic drugs. *See* Neuroleptics
Antisocial behavior
  clinical conceptualizations, 106, 107
  comorbidity, 56
  depression and, 91–92
  development, 113
  familial risk factors, 59
  psychosocial interventions, 142